PRINCIPLES AND APPLICATIONS OF CARDIORESPIRATORY CARE EQUIPMENT

Principles and Applications of Cardiorespiratory Care Equipment

DAVID H. EUBANKS, Ed.D., R.R.T.
Vice President, Program Development and Continuing Education
Professor of Allied Health
Medical College of Ohio
Toledo, Ohio

ROGER C. BONE, M.D.
President and Chief Executive Officer
Professor of Medicine
Medical College of Ohio
Medical College Hospitals
Toledo, Ohio

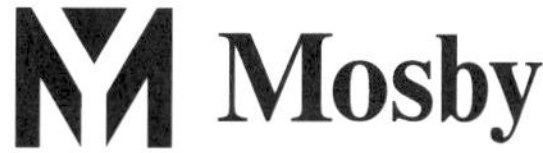

St. Louis Baltimore Boston Chicago London Madrid Philadelphia Sydney Toronto

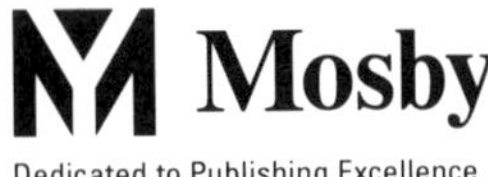

Dedicated to Publishing Excellence

Publisher: George Stamathis
Editor: James F. Shanahan
Developmental Editor: Jennifer Roche
Project Manager: Nancy C. Baker
Project Supervisor: Carol A. Reynolds
Production Editor: Jerry Schwartz
Proofroom Manager: Barbara M. Kelly
Designer: Carol A. Reynolds
Manufacturing Supervisor: Theresa Fuchs

Printed in the United States of America
Composition by Graphic World, Inc.
Printing/binding by Maple-Vail

Mosby–Year Book, Inc.
11830 Westline Industrial Drive
St. Louis, Missouri 63146

Library of Congress Cataloging in Publication Data

Principles and application of cardiorespiratory equipment / [edited by] David Eubanks, Roger Bone.
p. cm.
Includes bibliographical references and index.
ISBN 0-8016-7448-4
1. Cardiopulmonary system—Diseases—Patients—Rehabilitation—Equipment and supplies. 2. Respiratory therapy—Equipment and supplies. I. Eubanks, David H., 1937- . II. Bone, Roger C.
[DNLM: 1. Respiratory Therapy—instrumentation. 2. Respiratory Therapy—methods. 3. Ventilators, Mechanical. WB 342 P9565 1993]
RC702.P75 1993
615.8'36—dc20
DNLM/DLC
for Library of Congress 93-30441
CIP

1 2 3 4 5 6 7 8 9 0 98 97 96 95 94

To my wife, Jacquie, and my daughters Kathryn, Julie, and Jawnie, whose patience, understanding, and support helped me to keep going when times were tough.

D.H.E.

To my wife, Rosemary, and my daughters, Mary Catherine and Cynthia.

R.C.B.

CONTRIBUTORS

Russell A. Acevedo, M.D., F.C.C.P.
Associate Clinical Professor of Medicine and Critical Care
State of New York Health Science Center at Syracuse
Medical Director, Acute Care Area
Crouse Irving Memorial Hospital
Syracuse, New York

Thomas F. Anderson, Ph.D., M.Ed., B.S., R.R.T.
Professor
Associate Dean for Health and Natural Sciences
Waubonsee Community College
Sugar Grove, Illinois

Roger C. Bone, M.D.
President and Chief Executive Officer
Professor of Medicine
Medical College of Ohio
Medical College Hospitals
Toledo, Ohio

Pamela L. Bortner, B.S., R.R.T.
Anesthesia Clinical Associate/Patient Assessor
The Toledo Hospital
Toledo, Ohio

Neal J. Cohen, M.D., M.P.H., M.S.
Professor, Anesthesia and Medicine
University of California, San Francisco
Director, Intensive Care Unit
Moffitt-Long Hospital
San Francisco, California

David H. Eubanks, Ed.D., R.R.T.
Vice President, Program Development and Continuing Education
Professor of Medicine
Medial College of Ohio
Toledo, Ohio

Robert J. Fallat, M.D.
Associate Professor of Medicine
University of California at San Francisco
Medical Director, Division of Pulmonary Medicine
California Pacific Medical Center
San Francisco, California

James B. Fink, M.S., R.R.T.
Research Associate
Department of Medicine
Stritch School of Medicine
Loyola University Medical Center
Administrative Director, Respiratory Care Service
Edward Hines Jr. Veterans Administration Hospital
Hines, Illinois

Eric H. Gluck, M.D.
Associate Professor of Medicine
Rush University
Associate Director of Respiratory Care
Presbyterian St. Luke's Medical Center
Chicago, Illinois

Robert A. May, M.D., R.R.T.
Associate Director, Respiratory Care Program
University of Toledo
Medical Director, Department of Respiratory Care
The Toledo Hospital
Toledo, Ohio

Oscar A. Schwartz, M.D., F.C.C.P.
Clinical Assistant Professor
St. Louis University School of Medicine
Medical Director-Vencore Hospital
Director Pulmonary-St. Mary's Health Center
St. Louis, Missouri

Michael G. Snow, R.P.F.T.
Manager, Pulmonary Physiology and Research
California Pacific Medical Center
San Francisco, California

Joseph G. Sorbello, M.S.Ed., R.R.T.
Assistant Professor
Department of Respiratory Care and Cardiorespiratory Sciences
SUNY Health Science Center at Syracuse
Syracuse, New York

Barbara G. Wilson, M.Ed., R.R.T.
Research Associate
Pediatric Respiratory Care Services
Duke University Medical Center
Durham, North Carolina

PREFACE

Discussions leading to the writing of this book began 3 years ago when it became apparent to the authors and those in respiratory care practice and pulmonary medicine that a text was needed to discuss respiratory care equipment from a clinical as well as from a technical perspective.

This realization is the premise upon which this book was written. All contributors have written their chapters so that a functional, theoretical basis in the use of the equipment is developed, followed by a discussion of the operation and clinical application of equipment. Each author has included the necessary figures, tables, and charts to clearly explain theoretical operation of the equipment and its application to patients.

Indications and contraindications for the use of specific devices are discussed along with desired therapeutic efficacy. The combined education and clinical experience of the physician and therapist teams focuses each chapter on the most practical and clinically relevant information for each piece of equipment. Even the references were selected because of their appropriateness to clinical care. All chapters follow a standard format which makes them easy to read—the reader does not have to become familiar with a new writing style or format as he moves from chapter to chapter. Each chapter builds upon previously acquired knowledge so that in the last two chapters the combined knowledge is integrated into bedside monitoring and laboratory testing techniques through the use of case studies and other examples.

All the chapters contain the most current information possible about the equipment that is presented. As is the case with any equipment text, the biomedical industry is advancing so quickly that some of the equipment will have changed prior to the publication of this text. For this reason, each author also has included principles and theories that would enable the reader to apply this information to new equipment as it becomes available for clinical use. When writing their respective chapters, the contributors were instructed to assume that the reader would have at least minimal understanding of the basic sciences and respiratory care courses expected of any entry level practitioner. Consequently, this text is probably of most value to more advanced audiences such as respiratory therapists, nurses, medical students, physician assistants, nurse practitioners, practicing physicians, and others such as paramedics who wish to learn about the clinical applications of respiratory care equipment in a comprehensive yet succinct presentation.

The book is unique because it takes what could have been mundane technical information and makes it come alive by the authors who relate their own experiences and those of their colleagues. The book was enjoyable and educational to edit and we hope that it will be a useful resource to you as you care for your patients.

DAVID H. EUBANKS, Ed.D., R.R.T.
ROGER C. BONE, M.D.

ACKNOWLEDGMENTS

The authors wish to recognize the contributions of the many people who helped to make this book a reality.

We are especially grateful to Forrest Bird, M.D., Ph.D., Sc.D., of Percussionaire Corporation of Sand Point, Idaho, for his information about the Oscillation (r)-1 Amplifier and other Percussionaire products and to J.D. Mortensen, M.D. and Robert N. Schaap from Cardiopulmonomics, Salt Lake City, Utah, for their presentation of information on 1VOX.

We are also appreciative of Anne Buteyne, Mary Katherine Krause, and other members of our former staff at Rush Presbyterian-St. Luke's Medical Center for their assistance in word processing and proof reading materials.

We also wish to thank Donna Ash, Dr. Eubanks' administrative assistant at the Medical College of Ohio, for her help in coordinating the many phone calls and other details necessary to pull it all together.

Last, but not least, a special thanks to our editor, Jim Shanahan of Mosby–Year Book, without whose tenacity and talent this book would not have happened.

CONTENTS

1

Generation, Storage, and Control of Medical Gases

THOMAS F. ANDERSON, Ph.D., R.R.T.
OSCAR SCHWARTZ, M.D., F.C.C.P.

OBJECTIVES

- Describe the numerous mechanisms by which compressed gases are supplied to medical facilities.
- Differentiate among the types and styles of medical gas cylinders.
- Identify and explain distinguishing marks and/or labels on compressed gas cylinders.
- State the recommended methods for cylinder identification.
- Discuss the impact that the regulatory agencies have on the compressed gas industry.
- Compare and contrast the various compressed gas cylinder safety systems.
- Compute cylinder gas content.
- Classify medical gases.
- Compare and contrast the various methods by which oxygen is produced.
- Compare and contrast bulk oxygen storage systems.
- Identify and describe key components of a central piping system.
- Compare and contrast portable oxygen supply systems.
- Diagram the key internal mechanism of an air compressor.
- Trace the flow of gas through a pressure reducing valve and a flowmeter.
- Differentiate between a pressure reducing valve and a regulator.
- Distinguish between a pressure reducing valve and flow controlling devices.

Medical gas delivery is a crucial constituent in the daily practice of respiratory care providers. While many practitioners tend to focus primarily on patient needs, they must not take for granted safe and effective operation of medical support equipment. This is why it is meaningful for physicians and others to have knowledge of the mechanisms by which medical equipment operates. This chapter focuses on the structure, function, and safe and appropriate usage of medical gas cylinders, piping systems, air compressors, oxygen concentrators, pressure reducing valves, and flow regulating devices.[1, 2]

MEDICAL GAS CYLINDERS

There are two methods by which compressed medical gases can be delivered to a medical facility: (1) by compressed gas cylinders and (2) via a central piping system. Gas cylinders are a convenient and safe method by which to store and transport medical gases. Since their introduction in the late 18th century, time and technological advancements have not altered the need for and use of gas cylinders.[3]

Construction

Gas cylinder construction currently falls under the domain of both industrial standards and the Department of Transportation (DOT). Traditionally, gas cylinders have been constructed of highly tempered seamless steel that is nonreactive to their liquid or compressed gaseous content. Depending upon the specific construction methods, gas cylinders are classified as "3A" (non–heat treated) or "3AA" (heat treated).[4, 5]

In recent years, aluminum cylinders have gained in popularity. These cylinders are held to the same rigorous construction and inspection standards as are steel cylinders. However, an advantage to their use for respiratory care providers is that aluminum cylinders are much lighter and easier to handle than traditional steel cylinders.

Labeling

The DOT and the Compressed Gas Association (CGA) require each manufacturer to mark (stamped into the steel) all gas cylinders with specific identifying marks (Fig 1–1).[4] These markings provide pertinent information to respiratory care providers. Required information on each cylinder includes the DOT classification (3A, 3AA), maximum service pressure, serial number, ownership and manufacturer's mark, original test date, elastic expansion, and retest dates and inspector's mark. Following the 3A or 3AA classification, a maximum service pressure is listed in pounds per square inch (psi).

The normal service pressure limit for 3A or 3AA gas cylinders is 2,015 psi. This limit on oxygen and mixtures of oxygen/helium or carbon dioxide can be exceeded by 10%[5]. A 10% pressure increase would be approximately 2,200 psi, which is the usual maximum service pressure of a newly filled compressed gas cylinder.[4, 5]

The serial number links the gas cylinder to a specific origin, thus creating a reference point for length of service, durability, safety, and possible recall. The ownership and manufacturer's mark reference the original firms. These marks and firms are registered with the Bureau of Explosives.[4] The original hydrostatic test date indicates that the gas cylinder was subjected to a water-jacket test. This test determines the cylinder's wall thickness, as well as its elastic expansion (expressed in cubic centimeters). The higher the elastic expansion, the thinner the cylinder wall, and vice versa. Hydrostatic testing and internal inspection and cleaning are performed on a 5- or 10-year retest schedule. This schedule is determined by DOT regulation.

Identification

Every respiratory care provider must be able to properly identify every type of medical compressed gas cylinder. Currently, there are two recommended methods of identification and one supplementary method. Careful use of clear, unmarred labels and standardized valve outlet connections is the recommended system; color coding is a supplementary method of identifying cylinders.[6, 7]

As with all prescriptions (including prescriptions for medical gases), the Federal Drug Administration (FDA) regulates and sets standards for purity, potency, and quality of cylinder contents. These features must be indicated on the exterior of gas containers on clearly marked, unmarred labels.[6] Appropriate precautions or warnings should also be listed. According to the American National Standards Institute (ANSI), this is the only absolute way to determine the contents of compressed gas cylinders.[8]

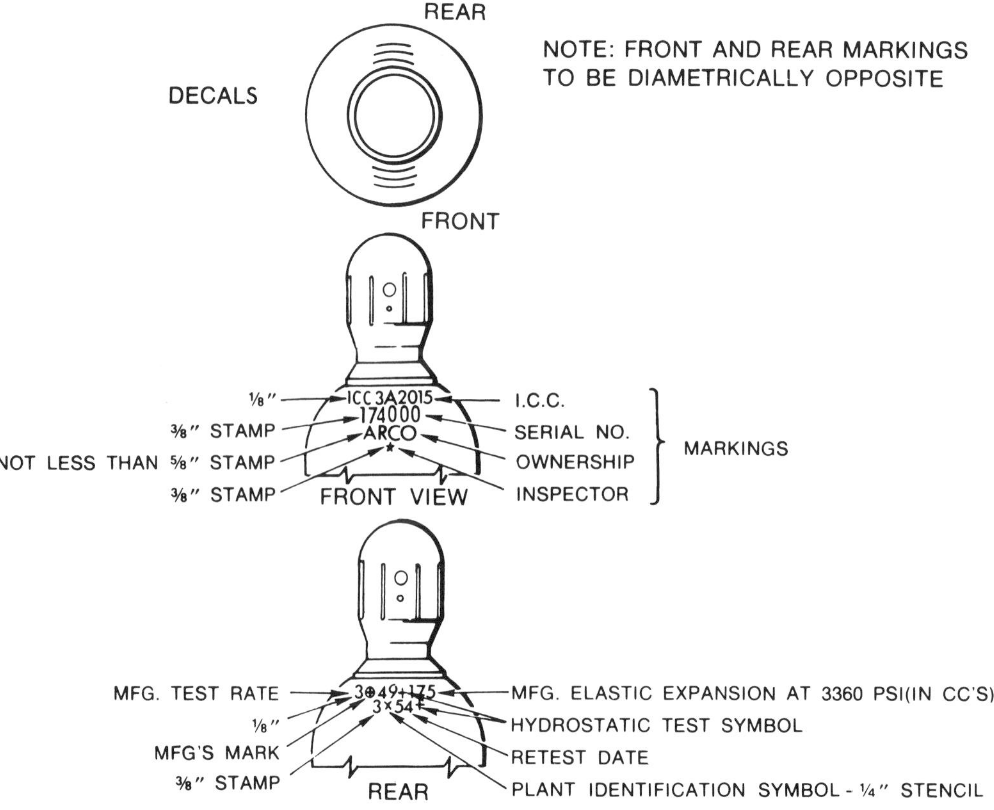

FIG 1–1
Permanent cylinder markings required for Interstate Commerce Commission (ICC) or Board of Transportation Commission for Canada (BTC) specifications. (Courtesy of Compressed Gas Association.)

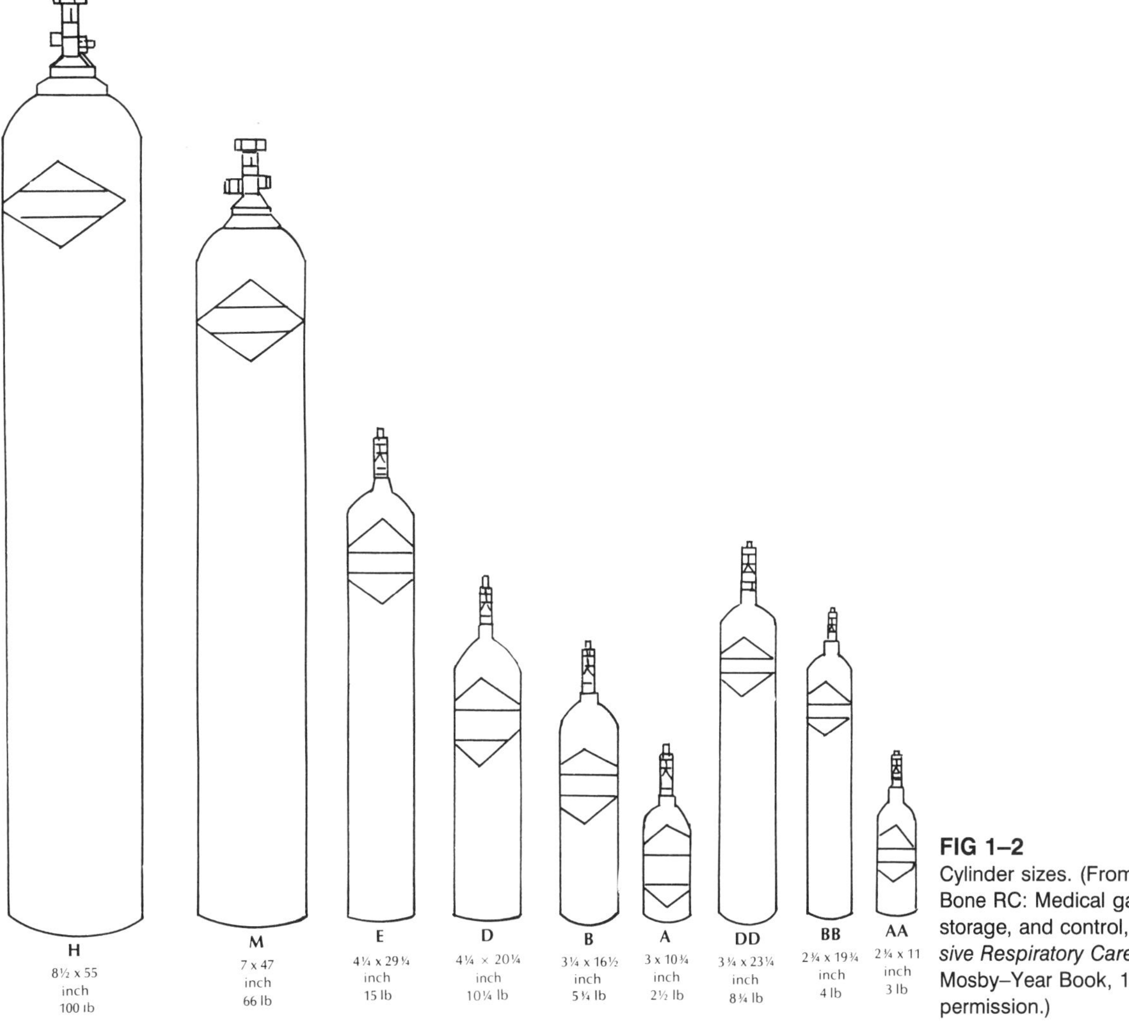

FIG 1–2
Cylinder sizes. (From Eubanks DH, Bone RC: Medical gases, production, storage, and control, in *Comprehensive Respiratory Care,* ed 2. St Louis, Mosby–Year Book, 1990. Used by permission.)

Standardized valve outlet connections are a second method used to identify gas cylinders. Since gas cylinders are available in a variety of sizes, letter designations have been given to each specific size (Fig 1–2). Small gas cylinders (designated by letters *AA* through *E*) utilize a standard valve outlet connection called a yoke; these cylinders are more convenient for portable gas administration or for low-use areas. Large gas cylinders (designated by letters *M* to *K*) utilize standard valve outlets with various types of internal and external threading. Since these gas cylinders are much larger and require wheeled carts to transport the cylinders from one area to another, these units are more appropriate for long-term administration or in high-use areas.

Although this system is not recommended, a third method sometimes used to identify gas cylinder content is the color code system (Table 1–1). Colors painted on a gas cylinder can be misinterpreted for a variety of physical and/or chemical reasons, so color identification should only be supplemental to reading cylinder content labels.

Unfortunately, even if all of the above methods of identifying gas cylinder contents are followed, accidents can still occur—cylinders may occasionally contain the wrong gas, or the assumed pure gas may be contaminated

TABLE 1–1
Medical Gas Color Codes

Gas	Color
Oxygen	Green (international: white)
Carbon dioxide	Gray
Nitrous oxide	Light blue
Cyclopropane	Orange
Helium	Brown
Ethylene	Red
Carbon dioxide	Gray and green
Helium and oxygen	Brown and green
Air	Yellow or black

by rusty water or other undesirable substances.[9–11] It is therefore recommended that practitioners periodically check cylinder contents with oxygen analyzers (to check the oxygen content) and white filter paper (to test for impurities). These checks should be conducted while the cylinder is in an inverted position.

Computing Compressed Gas Cylinder Contents

All newly serviced (full) medical gas cylinders contain approximately 2,200 psig (pounds per square inch as indicated on the pressure gauge) of gas. The most commonly used gas cylinders in a medical environment are the *E* (622 L), *G* (5,260 L), and *H* to *K* (6,900 L). A comparison of gas content in liters to other values may be calculated by using Table 1–2. To compute how long a cylinder will operate, a pressure-volume conversion factor is needed (Table 1–3). This factor can be calculated by using the following formula:

Volume/pressure = Conversion factor,

where the **volume** of the full cylinder is measured in liters and **pressure** is measured in pounds per square inch.

Prediction of the length of time that a cylinder will provide the medical gas flow desired is determined by three factors: (1) the volume (in liters) of gas remaining in the cylinder, (2) the pressure (pounds per square inch [gauge]) exerted by the compressed gas, and (3) the desired flow rate (in liters per minute). The following formula is most commonly used in determining the time remaining in a gas cylinder:

(Gauge pressure × Conversion factor)/Flow rate = Time remaining

where **gauge pressure** is measured in pounds per square inch (gauge), **flow rate** is measured in liters per minute, and **time remaining** is measured in minutes.

For example, if a half-full H cylinder at a flowrate of 5 L/min were selected, what would be the estimated time that this cylinder could be used before another cylinder would be needed? To compute the time remaining, multiply the gauge pressure reading (1,100 psig) by the conversion factor (derived from Table 1–3) and divide by the 5 L/min flow rate. The remaining time would equal 660 minutes, or approximately 11 hours.

Operating Compressed Gas Cylinders

The top portion (neck) of gas cylinders incorporates valve assemblies that are designed to allow operators to safely remove gas from the cylinders. There are two basic types of valve assemblies: direct-acting valves and indirect-acting valves.

Direct-acting Valves

Direct-acting valves (sometimes called needle valves) are found on both small and large cylinders.[6] A counterclockwise movement of the valve stem opens the valve. This movement displaces the valve from the seat and allows a portion of the compressed gas to escape. Fig 1–3 illustrates the basic action of the direct-acting valve assembly. Turning the valve stem counterclockwise moves the valve further from the valve seat, which exposes a larger opening for gas to escape. Conversely, turning the valve stem clockwise forces the valve into the valve seat, decreases the size of the opening, and inhibits the escape of gas. This type of valve assembly is recommended for cylinders rated higher than 1,500 psig.

Indirect-acting Valves

Indirect-acting valve assemblies (Fig 1–4) are designed to work on smaller compressed gas cylinders (those designed for pressures of 1,500 psi or less).[12] Operators manipulate the valve assembly in a similar manner as for direct-acting valves. These valves, however, have fewer moving parts and are often recommended for use in the administration of precise gas concentrations such as may be needed in laboratory settings or in anesthesia.

Safety Systems

To prevent the inappropriate administration of a medical gas, an intricate safety system has been developed through the CGA, the DOT, the National Fire Protection Association (NFPA), and the American Standards Association (ASA).[2, 13] The two safety systems utilized by manufacturers of cylinders are the pin index safety system

TABLE 1–2

Common Metric Equivalents

Liters	Cubic Feet	Gallons
1.0	0.035	0.264
28.3	1.0	7.48
3.785	0.132	1.0

TABLE 1–3

Pressure/Volume Conversion Factors for Cylinders

Cylinder Size	Conversion Factor
E	622.0 L/2,2000 psi = 0.28 or 0.3
G	5,260.0 L/2,200 psi = 2.39 or 2.4
H or K	6,900.0 L/2,200 psi = 3.0

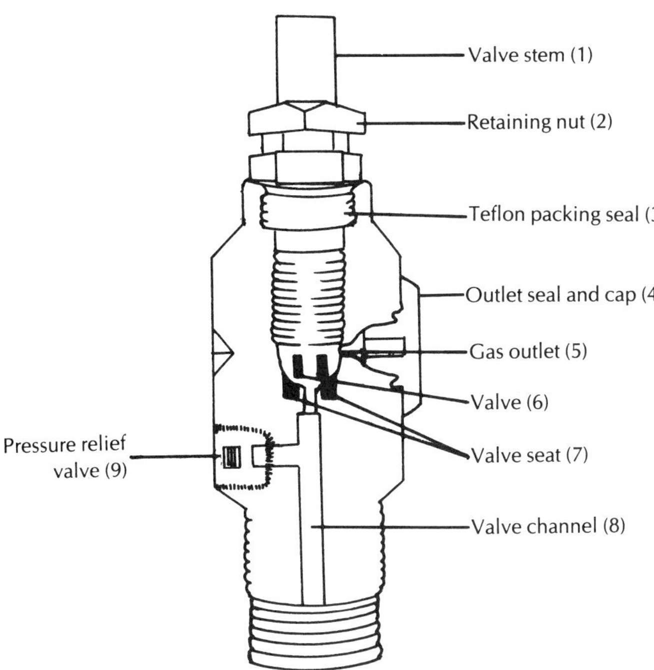

FIG 1–3
Components of a direct-acting valve as seen in cross section. (From Eubanks DH, Bone RC: Medical gases, production, storage, and control, in *Comprehensive Respiratory Care,* ed 2. St Louis, Mosby–Year Book, 1990. Used by permission.)

(PISS; designed for small cylinders) and the American standard safety system (designed for larger cylinders). Other significant safety systems used by manufacturers of accessories and/or attachments to cylinders are the diameter index safety system (DISS; designed for threaded gas connections) and the quick-connect systems (for rapid attachment to stationary wall or ceiling units). Both of these latter systems apply only in situations in which the working pressure is 200 psig or less. The DISS and quick-connect systems will be discussed in detail later in the section on piping systems.

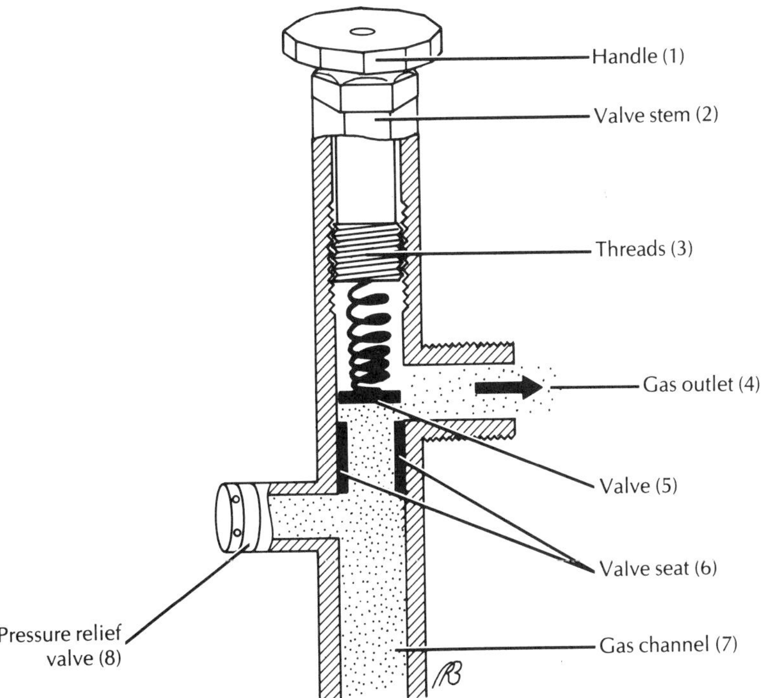

FIG 1–4
Components of an indirect-acting valve as seen in cross section. (From Eubanks DH, Bone RC: Medical gases, production, storage, and control, in *Comprehensive Respiratory Care,* ed 2. St Louis, Mosby–Year Book, 1990. Used by permission.)

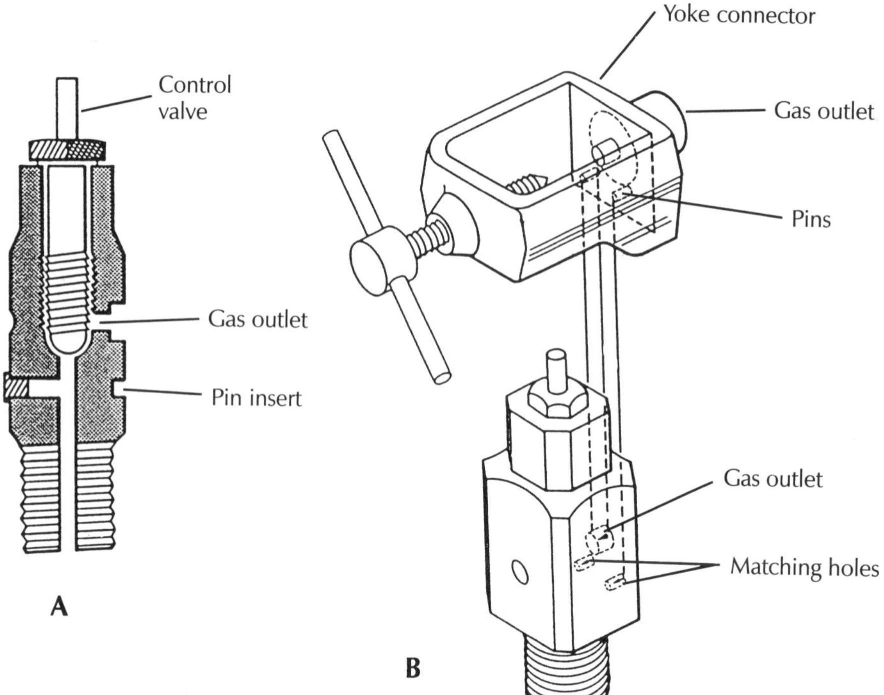

FIG 1–5
A, cross-section of a small yoke-type cylinder valve. **B,** yoke connector showing the regulator inlet and pin safety system. (From Barnes TA: Equipment for mixed gas and oxygen therapy, in *Respiratory Care Practice.* St Louis, Mosby–Year Book, 1988. Used by permission.)

Pin Index Safety System

The PISS is designed to prevent accidental attachment of a reducing valve specific for a particular gas to a cylinder with the wrong contents. This type of valve incorporates a system matching pins and holes (Fig 1–5). The yoke connector that is used to attach the regulator to the valve stem on the gas cylinder has two strategically positioned pins. The valve assembly on the cylinder has two matching holes to receive the pins on the yoke connector. When the yoke connector is attached to the valve assembly on the cylinder, the handle is twisted to tighten the aligned pins together. The gas outlet of both the yoke connector and valve assembly also fit together. This tight fit aided by a washer prevents leakage. The PISS has a total of six pin/hole positions, each representing a specific gas that can be incorporated into the valve assembly. A total of ten PISS positions are available, but only eight are currently assigned (Table 1–4); the PISS positions are numbered from left to right (Fig 1–6). For example, oxygen is assigned position 2-5; air is assigned 1-5.

TABLE 1–4
Gas Assignments for the Pin Index Safety System

Gas	Index position
Oxygen	2-5
Oxygen and carbon dioxide (up to 7%)	2-6
Oxygen and carbon dioxide (over 7%)	1-6
Oxygen and helium (up to 80%)	2-4
Oxygen and helium (over 80%)	4-6
Compressed air	1-5
Nitrous oxide	3-5
Ethylene	1-3
Cyclopropane	3-6

American Standard Safety System

The American standard safety system is designed to prevent inappropriate attachment of any device to large gas cylinders. This system is designed to work with large gas cylinders that are pressurized in excess of 1,500 psig. It employs a combination of right- or left-handed, internal/external, and varying thread type and size connectors with a variety of nipple and seal configurations (Fig 1–7).[7] Currently, 26 combinations are used for more than 62 listed gases.[14] This means that some gases use the same threaded connections. Medical gases are assigned right-handed threads; fuels (e.g., butane) are assigned left-handed threads.

CLASSIFICATION AND MANUFACTURE OF MEDICAL GASES

Classification

Medical gases are classified as (1) flammable (burn readily), (2) nonflammable (do not burn readily), or (3) nonflammable but support combustion.[15] Medical gases (and mixtures) most commonly used by respiratory care

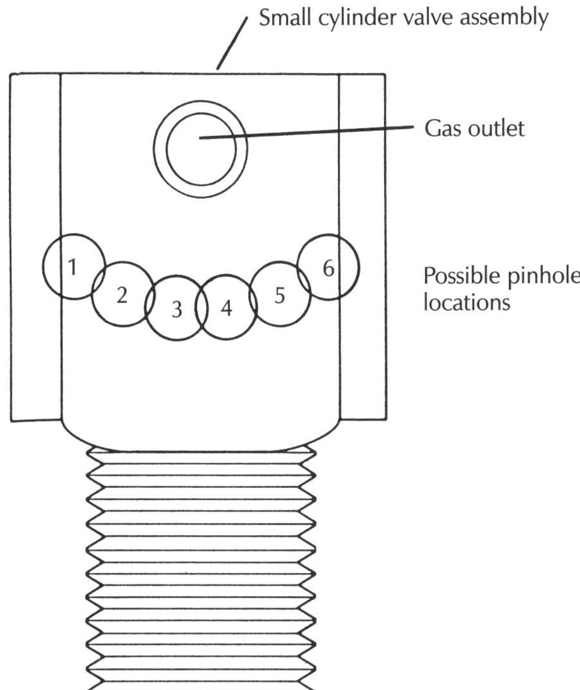

FIG 1–6
Possible PISS hole locations. (From Eubanks DH, Bone RC: Medical gases, production, storage, and control, in *Comprehensive Respiratory Care,* ed 2. St Louis, Mosby–Year Book, 1990. Used by permission.)

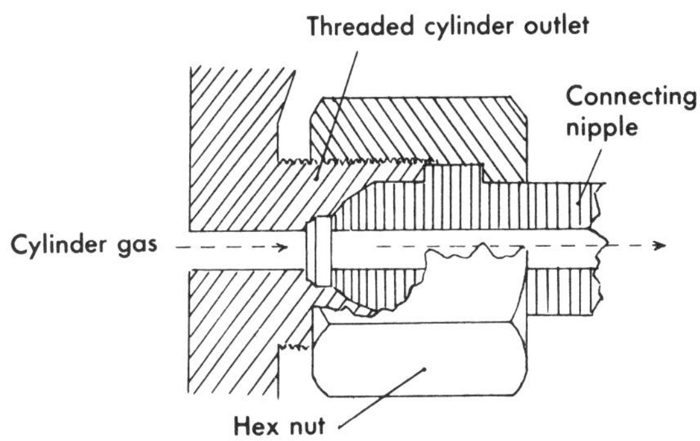

FIG 1–7
This sketch illustrates the structure of a typical American Standard connection such as might be used to attach a reducing valve to a large high-pressure cylinder. The hexagonal nut is held onto the nipple of the reducing valve by a circular collar, seen as a cross-sectional projection on the nipple. As the hex nut is tightened onto the threaded cylinder outlet, the end of the nipple is snugly seated into the conical outlet. (From Scanlan CL, Spearman CB, Sheldon RL: Production, storage, and delivery of medical gases, in *Egan's Fundamentals of Respiratory Care,* ed 5, St Louis, 1990, Mosby–Year Book; modified from Compressed Gas Association: *Connection No 540,* Pamphlet V-1, New York, Compressed Gas Association, 1987. Used by permission.)

providers are generally of the third category (e.g., oxygen, air, oxygen/helium, oxygen/carbon dioxide). Respiratory care providers must therefore develop a thorough understanding of the potential dangers associated with use of these agents and their associated equipment.

Fractional Distillation

The most common method of mass-producing oxygen is by fractional distillation. The process was first introduced in 1907 by Dr. Karl von Linde.[3] This technique provides a simple and economical method by which to convert atmospheric air into its many component gases (78.08% nitrogen, 20.95% oxygen, 0.93% inert gases, 0.03% carbon dioxide, and 0.01% hydrogen). Fractional distillation involves the entrainment of atmospheric air into a series of filters, compressors, heat removers, expanders, and heat absorbers. By systematically compressing and expanding atmospheric air, it is eventually converted to a liquid state (the Joule-Kelvin method).[8, 16] The liquified gas is then warmed. At specific critical temperatures and pressures, the various component gases return to their gaseous state; they are then individually captured in appropriate containers (Fig 1–8). The purity of the oxygen generated through this process exceeds the standards set by the FDA. Other methods of gas separation that can be used include electrolysis, chemical decomposition, and physical separation (which will be discussed in the section on oxygen concentrators).

BULK OXYGEN STORAGE SYSTEMS

Most medical facilities that use large quantities of oxygen make use of some type of bulk oxygen storage system. Bulk storage of oxygen is usually defined as any system capable of accommodating more than 13,000 ft^3 of gas ready for use.[17] There are two major types of storage systems: compressed gas cylinder banks and bulk liquid oxygen reservoirs. The system of choice for any institution depends upon the volume of gas used by the facility. Both systems require routine maintenance and oversight; these functions are usually handled by hospital engineering staff and medical gas suppliers. Whichever system is selected, materials must comply with the standards set forth by the NFPA.[17–19]

Compressed Gas Cylinder Bank

Compressed gas cylinder banks consist of a series of gas cylinders interconnected by pressure regulators, vaporizers, connecting tubing, and safety devices (Fig 1–9). These cylinders contain oxygen in either a liquid or a gaseous state. Cylinders may be contained within a manifold (from which the cylinders can be exchanged or rotated on a regular schedule), they may be permanently

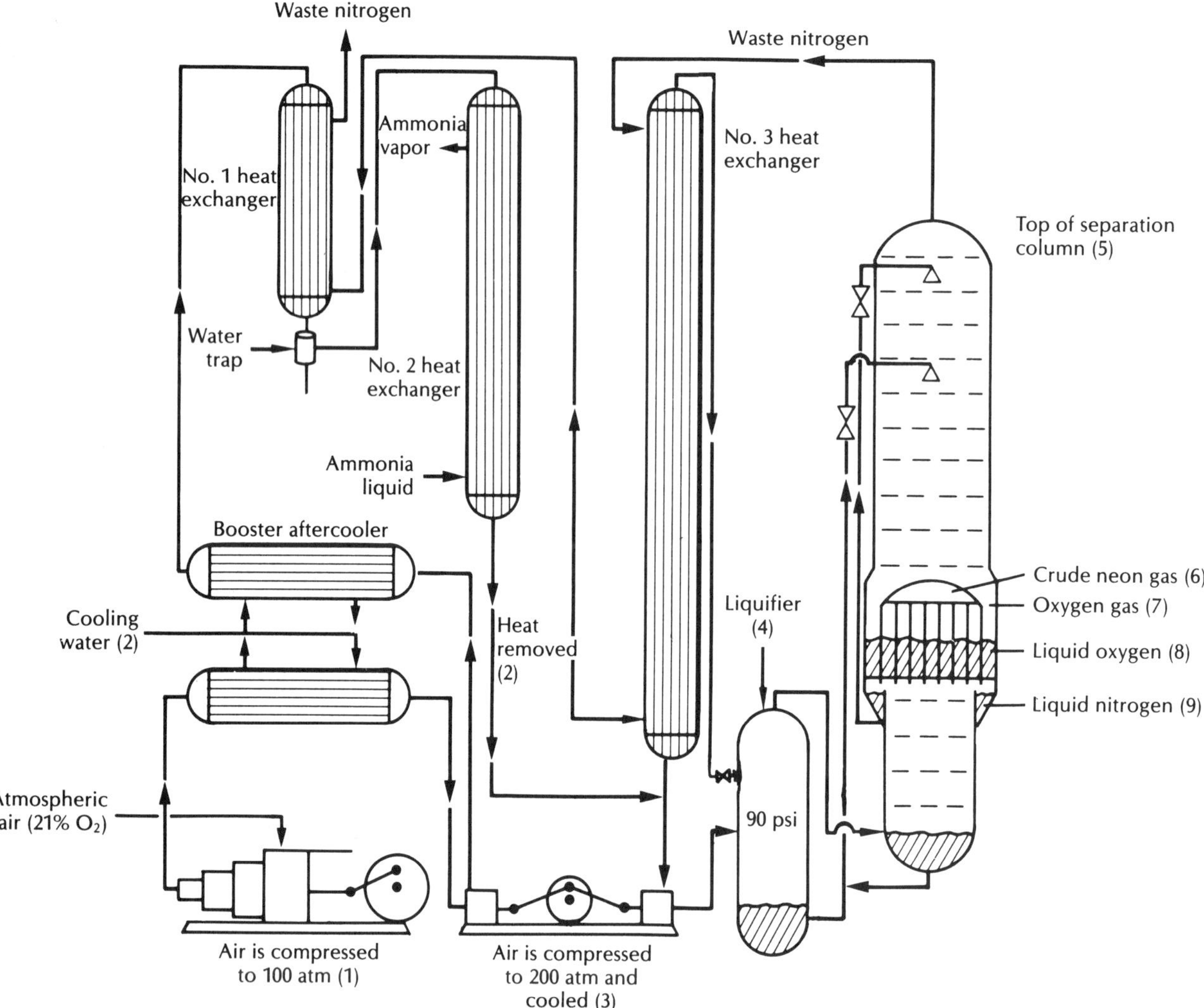

FIG 1–8
Fractional distillation of liquefied air. (From Eubanks DH, Bone RC: Medical gases, production, storage, and control, in *Comprehensive Respiratory Care,* ed 2. St Louis, Mosby–Year Book, 1990. Used by permission.)

fixed (each of the cylinders is refilled when emptied), or they may be permanently fixed on a trailer (the entire trailer is exchanged when necessary).[20] Whichever method is selected, the gas within the system is ultimately supplied to the medical facility through a central supply line.

Liquid Bulk Oxygen System

The majority of medical facilities (large volume users—>1,000 standard cubic feet per hour [SCFH]) find that a liquid bulk oxygen system is the most practical and economical system for bulk oxygen storage and accessibility. Liquid bulk oxygen systems use large "canisters" (called Dewar flasks) constructed in a manner similar to thermos bottles (Fig 1–10).[21] The liquid content of the canister is held at a pressure of less than 250 psig and is protected by a double (vacuum) insulated wall (Fig 1–11). This container keeps the liquid oxygen below its critical temperature of −181.4°F (−118.6°C). Above the surface of the liquid oxygen, gaseous oxygen rises and exits through a series of valves and a vaporizer before entering the institution's central piping system.

Hazards arising in bulk oxygen delivery systems occur frequently and are due primarily to a lack of awareness of design and function among hospital personnel (Table 1–5).[22] Clinically, the greatest hazards relate to a loss of oxygen supply to patients, overpressurization, and fire.

There are a number of basic rules that should be followed to prevent unnecessary problems in the use of bulk oxygen systems:

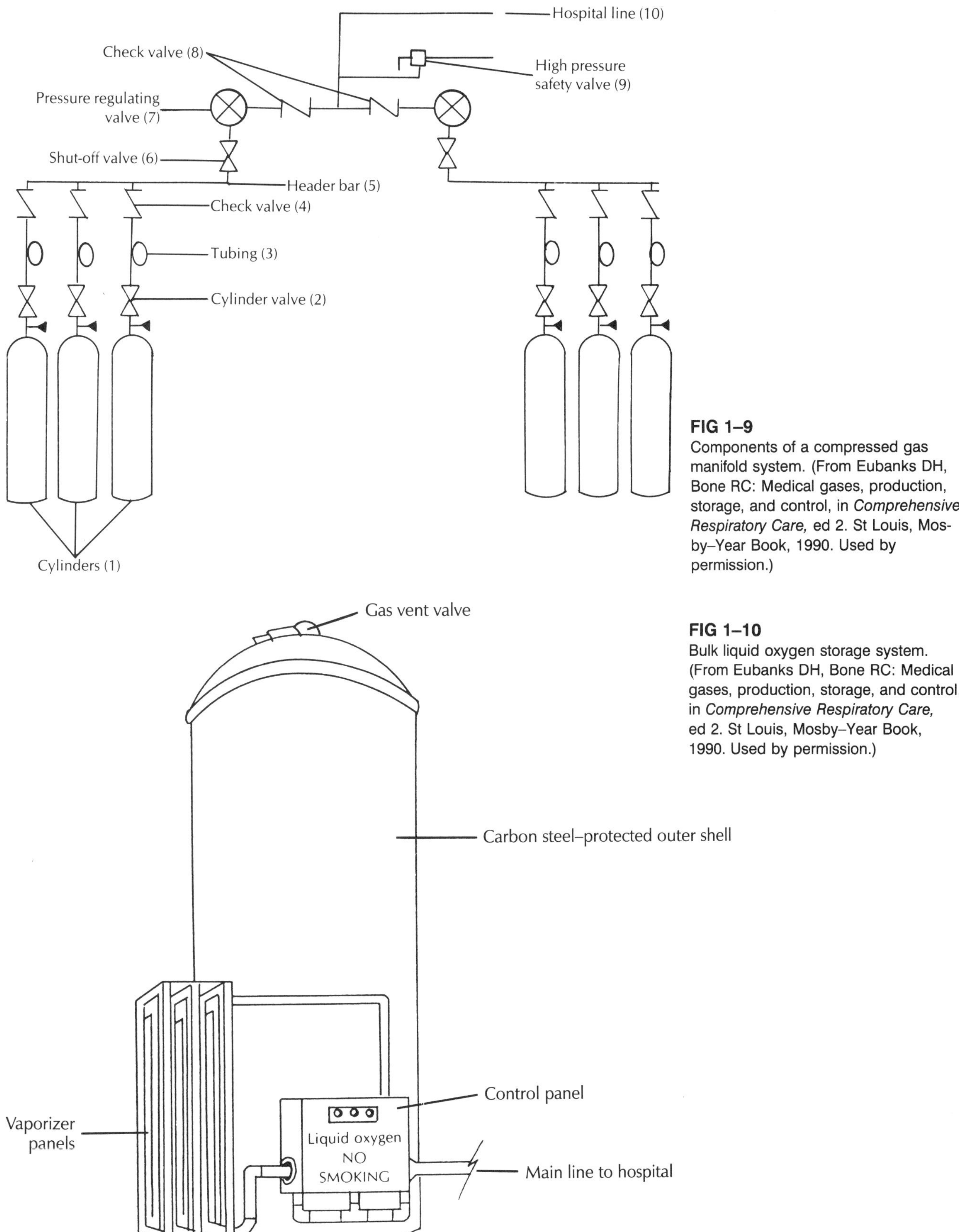

FIG 1–9
Components of a compressed gas manifold system. (From Eubanks DH, Bone RC: Medical gases, production, storage, and control, in *Comprehensive Respiratory Care,* ed 2. St Louis, Mosby–Year Book, 1990. Used by permission.)

FIG 1–10
Bulk liquid oxygen storage system. (From Eubanks DH, Bone RC: Medical gases, production, storage, and control, in *Comprehensive Respiratory Care,* ed 2. St Louis, Mosby–Year Book, 1990. Used by permission.)

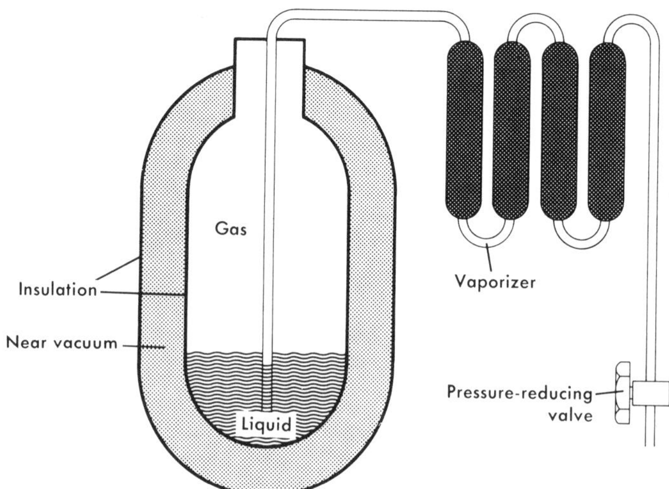

FIG 1–11
A liquid-oxygen stand tank (fixed station). (From McPherson SP, Spearman CB: *Respiratory Therapy Equipment,* ed 3. St Louis, Mosby–Year Book, 1985. Used by permission.)

- Always verify that a liquid oxygen storage tank in fact contains liquid oxygen.
- Periodically check the line pressure (40 to 60 psig) and oxygen purity (>99%) at wall outlets in various locations throughout the medical facility. Dirty oxygen causes line filters to clog, thereby decreasing the oxygen pressure at station outlets.
- Understand how the bulk oxygen system is to be shut down, how backup systems are utilized, and how control valves can be operated to isolate specific areas of the hospital.
- Understand how backflow alternatives may be introduced to provide adequate medical gases to patient areas in the event of isolated failure of the main oxygen system.
- Be aware of construction projects that could result in inappropriate placement of pressure reducing valves in the main gas piping system. Improperly placed reducing valves can cause undesirable decreases in gas pressure in the oxygen piping system, which in turn can prevent proper operation of ventilators and other gas-operated medical equipment.
- Be aware of any construction changes in the medical gas piping system that could result in either a reduction of the internal diameter of oxygen-carrying pipes or an increase in their length. Either of these changes (according to basic physical laws) will cause a significant decrease in gas flow to medical service areas.[23]

To prevent a sudden loss of oxygen in the central piping system, the NFPA requires the installation of a secondary or backup manifold system with a supply of oxygen that will last for 24 hours.[24, 25] This emergency system must be compatible with and connected to the primary bulk oxygen delivery system. For this reason, all respiratory care departments should have a contingency plan in place so that every respiratory care provider is prepared to respond to any unexpected interruption of the entire bulk oxygen supply system and its emergency backup system.

TABLE 1–5
Reported Hazards in Bulk Oxygen Delivery at Beth Israel Hospital: 1978–1979*

Inappropriate and unilateral adjustment of the main line pressure regulators resulting in a reduction in line pressure to the hospital
Cessation of flow from the main supply vessel because of inapprorpiate manipulation of the main supply control valve
Unsignaled activation and depletion of the reserve supply
Excessive depletion of the reserve supply because of pressure imbalance in the system
Excessive depletion of the reserve supply because of failure of the vacuum seal on the reserve supply vessel
Leaking of oxygen from ruptured piping connnecting the reserve supply to the main system
Leakage of oxygen from the reserve supply through a loose packing gland on a valve
Leaking seat in the main line pressure regulator
False alarms resulting from calibration drift in line pressure sensors
Failure of a line pressure sensor because of occlusion of the pressure fitting with foreign material (welding flux)
Failure of monitoring personnel to notify the appropriate clinical service

* From Bancroft LM, du Molin GC, Hedley-Whyte LH: *Anaesthesia* 1980; 52:504–510. Used by permission.

PRIMARY AND EMERGENCY BACKUP PIPING SYSTEMS

Piping systems to dispense medical gases in a facility are as diverse and unique as the number that are in operation. There are several factors that must be taken into consideration when discussing supply systems. First, each facility must determine the kind(s) of gas(es) it will be using and the anticipated volume of each (usually predicted on a monthly basis and then converted to a fiscal-year estimate). Second, a decision must be made as to what type of bulk oxygen storage system will provide an ample supply. Third, compliance with NFPA codes and other federal, state, and local regulating agencies concerned with the safe handling and storage of gases must be ensured.[17–19] Finally, the fiscal factor(s) that apply to the system of choice must be taken into account.

Central Piping Systems

Central piping systems (Fig 1–12) carry medical gases to locations within medical facilities where they are ultimately used. Piping systems must follow strict NFPA standards as to the type of materials utilized and the manner in which the materials are installed.[3, 8, 26] To maintain a constant pressure (50 psig) at the station outlets, a variety of tube diameters and riser valves are incorporated into centralized piping systems. Since oxygen is classified as a nonflammable gas (but supports combustion), zone valves are strategically placed such that specific areas of a building can be shut down and isolated in case of emergency.

Station outlets located in patient rooms and other locations throughout hospitals incorporate diameter index and the quick-connect safety systems.

Diameter Index Safety System

The DISS, like the PISS described earlier, prevents accidental attachment of the wrong equipment to exposed, threaded connections. The DISS is different from the two safety systems described earlier in that it is designed to work on pressurized systems of 200 psig or less. Respiratory care providers often encounter this type of safety equipment when working with flowmeter outlets such as the one shown in Fig 1–13. Both the DISS and American standard safety system use a threading mechanism to prevent inappropriate connection of medical equipment (Fig 1–14). The threads and hex nuts of the DISS are characteristically much smaller than those of the American standard safety system. The CGA and many compressed gas companies can be contacted for specific gas and assigned safety system number and/or design.[27]

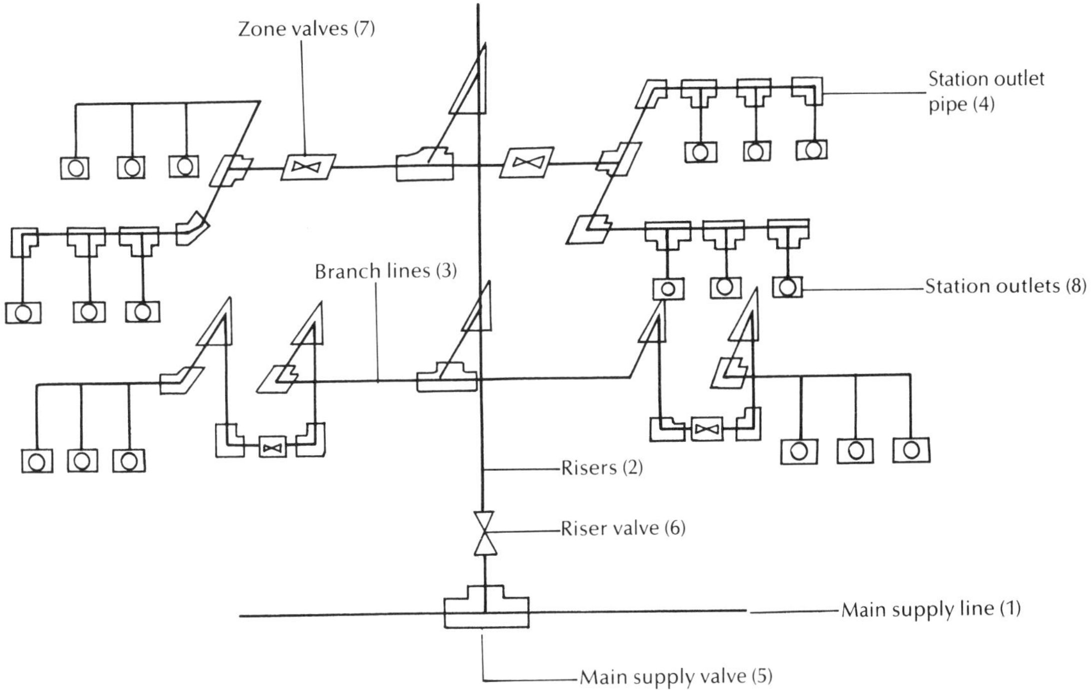

FIG 1–12
Hospital gas piping system. (From Eubanks DH, Bone RC: Medical gases, production, storage, and control, in *Comprehensive Respiratory Care,* ed 2. St Louis, Mosby–Year Book, 1990. Used by permission.)

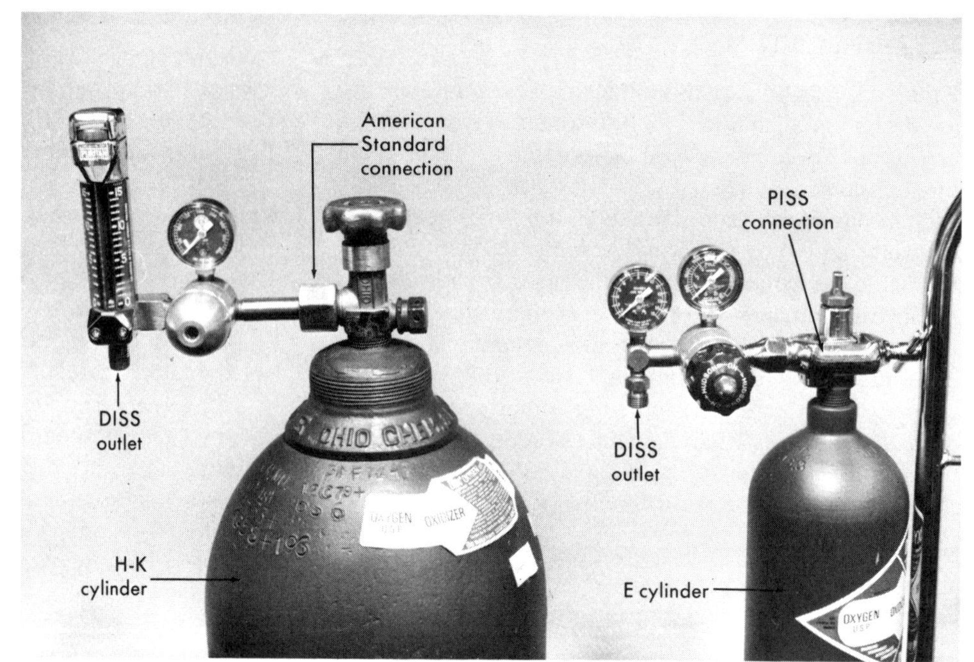

FIG 1–13
Comparison of safety systems used for compressed gases. Note that the DISS connections are for outlets having reduced pressures (less than 2,200 psig), whereas the American Standard connection is shown for a large cylinder and the PISS connection is shown for a small cylinder. (From Spearman CB, Sheldon RL, Egan DF: *Egan's Fundamentals of Respiratory Therapy,* ed 4. St Louis, 1982, Mosby–Year Book, 1982. Used by permission.)

Quick-Connect System

The quick-connect system is designed to allow the connection of low-pressure units to wall, ceiling, and other stationary outlets that receive gas from central piping systems.[26] Typically, flowmeters and high-pressure hoses from ventilators utilize quick-connect systems. The surface mount of a quick-connect coupling has a female connection (receiver) designed to stop the flow of gas when the equipment is not in use (Fig 1–15). A rapid push on the "male" adaptor secures the coupling and activates the line, which then pressurizes the attached medical equipment. Each outlet/connector is designed and manufactured to prevent inappropriate connections (i.e., oxygen to air).

To disengage equipment from the gas outlet, there is a small knob to turn, button to push, or some other quick-release control to manipulate. Similar to the other safety systems described, the quick-connect system uses different configurations, colors, and printed labels to identify sundry types of compressed gases or vacuum. These safety systems draw the attention of the respiratory care provider, prevent inappropriate connection of equipment, and ultimately, render safe the administration of medical gases to patients.

Portable Oxygen Supply Systems

Portable oxygen supply systems are based on either compressed gas or liquid gas systems.

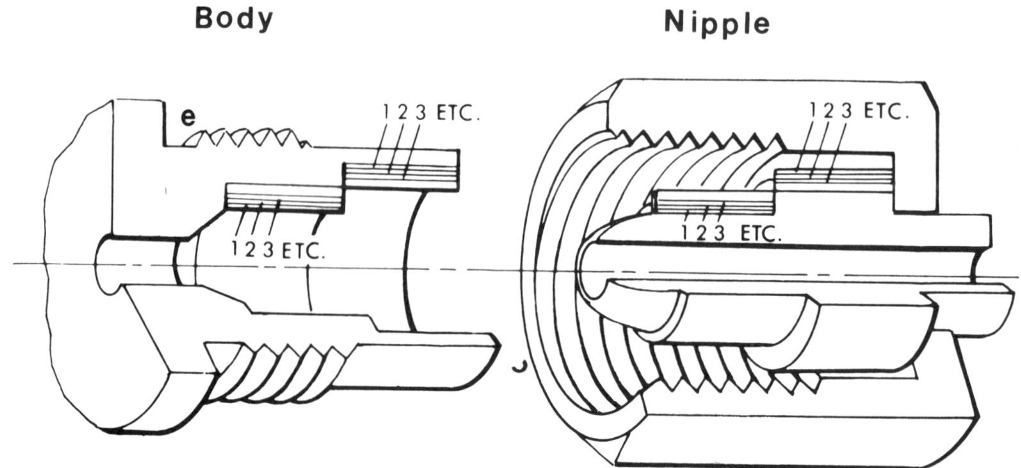

FIG 1–14
The DISS standard low-pressure connection for medical gases, compressed air, and suction. The small bore in the body mates with the small diameter of the nipple, and the large bore in the body mates with the large diameter of the nipple. (Courtesy of Compressed Gas Association.)

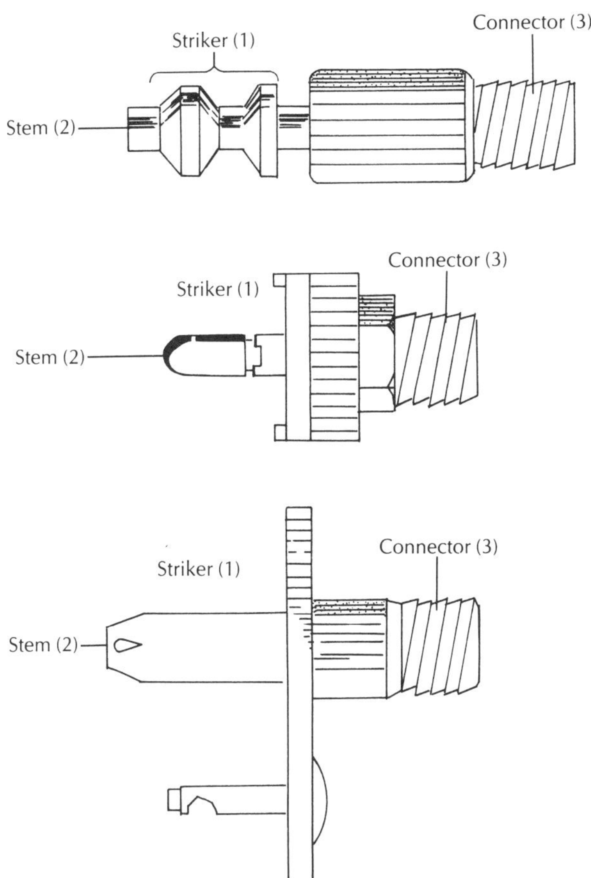

FIG 1–15
Quick-connect adapters for attachment of equipment to patient station outlets. (From Eubanks DH, Bone RC: Medical gases, production, storage, and control, in *Comprehensive Respiratory Care,* ed 2. St Louis, Mosby–Year Book, 1990. Used by permission.)

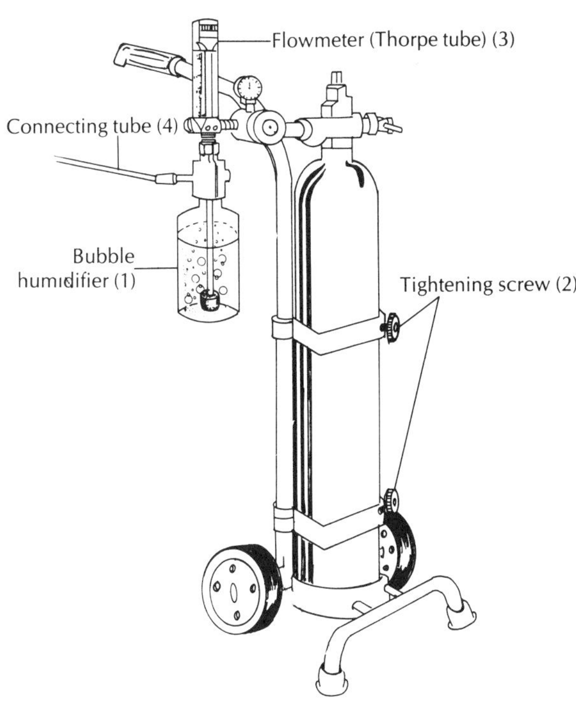

FIG 1–16
"E" size oxygen cylinder mounted in a small wheeled stand. (From Eubanks DH, Bone RC: Medical gases, production, storage, and control, in *Comprehensive Respiratory Care,* ed 2. St Louis, Mosby–Year Book, 1990. Used by permission.)

Compressed Gas Systems

Compressed gas systems (discussed earlier) are portable systems that utilize an "E" (or smaller size) gas cylinder (Fig 1–16), which can be placed on a portable cart, wheelchair, or a patient transfer bed (Fig 1–17). The E cylinder provides a 2,200-psig gas source that when used in conjunction with a regulator, reduces the high-pressure gas source to a lower working pressure of 50 psig. Compressed gas systems are the systems of choice for short-term use in a medical environment. This type of system affords an excellent source of compressed (low pressure) gases to support any respiratory care equipment/apparatus in transport.

NOTE: If a Thorpe tube–type flowmeter is used with the portable cylinder, it should not be used in the horizontal position because the flow indicator (ball) is gravity dependent and must be in a vertical position to indicate the flow rate.

Portable Liquid Oxygen Supply Systems

Portable liquid oxygen supply systems are generally chosen for use in the home environment. These units are miniature versions of the bulk liquid oxygen supply systems discussed previously. Several manufacturers produce portable liquid supply systems; each product varies slightly in style, but all provide basically the same level of service for the patient. Portable units incorporate both a bulk storage unit and a portable, refillable, lightweight carrying container. The storage unit is normally filled with 40 lb of liquid oxygen (24,368 L of gaseous oxygen) and provides a low working pressure between 20 and 90 psig. Controls on the portable liquid oxygen container enable the patient to select oxygen flow rates suitable for use with a nasal cannula, transtracheal catheter, mask, or other oxygen therapy modality.

Customarily, the larger liquid oxygen storage unit remains in a permanent place in the home, and the carrying container is filled from the storage unit as necessary (Fig 1–18). When full, the portable liquid carrying container weighs between 6 and 11 lb and provides approximately 1,025 L of gas (Fig 1–19).[28] Portable systems allow patients who require oxygen the freedom to move about in their homes and communities (Fig 1–20). Respiratory care providers are responsible for

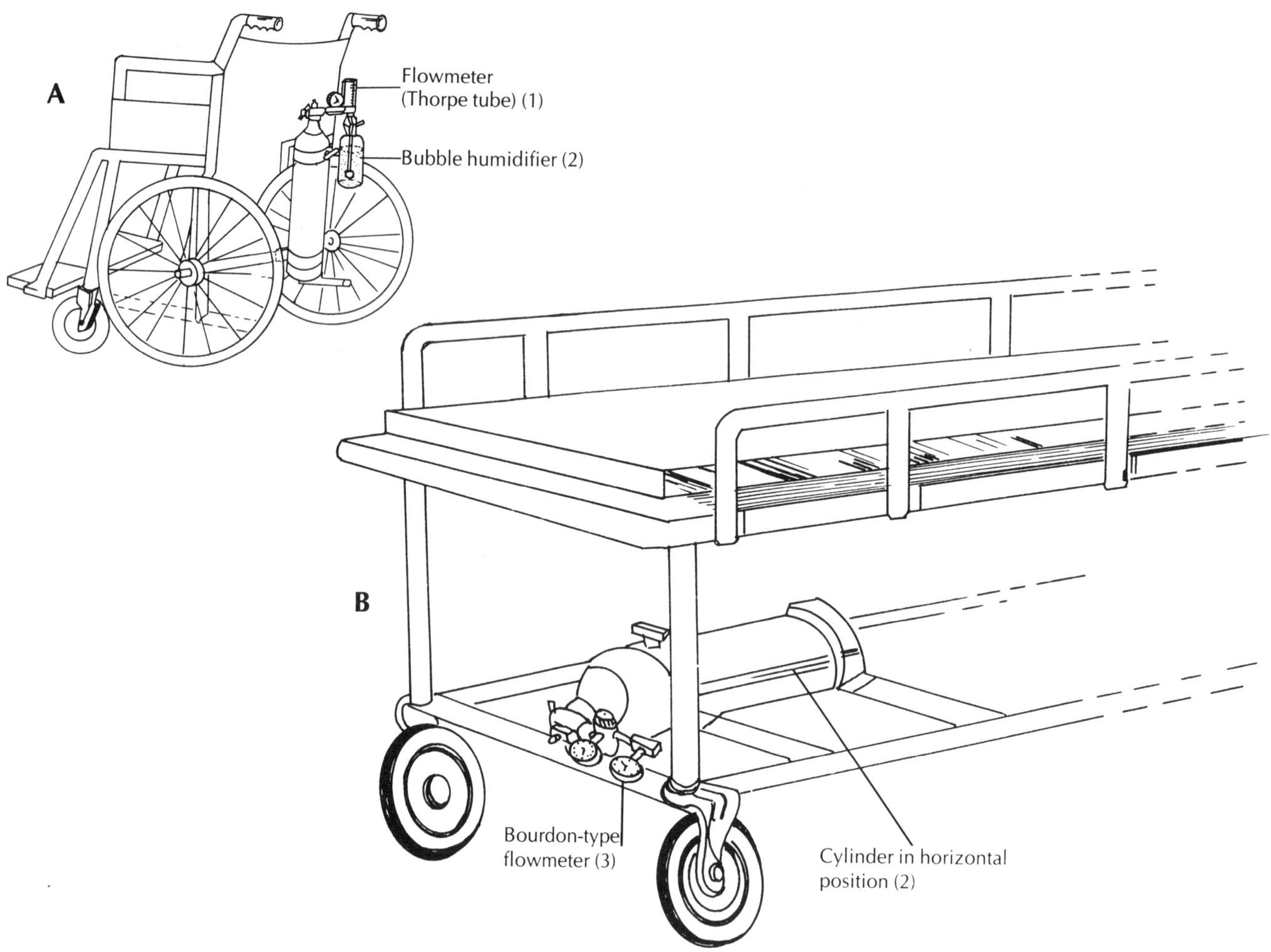

FIG 1–17
Special retainer for transporting an oxygen cylinder on a wheelchair **(A),** a nd a stretcher **(B).** (From Eubanks DH, Bone RC: Medical gases, production, storage, and control, in *Comprehensive Respiratory Care,* ed 2. St Louis, Mosby–Year Book, 1990. Used by permission.)

ensuring that both patients and their families are thoroughly informed and aware of the hazards and safety precautions associated with the storage and usage of liquid oxygen containers and supplies.

AIR COMPRESSORS

As previously mentioned, the earth's atmosphere is made up of a gas mixture containing nitrogen, oxygen, inert gases, carbon dioxide, and hydrogen. An air compressor is a motor-driven unit with a storage reservoir that draws in room air, pressurizes it, and stores it for subsequent use. This compressed air can be administered directly to a patient or provided at a low working pressure to operate a specific piece of equipment. A variety of types and styles of air compressors are available to accomplish this aim.

Large commercial compressors incorporate large reservoirs, filters, and drying systems to provide a 50-psig working pressure to hospital central piping systems (Fig 1–21). Smaller and more portable units (not shown) contain no reservoirs but can provide compressed air to locations where central piping systems are unavailable. Both types of air compressors employ an electric power source to operate a piston, a diaphragm, or a rotary mechanism that ultimately draws in, compresses, and stores atmospheric air for later use. (Note: It is critical that compressed air for medical purposes be free of environmental contaminants such as dust or oil droplets that can be released by the compressor. For this reason, air compressors must use water-sealed or other components to protect the air against oil droplets.)

Fig 1–22 illustrates a piston compressor; Fig 1–23, a diaphragm; and Fig 1–24, a rotary mechanism. Each mechanism entrains filtered atmospheric air into an enclosed space. Both the piston and diaphragm pumps

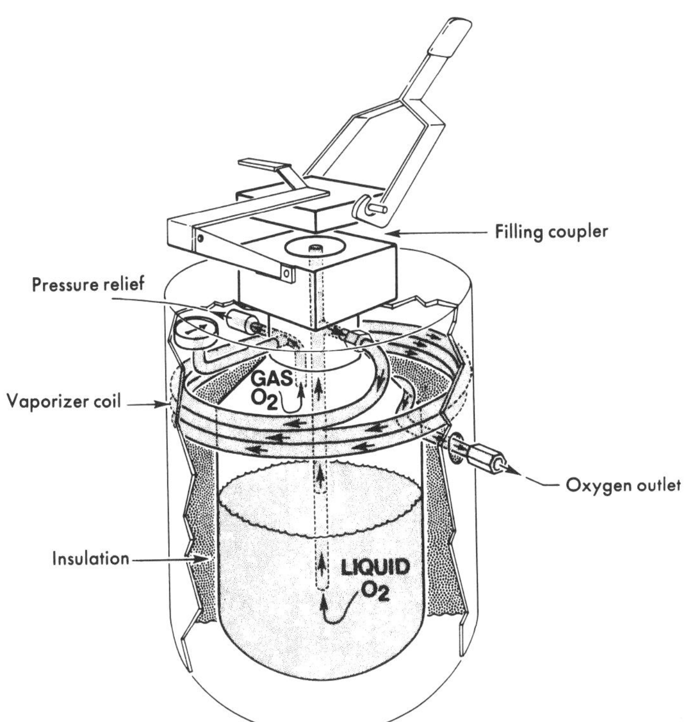

FIG 1–18
Diagram of a Linde Walker system reservoir. (From Lampton LM: Home and outpatient oxygen therapy, in Brashear RE, Rhodes ML (eds): *Chronic Obstructive Lung Disease.* St Louis, Mosby–Year Book, 1978. Used by permission.)

make use of a series of one-way valves. As the piston or diaphragm descends, filtered air is pulled into a chamber through the one-way valve (inlet). When the piston or diaphragm ascends, the air in the chamber is compressed and forced through the second one-way valve (outlet), drier, and reducing valve (discussed later) to the appropriate service area.

A rotary mechanism, such as is illustrated by the water-sealed pump shown in Fig 1–24, is composed of a rotor with attached blades that spin freely inside a housing that contains water. The spinning blades force water against the walls to form a leak-proof seal. As air is drawn in through the main inlet it is compressed by the spinning blades and discharged through the exit port. A small amount of water must be constantly added to the pump to maintain the required seal.

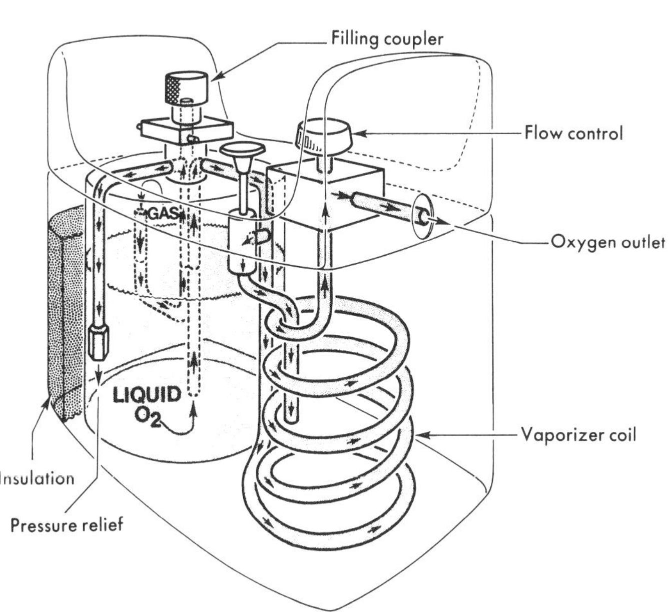

FIG 1–19
Diagram of a Linde Walker portable unit. (From Lampton LM: Home and outpatient oxygen therapy, in Brashear RE, Rhodes ML (eds): *Chronic Obstructive Lung Disease.* St Louis, Mosby–Year Book, 1978. Used by permission.)

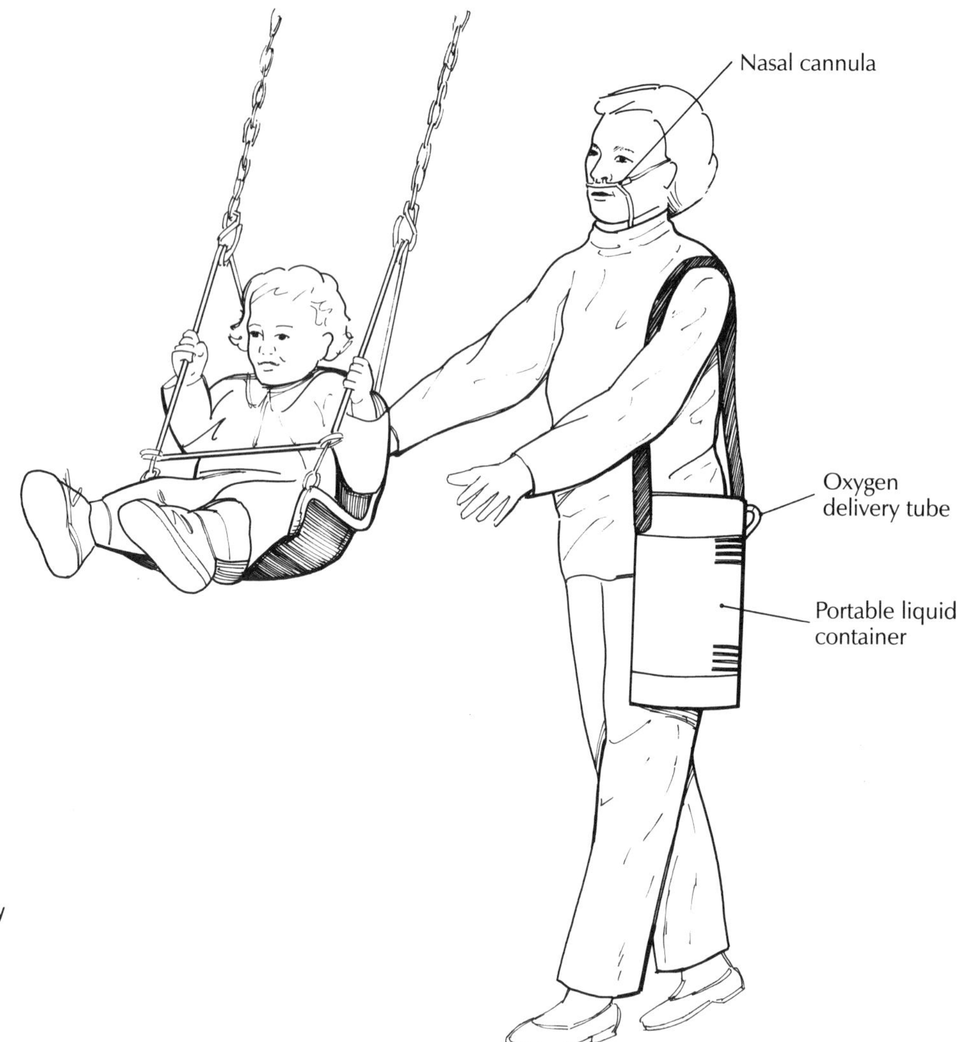

FIG 1–20
The portable liquid oxygen stroller by Cryogenic Associates weighs 9½ lb (full) and lasts up to 8 hours at 2 L/min of gas flow. (Courtesy of Cryogenics Associates, a division of Beatrice Foods, Indianapolis.)

OXYGEN CONCENTRATORS

The purpose of an oxygen concentrator is to provide patients with an enriched oxygen supply (greater than 21% oxygen at a flow rate of 1 to 10 L/min). Low- to moderate-flow oxygen delivery devices are used with concentrators in the home environment. Oxygen concentrators are designed to entrain atmospheric air and then physically separate the oxygen and nitrogen. This process is accomplished by one of two methods: molecular sieves or semipermeable membranes.[3]

Molecular Sieves

Molecular sieves provide users with an oxygen concentration in excess of 90% when set at a low flow rate (1 to 2 L/min). If higher flow rates are desired, the oxygen concentration declines significantly. Oxygen is physically separated from the atmospheric gas through the use of an air compressor and inorganic sodium/aluminum silicate pellets. The pellets are placed in a pair of sieves that are in line with the flow of filtered, compressed air (Fig 1–25). The pellets absorb both water vapor and nitrogen from the compressed air, so the gas exiting from the sieves is enriched in oxygen. The exiting gas is held in the reservoir until it is diverted to the patient outlet. Manufacturers recommend that humidifiers be used in conjunction with this type of system to replace some of the water vapor removed in the filtering process.

Water vapor and nitrogen (that have been physically removed from atmospheric air) are periodically removed from the pellets through a backwashing process. Depending upon usage, the backwashing process reactivates the pellets for some time. Manufacturers of molecular sieves recommend that the pellets be replaced routinely or the anticipated final oxygen concentration may be less than desired.

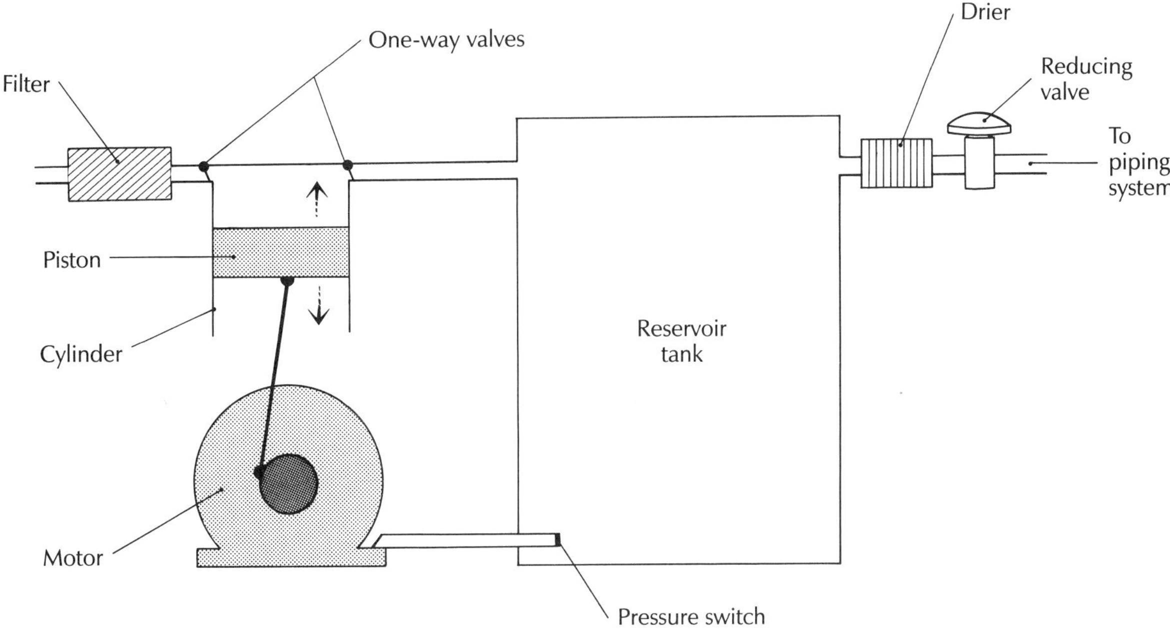

FIG 1–21
Large air compressor system for a piping system. The compressor sends gas to the reservoir at higher than line pressure. When the preset pressure level is reached, the pressure switch shuts the compressor off. Gas leaves the reservoir and passes through the dryer to remove moisture, and the reducing valve reduces gas to the desired line pressure. When the reservoir pressure has dropped to near line pressure, the pressure switch turns the compressor back on. (From McPherson SP, Spearman CB: *Respiratory Therapy Equipment,* ed 3. St Louis, Mosby–Year Book, 1985. Used by permission.)

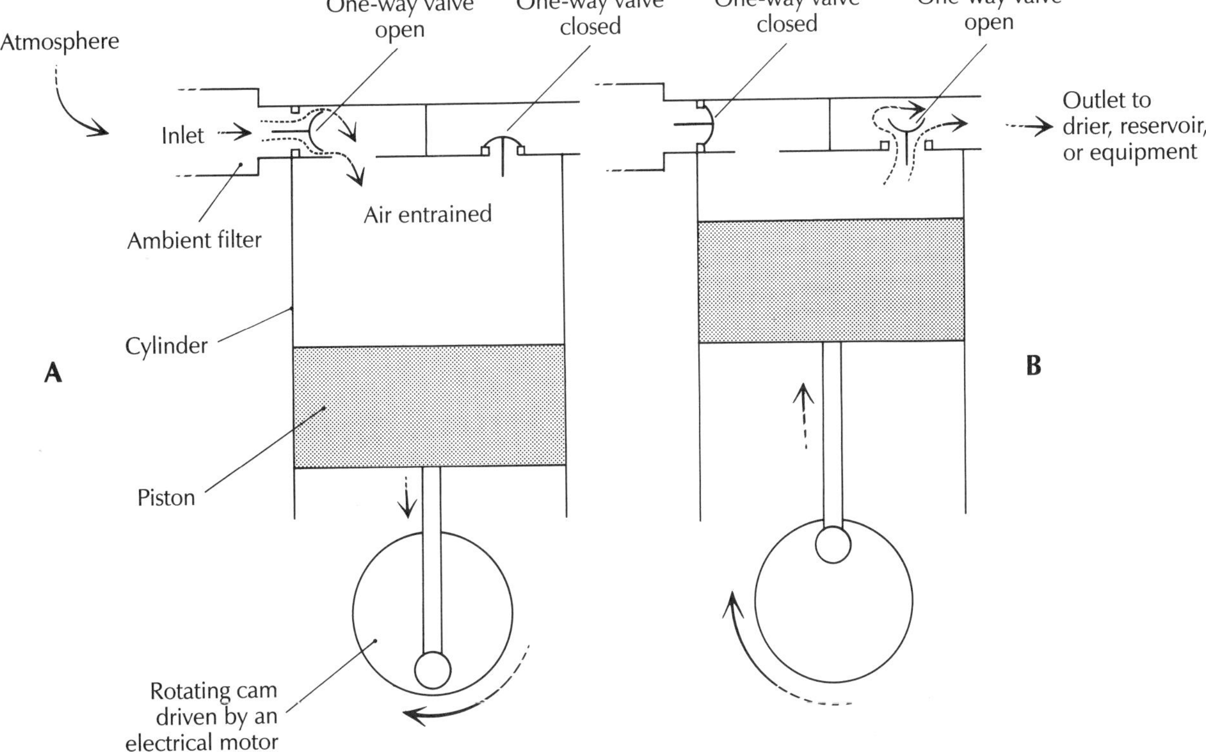

FIG 1–22
Piston compressor. **A,** the descending piston entrains filtered room air via the one-way valve into the chamber. **B,** the ascending piston forces the compressed air out the one-way valve into the pressurized system.

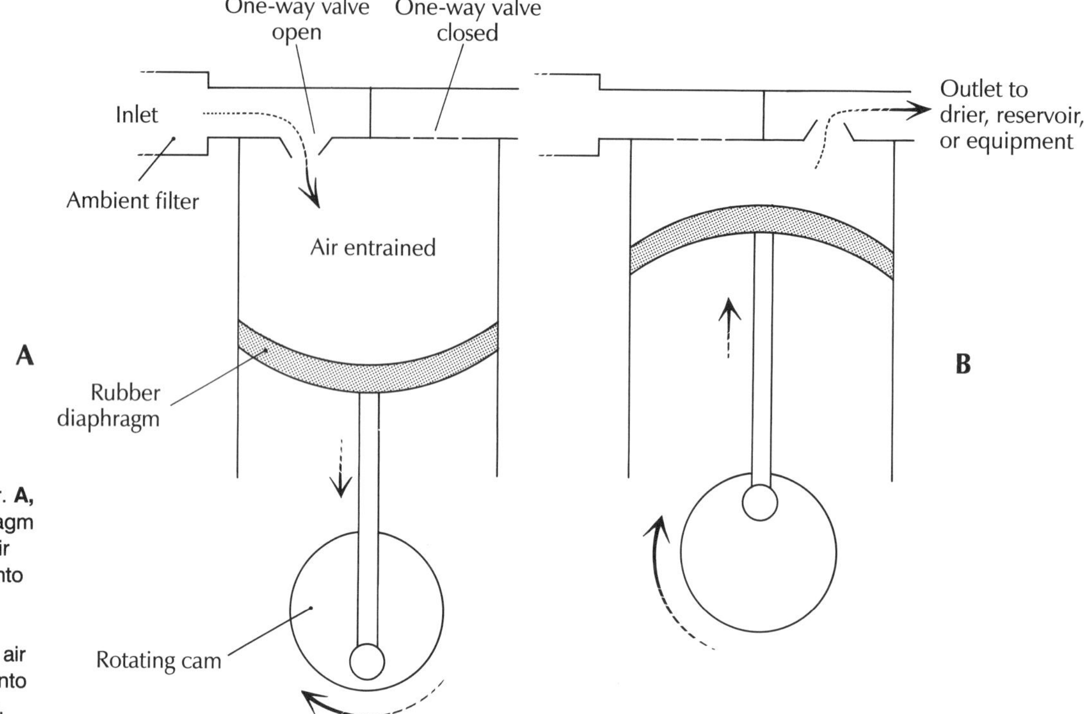

FIG 1–23
Diaphragm compressor. **A,** the descending diaphragm entrains filtered room air via the one-way valve into the chamber. **B,** the ascending diaphragm forces the compressed air out the one-way valve into the pressurized system.

Semipermeable Membranes

Semipermeable membranes are another physical means by which oxygen can be separated from other atmospheric gases (Fig 1–26). This type of oxygen concentrator generates a constant 40% enrichment at either a low (1 to 2 L/min) or high (8 to 10 L/min) flow rate. A vacuum pump provides a negative pressure gradient across the membrane.[3] Since the diffusion rate is slower for nitrogen, water vapor and oxygen diffuse more rapidly across the membrane and are collected on the opposite side. Although enough water remains in the gas to eliminate the need for a humidifier, a large proportion of the water vapor is removed from the oxygen-enriched gas by a condenser.

Most manufacturers recommend that this type of enricher be operated at three times the flow rate used

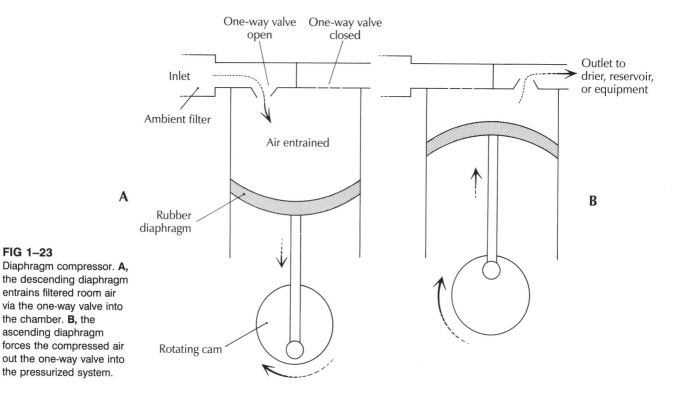

FIG 1–24
Rotary compressor. A series of rotating blades entrain *(inlet)* filtered room air through a one-way valve into the central chamber. As the blades rotate, the space between the blades and the chamber wall becomes smaller, and water is forced against the housing wall to form a seal. The compressed air exits through the one-way valve *(outlet)* to the pressurized system. (Courtesy of OHIO Medical Products, Madison, Wisc.)

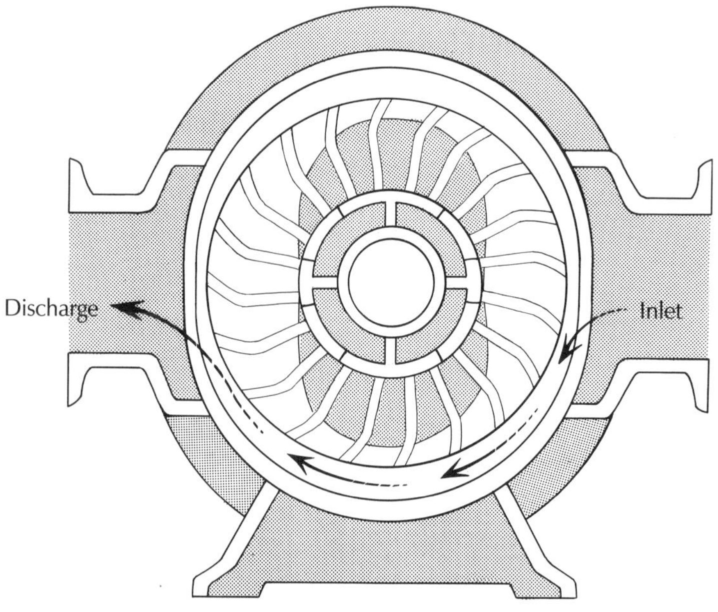

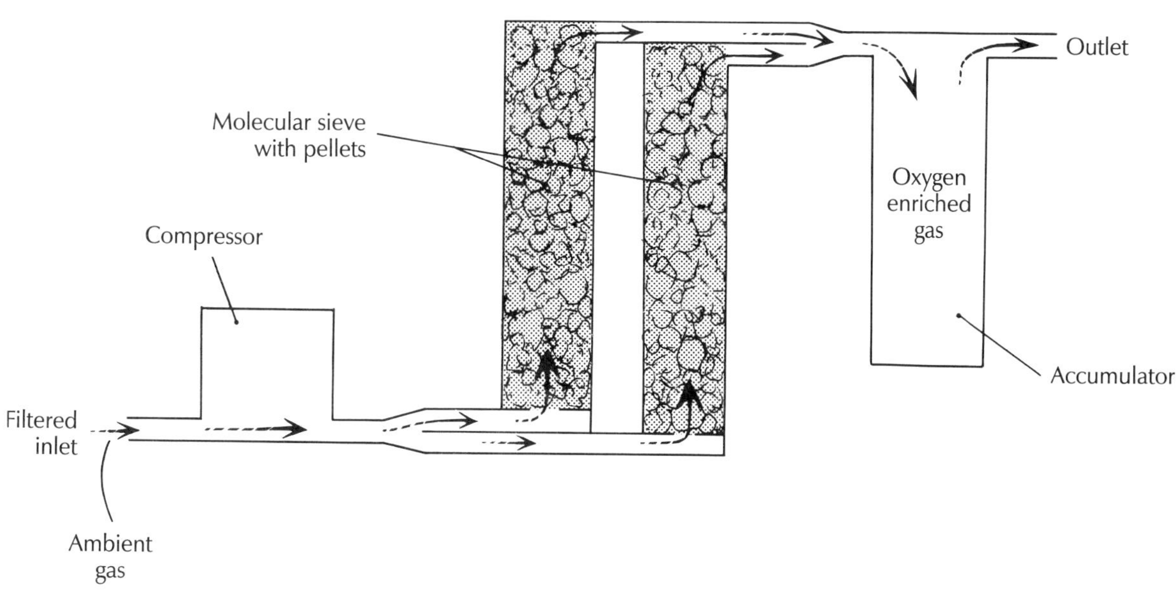

FIG 1–25
Molecular sieve. Filtered compressed air enters the pellet-filled molecular sieve where water vapor and nitrogen are absorbed. Dry, oxygen-enriched air remains in the accumulator until needed.

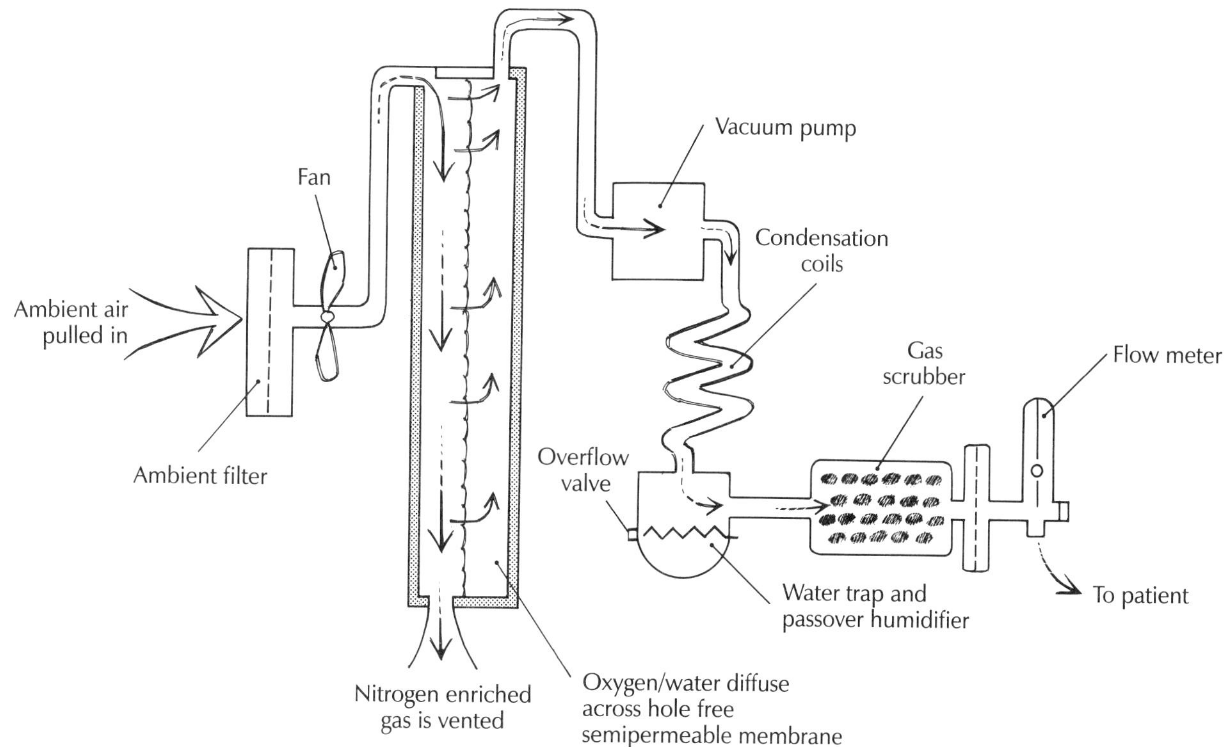

FIG 1–26
Semipermeable membrane concentrator (enricher). Ambient air is pulled into the unit where oxygen and water vapor are separated from nitrogen by diffusion across a semipermeable membrane.

with a 100% oxygen source. For example, to deliver inspiratory oxygen (F_{IO_2}) to a level of 28% from a 100% oxygen cylinder, the flow rate would be adjusted to 2 L/min. With an enricher, the flow rate would need to be set at 6 L/min to deliver a 28% oxygen concentration.*

Continuous Vs. Intermittent Oxygen Use

Clinically, oxygen concentrators and enrichers are making continuous oxygen therapy at home more convenient and less hazardous than was the use of traditional cylinders and liquid oxygen containers. The medical benefits realized by the patient receiving nearly continuous oxygen therapy (12 hr/day) as compared with when only nocturnal oxygen is used were well documented in the nocturnal oxygen therapy trial[29](NOTT) conducted in North America. Clinical benefits of long-term oxygen therapy include improved survival, improved neuropsychological function, reduced pulmonary artery pressure and pulmonary vascular resistance, and slowed progression of pulmonary hypertension.[30]

More recent studies involving patients who received continuous oxygen (24 hr/day) by transtracheal catheter have shown additional clinical benefits to those who receive oxygen via nasal cannula.[30] The medical literature offers mounting documentation of the benefits of receiving long-term continuous oxygen therapy. One of the most impressive outcomes from the many long-term oxygen trials is that oxygen may have a significant reparative effect.[30]

This revelation has created a debate among care givers as to whether or not the repair is permanent and, if so, should oxygen therapy be discontinued or reduced to decrease costs? This question has not been answered and undoubtedly will remain a topic of investigation and debate in the coming years.

PRESSURE REDUCING VALVES AND REGULATORS

Pressure Reducing Valves

Pressure reducing valves are attached to both compressed gas cylinders and bulk oxygen systems. These valves provide a mechanism to convert the high storage pressure of 2,200 psig to a workable pressure of approximately 50 psig. It is important to not mistake pressure reducing valves for regulators and vice versa. The function of a regulator is twofold—to reduce gas pressure to a workable level and to control and indicate the flow of gas leaving the unit. The device that controls and indicates the flow rate is called a flowmeter (discussed in the next section). Most respiratory care providers take for granted the ready availability of a 50-psig working pressure gas source. This low working pressure activates a large variety of respiratory care equipment, so the significance of a pressure reducing valve should not be minimized.

There are a variety of reducing valves on the market; each of them is composed of a series of chambers, springs, a rubber diaphragm, pressure relief (pop-off) ports, inlets, and outlets. The configuration of these features varies among manufacturers. Typically, as shown in Fig 1–27 and explained below, pressure reducing valves work on the principle of gas pressure vs. spring tension.

Fig 1–27 illustrates the basic design of a simple one-step (single-stage), adjustable pressure reducing valve that has been set to deliver 50 psig. The source gas (2,200 psig) enters an inlet *(C)* and closed reduction chamber *(B)*. The pressure exerted by the gas pushes on the surface of the flexible rubber diaphragm *(2)*. In turn, the tension exerted by the diaphragm spring(s) *(5)* in the ambient chamber *(A)* defines the excursion of the flexible rubber diaphragm. This limitation created by the diaphragm spring(s) directly affects the valve *(9)* position, the volume, the gas pressure in the closed reduction (pressurized) chamber *(B)*, and the gas pressure at the outlet port *(11)*. In this illustration, the pressure of gas exiting the outlet port *(11)* is determined by the amount of tension created by the adjustment made on the screw handle *(3)*. As the screw handle *(3)* is tightened, the tension on the spring increases, and the amount of pressure to counter the tension on the spring increases; the reverse applies to lowering the pressure.

As stated above, Figure 1–27 illustrates an adjustable pressure reducing valve. An adjustable reducing valve enables the user to select a wide range of working pressures, from 5 psig to as high as 2,200 psig (from a full cylinder). Preset pressure reducing valves do not have a screw handle *(3)* and deliver only the pressure selected by the manufacturer. Preset pressure reducing valves, which are normally set by manufacturers to 50 psig ± 5 psig, are the most common valve found in respiratory care departments.

Pressure reducing valves are also distinguished as to whether they are single-stage or multiple-stage units. Single-stage (or one-step) valves are designed to reduce the source gas pressure in a full cylinder (2,200 psig) directly to a desired working pressure. These types of valves are found on both central piping systems and compressed gas cylinders. Multiple-stage reducing valves (which can have two or more stages) reduce the source gas to a midrange pressure in each stage until a desirable final pressure is reached. Multiple-stage pressure reducing valves are most applicable for precision work and are

*Large concentrators are available for use as institutional supply systems.

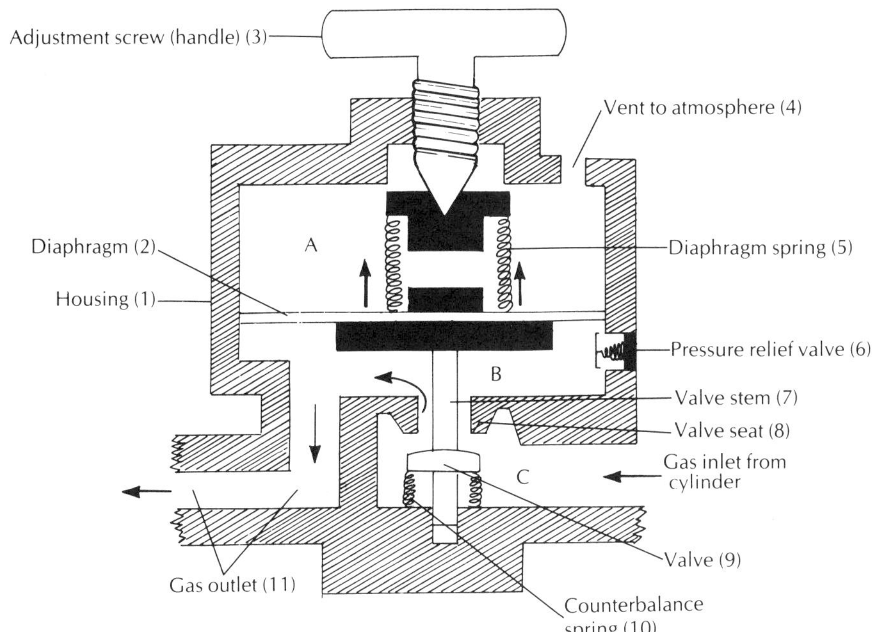

FIG 1–27
Components of a single-stage reducing valve as seen in cross section. (From Eubanks DH, Bone RC: Medical gases, production, storage, and control, in *Comprehensive Respiratory Care,* ed 2. St Louis, Mosby–Year Book, 1990. Used by permission.)

typically found in research laboratories; they are generally not found on central piping systems.

Despite the fact that all pressure reducing valves possess similar exterior physical characteristics (e.g., size, weight, general appearance), there is a simple method by which a user can distinguish among a group of pressure reducing valves. Each pressure reducing stage chamber must have a relief valve (Fig 1–27)*[6]*) to provide for the release of excess pressure. This is a safety component to prevent rupture of a pressure reducing valve when exposed to excessive pressure. Respiratory care providers need only count the number of pressure relief valves (Fig 1–27 *[6]*) found on the external housing of each unit to accurately determine whether the unit is a single- or multiple-stage pressure reducing valve.

Regulators

As described earlier, a regulator is a combination of a pressure reducing valve and a flowmeter. In order for a respiratory care provider to know exactly what pressures are being used, a pressure gauge is attached to all regulators. Pressure gauges indicate the pressure remaining in a compressed gas cylinder and, if an adjustable reducing valve is used, the pressure within the closed reduction chamber.

Bourdon Pressure Gauge

Figure 1–28 illustrates the components of a Bourdon pressure gauge. The Bourdon pressure gauge is attached to a pressure source (usually a pressure regulator or reducing valve). The source pressure is exerted onto the interior surface of a hollow, crescent-shaped tube; the pressure alters its shape (straightens the tube to some degree) and thereby moves the gear mechanism.[28] The calibrated gear mechanism, in turn, is attached to a needle indicator that reflects the amount of pressure within the system. As the pressure changes within the hollow tube, the calibrated gear mechanism readjusts, and the indicator moves accordingly.

Respiratory care providers must be aware of the difference between a Bourdon pressure gauge and a Bourdon flowmeter. Both mechanisms are identical to the mechanism described in Figure 1–28. The major physical difference is that the pressure gauge faceplate reads in pounds per square inch and the flowmeter reads in liters per minute. Bourdon flowmeters also have an adjustable needle valve (described in the next section).

FLOWMETERS

A flowmeter is designed to control and indicate the flow rate of a gas. Since medical gases are prescribed, respiratory care providers must be able to differentiate among the various types of flowmeters available. Flowmeters can be permanently attached to a pressure reducing valve to create a regulator, or they can be used independently and affixed via a quick-connect adaptor to a central piping system station outlet. This arrangement enables practitioners to administer low-pressure–system gases in liters per minute. Flowmeters are labeled on their housings as to the specific type of gas each unit is

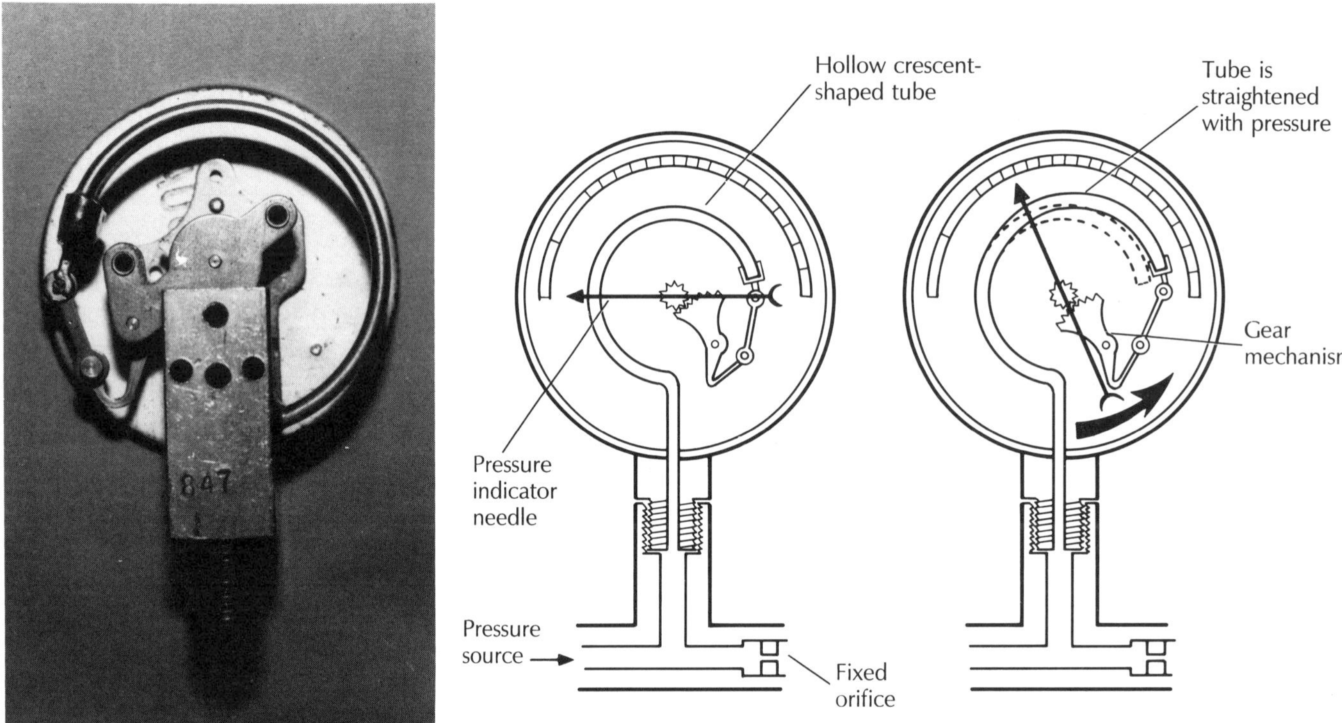

FIG 1–28
Components of a Bourdon pressure gauge. As gas enters from the source, a backpressure is created by the fixed orifice. This backpressure is reflected throughout the hollow, crescent-shaped tube and causes it to straighten and move the indicator needle along a pressure scale. (From Barnes TA: Equipment for mixed gas and oxygen therapy, in *Respiratory Care Practice.* St Louis, Mosby–Year Book, 1988. Used by permission.)

designed to control. Flow indicators (ball, bobbin, or rod) rise as the control valve is opened and display the gas flow along a graduated scale in units of liters per minute. Flowmeters employ a variety of quick-connect and DISS to ensure safe administration of appropriate medical gases.

Flowmeters are categorized by their physical characteristics as flow restrictors, Bourdon gauges, or Thorpe tubes.[31]

Flow Restrictor

Flow restrictors are simple devices that allow a low constant pressure (50 psig) to be exposed to a permanent orifice (Fig 1–29). The pressure gradient established at the orifice controls the exiting flow. The only way the flow will change is if an unnatural pressure drop occurs. The physical design of the flow restrictor prevents inappropriate flow rates from being delivered to the patient. Furthermore, flow restrictors are not affected by gravity and function equally well in upright, horizontal, and upside-down positions.

Bourdon Gauge Flowmeter

The Bourdon gauge flowmeter functions in the same manner as the Bourdon pressure gauge described earlier (see Fig 1–28). In this particular application, the needle indicator identifies a particular flow rate (in liters per minute) rather than a pressure. Figure 1–30 illustrates how the Bourdon gauge is attached to a permanent orifice. As the low (50 psig) pressure source gas *(4)* enters the unit, the permanent orifice *(2)* restricts the flow of gas that can exit the outlet *(6)*. A common characteristic shared between the flow restrictor and the Bourdon gauge is that gravity has no effect on the operation of the Bourdon gauge flowmeter. That is, the Bourdon gauge flowmeter functions satisfactorily in any position.

Enlarging the permanent orifice of a Bourdon gauge flowmeter allows more gas to flow through the gauge than is indicated by the needle; the Bourdon gauge becomes "noncompensated." Noncompensation implies that if a restriction is placed over the outlet *(6)*, a backpressure (higher pressure) is created proximal to the orifice; this pressure change causes the hollow crescent tube to straighten and alters the gear mechanism. The

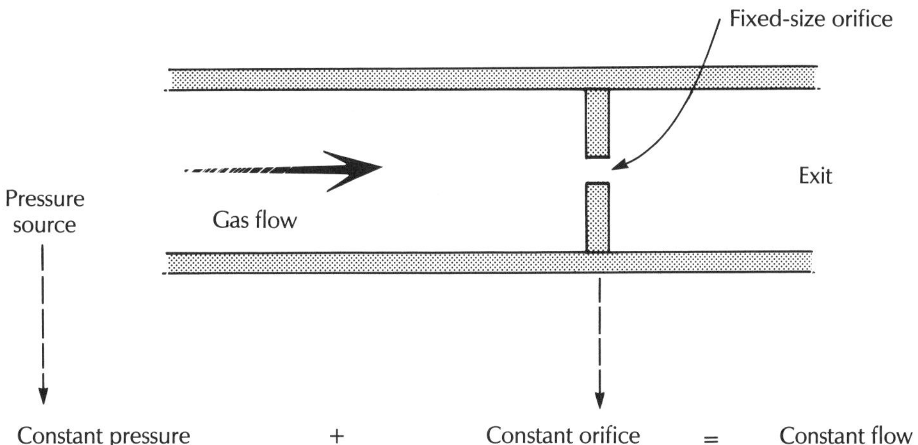

FIG 1–29
Flow resistor–type flowmeter. Gas flow at the exit point is determined by the pressure drop created across the fixed orifice.

needle indicator then registers a higher flow (liters per minute) than is actually exiting the unit.[28] That is, if the oxygen connecting tube becomes pinched such that little or no oxygen is flowing to the patient, the needle indicator (because of the high backpressure) reads higher than the actual flow. Thus, the patient does not receive the prescribed amount of oxygen and may be placed in jeopardy.

Thorpe Tube Flowmeter

The physical characteristic that differentiate a Thorpe tube flowmeter from the other flowmeter described above is that a Thorpe tube flowmeter (Fig 1–31) has a variable orifice size[28] that is controlled by a flow-control knob *(13)*. A 50-psig source gas enters the flowmeter via the gas inlet *(3)* and continues to the gas flow tube *(9)*. The pressure gradient generated proximal to the orifice fluctuates according to the size of the variable orifice. The wider the opening, the lower the pressure resistance and the higher the exiting flow. As the outlet is closed, the pressure resistance increases and the flow exiting the unit decreases. On a standard Thorpe tube flowmeter, the flow rate scale *(8)* ranges from 1 to 15 L/min. However, if the control knob *(13)* is opened to the maximum or "flush" setting, the flowmeter can deliver flows greater than 60 L/min.[31]

A second differentiating characteristic between the Thorpe tube and other types of flowmeters is the necessity of having the Thorpe tube in an upright position. The indicator ball *(7)* in the conical gas flow tube *(9)* uses gravity in opposition to lift to represent the flow rate. At higher flow rates, the velocity of the moving gas supports the indicator ball. If the Thorpe tube is placed in any position other than upright, even though the flow rate remains constant, the indicator ball will not

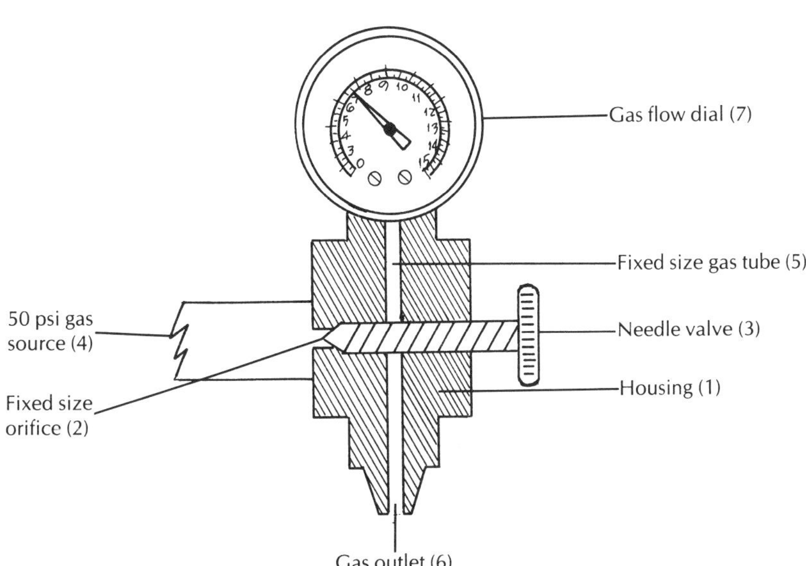

FIG 1–30
Bourdon gauge flowmeter. The flow rate at the gas outlet is controlled by moving the control valve in and out of its seat. (From Eubanks DH, Bone RC: Medical gases, production, storage, and control, in *Comprehensive Respiratory Care,* ed 2. St Louis, Mosby–Year Book, 1990. Used by permission.)

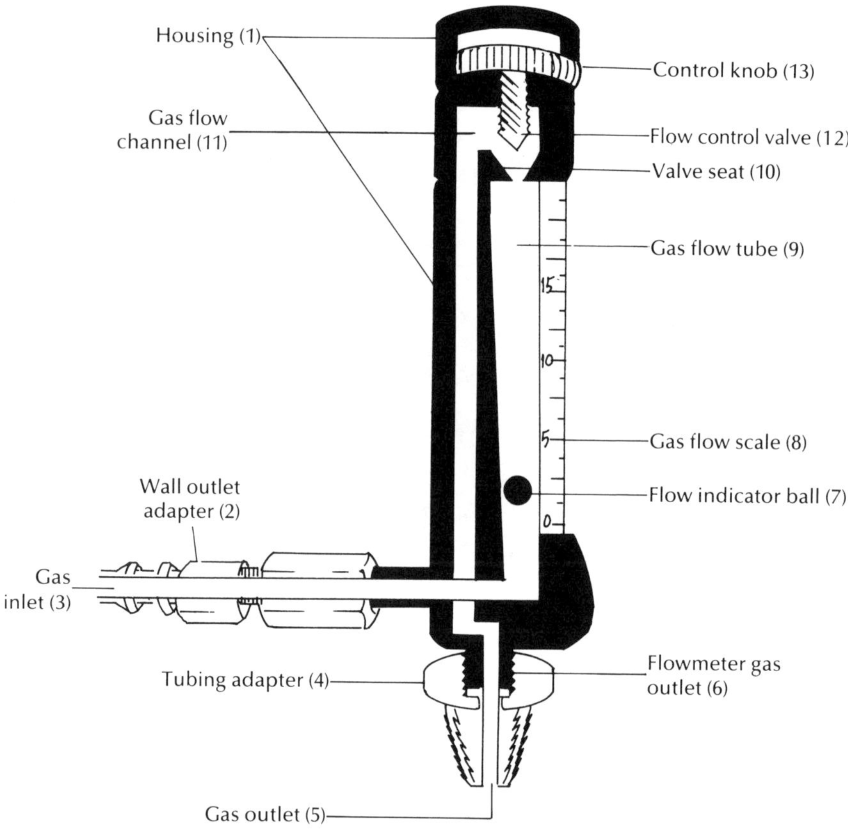

FIG 1–31
Thorpe tube flowmeter showing the location of the control valve distal to the flow tube. (From Eubanks DH, Bone RC: Medical gases, production, storage, and control, in *Comprehensive Respiratory Care,* ed 2. St Louis, Mosby–Year Book, 1990. Used by permission.)

reflect the actual flow of gas through the tube. For this reason, the Thorpe tube flowmeter is not the flowmeter of choice when transporting a patient.

Third, unlike earlier models, the majority of Thorpe flowmeters in use today are considered to be compensated for backpressure (this means that the indicator ball accurately reflects the flow being delivered to the patient). They are considered to be compensated because the control knob *(13)* is placed distal to the conical flow tube *(9)*. When the control knob is opened, the entire flow tube is exposed to 50-psig pressure and is therefore unaffected by backpressure (which can never exceed line pressure) (50 psig).

BASIC SAFETY RULES

In order to prevent unnecessary problems with the use of flowmeters it is recommended that the following be observed:

- Flowmeters should not be used with mechanical devices that incorporate regulators (i.e., devices that require 50-psig operating pressures). Novel approaches to the adaptation of regulators to flowmeters inappropriately decrease the flow to the regulator and are therefore not considered usual and customary treatment in mechanical ventilation or other settings.
- Novel approaches to the storage of "E" cylinders during transport affect regulation and alter gas flow. Therefore only standard storage protocols should be used.
- Flowmeters should not be repaired by other than factory-trained and authorized personnel.
- Flowmeters should be used only for the gas for which it was manufactured. NOTE: If a gas mixture is administered by using a standard oxygen flowmeter, correction factors should be applied to determine the accurate flow rate.

SUMMARY

Issues related to the delivery and storage of medical gases have changed considerably in recent years and now offer considerable challenge. Because there are many types of delivery systems, the ability to differentiate among types and styles of equipment becomes important. Diversity in flowmeters and regulators and the ability to understand the appropriate function of each of these devices are cornerstones to their safe and effective use. The assurance of being able to safely deliver what is prescribed becomes one of the most significant quality assurance issues. Safe usage of compressed gas in institutions requires sufficient knowledge of medical gas bulk systems and the relevant quality assurance issues pertinent to identifying leaks and potential hazards in construction, as well as having the ability to deal with gas contamination. Respiratory care providers and medical directors play integral roles in quality assurance by providing rapid intervention in case of problems. Periodic review of shut-off valves, piping concerns, and bulk gas storage systems needs to be integrated into quality assurance assessment and should be monitored routinely.

The safe use of medical gases and their delivery systems requires a thorough knowledge of the gases and systems being employed. Improper handling, faulty assembly of equipment, or improper maintenance of gases may cause considerable hazard or injury. Numerous systems are designed to ensure that easy recognition, maintenance, and utilization of equipment and standardization of storage systems for medical gases, as well as regulators and flowmeters, help facilitate the ease and safety of operation. These systems, however, are only as good as the people who use them and whose obligation it is to use them responsibly—respiratory care providers.

REFERENCES

1. Bancroft ML, Steen JA: Health device legislation: An overview of the law and its impact on respiratory care. *Respir Care* 1978; 23:1179.
2. Compressed Gas Association: *Characteristics and Safe Handling of Medical Gases,* Pamphlet P-2, Arlington, Va, Compressed Gas Association, 1984.
3. McPherson SP: *Respiratory Therapy Equipment.* St Louis, Mosby–Year Book, 1990.
4. Compressed Gas Association: *Handbook of Compressed Gases.* New York, Van Nostrand Reinhold, 1985.
5. Code of Federal Regulations: Title 49, Parts 1 to 199. Washington, DC, US Government Printing Office, 1973.
6. Compressed Gas Association: *Characteristics and Safe Handling of Medical Gases.* New York, Compressed Gas Association, 1984.
7. Compressed Gas Association: *Characteristics and Safe Handling of Medical Gases,* Pamphlet P-1, Arlington, Va, Compressed Gas Association, 1965.
8. Burton GG, Hodgkin JE, Ward JJ: *Respiratory Care: A Guide to Clinical Practice.* Philadelphia, JB Lippincott, 1991.
9. Boon PE: Correspondence C-size cylinders. *Anaesth Intensive Care* 1990; 69:586–587.
10. Coveler LA, Lester RC: Contaminated oxygen cylinder. *Anaesth Analg* 1989; 69:674–676.
11. Jawan B, Lee JH: Cardiac arrest caused by an incorrectly filled oxygen cylinder: a case report. *Br J Anaesth* 1990; 64:749–751.
12. Puritan Compressed Gas Corporation: *Puritan Medical Gases, Cylinder Color Chart.* Los Angeles, Puritan-Bennett Corp, 1989.
13. National Fire Protection Association: *Inhalation Therapy,* NFPA Publication No 56B, Quincy, Mass, National Fire Protection Association, 1982.
14. Scanlan CL, Spearman CB, Sheldon RL: *Egan's Fundamentals of Respiratory Care.* St Louis, Mosby–Year Book, 1990.
15. National Fire Protection Association: *Basic Classification of Flammable and Combustible Liquids,* NFPA Publication No 321, Quincy, Mass, National Fire Protection Association, 1991.
16. Thalken FR: Production storage and delivery of medical gases, in Scanlan CL, Spearman CB, Sheldon RL (eds): *Egan's Fundamentals of Respiratory Care.* St Louis, Mosby–Year Book, 1990.
17. National Fire Protection Association: *Bulk Oxygen Systems at Consumer Sites,* NFPA Publication No 50, Quincy, Mass, National Fire Protection Association, 1990.
18. National Fire Protection Association: *Flammable and Combustible Liquids Code,* NFPA Publication No 30, Quincy, Mass, National Fire Protection Association, 1990.
19. National Fire Protection Association: *Uniform Coding for Fire Protection,* NFPA Publication No 901, Quincy, Mass, National Fire Protection Association, 1990.
20. Compressed Gas Association: *Handbook of Compressed Gases,* New York, Van Nostrand Reinhold, 1981.
21. National Fire Protection Association: *Storage of Liquid and Solid Oxidizing Materials,* NFPA Publication No 43A, Quincy, Mass, National Fire Protection Association, 1980.
22. Bancroft LM, du Molin GC, Hedley-Whyte LH: Hazards of hospital bulk-oxygen delivery systems. *Anaesthesia* 1980; 52:504–510.
23. Mushin WW, Jones PL: *Physics for the Anaesthetist.* Boston, Blackwell, 1987.
24. National Fire Protection Association: *Respiratory Therapy,* NFPA Publication No 56B, Quincy, Mass, National Fire Protection Association, 1973.
25. National Fire Protection Association: *Bulk Oxygen Systems,* NFPA Publication No 50, Quincy, Mass, National Fire Protection Association, 1974.
26. National Fire Protection Association: *Noninflammable Medical Gas Systems,* NFPA Publication No 56F, Quincy, Mass, National Fire Protection Association, 1983.
27. Compressed Gas Association: *Diameter Index Safety System,* Pamphlet V-5, Arlington, Va, Compressed Gas Association, ed 3. 1989.

28. Eubanks DH, Bone RC: *Comprehensive Respiratory Care.* St Louis, Mosby–Year Book, 1990.
29. Nocturnal Oxygen Therapy Trial Group: Continuous or nocturnal oxygen therapy and chronic obstructive lung disease: A clinical trial. *Ann Intern Med* 1980; 93:391–398.
30. O'Donahue WJ Jr: New concepts in long-term oxygen therapy. *RT* 1992; 5:47–53.
31. Ward JJ: Equipment for mixed gas and oxygen therapy, in Barnes TA (ed): *Respiratory Care Practice.* St Louis, Mosby–Year Book, 1988.

2

Administration of Oxygen and Other Medical Gases

BARBARA G. WILSON, M.Ed., R.R.T.
ROGER C. BONE, M.D.

For life, nothing is more important than oxygen supply.
J.W. Severinghaus and P.B. Astrup, 1986[1]

OBJECTIVES

- Compare and contrast the principles of operation of low- and high-flow oxygen systems.
- List the performance characteristics and clinical application of the various types of oxygen devices.
- Discuss the benefits and disadvantages of using an electronic demand oxygen delivery system.
- Point out possible complications of using transtracheal oxygen as compared with other oxygen therapy modalities.
- Compare and contrast the method for providing humidity or aerosol therapy with the various oxygen devices.
- Explain the clinical advantages and disadvantages of using molecular humidity and aerosol to condition inspired gas.
- Appraise the clinical benefits of breathing helium/oxygen (heliox) and carbon dioxide/oxygen (carbogen) gas mixtures.
- Describe the hazards and complications of oxygen administration.

Oxygen and medical gas administration are standard treatment modalities for patients with respiratory and/or cardiac disease. Delivery methods logically vary with the acuity of the patient condition and the care setting. Although medical gas therapy is common medical practice, devices used to administer medical gases continue to develop and change as technologies advance. Health care practitioners must have a thorough understanding of the principles of oxygen and medical gas therapy and be able to select the device(s) that deliver the desired gas concentration at the required inspiratory flow while allowing for maximum patient comfort, mobility, and treatment compliance. The selection of any device should be based upon its performance characteristics (i.e., delivered flow rate, F_{IO_2}, relative humidity), the desired clinical goal(s), and patient tolerance. This chapter will discuss the administration of oxygen and other medical gases and focus on current methods and techniques and the clinical usefulness of each device.

PRINCIPLES OF OXYGEN ADMINISTRATION

Oxygen is a drug and should only be administered following a physician's prescription. Like most drugs, oxygen has toxic effects at higher or prolonged doses; therefore the goal of oxygen therapy is to administer the lowest fraction of inspired oxygen (F_{IO_2}) for the shortest period of time to maintain normal oxygen delivery for the patient. This requires careful analysis of the medical gas administered and assessment of adequate oxygen delivery in the patient. Medical gas analyzers and metering devices (see Chapters 1 and 7) are readily available to measure the oxygen concentration or the precision of gas flow administered to the patient.

Oxygen delivery is a function of the following relationship:

$$\textbf{Oxygen delivery} = \text{Arterial } O_2 \text{ content } (Ca_{O_2}) \times \text{Cardiac output,}$$
$$\text{where } Ca_{O_2} = 1.34 \times \text{g Hgb} \times Sa_{O_2} + Pa_{O_2} \times 0.003.$$

An assessment of oxygenation that focuses solely on the adequacy of Pa_{O_2} levels is an incomplete picture of tissue oxygenation. Pa_{O_2} represents the amount of oxygen dissolved in blood plasma and contributes the smallest proportion (0.3 mL/dL at a Pa_{O_2} of 100 mm Hg) of oxygen carried to the tissues. Saturation of available hemoglobin levels accounts for the largest portion of oxygen delivered to the tissues (20.1 mL/dL at 100% saturation and 15 g hemoglobin). Practitioners should be careful to assess arterial saturation, hemoglobin levels, and cardiac output to determine tissue oxygenation for any given patient scenario. Laboratory as well as clinical assessment of tissue oxygenation will provide the most comprehensive information for the development of oxygen dosing strategies. Clinical assessment of adequate tissue oxygenation is demonstrated by normal vital signs, patient color, capillary refill time, urine output, and the absence of metabolic acidosis. These signs coupled with laboratory measurements provide a comprehensive picture of a patient's oxygen delivery.

Patients receiving low-flow oxygen therapy should be monitored by appropriate respiratory care personnel at least once per day to assess equipment function and appropriateness of the oxygen prescription. More frequent assessment should be performed for those patients receiving an F_{IO_2} greater than 0.50, heated gas mixtures, or blended high-flow oxygen systems or for patients who have artificial airways.[2] The standard of practice for newborns requires continuous analysis every 4 hours, but data to support this practice are not available.

OXYGEN ADMINISTRATION DEVICES

Oxygen devices have classically been described by two different sets of terms: low-flow, high-flow systems or fixed-performance, variable-performance systems[3–5] (see Table 2–1). We prefer to use a combination of these classifications and divide oxygen devices into two functional groups: low-flow (variable-performance) and high-flow (fixed-performance) systems to best describe their principles of operation. *Low-flow devices* supply a set flow of oxygen that is a portion of the patient's total inspired gas. The performance of these devices varies in that the concentration of oxygen or the fraction of inspired oxygen (F_{IO_2}) administered changes as the total minute ventilation or peak inspiratory flow rate of the patient changes, that is, as minute ventilation or the peak inspiratory flow rate increases, the F_{IO_2} administered with a low-flow device will decrease.[6, 7] Low-flow systems provide lower oxygen concentrations because of room air entrainment, usually 0.21 to 0.40, and are best suited to patients with a stable respiratory status and oxygen requirements. The lower delivered oxygen flows and design simplicity of these devices make them more cost-effective than other oxygen devices from supply and personnel perspectives.

Reservoir systems provide a set flow of oxygen to the patient plus a volume of gas contained in an appliance reservoir. These devices may be considered variable- or fixed-performance systems. If the volume of gas contained in the reservoir plus the set flow rate is sufficient to meet the patient's minute ventilation or peak inspiratory flow rate without entraining room air, a reservoir device is considered a fixed-performance, high-flow device because the delivered F_{IO_2} does not vary with spontaneous breathing. If set flow rates plus the volume of the reservoir do not meet spontaneous inspiratory demands and the patient entrains room air during breathing, the reservoir device is considered a variable-performance, low-flow device, and the delivered F_{IO_2} will vary. Reservoir devices provide medium to high concentrations of oxygen, usually greater than 0.50, and are best suited for short-term administration of oxygen in emergency situations, where high F_{IO_2} delivery and ease of operation are important.

High-flow oxygen devices supply a total flow rate that exceeds the patient's minute ventilation and peak inspiratory flow demands. The performance of these devices is fixed in that the F_{IO_2} delivered is independent of the patient's minute ventilation and inspiratory flow demands. High-flow devices provide a broad range of oxygen concentrations from 0.21 to 1.00 and are indicated for patients who have changing spontaneous ventilatory needs. High-flow devices are structurally more

TABLE 2–1

Comparison of Low-Flow, Reservoir, and High-Flow Oxygen Devices

Feature	Low Flow	Reservoir	High Flow
Cost	Inexpensive	Inexpensive	Costly
F_{IO_2}	Variable, low F_{IO_2}	Variable, moderate	Precise, 0.21-1.00
Patient compliance	Patient can eat and ambulate	Hot, patient cannot eat or wear glasses, difficult to ambulate	Patient cannot eat or wear glasses, difficult to ambulate
Ease of use	Easy to use	Easy to use	Higher skill required for safe use
Humidity	Low relative humidity	Low relative humidity	Body humidity
Gas flow	Conserves gas flow	Conserves gas flow	Requires high gas flows
Patient respiratory status	Minute ventilation and peak flow demands must be stable	Increased risk for aspiration. Respiratory parameters must be stable	Meets all minute ventilation and peak flow demands

complex, consume higher gas flows, and require more technical skill and expertise to function effectively, which makes them the most costly oxygen administration devices.

Medical gases are dried during the manufacturing process (see Chapter 1) to enhance the purity of the end product gas. Supplemental humidification has traditionally been recommended for all oxygen and medical gas devices to reduce the humidity deficit created in the respiratory tract by the administration of dry medical gases. Minimizing the humidity deficit is thought to reduce mucosal damage, prevent drying of secretions, and increase patient comfort and compliance. It is desirable that the condition of inspired medical gas mimic the conditions present in the respiratory tract during normal breathing from the atmosphere. Chatburn and Primiano have suggested that the relative humidity and temperature output of any medical gas delivery system meet the inspiratory conditions occurring *at the point of entry* into the respiratory tract.[8] These conditions vary with the location in the respiratory tract.

Medical gas delivered to the nose should be heated and humidified to room air conditions: 22°C and 50% relative humidity. Gas delivered to the oropharynx should be heated and humidified to 29 to 32°C and 95% relative humidity. Gas administered below the upper airway via endotracheal or tracheostomy tubes should be delivered at 32 to 34°C and 100% relative humidity.[8] Practitioners should be aware of these humidification standards and select the humidification and oxygen systems appropriate to deliver the prescribed F_{IO_2}, inspiratory flow rate, and relative humidity to achieve the mutual goals of oxygenation and humidification. (See Chapter 3 for an extensive discussion of this subject.)

Humidification methods vary with the type of oxygen delivery device selected. Low-flow and reservoir devices are usually humidified with unheated bubble humidifiers that deliver 30% to 40% relative humidity at room temperature.[9] In a stable patient with a normal-functioning upper airway, low-flow oxygen therapy may not require additional humidity. This type of patient may be capable of humidifying low-flow inspired gas without supplemental humidification.[10, 11] Recent studies have shown that patients with exercise-induced asthma and increased minute ventilation benefit from supplemental humidification of inspired gases during periods of respiratory distress.[11, 12] This is perhaps the patient population that may benefit the most from humidification of low-flow gas therapy. High-flow oxygen systems usually require heated humidification or aerosol therapy because of the high inspiratory flow rate produced by these devices and the location within the respiratory tract where the gas is delivered.

Infection Control

Oxygen devices today are made of disposable plastic and designed for single-patient use. Humidifiers and nebulizers are also sterile prefilled disposable devices. Reusable humidifiers and nebulizers should be cleaned and sterilized according to hospital policy. Centers for Disease Control (CDC) guidelines recommend that oxygen devices be changed every 48 hours to prevent nosocomial infection.[13] Many hospitals have conducted their own infection control studies that indicate that this equipment change interval can be increased; however, it is incumbent upon the institution to document infection rates and equipment procedures to justify varying from CDC recommendations. Humidifiers that deliver water vapor have the lowest risk for nosocomial infection because pathogens are transmitted via particulate water. Water condensate that accumulates in nebulizer delivery tubing should *never* be drained back into the nebulizer reservoir because this could contaminate the reservoir and deliver pathogens via the aerosol to the patient's airway. Heated nebulizers should be changed every 24 hours for this reason.

Low-Flow (Variable) Devices

Nasal Catheter

Oxygen administration via nasal catheter has been used since the early 1900s. It is a soft plastic tube with small gas flow ports at the tip that is inserted into one of the nares of the nose and passed to the back of the nasopharynx into the oropharynx just behind the uvula.* Nasal catheters are available in several sizes and categorized by outer diameter (OD) of the catheter. Adult catheters are usually 12 to 14 F and pediatric catheters, 8 to 10 F.

A nasal catheter should be lubricated with water-soluble gel before insertion to facilitate passage into the nasopharynx and prevent trauma and adherence to delicate nasal mucosa. Catheter placement should be changed to the opposite nare every 8 to 12 hours to reduce mucosal crusting and adherence. Nasal catheters are commonly attached to small-bore oxygen tubing and a simple bubble humidifier and flowmeter. Nasal catheters can provide variable low F_{IO_2} delivery (0.28 to 0.45) at flow rates of 1 to 8 L/min. Direct measurement of F_{IO_2} is not practical in a clinical setting. Several authors have published F_{IO_2} predictions at set flow rates.[14, 15] F_{IO_2} predictions are a function of the delivered oxygen flow rate, patient minute ventilation, peak inspiratory flow demands, and nose vs. mouth breathing. The F_{IO_2}

*Use is counterindicated in patients with facial trauma or patients with a basilar skull fracture.

remains consistent only when the patient's respiratory parameters are stable. Ideally, oxygen flows should be titrated to the desired level of tissue oxygenation. Practitioners should begin oxygen flow at 1 L/min and increase in half-liter (0.5 L/min) increments until pulse oximetry (Spo_2) or Pao_2 values are acceptable.

Nasal catheters are not widely used today because of patient discomfort. Patient compliance is poor with this device because insertion and frequent repositioning are uncomfortable or painful. Patients frequently complain of dry, sore throats and comply with this method of oxygen administration for only short periods of time. Gastric inflation and resultant vomiting and aspiration may also occur if catheter placement is deep in the oropharynx or esophagus and the gas flow is high. Recommended clinical applications include short-term oxygen therapy during diagnostic fiber-optic bronchoscopy or postanesthesia recovery.

Nasal Cannula

A nasal cannula is a set of soft plastic prongs that fit a short distance (< ½ in.) into the nares and have adjustment straps that go over the ears and around the back of the head (elastic) or over the ears and under the chin (bolero style). Several cannula designs currently exist. Conventional nasal cannulas are variable-performance, low-flow oxygen devices that are available with straight, curved, and flared prongs. Reservoir/pendant cannulas incorporate small-volume reservoirs to conserve gas flow and are commonly recommended for home care use. Demand-flow cannulas sense patient inspiratory efforts and deliver adjustable bursts of oxygen only during inspiration, also an attempt to conserve gas flow. Each design has its clinical application and advantages and disadvantages and will be presented separately (see Table 2–2).

Conventional nasal cannulas are the most common oxygen delivery device used today. Available in adult, pediatric, and infant sizes, the nasal cannula is the standard for stable respiratory patients because of the ease of oxygen administration and the high degree of patient compliance. Patients may eat, talk, and wear eyeglasses while receiving supplemental oxygen via nasal cannula. Nursing care and ambulation are also facilitated by this device's simple design. Figure 2–1 illustrates the bolero-style nasal cannula for an adult. In this figure the patient's mouth is opened to demonstrate the point that was made by Kory et al. in 1962 that an open mouth does not lower the Pao_2 as long as the nasal passages and pharynx are patent.

As a variable-performance, low-flow oxygen device, it is difficult to predict and control inspired oxygen concentrations with a nasal cannula. Therefore, it is applicable for short- or long-term oxygen therapy in patients of all ages with stable respiratory parameters who require low oxygen concentrations. The maximum recommended flow rate is 6 L/min (0.40 to 0.44 Fio_2). It is essential that practitioners understand that there is no appreciable increase in patient oxygenation at gas flows in excess of 6 L/min with a conventional nasal cannula. The small anatomic gas reservoir provided by the nasopharynx is filled at these flow rates, and any additional increase in oxygen flow spills out of the nose into room air. Low-flow flowmeters calibrated in increments of 25, 100, or 250 mL instead of liters per minute facilitate the titration of nasal oxygen to desired levels of tissue oxygenation for children and infants. If a regular flowmeter is used, newborn and infant cannula flows should be limited to a maximum of 2 L/min (0.25 to 0.28 Fio_2).[16, 17] The selection of a bubble humidifier with a nasal cannula may depend on the duration of gas therapy and the set flow rate. Oxygen supplied to adults via nasal cannula at flow rates less than 4 L/min need not be humidified.[18] Patients requiring long-term oxygen therapy may prefer the use of a bubble humidifier to prevent

TABLE 2–2
Advantages and Disadvantages of Nasal Oxygen Devices

Device	Advantages	Disadvantages
Nasal catheter	Difficult to dislodge with active patients; useful during fiber-optic bronchoscopy; disposable	Requires frequent repositioning; uncomfortable, drying: gastric inflation may occur; low relative humidity
Conventional nasal cannula	Easy to use, comfortable; patient may eat, talk, wear eyeglasses with device; unobtrusive appearance; allows for ambulation; good patient compliance; low-cost device; disposable	Respiratory status must be stable and predictable; administers only low concentrations of oxygen; low relative humidity; obtrusive appearance
Reservoir/pendant nasal cannula	Conserves gas flow; allows for ambulation; excellent for home care; economical; disposable	More obtrusive appearance; cosmetic considerations; not practical for acute care
Demand-flow cannula	Conserves oxygen flow; disposable	Potential for mechanical malfunction; less portable for ambulation/home care

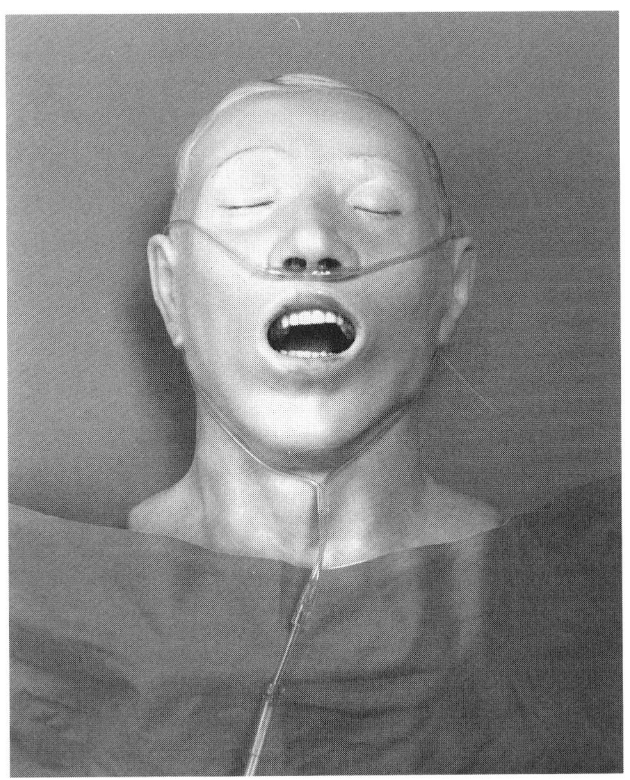

FIG 2–1
Nasal cannula.

drying of nasal mucosa at flows greater than 4 L/min.

Reservoir/pendant nasal cannulas incorporate small plastic appliance reservoirs (20 to 40 mL) into the standard cannula design to facilitate adequate oxygenation at lower set flow rates, conserve oxygen supplies, and reduce costs. A reservoir cannula set at 0.5 L/min can provide arterial oxygen saturations equivalent to that available with a standard cannula at 2 L/min. Figure 2–2 illustrates the reservoir nasal cannula, which results in as much as a 50% to 75% savings in oxygen flow.[19] The reservoir cannula has the appearance of a large plastic mustache, whereas the pendant cannula hangs the reservoir under the chin on the anterior of the chest like a necklace. Performance characteristics are comparable for both systems.[20, 21]

Again, the delivered F_{IO_2} will vary with these devices as spontaneous respiratory demands of the patient change. Practitioners should remember that the reservoir/pendant nasal cannulas incorporate an appliance reservoir to conserve gas flow, not increase the delivered F_{IO_2}, as is the case with other oxygen devices. Cosmetically, patients may or may not be receptive to these designs, because they are more noticeable than conventional cannulas. However, the cost savings to patients receiving home oxygen therapy are significant and warrant consideration of these devices.[22] The use of a bubble humidifier with reservoir/pendant cannulas is probably unnecessary because of the significant reduction in delivered flow rates. However, patients may request humidification for comfort reasons.

Demand-flow cannulas incorporate a conventional nasal cannula with a demand oxygen delivery system (DODS) to administer oxygen in controlled bursts during inspiration only. A sensing valve determines the beginning of inspiration and activates a solenoid valve to administer a burst of oxygen. The volume of oxygen delivered, equated to flow in liters per minute, may be adjusted by changes in the length of the oxygen burst, or the breath interval of the burst may be adjusted to titrate oxygen delivery to provide adequate oxygenation and conserve gas usage by 50% to 60%.[23, 24] This device may be prone to mechanical failure because of the complexity of its design and is not as portable as the other types of nasal cannulas.[25] Manufacturers of the DODS include

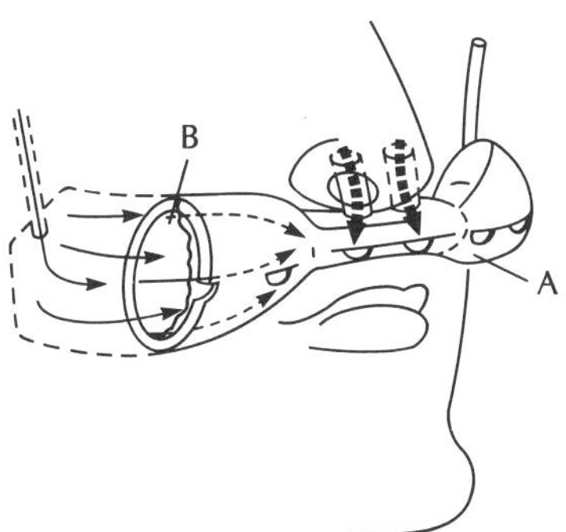

WHILE PATIENT IS EXHALING, oxygen is accumulating in the reservoir (A) formed by the inflated diaphragm (B) and the back wall of the Oxymizer.

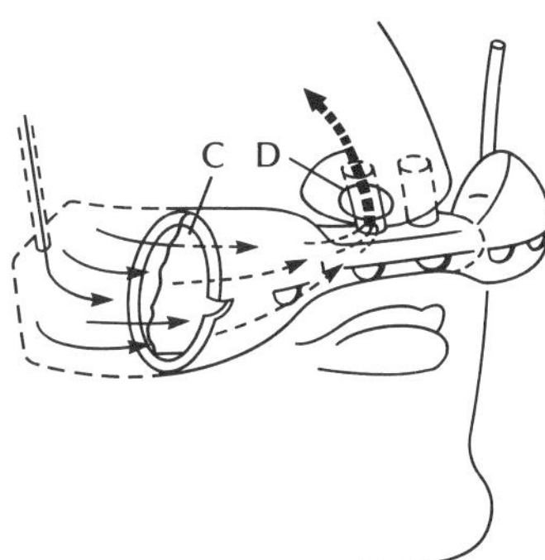

WHEN PATIENT INHALES, the diaphragm (C) collapses, and the oxygen-enriched air from the reservoir is released to the patient (D).

FIG 2–2
Reservoir nasal cannula. (Courtesy of Chad Therapeutics, Chatsworth, Calif.)

Chad Therapeutics, Pulsair, Inc., John Bann Co., and Puritan-Bennett Corporation.

Transtracheal Oxygen Therapy

The newest method of delivering long-term low-flow oxygen therapy is the transtracheal oxygen (TTO_2) catheter, developed first by Heimlich in 1982[26] and then enhanced by Spofford and Christopher in 1986.[27] The TTO_2 system bypasses the nose and mouth as a route of oxygen administration by surgically placing a soft, large-bore catheter directly into the trachea between the second and third tracheal rings (Fig 2–3). The catheter is secured at the base of the neck with a bead-chain necklace (Fig 2–4). Oxygen is delivered through standard connecting tubing and a flowmeter. A bubble humidifier may be used at home for supplemental humidification. This may be an individual decision by the patient and physician. Bubble humidifiers are not commonly recommended with portable liquid systems outside the home because of difficulty with water spillage into the connecting oxygen tubing as the patient ambulates.

The TTO_2 device combines the function of a variable-performance low-flow oxygen device and a reservoir system that may or may not incorporate a DODS.[28, 29] The placement of the transtracheal catheter allows the upper airways and the trachea to act as an expanded anatomic reservoir for oxygen during expiration. The delivered F_{IO_2} is therefore increased at any given flow. As much as a 50% to 72% reduction in oxygen flow has been reported to achieve comparable oxygenation with a nasal cannula.[30, 31] Like the nasal cannula, once the anatomic reservoir is full during expiration, additional increases in oxygen flow will not result in direct increases in oxygen saturation. This device not only decreases oxygen usage but also affords the oxygen-dependent patient increased exercise tolerance, reduced dyspnea, improved ability to smell and taste, and improved oxygenation in those patients with refractory hypoxemia.[32, 33] The device is also more cosmetically appealing because the catheter can be concealed under clothing, which contributes to greater patient compliance. Improvements in polycythemia and cor pulmonale have also been reported with TTO_2 therapy.[34]

Potential risks of the transtracheal procedure include bleeding, abscess, subcutaneous emphysema, pneumothorax, bronchospasm, airway obstruction, and pneumonia.[32, 35, 36] One group has reported that in a 2-year experience ($n = 100$), no cases of bleeding, abscess, or pneumothorax occurred. Subcutaneous emphysema (3%) and bronchospasm (2%) were uncommon.[37, 38] The transtracheal device is compatible with all conventional home oxygen equipment. No definitive cost analysis studies have been published, but preliminary reports suggest that oxygen therapy cost to the patient is reduced

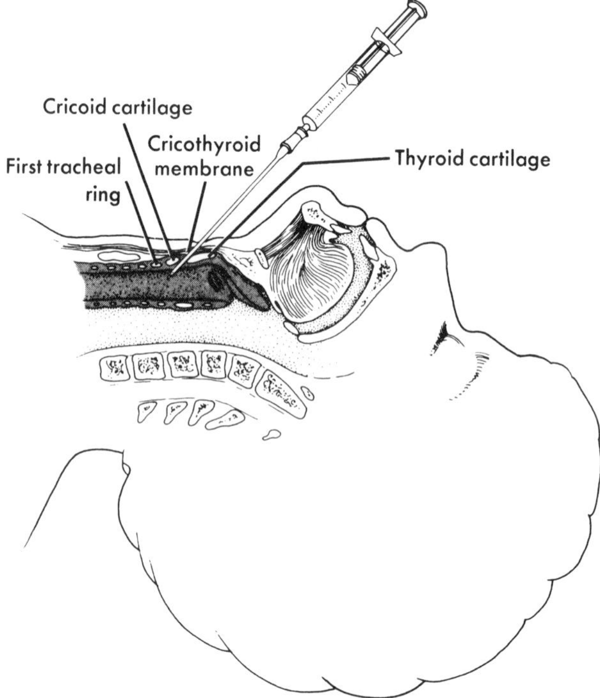

FIG 2–3
Drawing of SCOOP catheter placement.

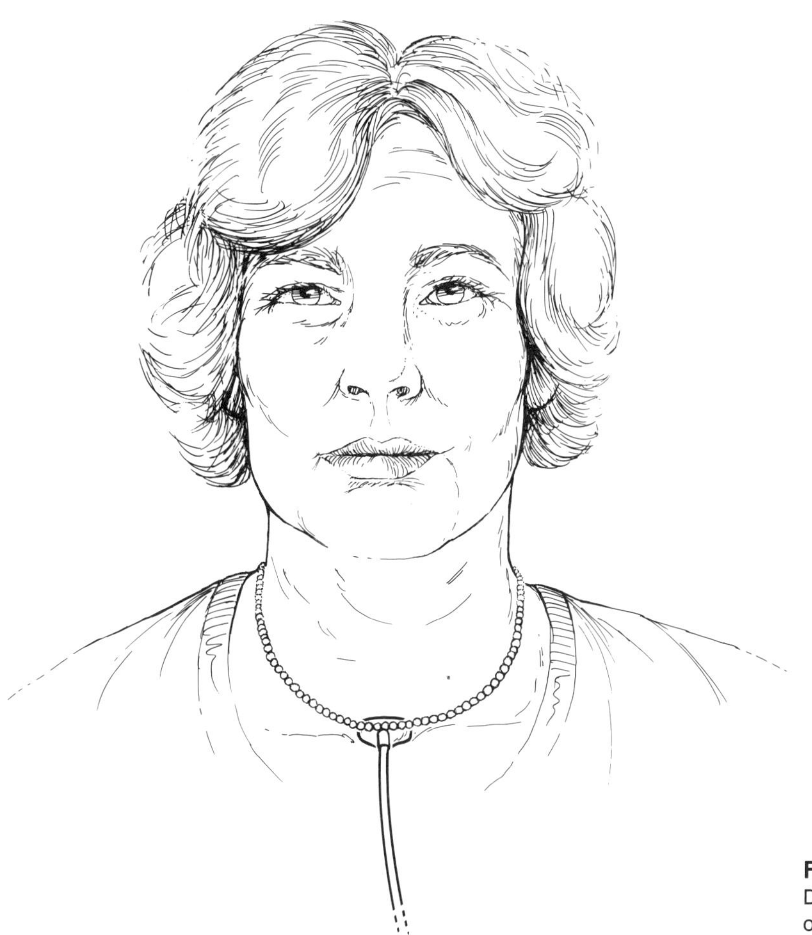

FIG 2–4
Drawing of an adult wearing a SCOOP transtracheal oxygen catheter.

and that fewer patient hospital days per year further reduce health care costs with TTO_2 therapy.

A patient's ability to provide self-care is key to the successful use of a transtracheal catheter. Patients are expected to routinely clean and replace the catheter at home, assess the catheter stoma, and alert health care professionals if signs of inflammation or other abnormalities are present. Patients who receive TTO_2 therapy are encouraged to have a friend or family member equally as proficient in the care of the transtracheal catheter available to assist the patient if difficulty arises at home.

Oxygen Masks

Masks are soft plastic devices that cover the nose and mouth. They may be classified as low-flow (reservoir) or high-flow oxygen systems, depending on the design and principle of operation. Reservoir masks add an appliance (mechanical) reservoir to the patient's anatomic reservoir to hold a volume of gas that supplements the set oxygen flow during inspiration. In general, the larger the appliance reservoir, the higher the FIO_2 delivered with this type of mask. The FIO_2 produced by a reservoir mask is a function of the set oxygen flow rate, the size of the reservoir, patient minute ventilation, peak inspiratory flow, and leaks around the mask and face. High-flow mask designs incorporate a method of producing total gas flows that match or exceed the spontaneous respiratory demands of the patient. Gas flow may be produced as a function of the mask design (e.g., venturi masks) or by an additional device to which the mask is attached (e.g., large-volume nebulizer).

All masks used for medical gas and oxygen therapy should be soft, pliable, disposable, and transparent. Transparent masks allow health care providers to identify secretions or vomitus collected in the mask and minimize or prevent aspiration. Masks are not recommended for patients who cannot cough or protect their airway and are most successful if used to deliver moderate to high FIO_2 for short periods of time, for example, emergency care or patient transport. Adult patients frequently complain that masks are hot and that eating or wearing eyeglasses is impossible, and this results in marginal patient compliance. Young children do not tolerate oxygen masks; they are continually taking them off and

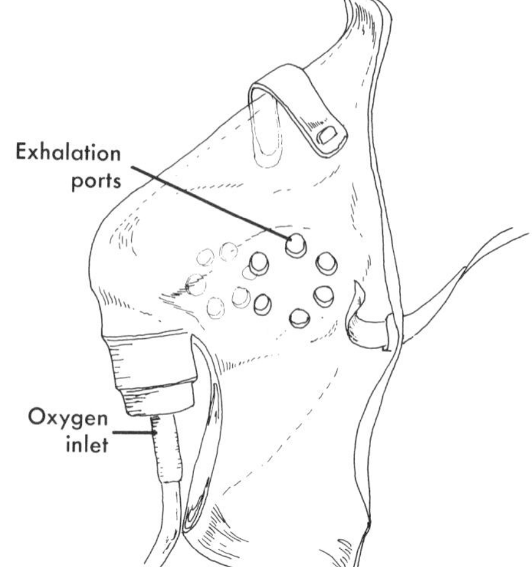

FIG 2–5
Simple oxygen mask. (From McPherson SP: Gas regulation, administration, and controlling devices, in *Respiratory Therapy Equipment,* ed 3, St Louis, Mosby–Year Book, 1985. Used by permission.)

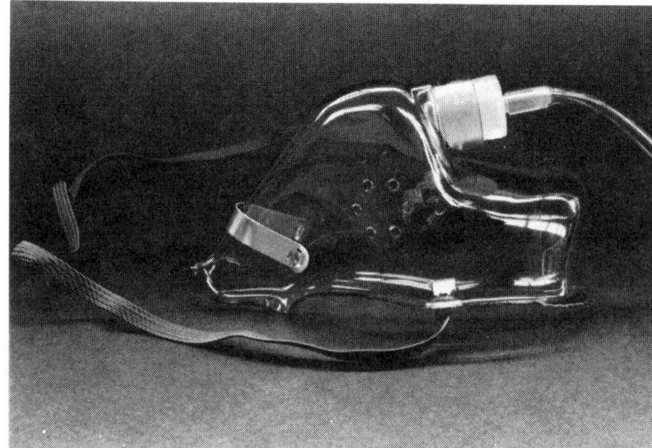

fighting care givers as they attempt to replace them. Masks for infant oxygen therapy may actually occlude an infant's airway and are considered dangerous. Patients who require continuous oxygen therapy and who wish to take off their mask to eat should have a nasal cannula set up at the bedside at an equivalent liter flow to supply adequately oxygenation during this activity. Humidification via bubble humidifier is not practical with masks because gas flows over 6 to 8 L/min cause the 2-psig relief valve on the humidifier to open and vent gas into the atmosphere away from the patient. The following oxygen reservoir masks will be discussed individually: simple, partial rebreather, and nonrebreather. Venturi and aerosol masks will be discussed with high-flow oxygen devices.

A *simple mask* is used for the administration of moderate F_{IO_2} (Fig 2–5). It is a low-flow, variable-performance device that incorporates a small gas reservoir, and the F_{IO_2} varies with changes in the patient's respiratory status. Estimated F_{IO_2} values range from 0.40 to 0.60 at oxygen flows of 5 to 10 L/min.[2] Small-bore oxygen tubing carries the set gas flow from the flowmeter to the center of the mask, near the patient's nose and mouth. This area forms a small gas reservoir that contributes volume to the set gas flow to increase F_{IO_2}. Holes are placed on the sides of the mask for room air gas entrainment and venting exhaled gas. A metal clip over the bridge of the nose and an adjustable elastic strap facilitate the fit to the patient's face and hold it in place. Although the appliance reservoir of a simple mask is small, a *minimum* flow of 5 L/min is recommended to prevent carbon dioxide buildup within the mask.[39] Simple masks are best for short-term oxygen therapy such as anesthesia recovery, emergency care, therapeutic bronchoscopy, and patient transport.

A *partial rebreathing mask* design is similar to the simple mask with the addition of a large-volume plastic reservoir bag (Fig 2–6). The bag is attached to a connector below the patient's nose where gas flow from the flowmeter enters the mask. The reservoir is filled during expiration by a portion of the patient's exhaled

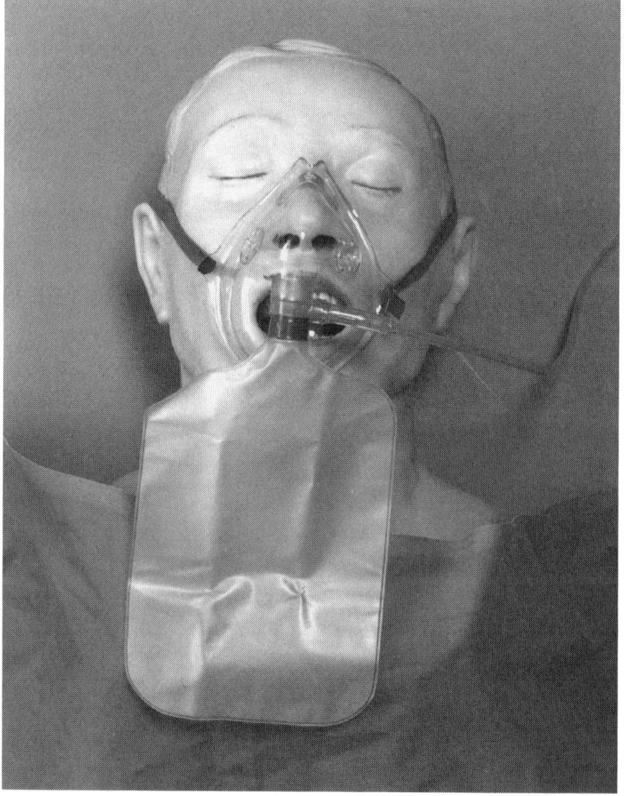

FIG 2–6
Partial rebreather mask.

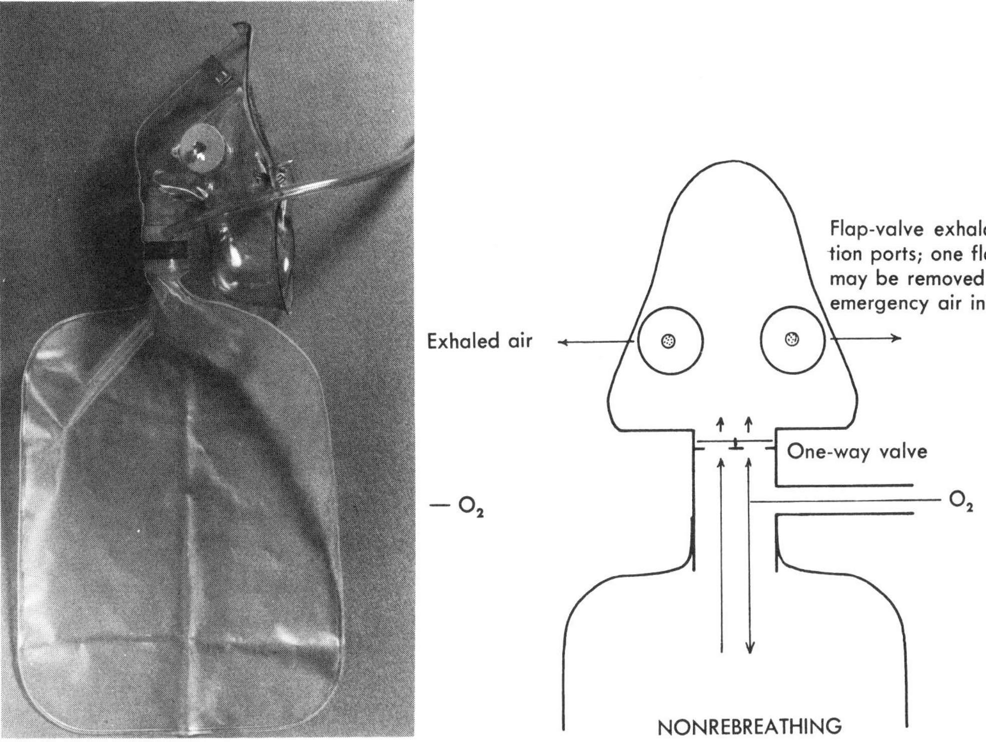

FIG 2–7
Nonrebreather mask diagram.

gas, presumably the first portion of expiration, low-CO_2 and high-F_{IO_2} gas from the patient's anatomic reservoir, plus the fresh flow of gas into the mask from the flowmeter. As the patient inspires, gas flow is drawn from the mask, the reservoir bag, and the set oxygen flow. Exhalation ports remain open in this mask during inspiration and provide a potential source of entrained room air. The partial rebreather is a variable-performance reservoir system where F_{IO_2} will vary with changes in the patient's respiratory status. The oxygen flow rate should be titrated to keep the reservoir bag partially inflated at peak inspiration to prevent entrainment of room air, which will dilute the delivered F_{IO_2}. The recommended *minimum* flow for this mask is 10 L/min to prevent carbon dioxide buildup. The predicted F_{IO_2} is 0.60 to 0.80 at 10 to 15 L/min.[2, 11]

A *nonrebreathing mask* adds one-way valves to the design of the partial rebreather to prevent rebreathing of gas and decrease room air entrainment. Leaflet valves are placed between the reservoir bag and the mask and at one of the exhalation ports. Closing both exhalation ports with leaflet valves is not recommended because of the risk of suffocation should the source gas to the mask become disconnected on a patient with altered consciousness. Source gas fills the reservoir bag from below the first valve as the patient exhales through the leaflet valve and the open exhalation port. During inspiration, the valve between the bag and the mask opens to entrain gas from the reservoir bag in addition to the set gas flow. The leaflet valve on the exhalation port closes to decrease room air entrainment and dilution of the delivered F_{IO_2}. Figure 2–7 demonstrates the ideal structure of a nonrebreathing mask with two leaflet valves in place at the exhalation ports. The open exhalation port on disposable nonrebreathing masks and the potential for the patient to breathe around the mask and face make this mask a variable-performance reservoir device that delivers an F_{IO_2} of greater than 0.80 at flow rates in excess of 15 L/min.[11]

Nonrebreathing masks should be used for the short-term emergency administration of high concentrations of oxygen. They are also recommended for the administration of other medical gas mixtures such as heliox (helium/oxygen) and carbogen (carbon dioxide/oxygen) because they are easy to use, conserve gas flow (as compared with high-flow systems), and provide the highest concentration of inspired gas of all simple oxygen devices.

High-Flow (Fixed Performance) Devices

A *venturi mask* employs an air entrainment system to provide accurate, reliable F_{IO_2} delivery at high total flow rates (Fig 2–8). A variable-size restriction is created in the

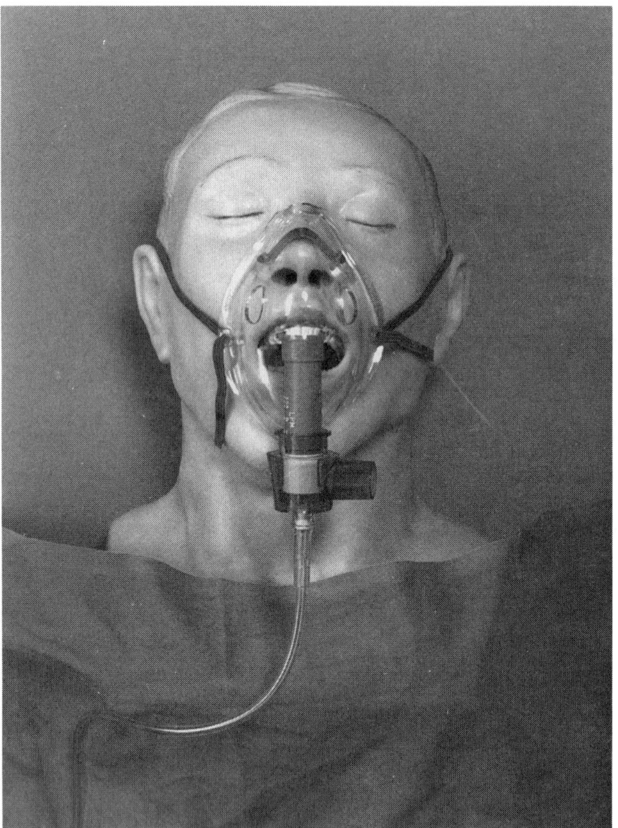

FIG 2–8
Entrainment (venturi) mask.

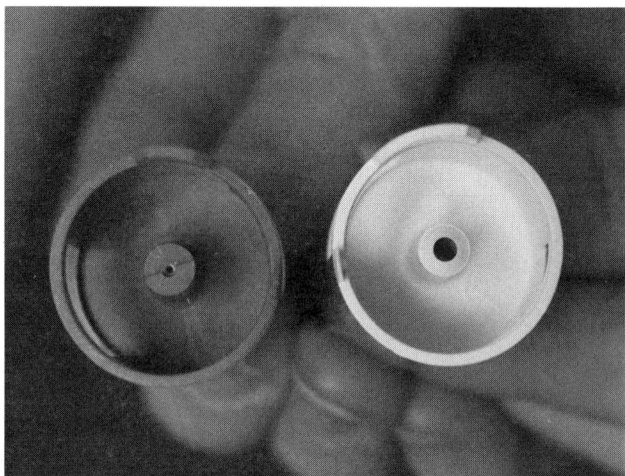

FIG 2–9
Restriction sizes for a commercially available entrainment mask.

source gas stream, and room air is entrained through openings to the side of the restriction proportionate to the velocity that the gas moves through the restriction. As the orifice size at the restriction decreases, the velocity of the source gas increases, room air entrainment increases, and F_{IO_2} decreases. Figure 2–9 illustrates two orifice sizes used in one commercially available mask. The smaller orifice entrains proportionately more room air and delivers a lower series of F_{IO_2} than the larger orifice. By regulating the size of the opening for room air entrainment, F_{IO_2} is controlled further: the larger the opening, the more room air is entrained and the lower the delivered F_{IO_2}.

Changes in the set flow of source gas with these masks will increase the total flow rate delivered to the patient but will **not** alter the delivered F_{IO_2}. Only changes in the size of the line restriction and the room air entrainment port will alter F_{IO_2} (Fig 2–10). Large-bore exhalation ports are placed on either side of the mask. Humidification is adequate without a bubble humidifier because of the high proportion of entrained room air as compared with dry source gas. Relative humidity can be increased further for those patients with thick secretions by administering aerosol via an attachment cup placed around the entrainment ports on the mask (see Fig 2–8). It is important to power such a nebulizer with compressed air, not oxygen, to preserve the delivered F_{IO_2}. Venturi masks may be easily adapted to tracheostomy collars for patient transport without the risk of water spills occluding tubing, as occurs with large-volume nebulizers.

Venturi masks are very cost-effective because they deliver high gas flows to the patient at low to average source gas settings. In Table 2–3 note the difference in the set flow rates as compared with the total flow delivered to the patient as a result of the air-to-oxygen entrainment ratios in these masks. At F_{IO_2} values less than 0.50, the venturi mask can easily match the peak inspiratory flows of an unstable patient with respiratory disease whose peak inspiratory flow rates can exceed 40 L/min.[40] High-flow oxygen systems should be assembled to deliver this flow rate as a minimum starting point, with the F_{IO_2} analyzed at the patient's nose and mouth to determine the presence of room air entrainment. Increases in the source gas flow rate can be made to further increase the total flow delivered without altering the F_{IO}^{2}.[41–43] Large-volume nebulizers also use an air entrainment device to produce the desired F_{IO_2} at high flow rates. The principle of operation and entrainment ratios are similar to the venturi mask. All previously discussed oxygen devices produce dry gas and depend on a second device to increase relative humidity. A large-volume nebulizer produces aerosol and humidity as part of its principle of operation and may be cool or heated to further increase delivered relative humidity (100% at body temperature). They are most useful with patients who have thick, tenacious secretions or require cool mist for upper airway edema or trauma. Heated nebulizers should have in-line temperature probes and should be adjusted to deliver gas at 31 to 34°C. Recommended flow rates are a *minimum* of 10 to 15 L/min at all F_{IO_2} settings.

Room air entrainment is easily identified with large-volume nebulizers by observing the stream of aerosol leaving the patient appliance throughout inspiration. If the aerosol output is interrupted at any point during inspiration, the total flow is insufficient, and room air is being entrained. The set flow rate should then be increased until aerosol billows continuously during inspiration. If the set flow cannot be increased further or the F_{IO_2} is greater than 0.50, two nebulizers should be combined via a tubing wye to double the potential flow available to the patient. These devices are presented in greater detail in Chapter 3 and will only be presented as oxygen devices in this chapter. Many patient attachments (appliances) may be used with large-volume nebulizers to deliver the prescribed F_{IO_2} and mist to the patient via large-bore aerosol tubing.

Aerosol face masks, tracheostomy masks, tee-pieces (Brigg's adapters), and face tents may be used with these nebulizers. An aerosol face mask is a soft, transparent mask similar to the simple mask, except for the large-bore tubing connection near the patient's nose and the large exhalation ports on each side of the mask. "Tusks," or short lengths of aerosol tubing, may be inserted into the exhalation ports to act as gas reservoirs to reduce room air entrainment and preserve the delivered F_{IO_2}. Figure 2–11 illustrates an aerosol face mask with gas reservoirs

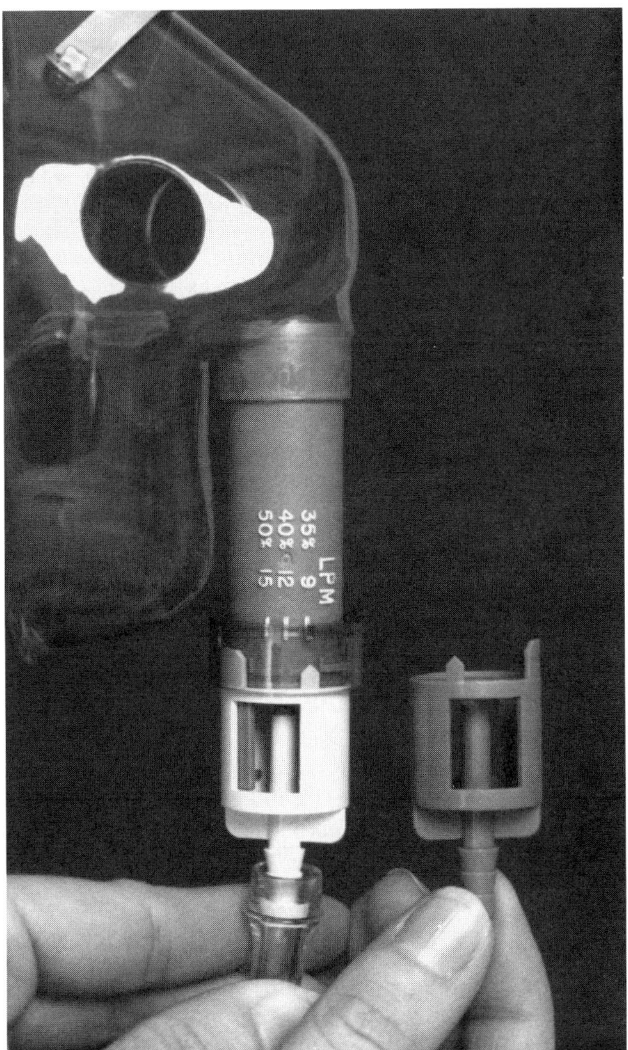

FIG 2–10
Entrainment (venturi) mask with attachments to limit the volume of entrained room air.

TABLE 2–3
Comparison of the Set Flow Rate to the Total Delivered Flow Rate With Venturi Masks

F_{IO_2}	Flow Rate (L/min)	Entrainment Ratio	Total Flow (L/min)
0.24	4	20:1	84
0.28	5	10:1	55
0.31	7	7:1	54
0.35	7	5:1	40
0.40	8	3:1	32
0.50	10	1.7:1	27

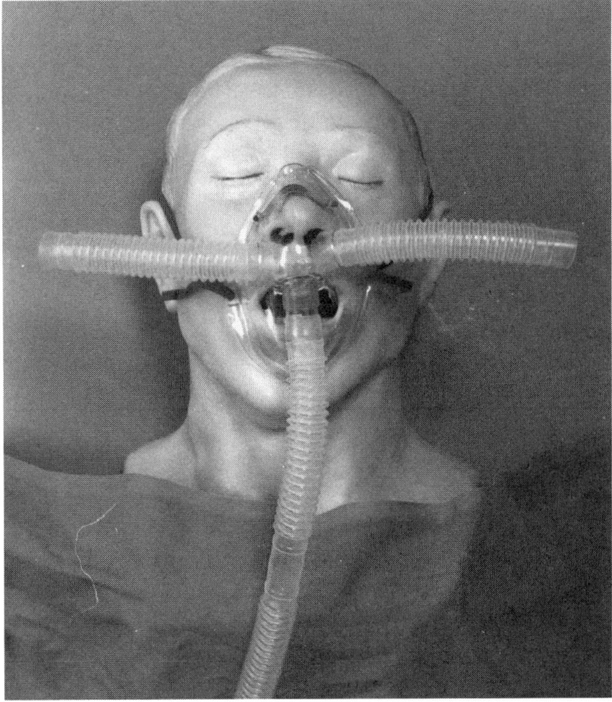

FIG 2–11
Aerosol face mask with reservoir tubing.

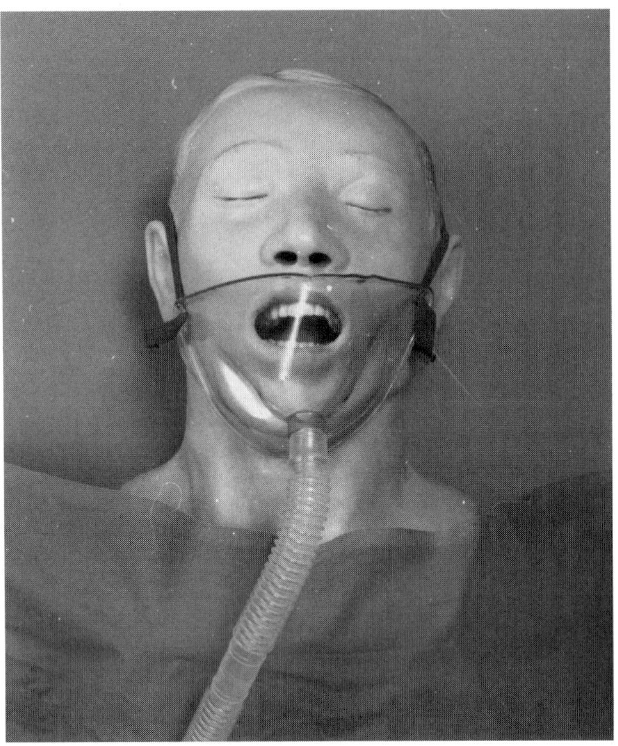

FIG 2–12
Aerosol face tent.

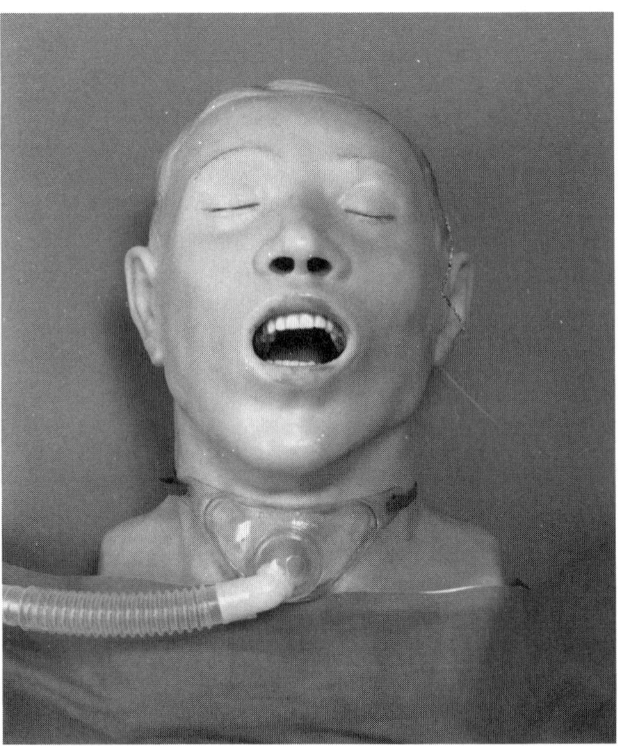

FIG 2–13
Aerosol tracheostomy mask.

attached. Face tents are large clear plastic masks that cup the chin and stand out from the face to direct gas flow upward toward the nose and mouth without actually touching the face (Fig 2–12). These devices are very helpful with patients who have facial injuries or burns and cannot tolerate an oxygen device touching their face or skin.

Tracheostomy masks are designed to hold large-bore tubing via a swivel adapter over the opening of a patient's tracheostomy tube with the support of an elastic strap around the patient's neck. "Trach" masks decrease the direct traction and pull on a tracheostomy tube and reduce the tracheal damage that other devices may cause (Fig 2–13). A tee-piece, or Brigg's adapter, is a 15-mm connection that fits directly onto the 15-mm connection of an endotracheal or tracheostomy tube. Reservoir tubing may be added to the tee to create an appliance reservoir and decrease room air entrainment from the open end of the tee-piece (Fig 2–14). The weight and size of a tee-piece connection with large-bore tubing and a reservoir attached may cause tracheal damage or dislocate a tracheostomy tube, so this is not practical for long-term use.

Intubated patients receiving oxygen therapy via tee-pieces are also at risk for progressive atelectasis and loss of functional residual capacity (FRC). Endotracheal intubation removes physiologic positive end-expiratory pressure (PEEP) from the upper airway and contributes to a progressive loss of lung volume. Intubated patients who are breathing spontaneously sometimes receive oxygen via continuous positive airway pressure (CPAP) in place of tee-piece oxygen therapy in an attempt to preserve the FRC of the lung.

With all these devices, the delivered F_{IO_2} and total flow rate are a function of the performance of the large-volume nebulizer. The appliance device is only the means of connecting the nebulizer to the patient and does not directly contribute to the production of F_{IO_2}. However, the fit of the appliance or tightness of the connection will affect the amount of room air that may be entrained by the patient. The practitioner should know that backpressure communicated to the air entrainment system by condensated water in the aerosol tubing or resistance to gas flow will decrease its efficiency and cause an increase in delivered F_{IO_2}. For this reason, all large-volume nebulizer setups should have water traps located in dependent areas to collect tubing drainout and preserve the F_{IO_2}.

Inspired oxygen may be regulated with large-volume nebulizers by adjusting the nebulizer collar setting, by bleeding in air or oxygen flows through a disposable connector, or by running the nebulizer at the 100% source gas setting off of an air/oxygen blender. Under these conditions, large-volume nebulizers are capable of delivering 0.21 to 1.00 FIO_2. The oxygen concentration should be analyzed at the patient's nose and mouth to accurately monitor inspired gas.

Environmental oxygen devices are high-flow reservoir devices that encircle a patient with a prepared atmosphere of medical gas, moisture, and temperature. Mist tents, isolettes (incubators), and oxygen hoods are common examples of environmental oxygen devices and are used primarily in neonatal and pediatric respiratory care. The use of environmental oxygen devices is limited to pediatrics because manipulation of a complete medical gas environment is more practical, controllable, and tolerable for infants and small children than for adults. Sicker children tolerate environmental devices better than oxygen masks, which produce feelings of claustrophobia and suffocation. Children often sleep and nap inside the tent canopy for extended periods of oxygen and moisture administration. However, some toddlers and young children (usually those who are less sick or recovering, with a stable respiratory status) tolerate these devices poorly because of isolation from their parents and the space limitation for play imposed by the device. Environmental devices become intermittent oxygen devices under these conditions, and patients who require continuous oxygen therapy would benefit from another oxygen device (e.g., a nasal cannula) with greater patient compliance.

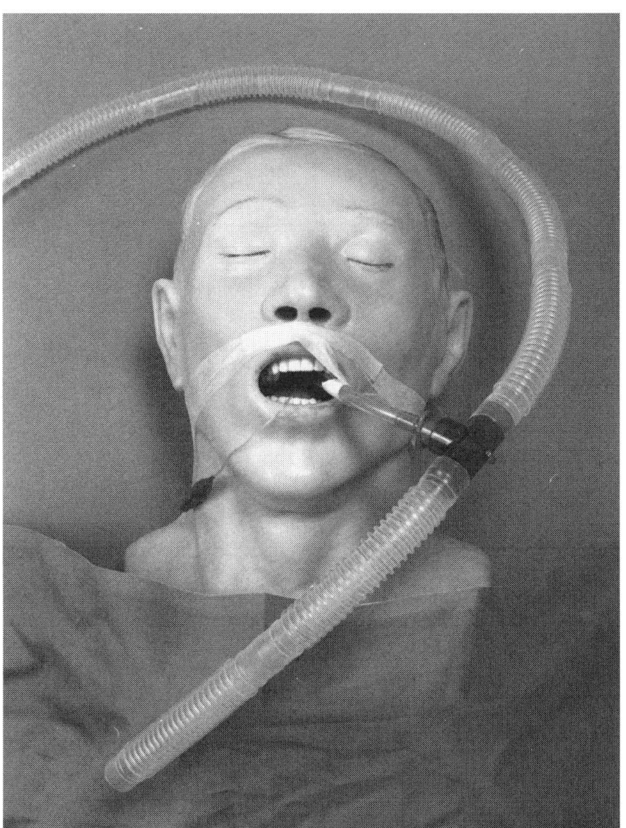

FIG 2–14
Tee-piece with reservoir tubing.

Mist or croup tents provide cool aerosol and low to moderate oxygen concentrations (0.21 to 0.50) for older babies and toddlers (Fig 2–15). The delivered FIO_2 of a mist tent is a function of the set gas flow, tent canopy volume, and tightness of the seal around the canopy. The FIO_2 should be analyzed continuously, as close to the child's face as possible. Flow rates greater than 10 to 15 L/min are required to prevent CO_2 buildup within the canopy. The internal canopy temperature can be lowered below room temperature via a cooling unit incorporated in the circulation unit of the tent. The amount of mist produced by a tent is a function of the nebulizer venturi and the total gas flow through the venturi. At lower FIO_2 delivery, the entrainment port is adjusted open, more room air is entrained per liter of set flow rate, the total gas flow is increased, and a greater density of aerosol is produced. As the density of the mist increases, pajamas and bedding must be changed frequently to keep the patient dry and comfortable.

Fig 2–15 illustrates the child adult mist (CAM) tent commonly used for the delivery of high-density mist therapy to an adult or pediatric patient. A high-density jet nebulizer delivers an aerosol mist into the tent canopy via large pipes. The circulation of gas within the canopy by the nebulizer flow causes gas to contact a metal plate with exposed coils. Chilled water is constantly circulated through the coils by inflow and outflow tubing to a refrigeration unit contained within the tent housing. The coils serve as a heat exchanger in which the warm air in the canopy is cooled by the chilled coils through the process of convection. This cooled air is recirculated through the tent to result in a controlled temperature within the canopy as determined by the refrigeration unit.

Health care providers and family should be instructed in the limitations and disadvantages of mist tents. Each time the canopy is opened for nursing or comfort care, the FIO_2 of the environment is sacrificed. Every effort should be made to coordinate care to limit the number of interruptions in oxygen delivery to the patient. Tents are most helpful for short periods of time when children require mist therapy to hydrate thick secretions and low to moderate concentrations of oxygen. Children are usually lethargic and sleep for long periods of time at this point in their respiratory illness. As soon as the child's energy and activity levels return, oxygen therapy should be changed to a device that allows normal parental interaction and movement for the child.

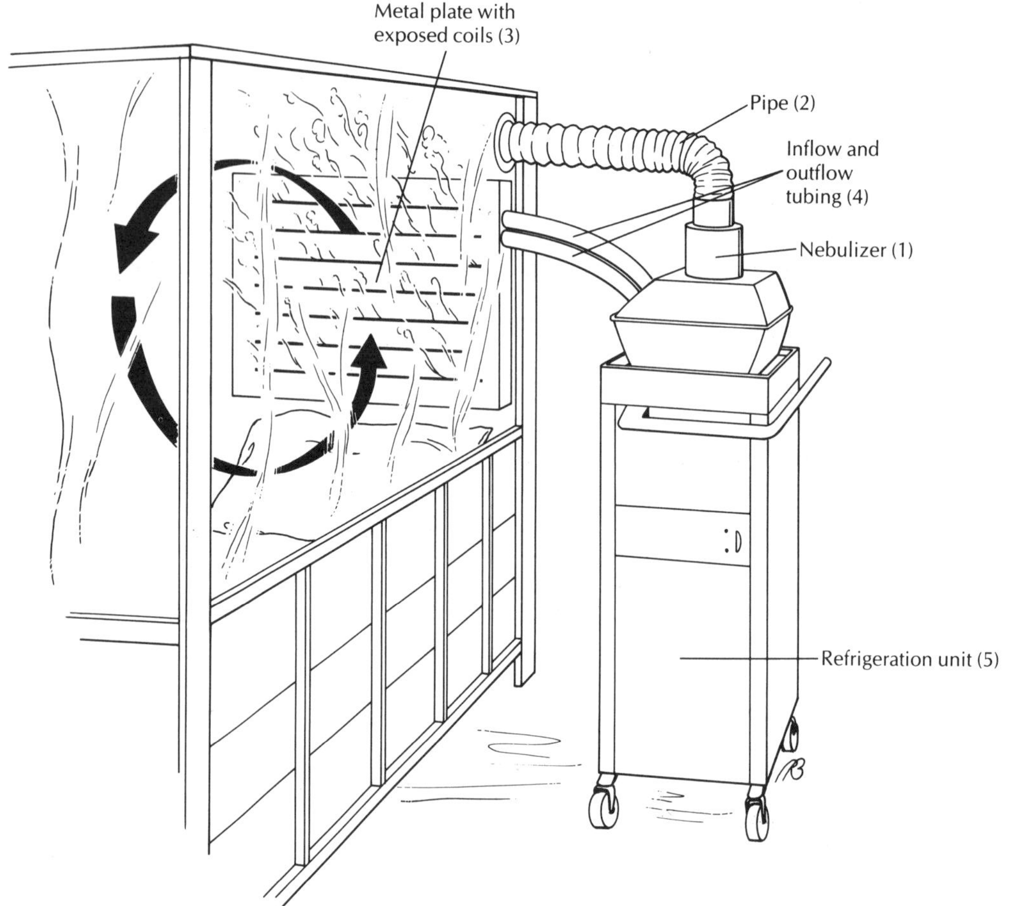

FIG 2–15
CAM tent. (From Bone R, Eubanks DH: Environmental therapy, in *Respiratory Therapy Equipment,* ed 3. St Louis, Mosby–Year Book, 1985. Used by permission.)

This will greatly improve treatment compliance and lower the anxiety of the child and parents.

Oxygen hoods, or *oxyhoods,* are clear Plexiglas chambers that deliver controlled oxygen concentrations to the head and face of neonates and small infants (Fig 2–16). Like an aerosol face mask, the oxyhood is a patient appliance that delivers a premixed gas flow to the patient. A second device, usually a large-volume humidifier or nebulizer, produces the desired gas mixture, humidity, and temperature. Oxygen concentrations inside an oxyhood are regulated best by setting the nebulizer or humidifier on 100% source gas and powering the device with an air/oxygen blender. This allows fine adjustment of the F_{IO_2} (1% to 2% increments) and reduces noise levels by inactivating the venturi mechanism.[44] Oxygen concentrations should be monitored continuously with high and low alarm limits set on the analyzer to prevent accidental hypoxia or hyperoxia in the newborn population. The total gas flow into a medium-sized hood should exceed 7 L/min to prevent CO_2 accumulation. The hood temperature should be

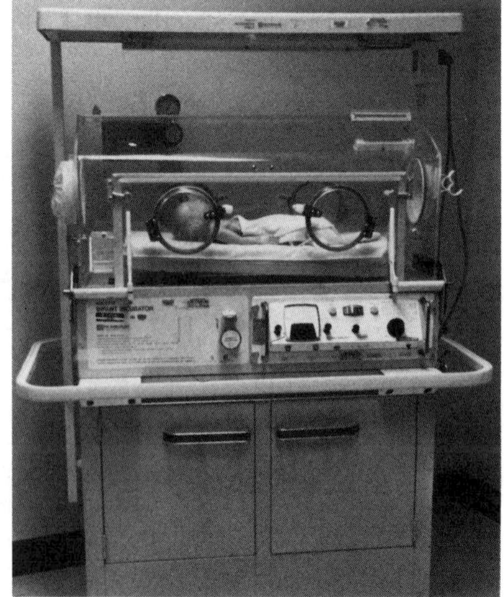

FIG 2–16
Isolette or incubator. (From Koff P., Eitzmann D., Neu J.: Oxygen therapy, in *Neonatal and Pediatric Respiratory Care,* ed 2, St Louis, Mosby–Year Book, 1993. Used by permission.)

maintained at 32 to 34° C and monitored continuously to prevent heat or cold stress in an unstable infant.

Oxyhoods allow nursing and comfort care for an infant without interrupting the delivered F_{IO_2}. They are most practical for newborns or small infants who require low to moderate oxygen concentrations, humidity, and temperature support. Oxyhoods can be well tolerated for extended periods of time while an infant's respiratory status stabilizes. Infants may then benefit developmentally from a change to a low-flow, variable-performance oxygen device that allows for hand-mouth stimulation and oral feeding.

Tables 2–4 to 2–6 compare oxygen delivery devices as well as their advantages and disadvantages.

Isolettes, or incubators, are most effective at providing a humidified neutral thermal environment for a newborn but are very poor as oxygen delivery devices. A neutral thermal environment allows an infant to maintain normal body temperature while expending minimal energy levels. The isolette servo regulates the environmental temperature inside the patient compartment via a probe taped to the infant's skin to maintain body temperature at 36.5 to 37° C. Humidity is produced by a heated passover humidifier to prevent skin drying and reduce insensible water loss. Oxygen may be administered via a standard flowmeter to the oxygen port at the back of the isolette. A pop-off valve limits the total gas flow into the isolette to 8 L/min unless a red flag attachment is raised and the room air entrainment ports are closed. The F_{IO_2} varies with the set flow rate of oxygen and any cracks or leaks in the patient compartment. Reliable oxygenation is best achieved by administering oxygen via oxyhood or infant nasal cannula inside the isolette[2] (Fig 2–17). In this way, body temperature is maintained, and F_{IO_2} is reliably administered and monitored while nursing care can be administered ad lib.

TABLE 2–4
Advantages and Disadvantages of Oxygen Masks

Advantages	Disadvantages
Deliver moderate to high F_{IO_2}	Increased risk of aspiration
Convenient and easy for patient transport	Masks are hot; patient cannot eat, wear glasses
Easy to assemble and maintain	Flow rate adjustment is vital to F_{IO_2} delivery
Can provide high inspiratory flow rates	Flow rate adjustment is vital to preventing CO_2 buildup
Nebulizers provide high relative humidity	Decreased patient compliance
Analysis of delivered F_{IO_2} is possible	Airway obstruction may be a problem in children
Disposable	Bubble humidifiers are not practical

TABLE 2–5
Comparison of Conventional Oxygen Delivery Devices

Oxygen Device	Delivered F_{IO_2}	Required Liter Flow (L/min)
Nasal catheter	Low, variable: 0.28–0.45	1–8
Nasal cannula	Low, variable: 0.40–0.44	≤6
Simple mask	Moderate, variable: 0.40–0.60	5–10
Partial rebreathing mask	0.60–0.80	>10
Nonrebreathing mask	0.90–1.00	>15
Venturi mask	0.24, 0.28, 0.31, 0.35, 0.40, 0.50, 0.60, 0.70	Variable by F_{IO_2}
Large-volume nebulizer	Moderate, variable	>10–15
Mist tent	0.21–0.50	>10–15
Incubator/isolette	Low, variable	<8, titrate to desired F_{IO_2}

TABLE 2–6
Comparison of Oxygen Conservation Devices

Oxygen Device	Delivered F_{IO_2}	Disadvantages
Reservoir nasal cannula	Low, variable, titrate to Sp_{O_2}	Obtrusive appearance
Pendant nasal cannula	Low, variable, titrate to Sp_{O_2}	Obtrusive appearance
Demand-flow cannula	Low, variable, titrate to Sp_{O_2}	Device most susceptible to technical failure; less portable
Transtracheal catheter	Low, variable, titrate to Sp_{O_2}	Requires minor surgery, skill to clean and change catheter

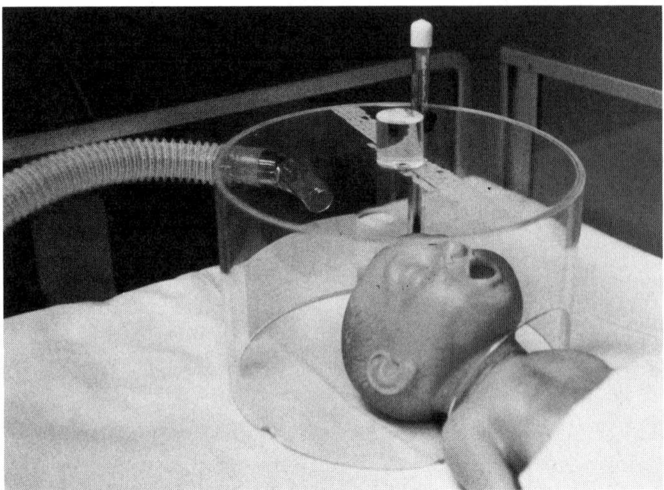

FIG 2–17
Oxyhoods. (From Koff, Eitzmann, Neu: Oxygen therapy, in *Neonatal and Pediatric Respiratory Care,* ed 2, St Louis, Mosby–Year Book, 1993. Used by permission.)

HYPERBARIC OXYGEN THERAPY

Hyperbaric oxygen (HBO) therapy is the administration of oxygen at greater than atmospheric pressure. During this procedure, a patient breathes 21% to 100% oxygen in an enclosed chamber capable of increasing ambient pressure. This chamber is known as a hyperbaric or decompression chamber. Increases in ambient pressure are measured in atmospheres of 760 mm Hg pressure. Most hyperbaric chambers are capable of administering a maximum of 3 atm of pressure to patients. Treatment schedules and tables have been developed by diagnosis to minimize the risk of oxygen toxicity and maximize therapeutic benefit. Duration of the dive, F_{IO_2}, atmospheric pressure level, and frequency of therapy may be varied according to the patient and diagnosis.

Throughout this chapter we have presented approaches to the treatment of hypoxemia that were directed at increasing the arterial saturation of hemoglobin through the administration of oxygen. As previously stated, arterial oxygen content is increased most efficiently by maintaining a normal hemoglobin level for the patient and by increasing arterial oxygen saturation via oxygen therapy. Increases in dissolved oxygen contribute little to the arterial oxygen content at normal barometric conditions. For example, a Pa_{O_2} of 600 mm Hg would increase the arterial oxygen content by 1.8 mL/dL, as compared with a 6.7-mL/dL increase when hemoglobin levels are increased from 10 to 15 g/dL or a 5-mL/dL increase, which occurs when arterial saturations are increased from 75% to 100% with oxygen therapy. As normal hemoglobin levels become fully saturated, no significant increase in arterial oxygen content is possible at normal atmospheric pressure.

This is the point when the amount of oxygen dissolved in plasma under hyperbaric conditions becomes a significant contributor to tissue oxygenation. Generally, Pa_{O_2} increases 700 mm Hg for each atmospheric increase in pressure during the administration of 100% oxygen. This represents a linear 2-mL/dL increase in arterial oxygen content for every atmosphere of breathing 100% oxygen.[39] The primary physiologic effects of increased arterial oxygen tension include new capillary bed formation and alterations in the metabolism and growth of anaerobic and aerobic organisms. Hyperbaric oxygen therapy can be used to successfully treat disease states where there is a decrease in oxygen carrying capacity. Conditions for which HBO therapy is currently recommended by the Undersea Medical Society[46] include the following:

- Air or gas embolism
- Carbon monoxide poisoning
- Traumatic ischemia (crush injuries)
- Cyanide poisoning
- Decompression sickness
- Selected wound healing
- Anemia
- Gas gangrene
- Necrotizing soft-tissue infections
- Refractory osteomyelitis
- Compromised skin grafts or flaps
- Radiation necrosis
- Selected anaerobic infections
- Thermal burns

There are two types of HBO chambers: monoplace (one person treated per chamber) and multiplace (more than one person treated per chamber). Monoplace chambers are somewhat portable, with a sliding stretcher system for moving the patient inside the chamber. These chambers can be flooded with 100% oxygen and do not require the patient to wear a mask or head tent. Multiplace chambers (Fig 2–18) are available in large centers and can accommodate many patients who require continuous nursing care from an attendant or require mechanical ventilatory support. These chambers often have air locks attached that can be entered, pressurized, and then opened into the primary chamber to provide assistance, deliver supplies, or administer medications. Some multiplace chambers may be equipped to function as a full-service operating room. Patients who require 100% oxygen in a multiplace chamber must wear tight-fitting nonrebreather masks or head tents (Fig 2–19). A chamber operator is essential to the safe operation of any hyperbaric chamber and

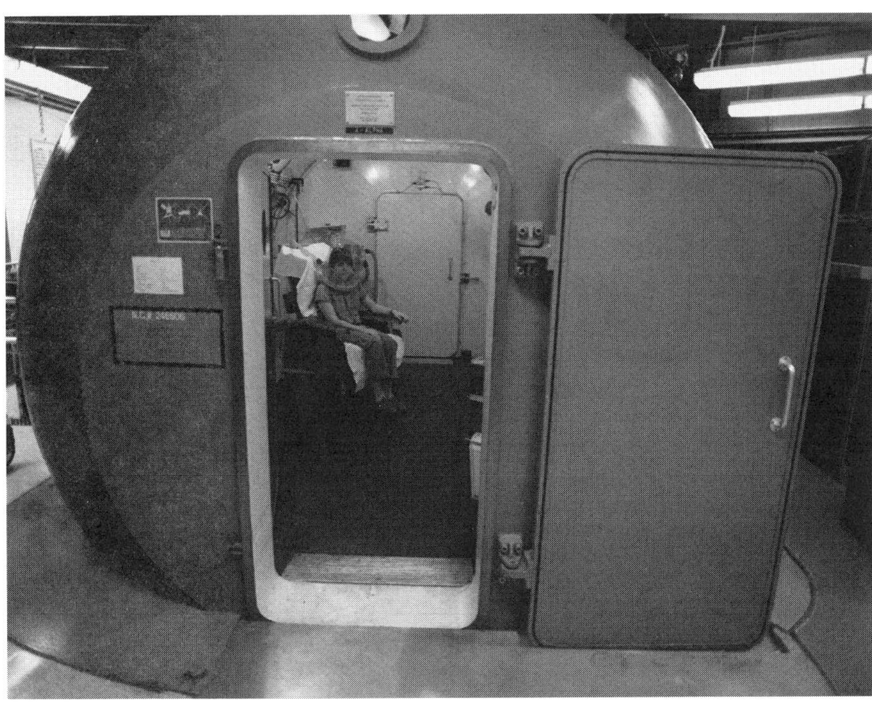

FIG 2–18
Multiplace hyperbaric chamber.

must be in attendance outside the chamber throughout the duration of any dive to monitor the system, communicate with the patient and/or attendant, and perform changes in the treatment protocol based upon patient response.

Middle ear barotrauma is a common side effect of hyperbaric therapy. Patients should be taught to clear their ears by performing repeated Valsalva maneuvers to reduce the pressure effects until comfortable. Intubated patients on ventilators should have myringotomies before decompression in the chamber. Oxygen toxicity may also be a complication of hyperbaric therapy. Common symptoms of O_2 toxicity during hyperbaric therapy include nausea, facial numbness or twitching, bradycardia, and unpleasant olfactory or gustatory sensations. Seizures may occur at higher atmospheric pressure (>3 atm). Central nervous system symptoms can be treated quickly by decreasing the F_{IO_2} or discontinuing oxygen therapy. After a short air break, oxygen may be instituted without further complications.[47]

Hyperbaric oxygen therapy is a high-flow oxygen delivery system and an intermittent therapy indicated for the diagnoses listed earlier. Treatment protocols are often time- and labor-intensive, sometimes requiring two to four dives per day for months to achieve the desired outcome. However, results may be dramatic and rewarding for patients as well as practitioners because they know that without hyperbaric therapy serious loss of limb or function would have occurred.

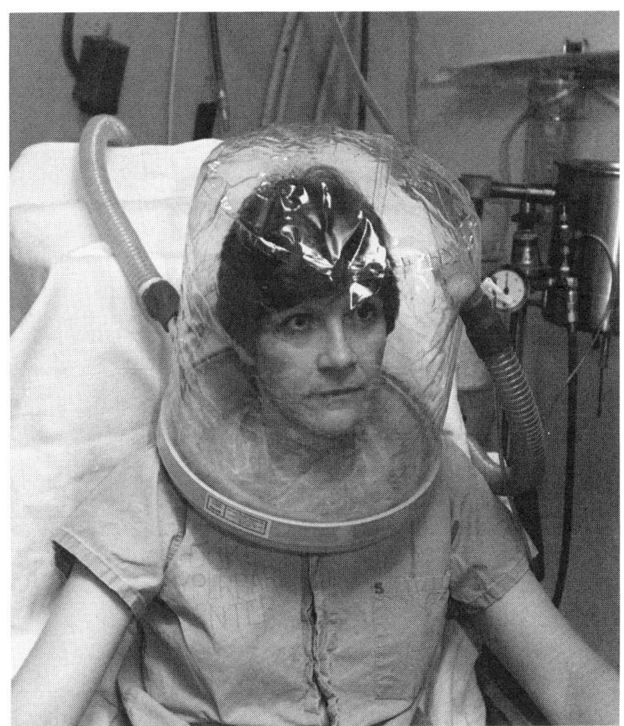

FIG 2–19
Head tent used with hyperbaric therapy.

OTHER MEDICAL GAS THERAPY

Helium/oxygen therapy, or heliox, is a commercially prepared gas mixture composed of 80% helium and 20% oxygen or 70% helium and 30% oxygen. Helium is odorless, tasteless, and chemically inert and does not affect any biologic processes in the body. In combination with oxygen, low-density helium becomes a therapeutic tool to decrease the work of breathing, increase oxygen delivery, and improve the distribution of ventilation for patients with upper airway obstruction. Helium is one third as dense (0.429 g/L) as room air (1.293 g/L) and should require one third the effort to deliver a volume of gas to the alveoli. Barach first described the rationale for heliox therapy[48–50] for asthmatics and patients with obstruction of the trachea and larynx. Mathewson most recently reviewed the current uses for helium.[51] Heliox is used today in pediatric respiratory care for infants and children with acute upper airway disease (epiglottiditis) or postextubation upper airway obstruction.

Practitioners should consider the following guidelines for heliox administration:

1. All helium/oxygen mixtures must have at least 21% oxygen to meet the patient's metabolic needs. Patients who require supplemental oxygen should receive the 70/30 heliox mixture. Gas regulators manufactured specifically for helium/oxygen mixtures must be used on heliox cylinders to ensure safe and accurate gas administration.

2. Helium has a high diffusibility and should be given via a closed system. Tightly fitting nonrebreathing masks are recommended to prevent dilution of the gas mixture.

3. Oxygen and air flowmeters will not accurately reflect heliox gas flow rates because of the differences in gas densities. Practitioners should be able to calculate predicted heliox flow rates to match set flows with patient minute ventilation demands. An 80/20 heliox mixture is 1.8 times more diffusible than oxygen, and 70/30 mixtures are 1.6 times more diffusible. For every 10 L/min of gas indicated on a standard flowmeter, 18 or 16 L/min of heliox at these concentrations will be delivered to the patient.[15]

4. Heliox therapy should be short-term therapy to get a patient through a tenuous clinical period. It is relatively expensive when compared with other medical gases, and its benefits are only available to the patient while breathing the gas mixture. Heliox therapy must therefore be continuous, not intermittent therapy. If patients appear to need extended (>2 days) heliox therapy, the underlying disease state and therapies should be reevaluated.

5. Heliox has a tendency to "layer out" in tents and oxyhoods with poor mixing of inspired gas. If an environmental oxygen device must be used because of a patient's age or size, a continuous oxygen analyzer should be placed as close to the patient's nose and mouth as possible and high and low alarm limits set to monitor inspired gas concentration changes.

Carbon dioxide/oxygen therapy is available commercially for medical gas therapy in 95%/5% and 93%/7% oxygen/carbon dioxide (carbogen) concentrations. At low concentrations it is a respiratory center stimulant. Very high concentrations of carbogen can result in respiratory center depression. Practitioners should be aware of the potential complications associated with carbogen mixtures, and any patient receiving CO_2/O_2 therapy should be monitored continuously. Elevated CO_2 levels may cause increases in arterial blood pressure, heart rate, and peripheral vasodilation. The toxic effects of carbogen therapy are easily recognized by alterations in vital signs and mental state. Therapy should be discontinued immediately if significant changes in any of these parameters occur. Carbogen therapy should be intermittent and treatment time limited to 10 to 15 minutes to minimize these side effects. Again, only gas regulators calibrated for CO_2 or CO_2/O_2 gas mixtures should be used to ensure precise administration of these potent mixtures.

CO_2/O_2 therapy is indicated for the following:

1. Cardiopulmonary bypass and extracorporeal membrane oxygenation (ECMO). Ninety-five percent/5% O_2/CO_2 mixtures are used to prevent total CO_2 washout by the artificial membrane lung.[52] Carbogen "sweep" flow is titrated across the membrane oxygenator to maintain the P_{CO_2} of the arterialized blood as it is returned to the patient.

2. Regional blood flow improvement. Carbon dioxide is a cerebral vasodilator. Low concentrations of inspired CO_2 may increase blood flow during administration and produce a therapeutic increase in perfusion; for example, ophthalmic artery occlusion may be dilated with carbogen therapy.

3. Manipulation of the distribution of blood flow between the pulmonary and systemic circulations. Carbon dioxide is a pulmonary vasoconstrictor. Infants with congenital heart disease involving a single ventricle and a connection between the aorta and pulmonary arteries (Norwood correction) may benefit from manipulating the distribution of blood flow away from the pulmonary vascular bed to the systemic vascular bed by increasing resistance to flow in the pulmonary circuit via administration of low concentrations of CO_2 (1% to 4%).[53] An in-line capnograph with alarm limits closely set must be used continuously to monitor inspired CO_2 concentrations. Continuous monitoring of respiratory and hemodynamic parameters is also recommended to ensure a safe balance of therapeutic effect vs. adverse responses.

Rossaint et al. first reported the long-term administration of *inhaled nitric oxide* in a concentration of 5 to 20 ppm to seven patients from 3 to 53 days for the treatment of adult respiratory distress syndrome.[54] In this study all seven patients survived. An editorial on this study explained the benefits of this technique to be the fact that vasodilatation and perfusion are increased only in the aerated regions of the lung, which reduces the overall mismatch between ventilation and perfusion and elevates the Pa_{O_2} for a given inhaled oxygen percentage (F_{IO_2}). It was also noted that inhaled nitric oxide may offer the additional benefit of inhibiting platelet aggregation and adhesion and retarding mitogenesis.[55]

However, this technique is still investigative and will need further study in a large-scale clinical trial before it can be accepted as practice.

HAZARDS AND COMPLICATIONS OF OXYGEN ADMINISTRATION

Oxygen and medical gas mixtures, like other drugs, have reported toxic effects. The toxic effects of helium/oxygen and carbon dioxide/oxygen mixtures were discussed in their respective sections of this chapter. The toxic effects of oxygen include oxygen toxicity, retinopathy of the newborn, oxygen-induced hypoventilation, and absorption atelectasis. A restatement of the goal of oxygen therapy should be to relieve hypoxemia and improve oxygen delivery while minimizing the toxic effects of oxygen therapy. This requires strict adherence to a medical care plan where the homeostasis of the patient is maintained and therapy is optimized to minimize toxic effects to the patient.

The degree of *oxygen toxicity* any patient experiences is a function of host tolerance, Pa_{O_2}, and the length of time of oxygen administration. Gestational development, age, and nutritional status also have an impact on host tolerance. Classic oxygen toxicity results in death of type I pneumocytes and destruction of the basement membranes. Final stages involve obliteration of the capillary beds and the formation of hyaline membranes and fibrosis. This results in a significant ventilation/perfusion mismatch compounding the hypoxemia already present.

Retinopathy of prematurity (ROP) develops when premature infants experience a Pa_{O_2} to the retina in excess of 100 mm Hg. Immature blood vessels of the retina constrict in response to an elevated Pa_{O_2}. If the hyperoxemia goes undetected and the vasoconstriction is prolonged, damage to the retina becomes irreversible, and eyesight is damaged.

Oxygen-induced hypoventilation may occur in patients with chronic CO_2 retention. These patients have altered ventilatory responses in the face of chronic hypercapnia that stimulate the respiratory centers of the brain to respond to changes in Pa_{O_2}, not Pa_{CO_2}. If oxygen administration increases Pa_{O_2} levels above 60 mm Hg, patients will have decreased stimulation to breathe and will hypoventilate. Oxygen therapy should be conservative in patients with chronic hypercapnia, and target Pa_{O_2} levels of 55 mm Hg should be adequate oxygenation for this population.

Absorption atelectasis results from prolonged administration of 100% oxygen. At lower F_{IO_2} delivery, nitrogen is inert and occupies alveolar space to prevent alveolar collapse. Prolonged administration of 100% oxygen washes all nitrogen from the alveoli and removes this space-occupying gas. It is recommended that attempts be made to wean any patient receiving 100% oxygen to a lower concentration as quickly as possible to prevent absorption atelectasis from contributing to further ventilation/perfusion mismatch.

SUMMARY

Successful administration of oxygen and other medical gases requires careful consideration of the patient's needs, care setting, and equipment performance. Patient needs include the determination of an F_{IO_2} that will provide adequate oxygen delivery to the tissues, adequate respiratory tract secretions and humidification, the ability to protect the native airway, and the degree of comfort and mobility the patient may experience with any oxygen device. The patient care setting will dictate the complexity of the gas therapy that the patient may receive. Acute care hospitals are prepared to administer and monitor any oxygen or medical gas device currently available. Home care settings, however, require technical simplicity so that the patient and family can manage the equipment with minimal education and training. Cost is a significant factor in the home setting, and devices that are simple to use and conserve gas are most cost-effective for long-term home use. Knowledge of equipment performance is key to successful gas therapy. A thorough understanding of the principles of the operation, performance limitations, and clinical indications of medical gas devices will facilitate selection of the most appropriate method of oxygen and medical gas administration. Practitioners who consider and weigh all these factors against each patient's clinical scenario will successfully achieve the goals of medical gas administration and provide quality respiratory care for their patients.

REFERENCES

1. Severinghaus JW, Astrup PB: History of blood gas analysis. VI. Oximetry. *J Clin Monit* 1986; 2:270–288.
2. American College of Chest Physicians, National Heart, Lung and Blood Institute: National Conference on Oxygen Therapy. *Chest* 1984; 86:234–237; published concurrently in *Respir Care* 1984; 29:922–935.
3. Shapiro BA, Harrison RA, Trout CA: *Clinical Application of Respiratory Care,* ed 2. St Louis, Mosby–Year Book, 1979.
4. Rarey KP, Youtsey JW: *Respiratory Patient Care.* Englewood Cliffs, NJ, Prentice-Hall, 1981.
5. Rau JL, Rau MY: *Fundamental Respiratory Therapy Equipment: Principles of Use and Operation.* Sarasota, Fla, Glenn Educational Medical Services, 1977.
6. Redding JS, McAlfie DD, Parham AM: Oxygen concentrations received from commonly used delivery systems. *South Med J* 1978; 71:169–172.
7. Goldstein RS, Young J, Rebuck AS: Effect of breathing pattern on oxygen concentration received from standard face masks, *Lancet* 1982; 2:1188–1190.
8. Chatburn RL, Primiano FP: A rational basis for humidity therapy,(editorial). *Respir Care* 1987; 32:249–254.
9. Darin J: The need for rational criteria for the use of unheated bubble humidifiers (editorial). *Respir Care* 1982; 27:945–947.
10. Estey W: Subjective effects of dry versus humidified low flow oxygen. *Respir Care* 1980; 25:1143–1144.
11. Deal EC, McFadden ER, Ingram, et al: Hyperpnea and heat flux: Initial reaction sequence in exercise-induced asthma. *J Appl Physiol* 1979; 46:476–483.
12. Chen WY, Horton DJ: Heat and water loss from the airways and exercise-induced asthma. *Respiration* 1977; 34:305–313.
13. Simmon BP, Wong S: Guideline for prevention of nosocomial pneumonia. *Am J Infect Control* 11(6):230-44, 1983.
14. Gibson RL, Comer PB, Beckham RW, et al: Actual tracheal oxygen concentrations with commonly used oxygen equipment. *Anesthesiology* 1976; 44:71–74.
15. Spearman CB, Sheldon RL, Egan DF: Gas therapy, in *Egan's Fundamentals of Respiratory Therapy,* ed 5. St Louis, Mosby–Year Book, 1990.
16. Vain NE, Prudent LM, Stevens DP, et al: Regulation of oxygen concentrations delivered to infants via nasal cannula. *Am J Dis Child* 1989; 143:1458–1460.
17. Fan LL, Voyles JB: Determination of inspired oxygen delivered by nasal cannula in infants with chronic lung disease. *J Pediatr* 1983; 103:923–925.
18. Campbell E, Baker D, Crites-Silver P: Subjective effects of oxygen for delivery by nasal cannula: A prospective study. *Chest* 1988; 86:241–247.
19. Tiep BL, et al: Evaluation of an oxygen-conserving nasal cannula. *Respir Care* 1985; 30:19–25.
20. Tiep BL, et al: A new pendant storage oxygen-conserving nasal cannula. *Chest* 1985; 87:381–383.
21. Gonzales SC, Huntington D, Romo R, et al: Efficacy of the Oxymizer pendant in reducing oxygen requirements of hypoxemic patients. *Respir Care* 1986; 31:681–688.
22. Tiep BL: Long-term oxygen therapy. *Clin Chest Med* 1990; 11:505–522.
23. Anderson WM, Ryerson G, Block AJ: Evaluation of an intermittent demand nasal cannula flow system with a fluidic valve. *Chest* 1984; 86:313–318.
24. Auerbach D, Flick MR, Block AJ: A new oxygen cannula system using intermittent-demand nasal flow. *Chest* 1978; 74:38–44.
25. Tremper JC, Campbell SC, Kelly SJ, et al: Reliability of the electronic oxygen conserver (abstracted). *Am Rev Respir Dis* 1987; 35:194.
26. Heimlich HJ, Carr GC: Transtracheal catheter technique for pulmonary rehabilitation. *Ann Otol Rhinol Laryngol* 1985; 94:502–504.
27. Christopher KL, Spofford BT, Brannin PK, et al: Transtracheal oxygen therapy for refractory hypoxemia. *JAMA* 1986; 256:494–497.
28. Tiep BL, Christopher KL, Spofford BT, et al: Pulsed nasal and transtracheal oxygen delivery. *Chest* 1990; 97:364–368.
29. Yaeger ES, Christopher KL, Goodman S, et al: Transtracheal and nasal oxygen and assessment of pulse and continuous flow (abstracted). *Chest* 1990; 98(suppl):21.
30. Christopher KL, Spofford BT, Brannin PK, et al: Transtracheal oxygen therapy for refractory hypoxemia. *JAMA* 1986; 256:494–497.
31. Spofford BT, Christopher KL: Tight control of oxygenation (abstract). *Chest* 1986; 89(suppl):485.
32. Spofford BT, Christopher KL, McCart D, et al: Transtracheal oxygen therapy: A guide for the respiratory therapist. *Respir Care* 1987; 32:345–352.
33. Wesmiller SW, Hoffman LA, Sciurba FC, et al: Exercise tolerance during nasal cannula and transtracheal oxygen delivery. *Am Rev Respir Dis* 1990; 141:789–791.
34. Heimlich HJ: Respiratory rehabilitation with transtracheal oxygen system. *Ann Otol Rhinol Laryngol* 1982; 91:643–647.
35. Burton G, Wagshul FA, Kine W, et al: Fatal mucus ball obstruction of the central airway in a transtracheal oxygen therapy patient (abstracted). *Respir Care* 1990; 35:1143.
36. Dewan NA, Bell CW, O'Donohue WJ, et al: Sequelae and complications during long-term follow-up of transtracheal oxygen therapy (TTO_2) (abstracted). *Am Rev Respir Dis* 1991; 143(suppl):78.
37. Christopher KL, Spofford BT, McCarty DM: The SCOOP catheter for transtracheal oxygen administration: two years experience—100 consecutive patients. Presented at The World Congress on Oxygen Therapy and Home Care, Denver, Feb 20, 1987.
38. Hoffman LA, Johnson JT, Wesmiller SW, et al: Transtracheal delivery of oxygen: efficacy and safety for long-term continuous therapy. *Ann Otol Rhinol Laryngol* 1991; 100:108–115.
39. Jensen AG, Johnson A, Sandstedt S: Rebreathing during oxygen treatment with face mask. The effect of oxygen flowrates on ventilation. *Acta Anaesthesiol Scand* 1991; 35:289–292.

40. McPherson SP: Gas regulation, administration, and controlling devices, in McPherson SP, editor: *Respiratory Therapy Equipment,* ed 4. St Louis, Mosby–Year Book, 1990.
41. Freidman SA, Weber B, Brisco WA, et al: Oxygen therapy: Evaluation of various air entraining masks. *JAMA* 1974; 228:474–478.
42. McPherson SP: Oxygen percentage accuracy of air-entrainment masks, *Respir Care* 1974; 19:658.
43. Friedman SA, et al: Effects of changing jet flows on oxygen concentrations in adjustable entrainment masks (abstract). *Respir Care* 1982; 25:1266.
44. Beckham RW, Mishoe SC: Sound levels inside incubators and oxygen hoods used with nebulizers and humidifiers. *Respir Care* 1982; 27:33–40.
45. Fife CE, Camporesi EM: Physiologic effects of hyperbaric hyperoxia, in *Problems in Respiratory Care: Clinical Application of Hyperbaric Oxygen,* Philadelphia, 1991, Lippincott.
46. Davis JC, Hunt TK: *Hyperbaric Oxygen Therapy.* Bethesda, Md, Committee Report, Undersea Medical Society, 1986.
47. Fife CE, Piantadosi CA: Oxygen toxicity, in *Problems in Respiratory Care: Clinical Application of Hyperbaric Oxygen,* Philadelphia, 1991, Lippincott.
48. Barach AL: The use of helium in the treatment of asthma and obstructive lesions of the larynx and trachea. *Ann Intern Med* 1935; 9:739.
49. Barach AL: The effects of inhalation of helium with oxygen on the mechanics of respiration. *Clin Invest* 1936; 15:47–61.
50. Barach AL: The therapeutic use of helium. *JAMA* 1936; 16:1273–1280.
51. Mathewson HS: Drug capsule: Helium—who needs it? *Respir Care* 1982; 27:1400–1401.
52. Mathewson HS: Drug capsule: Carbon dioxide: Therapeutic for what? *Respir Care* 1982; 27:1272–1273.
53. Guilquist SD, Schmitz ML, Hannon GD, et al: Carbon dioxide in the inspired gas improves early post operative survival in neonates with congenital heart disease following stage I palliation (Norwood) (abstract). *Circulation* 1992; 86(suppl):1435.
54. Rossaint R, Falke J, Lopeq F, et al: Inhaled nitric oxide for the adult respiratory distress syndrome. *N Engl J Med* 1993; 328:399–405.
55. Bone RC: A new therapy for the adult respiratory distress syndrome. *N Engl J Med* 1993; 328:431–432.

3

Humidity and Aerosols

NEAL COHEN, M.D.
JAMES FINK, M.S., R.R.T.

OBJECTIVES

- Describe the physiologic mechanisms for maintaining homeostasis of inhaled gases.
- Explain the physical components that determine humidity and aerosol production and deposition.
- Discuss clinical indications for humidity and aerosol therapies.
- State the general principles for delivery of humidity and aerosols.
- Point out the rationale for selecting various types of humidifiers, nebulizers, and metered dose inhalers for humidity control and drug administration.
- Distinguish between various procedures to prevent cross-contamination of patients and the environment from respiratory therapy procedures.

SUMMARY

The respiratory system is responsible for a number of functions in addition to gas exchange. One function of the upper airway is to ensure that inspired gases are warmed and adequately humidified. When the upper airway is bypassed, e.g., after placement of an endotracheal tube, humidification of inspired gases must be exogenously provided. The lung, in addition to providing a route for oxygenation and CO_2 elimination, can be used as a route of delivery of aerosols and medications. In order to appropriately deliver humidified gases and aerosols, the practitioner must understand the basic concepts of humidification and be knowledgeable about the available equipment and how to select and most effectively use it. This chapter will review how inspired gases are normally humidified, describe currently available techniques for providing humidification to patients whose normal airway mechanisms are compromised, and describe techniques for delivering aerosol therapy.

PHYSIOLOGIC CONTROL OF HEAT AND MOISTURE EXCHANGE

A primary function of the upper respiratory tract is to ensure heat exchange and humidification. A variety of mechanisms exist to accomplish these goals. Normal airways condition gas during both inspiration and exhalation. During inspiration the airway heats and humidifies gas. By the time that inspired gas reaches the lung parenchyma it is fully saturated to 100% relative humidity (RH) at body temperature. The point at which this occurs is called the *isothermic saturation boundary* (ISB).[1] Above the ISB, temperature and humidity decrease during inspiration and increase during exhalation. Below the ISB there are no fluctuations in temperature or RH. The point of ISB is normally approximately 5 cm below the carina at the level of the third-generation airways. A number of factors can cause the ISB to shift further down the airways. The ISB shifts distally with decreased environmental temperature and humidity, mouth breathing, and increased tidal volume and as a result of endotracheal intubation, which bypasses the upper airway completely. The ISB will, however, never fall to the level of the respiratory bronchioles or alveoli.

Normal Physiologic Control

Normal heat and moisture exchange within the airways is a complex mechanism.[2] During normal inspiration, turbulent flow of inspired gases ensures adequate contact of air with the mucosa. As inspired gas warms, water vapor is transferred to it by evaporation of fluid from the mucosal lining through the latent heat of vaporization, which results in humidity being added to the inspired gas. Warming and humidification continue until the inspired gas is fully saturated at body temperature. The latent heat of vaporization is dissipated in the water vapor and does not contribute to warming of gases. Loss of latent heat of vaporization causes the mucosa to cool. At the end of inspiration, the temperature of the nasal mucosa is 31°C[3] because of loss of heat by turbulent convection and loss of latent heat of vaporization.

During normal exhalation, heat is transferred to the cooler tracheal and nasal mucosa by convection. As gases cool, they hold less water vapor; condensation occurs and causes water to accumulate on the tracheal surfaces where it is reabsorbed by mucus. Heat is transferred back to the mucosa and results in warming and rehydration. Latent heat and water are held until the next inspiration.

The extent of heat exchange and humidification of inspired gases is influenced by the efficiency of the nose and mouth at accomplishing each function. During normal breathing, airflow in the nose is turbulent, and heat is transferred by turbulent convection over the turbinates and conchae and by direct contact of air with the respiratory mucosa. When breathing through the mouth, airflow is more laminar and requires heat transfer by radiation. Because air is a poor conductor of heat, the mouth is less efficient than the nose in heating inspired air.

The nose is also an active humidifier, whereas the mouth is not. The respiratory mucus layer in the nose is kept moist by secretions from mucous glands, goblet cells, and transudation of fluid through cell walls. The nasal mucosa, which has the greatest concentration of mucous glands and is quite vascular, provides an excellent source of heat and water capable of supplying nearly 1 L of fluid to inspired air each day. Heat is transferred from the rich capillary beds close to the mucosal surface. Because the nasal mucosa is cooled during inspiration, it is also able to reclaim significant quantities of heat and water on exhalation. The mucosa lining the sinuses, trachea, and bronchi also aid in heating and humidifying inspired gases.

The anatomy of the nose suggests that it has superior heat- and humidity-maintaining abilities. The nose can also function as an efficient organ of thermoregulation. Under conditions where the environmental temperature is greater than body temperature, the blood flow to the turbinates increases, and heat is lost through the nose. The actual benefits of nose breathing on heat and humidity, however, are probably overstated. Sara and Currie[4] evaluated the temperature and humidity of inspired gas in normal patients and those who had undergone tracheotomy. In the upper part of the trachea, gas inspired through the nose had a temperature of 34°C with an absolute humidity (AH) of 34 mg/L, as compared with gas inspired through a tracheotomy, which had a temperature of 31°C with an AH of 26 mg/L. Primiano et al.[5] measured temperature and water vapor continuously at the oropharynx during oral and nasal breathing of room air at 22°C with an RH of 15% to 39%. At the pharynx the temperature difference between inspired and expired gas was 4°C during nose breathing and 7°C during mouth breathing. Inspired gas increased 5°C during mouth breathing and 9°C during nose breathing. Expired gas temperature from the nose was 1 to 2°C less than body temperature, whereas that obtained during mouth breathing was 2 to 3°C less. During both mouth and nose breathing the difference between inspired and expired temperature was 10 to 11°C. During inspiration with nose breathing the RH was ≈95% at the oropharynx, whereas during mouth breathing the RH was ≈75%. On exhalation the RH values were similar between the two groups, ≈95% RH at the pharynx and ≈90% RH at the airway opening. These data suggest that the normal airway is capable of conditioning inspired gas to meet the needs of the lung no matter how it is delivered to the small airways. Medical gases delivered to the upper airway therefore do not require humidification beyond standard ambient conditions, although some authors have recommended otherwise.[6]

The upper airway and lungs also serve the function of protecting the airway by filtering particulates from inhaled gas as it travels to the lung parenchyma. The upper airway effectively filters out most particles greater than 10 μm. The nose offers more efficient filtering than does the mouth. Further filtration occurs at more distal levels within the tracheobronchial tree.

As with any mechanical system, the upper airway has limitations. It functions most efficiently under normal physiologic conditions. When presented with dry, cold inspired gases, as is the case when administering medical gases that contain no water vapor, the ISB is shifted further down the respiratory tract, which compromises the body's ability to heat and humidify gas. With a change in the ISB, ciliary function and mucus production are compromised. The lower gas temperature further down in the airways results in reduced ciliary activity within as few as 10 minutes. Once compromised, ciliary function can take several weeks to recover. Respiratory secretions become thicker and contribute to mucus plugging and an inability to maintain normal bronchopulmonary hygiene.

Definitions

Humidity

Humidity is defined in terms of the water content in air. The actual content or amount of water in a given volume of air is termed *absolute humidity* and is typically expressed in milligrams per liter.

Relative humidity is the content of water vapor expressed as a percentage of the maximum capacity of vapor that can be held at the same temperature. RH is calculated by dividing the amount of water in the air

TABLE 3–1
Capacity of Air to Hold Water at Different Temperatures

Temperature °C	°F	Content (mg/L)
0	32	4.9
10	50	9.4
15	59	12.8
20	68	17.3
25	77	23.0
30	86	30.4
35	95	39.6
37	98.6	43.9
40	104	51.1
45	113	65.6
50	122	83.2

(content) by the capacity (amount of water vapor that a gas can hold at any given temperature) of the air to hold water when totally saturated at a given temperature:

Relative humidity = Content/capacity.

At normal atmospheric pressure a gas cannot be more than 100% saturated. The greater the temperature of a gas, the greater its ability to hold water vapor. Table 3–1 shows the capacity of air to hold water at 100% saturation across a range of temperatures. As temperature decreases and capacity becomes less than content, water condenses or "rains out" of the gas and forms dew. This is called the dew point and indicates the point at which gas is 100% saturated. For example, on a hot summer day in Florida the temperature may be 34°C with 80% RH, which means that the water content, or AH, is 30 mg/L. This is the capacity of gas at 30°C. As the sun goes down and the air cools below 30°C, dew forms. The lower the temperature, the more water condenses from the air. As the temperature rises, the same AH results in a decreasing RH. The temperature-humidity curve becomes steeper above 20°C and allows relatively large volumes of water to be exchanged with relatively small changes in temperature (Fig 3–1).

Two heat exchange mechanisms are important in conditioning inspired air: heat transfer by evaporation and by convection. The heat loss by evaporation from the respiratory system is defined as the latent heat of vaporization of water. Energy is required for the water to change from a liquid to a vapor state. The specific heat of air is 1,008 J/kg. The specific heat of water is 4,200 J/kg, more than four times greater than that for air. The latent heat of vaporization (and latent heat of condensation) of water is 2,450 J/kg. Water is able to act as a heat reservoir in the respiratory tract because of these differences in energy requirement between heat of evaporation and heat of convection. Convection is the heat transfer from the mucosa to the inspired air. While both evaporation and convection cool the mucosa, heat loss resulting from

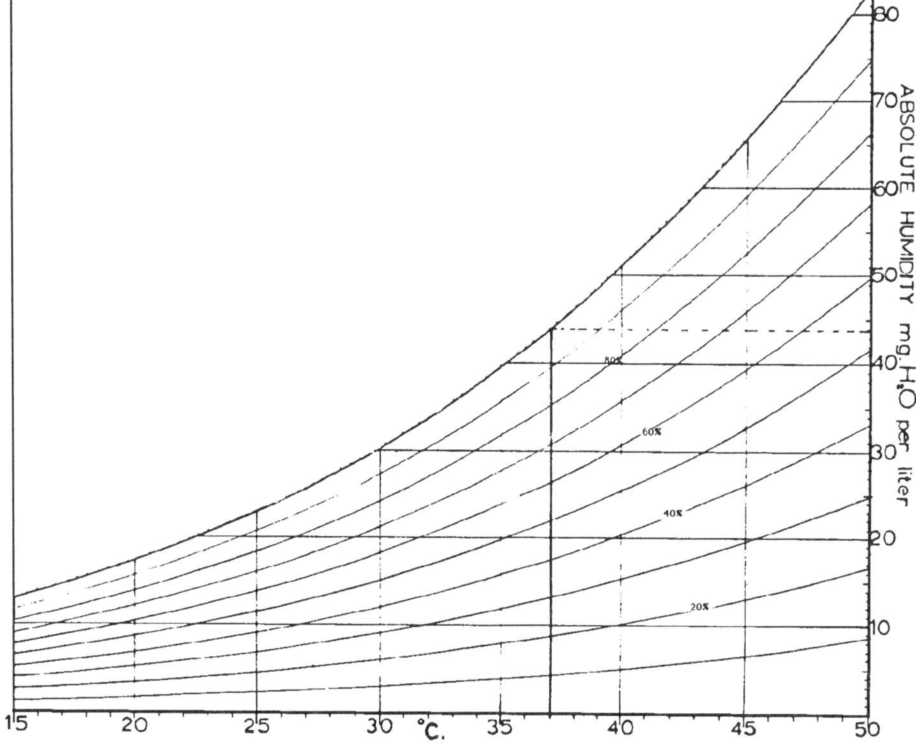

FIG 3–1
Psychometric nomogram demonstrating the water content of air over a range of temperatures. (Adapted from Burton GG, Hodgkin JE, Ward JJ (eds): *Respiratory Care: A Guide to Clinical Practice.* Philadelphia, JB Lippincott, 1991. Used by permission.)

evaporation of water is a bigger factor than the heat loss resulting from convection.

Under normal conditions about 250 mL of water and 1,470 J of heat are lost from the lung each day. Approximately 495 mL of water and 28,468 J of heat are required to change room air from its usual temperature of about 24°C and RH of 50% to alveolar conditions. In order to accomplish this, 245 mL of water and 27,000 J of heat must be reclaimed and returned to the upper respiratory tract every day[7]:

- At room temperature of 24°C and an RH of 50%, AH is approximately 11 g/m^3.
- At body temperature (37°C) and 100% RH, AH increases to 44 g/m^3.
- Respiratory volume for 24 hours is 15 m^3 (0.018 kg).
- Evaporative water loss is (44 − 11 g/m^3) × 15 m^3 = 495 g or approximately 495 mL.
- Energy required for evaporation = 0.495 kg × 2,436 J/kg = 1,205 J.
- Energy required for heating water = 0.495 kg × 4,200 J/kg × (37 − 24°C) = 27,027 J.
- Energy required for heating air = 0.018 kg × 1,008 J/kg × (37 − 24°C) = 235.9 J.
- Total energy requirement = 27,000 J.

Aerosol

An aerosol is a suspension of solid or liquid particles that can vary by shape, density, or size. Aerosols exist all around us as pollen, spores, dust, smoke, smog, fog, mist, and viruses (Fig 3–2). We can also create aerosols for therapeutic uses by physically shattering matter or liquid into small particles and dispersing it into a suspension. This can be accomplished by using gas jets, spinning disks, ultrahigh-frequency sound, or discharge of small quantities of Freon.

The particle size of an aerosol is dependent on the device used to generate it and the substance being aerosolized. The equipment used to produce aerosols (nebulizers) generally produce aerosols consisting of particles of varying diameters and shapes that are referred to as heterodisperse. The aerosol generators can be defined in terms of the characteristics of the particles created. The mean mass aerodynamic diameter (MMAD) defines the distribution of particle sizes generated; the MMAD is the particle diameter around which the mass of particles is equally distributed with 50% of particles heavier and 50% lighter. The geometric standard deviation (GSD) is a measure of the variability of the particle diameters within the aerosol; the higher the GSD, the more frequently larger and smaller particles are present. As the GSD increases, the MMAD increases because the larger particles carry more mass.[8]

Optimal delivery of aerosol to the lung depends on the inhalation technique and pulmonary function of the patient. Under the best of circumstances, aerosols administered to the lung cause less than 20% deposition. Aerosol droplets with an MMAD of 5 μm or less are deposited in the lung. Most particles greater than 5 μm impact on the upper airway. The depth of penetration into the bronchial tree is inversely proportional to particle size down to a size of less than 1 μm. Particles less than 1 μm carry a small volume and are so light and stable that many are not deposited in the lungs. Even when they do settle in the lung, these particles carry very small quantities of medication.

Most therapeutic aerosols target airways with a particle size range from 1 to 5 μm.

Size (μm)	Relative Volume
1	1
2	8
3	27
4	64
5	125
10	1,000

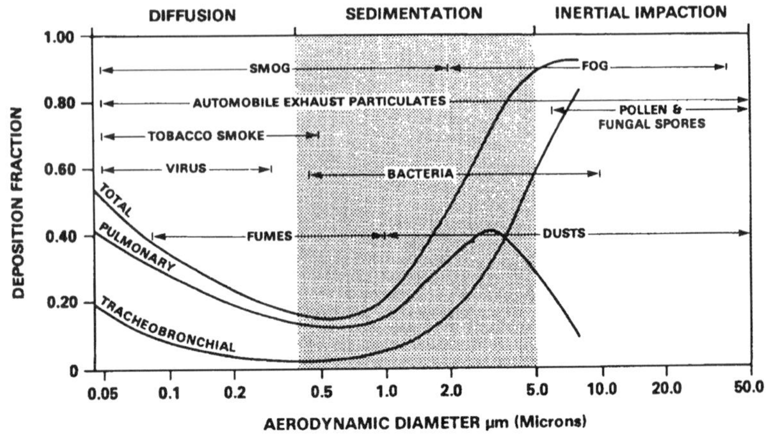

FIG 3–2
Size deposition relationships for stable particles with an aerodynamic diameter of 0.1 to 8 μm for the tracheobronchial and pulmonary compartments of the adult lung. The total curve is the sum of values for these two compartments of the lung. The range of particle diameters over which diffusion, sedimentation, and inertial impaction are most important are shown, as well as approximate size ranges of some of the commonly encountered aerosols. (Adapted from Newhouse MT, Dolovich M: Aerosol therapy in children, in *Basic Mechanisms of Pediatric Respiratory Disease: Cellular and Integrative.* Toronto, BC Decker, 1991. Used by permission.)

Aerosols with an MMAD of 0.8 to 2.0 μm are well targeted into the lung parenchyma. Particles less than 0.8 μm are often exhaled and of such small volume that they contribute little to the therapeutic effect.

Aerosol particles may change size because of evaporation or hygroscopic properties. Small particles get even smaller when inhaled with ambient gas at room temperature as the inspired air is heated en route to the lungs. Aerosols introduced into a heated ventilator circuit may grow because of hygroscopic properties and a change in temperature en route to the patient.

The respiratory care practitioner often assesses the adequacy of delivery of aerosol to a patient by visually observing the mist distributed by a nebulizer. Because of the size of particles generated, the unaided human eye cannot identify particles less than 1,000 μm in diameter (equivalent to a medium-sized grain of sand). What is identified when observing the output of a nebulizer is the defraction of light as it passes through the particles rather than the particles themselves.

Physics of Humidity and Aerosol Delivery

Mechanisms of Deposition

Deposition of inhaled particles within the lung is caused by a combination of mechanisms, including impaction because of inertia, sedimentation because of gravity, and diffusion because of brownian motion. The relative importance of each factor is dependent on the size, location, and motion of the particle.

Inertial impaction is the deposition of particles by collision with a surface. This is the primary mechanism for deposition of particles *over* 5 μm in diameter. The larger the particle size, the greater the inertia. Turbulent flow, complex convoluted passageways, bifurcation of the airways, and inspiratory flows greater than 30 L/min increase the impaction of particles in the larger airways. Most particles over 10 μm in diameter are deposited in the nose or mouth. Particles over 5 to 10 μm in diameter tend to be deposited in proximal airways before reaching bronchioles 2 mm or less in diameter. High inspiratory flow rates (greater than 30 L/min) tend to deposit more particles in the upper airway.

Gravitational sedimentation occurs when particles slow and settle out of suspension. Gravitational sedimentation is a time-dependent mechanism affecting particles down to 1 μm in diameter. Sedimentation is the primary mechanism for deposition of particles 1 to 5 μm in diameter in the central airways. Breath holding, by increasing residence time in the lung, affects deposition, especially in the last six generations of the airway. A 10-second breath hold has been reported to provide optimal particle deposition when compared with other breath-holding times.[9, 10]

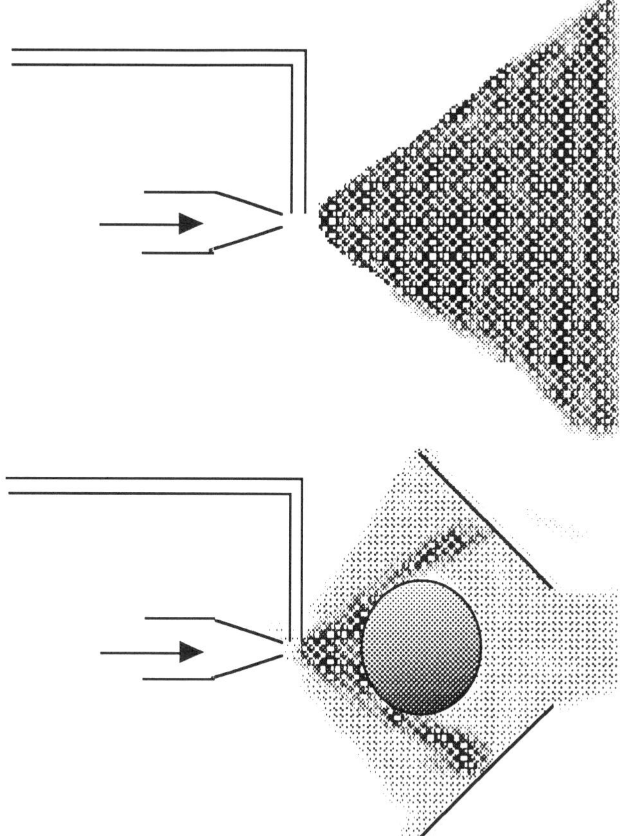

FIG 3–3
Jet nebulizers illustrating the use of baffles.

Diffusion and *brownian movement* are primary mechanisms for deposition of particles less than 3 μm in diameter into the lung parenchyma. Particle deposition is reported to be divided between central and peripheral airways.[11] Optimal deposition of particles smaller than 3 μm in diameter is suggested to occur when the inspiratory flow rate is less than 60 L/min and the tidal volume is less than 1 L. The overall significance of tidal volume to aerosol deposition has, however, not been well established. Bigger breaths theoretically capture more aerosol, but this relationship has not been conclusively demonstrated.

Influence of Nebulizer Design

Design characteristics of nebulizers affect the size and density of particles generated. Aerosol particle size can be reduced by incorporating baffles (surfaces that remove aerosol particles from suspension by inertial impaction) into the design of the nebulizer. Baffles are engineered to produce optimal-size particles by allowing large particles to impact on the baffle surface (Fig 3–3). The baffles can be created by the internal walls of the nebulizer, an object placed in line with the jet gas flow, the

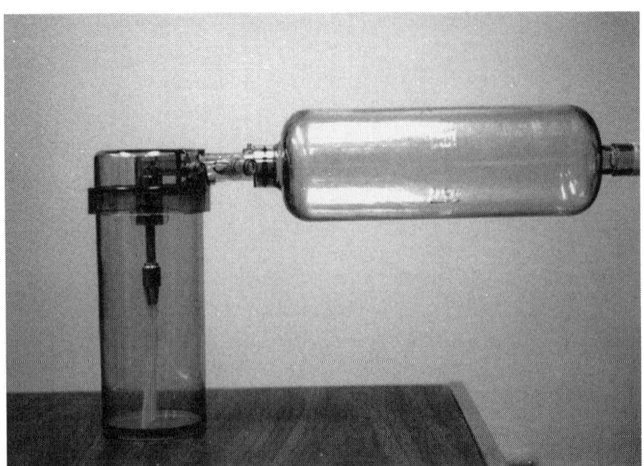

FIG 3–4
Nebulizer and drying chamber from the ICN SPAG-2 6000 series is an example of a settling chamber system that produces an almost monodisperse aerosol.

surface of a one-way valve, or the internal walls of a spacer or drying chamber. Well-designed baffle systems add to the efficiency of jet and mechanical nebulizers by allowing large particles to be removed from suspension to coalesce and return to the reservoir to be renebulized.

Baffles can also occur unintentionally and affect aerosol output and deposition. Unintentional baffles can be created by the angles within the aerosol tubing, by interfaces with other devices outside of the aerosol generator, and from the surfaces of the upper airway itself. Tubing, settling chambers, and one-way valves placed between the nebulizer and the patient also allow sedimentation of larger particles and reduce MMAD and output of the aerosol. The drying chamber used in the ICN Pharmaceutical Small Particle Aerosol Generator (SPAG) shown in Fig 3–4 produces a consistent small MMAD with a very low GSD. Large particles that are not baffled by the nebulizer or connecting tubing will be deposited in the upper airway.

Factors Affecting Drug Distribution

The goal of aerosol delivery of medication is to use the physical properties of gas exchange to deliver a known concentration of drug to the lung. Dosing of aerosolized medication to the lung is unfortunately an imprecise science. In vitro and in vivo models have been established to define the deposition of particles of various size within the lung. These models establish the relationship between particle size and aerosol deposition under optimal circumstances. It is less clear how much, if any, drug is delivered to the targeted areas of the lung in disease states and during acute exacerbations of underlying lung dysfunction. The factors that affect delivery of drug to the lung by aerosol generators include the inspiratory flow rate, the respiratory rate, the caliber of intrinsic airways, nose vs. mouth breathing, mask vs. mouthpiece delivery, the type and ease of use of the nebulizer, the drug formulation, humidity, the temperature of the gas stream environment, and patient characteristics including age, the ability to coordinate inspiratory effort, and comprehension.

Inspiratory flow rate. High inspiratory flow rates are associated with greater deposition of drug within the upper airways. This occurs as a result of increased impaction. In addition, high flow rates result in preferential distribution of gas to the upper lobes. Decreased inspiratory flow rates can affect the actuation of dry powdered inhalers (DPIs) and result in reduced drug available for inhalation.

Respiratory rate. Tachypnea reduces residence time of drug within the lung, thus allowing less opportunity for deposition.

Airway caliber. Decreased size of the airways, as occurs in patients with severe bronchospasm for whom the treatment is desired, restricts the flow of aerosol to targeted distal airways. Under this circumstance, the aerosol is deposited into the larger, more proximal airways, and larger doses of drug may be required.

Inhalation by mouth vs. nose. The nose is a more effective filter than the mouth; as a result, nasal inhalation filters most particles greater than 10 μm. Mouth breathing allows greater deposition of aerosol within the lung.

Mask vs. mouthpiece delivery. Inhalation through the mouth provides more respirable particles to the lung than does inhalation through the nose. This characteristic of optimal drug delivery, however, is probably overshadowed by the importance of patient comfort to optimal drug delivery. The choice of mask or mouthpiece should be based on patient comfort rather than considerations about aerosol deposition, even when the patient is primarily mouth-breathing.

Nebulizer type. Continuous nebulization, which produces aerosol continuously throughout the patient's respiratory cycle, is not very efficient in delivering medication to the patient because aerosol that is produced between inspirations is largely lost to the atmosphere. Demand nebulizers, which actuate the device in coordination with inspiration, are more efficient in delivering medication but increase the nebulization time as much as fourfold for the same volume of medication.

The ease or difficulty of use of the aerosol delivery system affects the speed and reliability of self-administration. Systems with multidose convenience appear to be the easiest for patients to use.

Drug formulation. The drug formulation can have an influence on drug delivery. Almost any solution can be nebulized, but the physical characteristics of the solution can affect particle size and nebulizer output. Formulations of dry powders are limited to only a few preparations. Metered dose inhalers (MDIs) have a greater variety of available formulations, but incorporating new drugs into MDIs is a lengthy process; therefore the drugs are not always available in the most desirable or therapeutically optimal form.

Humidity. Humidity affects both wet and dry aerosols. Droplets of solutions can either evaporate or grow depending on the water content and temperature of the gas around them. Powder will clump or aggregate in high humidity, thereby reducing delivered doses.

Patient characteristics. Small infants are obligate nose breathers; have tiny airways, small inspired volumes, and high respiratory rates; and are unable to cooperate to achieve ideal drug delivery (for example, by using breath-holding techniques). Older children are also often unable or unwilling to cooperate. Elderly patients may not be able to physically manipulate devices or to understand or cooperate with techniques to optimize aerosol delivery.

Actuation of the aerosol device during inspiration is mandatory with some nebulizers, particularly MDIs. Poor patient coordination will drastically reduce the delivered dose of medication.

The patient's ability to understand the therapy and its goals significantly affects the therapeutic efficacy of any treatment. Patients not only must understand the basic administration technique but must also be able to keep track of dosing requirements and recognize undesirable side effects and techniques to reduce them.

CLINICAL INDICATIONS FOR HUMIDITY AND AEROSOL THERAPIES

Humidity and aerosol therapy is provided both to ensure maintenance of normal physiologic conditions and as therapy for pathologic conditions.

Maintaining Normal Physiologic Conditions

The primary goal for humidity therapy is to provide adequate humidification and heat to inspired gas to approximate normal inspiratory conditions at the point of entry into the airway. Heat and humidity ensure normal operation of the mucociliary transport system. The circumstances under which the gas administered to a patient should be humidified and warmed are numerous:

Indications for humidifying inspired gas

- Administration of medical gases
- Delivery of gas to the bypassed upper portion of the airway
- Thick secretions in nonintubated patients

Indications for warming inspired gases

- Hypothermia
- Reactive airway response to cold inspired gas

Inspired gases should be humidified to ensure normal physiologic conditions, as well as to treat abnormalities of the respiratory tract. The most common situation in which gases should be humidified is during the administration of medical-grade gases. Administration of these dry gases to the airways is known to be a hazard because it causes heat and water loss and, if prolonged, structural damage.

As the airway is exposed to relatively cold dry air from the ambient environment, ciliary motility is reduced, airways become more irritable, mucus production increases, and pulmonary secretions become thick and encrusted in the airways. The hazard is particularly great when the normal humidifying capability of the airways is lost or bypassed, as occurs after endotracheal intubation.[12] Cytologic studies demonstrate damage to tracheal epithelium within 2 hours of the administration of dry gases via endotracheal tube, whereas gases at 60% RH produce no damage.[13] Even when room air is being breathed through an artificial airway, extrinsic humidification of the inspired gas should be ensured. The loss of the humidifying capabilities of the upper airway causes the ISB to shift to the lower airways, particularly when differences of as much as 10°C exist between ambient and tracheal temperatures. These more distal airways are less capable of adequately humidifying inspired gases.

The appropriate level of humidification and temperature to achieve during the administration of medical gases varies according to the method of delivery. Gas delivered to the nose or mouth should be heated and humidified to conditions equivalent to 50% RH (AH of 10 mg/L at 22°C). Gas delivered to the hypopharynx, such as when administered by nasal catheter, should be at 95% RH (AH of 28 to 34 mg/L with a temperature of 29 to 32°C).[14] When gas is delivered directly into the trachea through an endotracheal tube or tracheostomy tube, it should be warmed to 32 to 35°C and have 100% RH (AH of 36 to 40 mg/L).

Treating Pathologic Processes

The delivery of warmed, humidified inspired gases can also be used to prevent and treat a variety of pathologic conditions. Heated and humidified inspired gas is advocated for the treatment of upper airway inflammation,

TABLE 3–2
Range of Pharmaceuticals Delivered via Aerosol*

Nasal Delivery		Lung Delivery	
Clinical Indication	Drug	Clinical Indication	Drug
Allergies	Steroids	Asthma	Steroids, cromolyn Na, atropine, bronchodilators
Osteoporosis	Calcium	Influenza, RSV†	Ribavirin
Diabetes	Insulin	Pneumocystis	Pentamidine
Bone disease	Calcitonin	Fungal infection	Amphotericin
Hormone deficiency	Growth hormone	Cystic fibrosis	Aminogycloside, antibiotics
HIV†-related neuropathy	Peptide T		
Migraine	Ergotamine	Immunization	Vaccines
Postoperative pain	Butorphanol	Sarcoidosis	Steroid

* Adapted from Dolovich M: *Aerosol Med* 1989; 2:171–186.
† RSV = respiratory syncytial virus; HIV = human immunodefiency virus.

hypothermia, airway hyperactivity associated with breathing cold dry gases, and prevention and treatment of thick, tenacious pulmonary secretions.[15]

Upper Airway Inflammation

The use of cold humidified gases, often with bland aerosols, is advocated in the treatment of upper airway inflammation resulting from croup, epiglottiditis, postextubation swelling, etc.[16] The cool mist is thought to promote localized peripheral vasoconstriction, reduce swelling, and relieve the discomfort associated with upper airway inflammation.

Hypothermia

Delivery of warm (39 to 41°C) humidified gases can also be used to treat hypothermia. For a hypothermic patient, rewarming and reduction of further heat loss can be facilitated in part by heating the inspired gases.[17]

Airway Hyperreactivity to Cold Inspired Gas

Many patients react with severe bronchospasm to breathing cold inspired gas. For example, there is evidence that some asthmatics have increased airway resistance when breathing cold air.[18] The cause of the bronchospasm is most likely due to a shift of the ISB to more distal airways with associated stimulation of mast cells in that area. This response can be reduced by warming the inspired gases and may also be reduced in some patients by providing gas humidified with greater than 20 mg/L H_2O at 23°C.[2]

Treatment of Thick Secretions

Humidification of inspired gas has been advocated in patients with thick, tenacious secretions, whether they have intact upper airways or not. Currently no studies have been reported that document the role of external humidifiers in improving the character and mobilization of thick secretions. The most effective method for improving the character of pulmonary secretions is systemic hydration. Nonetheless, humidification has been advocated for patients with tenacious secretions that are difficult to clear.[18] The addition of heat to the humidifier system may also aid in improving the character and expectoration of the secretions.[19]

In addition to humidification, aerosol therapy with bland solutions such as distilled water and hypertonic saline is used to stimulate coughing as well as for secretion production. Such therapy has been used for diagnostic sputum induction.

Aerosol therapy is also used to deliver pharmacologically active agents to the airway. The indication for the aerosol is largely based on the indications for the drug and the targeted site of delivery. Table 3–2 lists the wide variety of drugs and current clinical indications for aerosol drug delivery.

GENERAL PRINCIPLES OF EQUIPMENT OPERATION

An understanding of the available techniques to humidify inspired gases is essential to the respiratory therapist. The first concept that must be understood is the difference between a humidifier and a nebulizer. A *humidifier* is a device that adds molecular water to gas. In contrast, a *nebulizer* is a device that produces an aerosol or suspension of particles in gas. Although the theoretical difference between humidifiers and nebulizers is clear-cut, the clinical selection of one type of device vs. another has significant overlap and is not based on definitive scientific data. Some humidifiers create aerosols, whereas some nebulizers add humidity to gas. Nebulizers have been employed to humidify gas, and in the case of anesthesia devices, humidifiers or vaporizers have been used to administer anesthetic agents.

Humidifiers

General Principles

Three functional variables affect the ability of a device to humidify gas: temperature, surface area, and time of contact. These factors are applied to various degrees in the design of commercially available humidification devices.

Temperature. Temperature is a very important factor for effective humidification. The greater the temperature, the more water vapor gas will hold. Failure to heat a humidifier will significantly reduce its efficiency and output. As evaporation occurs within the humidifier, the water at ambient temperature in the reservoir of the humidifier cools. As compressed gas delivered through the humidifier expands, it cools. These effects combine to significantly reduce the temperature in humidifiers that are not actively heated.

Unheated humidifiers can operate at temperatures more than 10°C below ambient temperature. Fig 3–5 illustrates that under these circumstances gas leaving a 10°C humidifier at 100% RH (AH of 9.4 mg/L) may provide only 43% RH at a room temperature of 24°C, or 21% RH at body temperature. Heated humidifiers actively replace heat lost from vaporization and compensate for cooling from gas expansion as shown in Fig 3–6.

A small surface area or short time of contact can reduce the beneficial effects of heating humidifiers. If enough heat can be added to the humidifying system, however, the effects of surface area or contact time can be overcome.

Surface area. The greater the surface area available for direct contact between water and gas, the greater the opportunity for evaporation. The greater the ratio of surface content area to gas volume, the more efficient the humidifier. Several strategies are utilized to optimize the surface area in humidifiers. These include bubble diffusion, aerosol generation of water droplets, and passover or wick technologies.

The bubble diffusion technique causes the gas to bubble through a column of water and results in diffusion of water into the gas. The smaller the gas bubble, the greater the ratio of surface area to relative gas volume, thus bringing more gas into contact with water. Although a large bubble has a greater surface area than a small bubble, a smaller relative volume of the gas in the bubble comes in contact with the water.

A second technique is to create an aerosol of water droplets in the gas stream. The smaller the particles and the greater the mist density (number of particles per volume of gas), the more surface area that is available for contact and subsequent evaporation.

Finally, passing gas over the surface of water will increase the humidity in the gas (Fig 3–7). The device utilized can be as simple as blowing the gas over a pan of water or as elaborate as those that incorporate vanes or wicks to optimize the surface interface. The larger the gas volume above the surface of the water and the smaller the

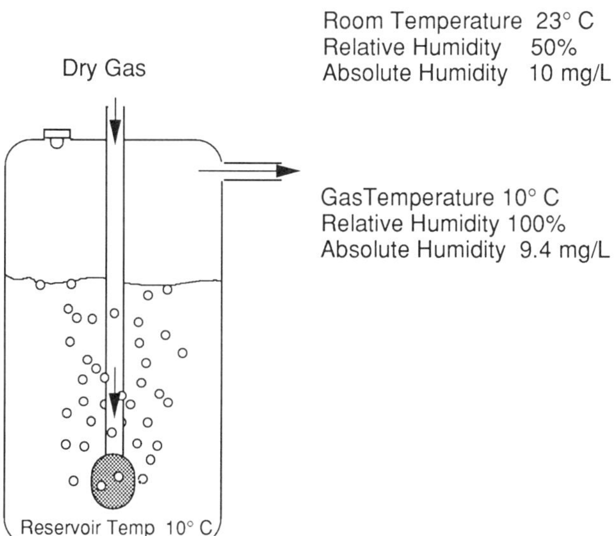

FIG 3–5
Effects of decreasing reservoir temperature on humidity output in an unheated bubble-type humidifier.

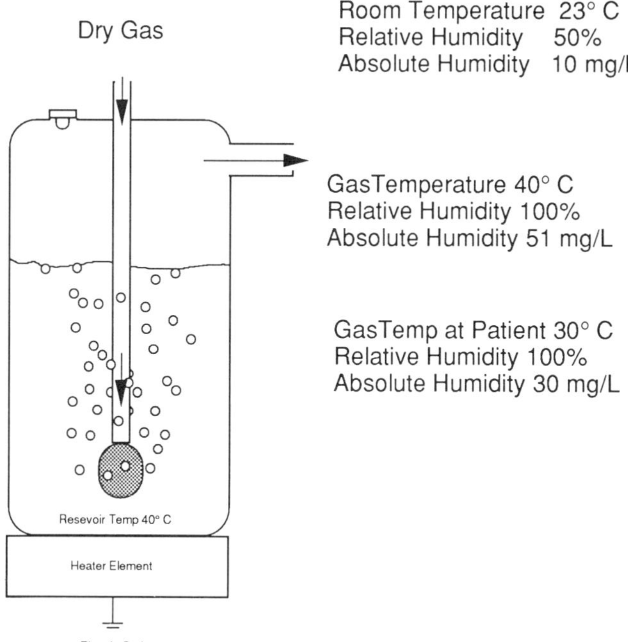

FIG 3–6
Effects of heating the reservoir of a humidifier.

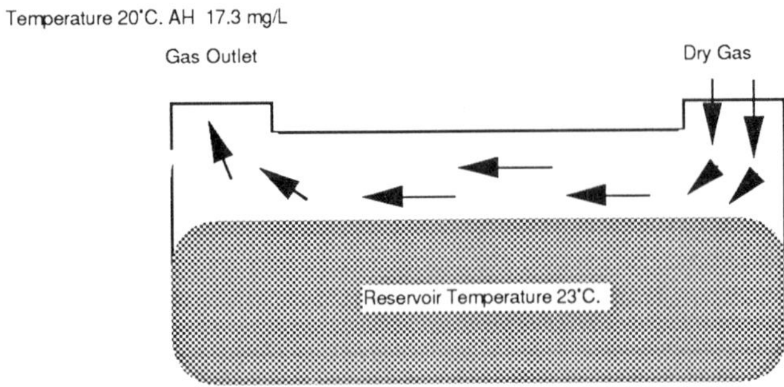

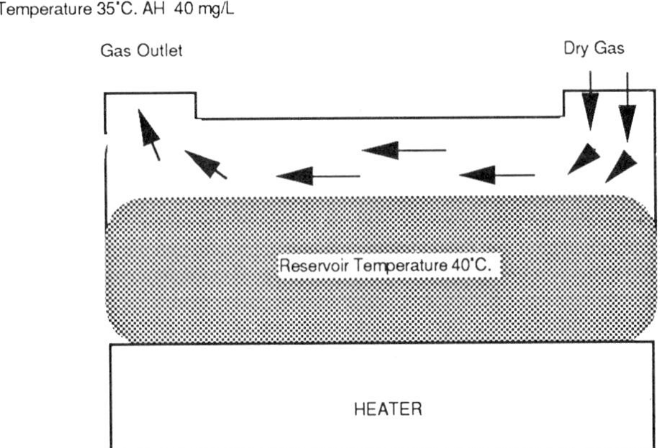

FIG 3–7
A simple passover humidifier and the effect of increasing the temperature of the reservoir.

surface area of the reservoir, the less efficient the humidifier because of the low ratio of surface area to volume. The wick-type humidifier, a variant of the passover humidifier, uses a porous absorbent paper (wick) extending above the surface of the water reservoir. Gas comes in contact with the water-saturated wick as well as the surface of the water.

Hygroscopic condenser humidifiers, also known as heat and moisture exchangers (HMEs), incorporate a large network or surface of hygroscopic paper, wire mesh, or filter material to bring the stream of gas into contact with water-laden surfaces of the filter material and create a very high surface-to-volume ratio.

Contact time. The longer the gas is in contact with water, the greater the opportunity for evaporation to occur. For the bubble diffusion humidifier, the deeper the water above the gas outlet, the greater the time of contact as the bubbles rise to the surface. As soon as the gas escapes from the water reservoir and ends contact with the fluid surface, humidification ceases. Low gas flow rates through the humidifier tend to provide greater contact time than high flow rates do. Aerosols suspended in the gas stream have extended contact (and opportunity

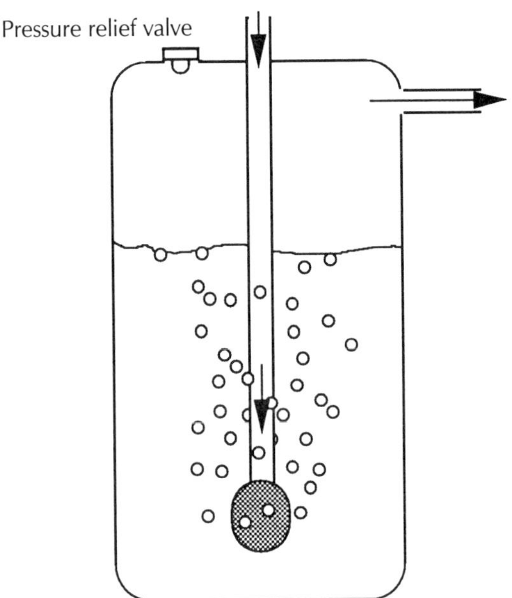

FIG 3–8
A simple bubble-type humidifier.

for evaporation) as the gas travels to the patient and enters the lungs.

Types of Humidifiers

Humidifiers can be classified into three general types defined primarily by the method of contact between the water and gas. Humidifier types include bubble-type humidifiers (BTHs), passover humidifiers, and jet nebulizer-humidifiers. HMEs are also classified as humidifiers.

Bubble-type humidifier. As previously described, in a BTH gas is directed under the surface of water and diffused to form bubbles (Fig 3–8). The larger the bubble, the greater the surface contact for the individual bubble, but the lower volume of gas actually in contact with the water. The deeper the water, the longer the contact. BTHs are commonly used with simple oxygen administration devices (i.e., cannulas, catheters, simple masks, reservoir rebreathers, and high-concentration venturi masks) and without heaters to bring gas to ambient levels of humidity. The dry medical gas is directed into a water-filled reservoir where the stream of gas is broken up (diffused) into bubbles that gain humidity as they rise through the water. While some designs use series of small holes in a tube running beneath the surface of the water, others incorporate some form of diffuser. The diffusers can be made of plastic foam, sintered metal, or mesh.

BTH devices are most efficient when used with gas flows of 5 L/min or less. They produce a content of water vapor ranging from 10 to 20 mg/L.[20] The higher the flow rate, the lower the vapor content secondary to the reduced temperature of the reservoir that occurs as a result of cooling from evaporation and the expanding gas. Although heating the reservoir might improve the efficiency of these units, the devices are generally connected to small-bore tubing that can be readily obstructed by condensate as the humidified gas cools en route to the patient. The condensate in the tubing counteracts any efficiency gained by heating.

To protect against obstructed or kinked tubing, bubble humidifiers should incorporate a pressure relief valve that provides an audible and visible alarm when high pressures (approximately 2 psi or 40 mm Hg) develop in the humidifier. The alarm serves the dual purpose of indicating that the flow of gas from the device has been interrupted and protecting the humidifier from being damaged by the excessive pressure. The pop-off device is often a gravity or spring-loaded valve that releases pressures above 2 psi. The pop-off valve should automatically resume normal position when pressures return to normal.[21]

At high flow rates bubble humidifiers produce particulates that can transmit or carry bacteria such as *Pseudomonas aeruginosa* from the reservoir of the humidifier to the patient.[22–30] The aerosol droplets carry the bacteria[31, 32]; the molecules of water cannot carry bacteria. Any device that produces aerosols must therefore be changed or cleaned regularly during routine use and consistently between patients to ensure that pathogens in the reservoir do not contaminate the patient.[33]

Passover-type humidifier. A passover-type humidifier directs gas over the surface of a body of water. A passover wick-type humidifier incorporates a wick saturated with water. Absorbent paper or cloth is used as the wick to draw water from the reservoir and saturate the fabric or paper, which then contacts the gas stream. A passover/barrier humidifier uses a hydrophobic barrier allowing water molecules to cross from the water reservoir into the gas stream. This type of passover humidifier has only been used with heated systems.

Jet nebulizer. Jet humidifiers incorporate a large reservoir nebulizer designed with baffles to minimize aerosol production exiting the humidifier while using the aerosol in the device to maximize surface contact with the gas. Some devices, as shown in Fig 3–9, direct the mist into the water reservoir's surface and use it as a baffle.

Jet nebulizers as humidifiers can deliver between 26

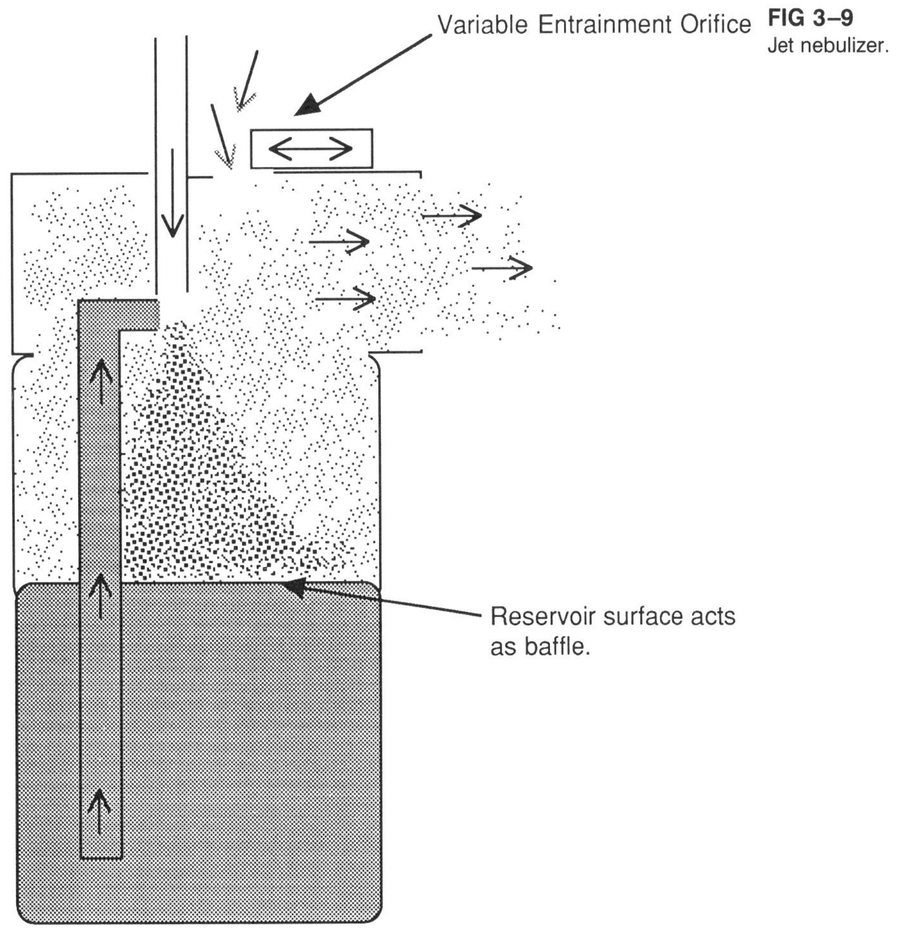

FIG 3–9
Jet nebulizer.

and 35 mg H_2O/L when unheated. Heated nebulizers can deliver 33 to 55 mg H_2O/L.[34–37] Although jet humidifiers can increase the water content, they pose an increased risk of infection from bacteria that might colonize the reservoir. Consequently, these devices should always be filled with sterile fluids or medications that are changed daily.[33]

One commercially available jet nebulizer, the Puritan Bubble/Jet humidifier, is adjustable to function as a bubble humidifier or jet humidifier. The dry source gas is directed either through the connecting tubing to the diffuser at the bottom of the reservoir or through a jet that draws fluid from the reservoir to create a mist. As a bubble humidifier, an adapter is used to connect to small-bore oxygen tubing. The large-bore outlet without the adapter fits the aerosol tubing and is typically used with the jet humidifier to avoid obstruction from rainout. These and other jet devices will be discussed more thoroughly in the discussion of nebulizers.

Heat and moisture exchanger. HMEs are also classified as humidifiers. They are often referred to as "artificial noses." Like the nose, HMEs capture exhaled heat and moisture and use it to heat and humidify the next inspiration. Unlike the nose, HMEs are passive humidifiers that do not add heat or water to the system. The role of the HME is to conserve heat and moisture from expired gas and to return them to the patient during the next inspiration. The ideal HME should have a low compliance, add little dead space to a ventilator circuit, add minimal weight, incorporate standard connections, add minimal resistance to flow, and operate at 70% efficiency, defined as the ratio of the AH of exhaled gas to the humidity returned to the patient by the HME.[20, 37]

Heated moisture exchangers have been in clinical use since the 1950s. They work in one of three ways. *Condenser humidifiers* allow expired water vapor to condense onto the relatively cool surface of the condenser. The condenser element is usually constructed of metallic gauze, corrugated metal, or parallel metal tubes to provide high thermal conductivity. On inspiration air cools the condenser to room temperature. On exhalation the fully saturated gas cools as it enters the condenser, and water rains out. The air then has 100% RH at a considerably lower temperature; the temperature of the condenser itself is increased. On the next inspiration, cool dry air is warmed by the condenser by evaporation of water from the surface. Condenser humidifiers are usually only about 50% efficient under ideal conditions.

Hygroscopic condenser humidifiers (Fig 3–10) contain materials such as paper, wool, or foam that are of low thermal conductivity. The material is then impregnated with a hygroscopic chemical such as calcium chloride or lithium chloride. The chemicals help to capture the

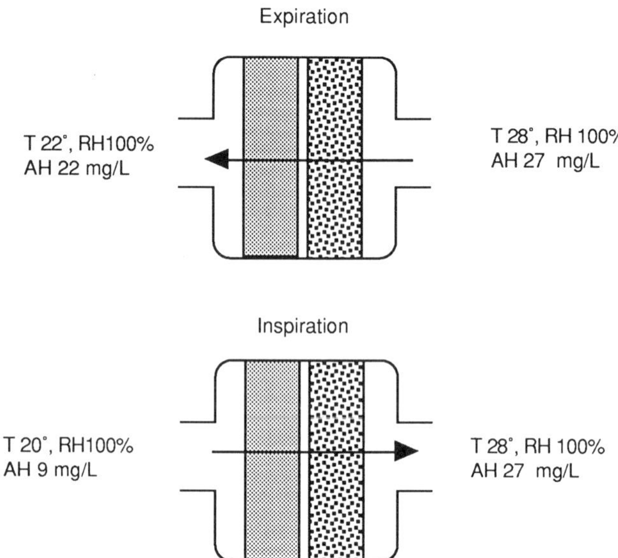

FIG 3–10
Hygroscopic humidifiers with changes in temperature and absolute humidity during inspiration and expiration.

exhaled water on expiration and reduce the RH of the exhaled gas to less than 100%; more water is available to humidify the next inspiration. During exhalation, warm saturated gas precipitates water on the cool condenser element, and water molecules bind to the salt without transition from the vapor to the liquid state and therefore without generation of latent heat. During inspiration the lower water vapor pressure in the inspired gas liberates water molecules from the hygroscopic compound without a fall in temperature because of vaporization. The efficiency of these devices can be as high as 70%.

Hydrophobic condenser humidifiers (Fig 3–11) use a water-repellent element with a large surface area and low thermal conductivity. Low thermal conductivity means that heat from conduction and the latent heat of condensation are not dissipated. During exhalation the condenser temperature rises to about 25°C because of conduction and the latent heat of condensation. On inspiration, cool gas and evaporation cool the condenser down to 10°C. This large temperature change results in more water being conserved to be used in humidifying the next breath. These devices are about 70% efficient. Hydrophobic humidifiers can also act as efficient microbiological filters.

A number of characteristics of HMEs must be taken into account when selecting the device as a method to provide humidification of inspired gases. The efficiency of HMEs falls as tidal volume, inspiratory flow, or F_{IO_2} increases.[38] Resistance through the HME is also important. When the HME is dry, resistance across the device is minimal. After several hours of use, however, the

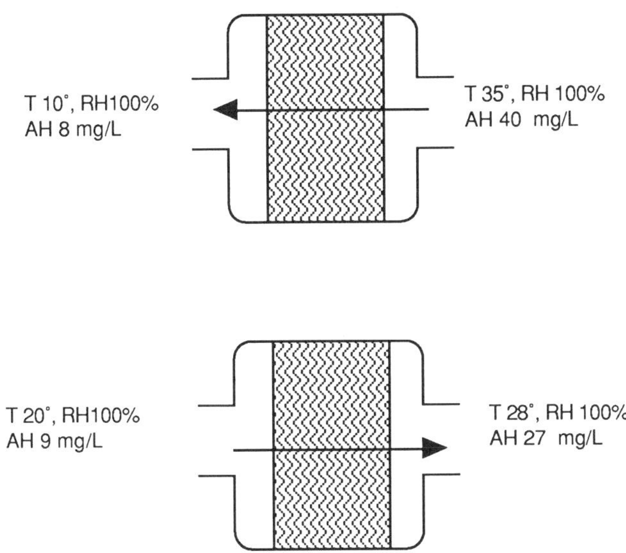

FIG 3–11
Hydrophobic condenser humidifier.

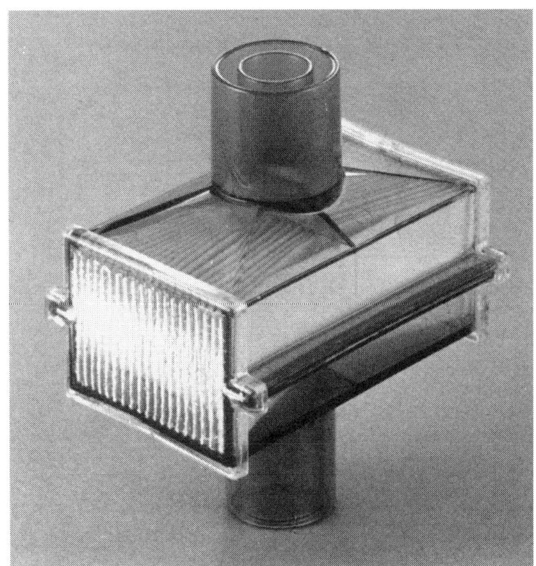

FIG 3–12
Pall HME 15-22 filter. (Courtesy of Pall Corp.)

resistance increases. It has been demonstrated that extended use of an HME in a lung model results in increased resistance as water is absorbed onto a hygroscopic HME.[39, 40] For some patients the increased work of breathing imposed by the HME may not be well tolerated, particularly for patients with underlying lung disease and inherently increased work of breathing.

HMEs are also considered bacteriostatic. They eliminate condensation from the ventilator circuit and *may* reduce the circuit as a potential source of infection. Several authors have shown that the Siemens hydrophobic condenser humidifier prevents the contamination of ventilator circuits and does not produce aerosols that could carry bacteria.[41] Other researchers who evaluated a number of HMEs were not able to confirm their safety with respect to nosocomial infection risk and demonstrated that many of the devices produced or passed aerosols that carry bacteria. Of the Siemens, Engstrom, Pall, and Portex hydrophobic condenser humidifiers, only the Pall humidifier (Fig 3–12) satisfactorily removed spores from the gas stream. Hedley et al. concluded that the pleated membrane filter provides a wider margin of safety than either hygroscopic or composite devices.[42]

Reservoir and Feed Systems

As the inspired gases are humidified, water must be added to the humidifier. The system used to replace the water in the humidifier should be designed to facilitate operation, to ensure continuity of therapy, and to minimize disruption of ventilatory support for those patients requiring mechanical ventilation. Continuous feed systems provide the most consistent replacement system; they are desirable because they allow water to be replenished without operator intervention and allow the use of sterile solutions with a decreased risk of contamination. The systems rely on gravity, usually with a pole-mounted reservoir external to the humidifier mechanism.

A number of methods are available for regulating continuous feed systems. They include flotation controls, level-compensated reservoirs, and optical sensors. For the flotation-type systems, as the water level rises, a float either occludes the flow of water or triggers a valve to close. Mauna Loa (Fig 3–13), 3M/Bird, and Fisher Paykel manufacture flotation-type systems. In the systems that control the water level by adjusting a reservoir (manufactured by Hudson/RCI and Marquest), an external reservoir is aligned horizontally with the humidifier to maintain relatively consistent water levels across the external reservoir to the humidifier chamber (Fig 3–14).

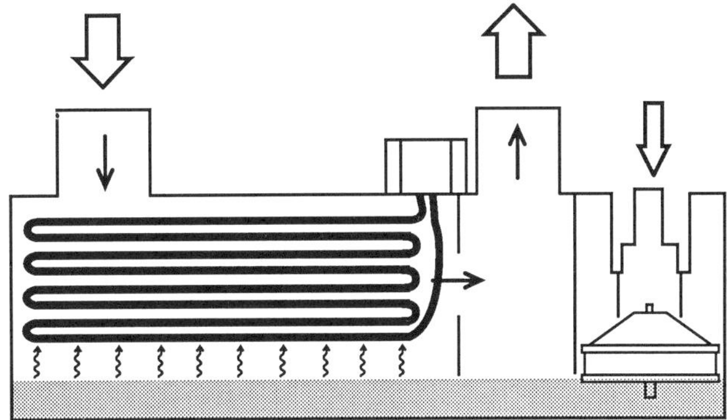

FIG 3–13
Mona Loa LavaPak uses a floatation device feed system.

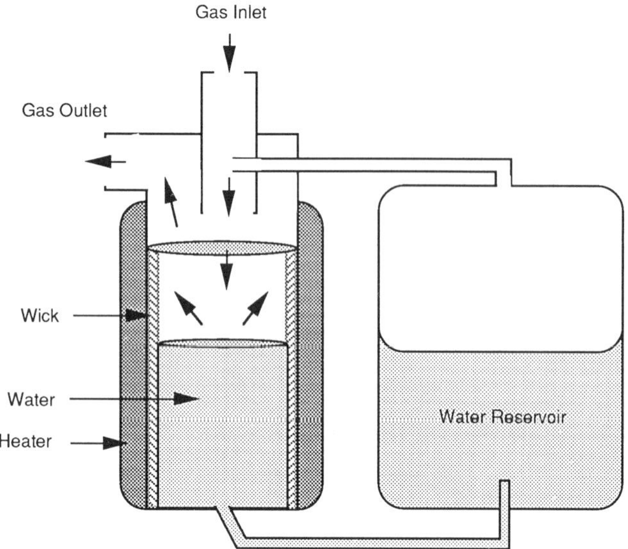

FIG 3–14
Schematic of the Hudson RCI Concha Column with a reservoir feed system.

Optical sensors can also be used to control the water level of continuous feed systems. Travenol markets a humidifier with a feed system that has an optical sensor incorporating a solenoid tube clamp. The optical sensor monitors the water level in the fluid chamber. As the water level falls, the system electronically opens a solenoid tube clamp and allows water to flow into the chamber. As the water level rises to the predetermined level, the sensor closes the clamp, and flow ceases. Another system (Inspiron) incorporates a hydrophobic barrier, a membrane that allows water vapor but not water to pass through it (Fig 3–15). With the barrier in place the chamber cannot overfill unless the barrier is disrupted or broken.

A number of intermittent feed systems are also available. The most common intermittent system uses a bottle of water that is poured into the humidifier. This type of system, as manufactured by Puritan Bennett and Fisher Paykel, requires discontinuation of humidifier operation (and interruption of mechanical ventilation, if used) to open the humidifier and pour water into the reservoir. One pour-type system does not require disruption of delivery. This exception is the Marquest chamber (Fig 3–16), which allows filling without interruption through the use of an internal level reservoir. The gravity water feed system also requires manual filling. The operator must periodically open a valve to feed water into the humidifier without disconnecting or interrupting humidifier operation.

Intermittent feed systems have several significant disadvantages over continuous feed systems. Those systems that are open are more susceptible to contamination of the reservoir. As the water level in manual feed systems falls, ventilator circuit compliance changes. Since gas is less compressible than water, changing the water volume in a fixed-volume container alters the compressible volume in both the humidifier and ventilator circuit. As a result, as the water level changes during use, so does delivered tidal volume. This problem is of greatest concern when used as part of the circuit for mechanically ventilated newborns and pediatric patients. Finally, the humidifier chamber can become empty if not checked regularly. For humidifiers that do not have alarms for low water levels, the humidity and temperature of gas delivered to the patient will be adversely affected.

Heating Systems

To improve the water output of the humidifiers, the water in the humidifier must be heated. Heated water humidifiers are particularly useful during long-term mechanical ventilatory support. Humidifier heaters use electricity to heat the water and gas. Three methods of heating the water are available. Heating elements can be located in the base of the humidifier, usually as a heating plate located under the reservoir. The heating element can also be "wrapped around" all or part of the humidifier chamber. Immersion heaters can also be used; in this system the heating element extends into the water reservoir. Some systems incorporate a combination of one or more heating technique.

All heaters have controllers that regulate electric power to the heater element. Heated humidifiers are defined as either servo-controlled or non–servo-controlled. Servo-controlled units monitor the temperature of gas delivered to the patient and adjust the power to the heater based on the temperature difference between the temperature setting of the humidifier and

FIG 3–15
Inspiron Vapophase humidifier with a hydrophobic membrane separating water from gas.

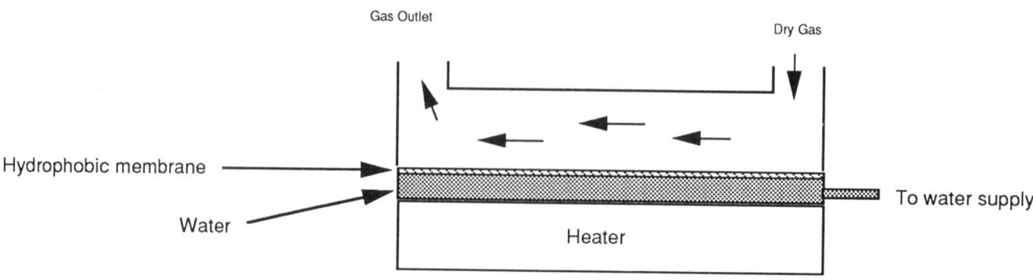

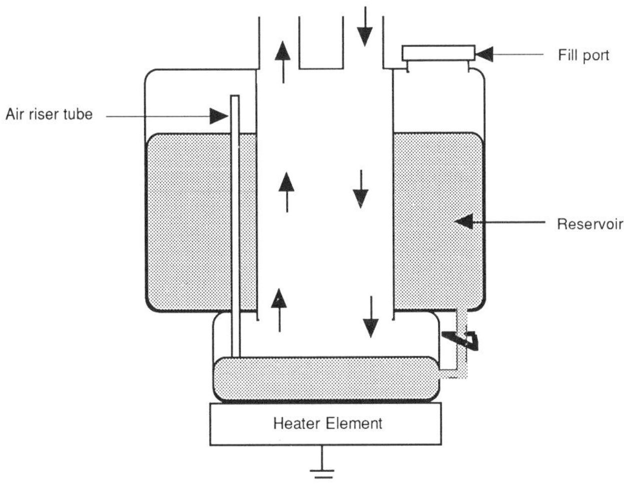

FIG 3–16
Feed system used with the Marquest SCT 2000 humidifier.

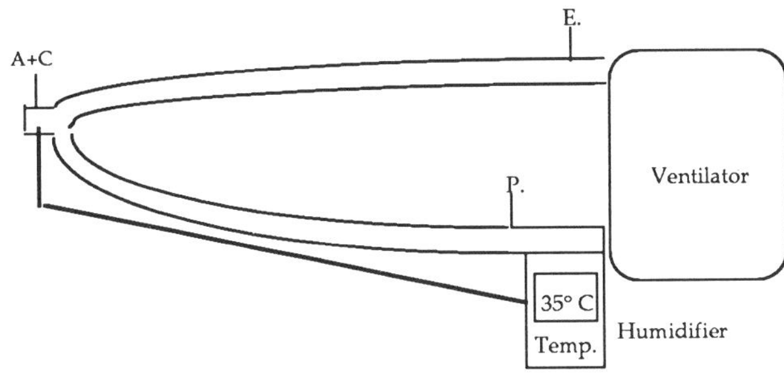

P. - Proximal Heater Output- 50°C. AH= 83 mg/L, RH=100%

A. - Patient Airway - 35C. AH = 40 mg/L, RH= 100%

Rainout from P to A = 43 mg/L

PL. - Patient Lungs - 37°C. AH= 44 mgL RH 100%

E. -Expiratory Limb -30°C. AH=30 mgL RH 100%

Rainout from PL to E =14 mg/L

FIG 3–17
Diagram of a conventional servo-controlled heated humidifier with a set temperature of 35°C measured at the airway. To accomplish this, the proximal heater output at *P* is 50°C. (See the text for a description.)

the distal temperature monitored by a thermistor probe placed downstream from the humidifier at or near the patient airway connection. When the set temperature of the heater is greater than the distal temperature, the controller applies more power to the heater. As the distal temperature nears or exceeds the set temperature, power is reduced. Thermistor probes at the airway are best placed in the inspiratory limb of the ventilator circuit. Placing the thermistor in this location reduces the influence of the exhaled gas temperature, which may be higher than that delivered by the humidifier.

Non–servo-controlled units monitor the temperature of the heater and provide power to the heater element based on the setting of the temperature control knob. The patient's airway temperature does not have an influence on the temperature of the heater. Both types of units have alarms and alarm-activated heater shutdown. Each individual heater has distinct advantages and disadvantages regarding performance, cost, safety, and ease of use that should be taken into account when selecting a system to purchase.

The American National Standards Institute (ANSI) standard Z-79.9 recommends that heated humidifiers have a water output level of at least 30 mg/L (100% RH at 30°C).[21] This level of humidity is considered to be the minimum required to avoid mucosal damage and inspissation of secretions for those patients whose upper airway has been bypassed by an endotracheal or tracheotomy tube. ECRI recommends that humidifiers have an output of 37 mg H_2O/L AH for inspired gas (85% RH at body temperature or 100% RH at 34°C).[43, 44]

One problem with heated humidifier systems is that once heated, the gas cools as it passes through tubing en route to the patient. With standard circuit tubing, the ambient environment conducts heat away from the tubing and gas and thereby reduces the temperature of the gas. As the gas cools, its ability to hold water vapor is reduced, and condensation ("rainout") occurs. The amount of condensate is proportional to the temperature differential and is affected by the ambient temperature, the gas flow, the selected patient airway temperature, and the length, diameter, and thermal mass of the breathing circuit.

One solution to the temperature drop and condensate in the tubing is to overheat the inspired gas as shown in Fig 3–17. Gas can be heated to as much as 50°C as it leaves the humidifier to provide 83 mg/L of water. If the gas temperature falls to 35°C at the patient connection, 40 mg/L water will be delivered. The remaining 43 mg/L of water, more than half of the total water coming out of the humidifier, will condense in the inspiratory limb of the circuit. The large amount of essentially "wasted" water carried in the humidified gas is costly; the delivery system is very inefficient. In addition to the direct cost of the lost water, the tubing must be frequently drained. The condensate in the circuit can also occlude the flow of gas through the circuit and inadvertently lavage or "drown" the patient, and it often becomes contaminated with bacteria from the patient's sputum.[45] When draining the tubing, it should be positioned so that the drainage is away from the patient's airway to avoid accidental lavage.

The condensate also poses a risk to the staff. As the circuit is disconnected, the practitioner can be sprayed with contaminated fluid in the eyes or other mucous membranes. When these systems are used, universal infection control practices must be observed: the use of gloves and goggles as splash guards to minimize the risk of exposure to contaminated secretions.[46, 47]

Water traps in both the inspiratory and expiratory limbs can be used to facilitate drainage of condensate from the ventilator circuit. The water trap should be located at a dependent point in the circuit so that it will drain by gravity. The traps selected should minimize changes in circuit compliance and allow emptying without disrupting ventilation of the patient.

Another approach is the use of a condensate drainage system such as the Nova Ventrx Criterion I.V. Drain Module shown in Fig 3–18. With this system condensate drains from both limbs of the circuit through the module, which is anchored to the ventilator. Condensate is collected in a closed bottle that needs to be emptied only once or twice in a 24-hour period, without disruption of ventilation.

Several mechanisms can be used to minimize condensate formation within the circuit. The best way to deal with condensate is to keep it from forming by maintaining a constant temperature of the gas within the circuit itself. Several mechanisms can be used to accomplish this, including increasing the thermal mass of the circuit itself, using a coaxial circuit with the inspiratory limb surrounded by the expiratory limb of the circuit, or adding heated wires to the circuit. Increasing the passive thermal mass of the circuit serves to insulate the gas inside the tubing from the cool ambient air outside. This is done by using thicker-walled tubing or wrapping the tubing with insulating material. These systems tend to reduce temperature drop but fail to eliminate significant condensate formation.

An alternative is to surround the inspiratory limb of the circuit with the expiratory limb in a coaxial manner. This technique uses the patient's warm exhaled gases to create a heated air bath surrounding the inspiratory limb. This principle is the basis of the Baines-type anesthesia circuit, which has limited application for ventilator circuits used for long-term support because of concerns about potential increases in imposed airway resistance and work of breathing.

The most practical method to prevent condensation is to install heated wires in the inspiratory limb of the circuit. This has become the most common approach to reduce condensation with standard heated water humidifiers. Reusable or disposable heated wire loops are inserted into the tubing to heat the gas and reduce the temperature differential between the humidifier and patient. Most heated wire circuits use dual servocontrols with two temperature probes, one monitoring the temperature of gas leaving the humidification chamber and the other placed at or near the patient airway as illustrated in Fig 3–19. The controller regulates the differential between the humidifier output and the patient airway. When heated wire circuits are used, the humidifier does not have to be set to as high a temperature as with conventional circuits. The reduction in condensate in the tubing results in lower sterile water use, a reduced need for drainage of the tubing, and less infection risk for both patients and workers.

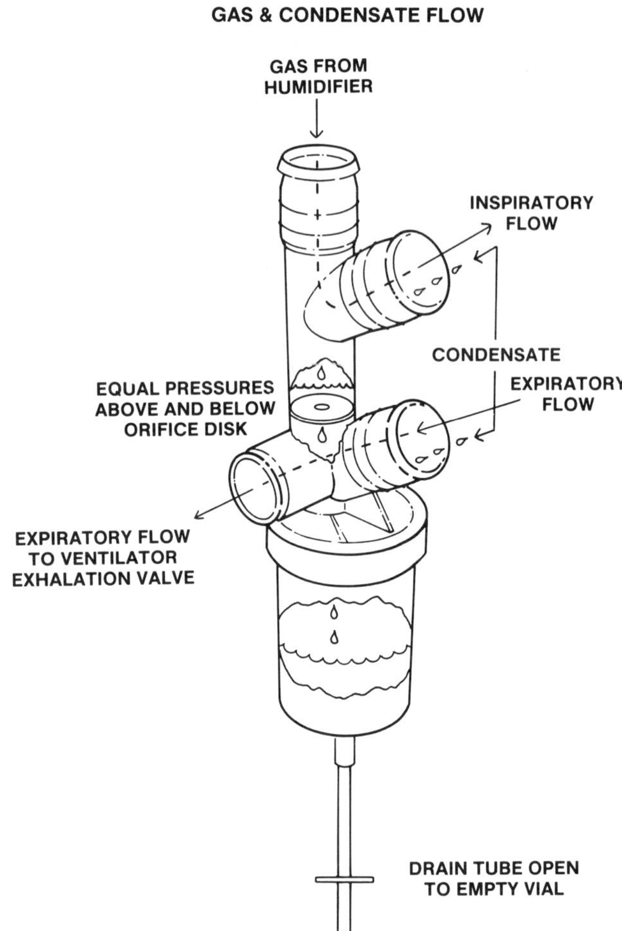

FIG 3–18
NovaVentrx Criterion I.V. drain module.

The Isothermal Servo-Pak IV servo temperature controller (Fig 3–20) is a device that could be used with conventional heated humidifiers that do not have heated wire capability. A thermistor probe at the airway is compared with the desired temperature setting, and power to the heater is regulated as appropriate.

Many humidifiers with heated wire capability include a "relative humidity" control that regulates the temperature differential between the humidifier and the circuit. It is important to realize that in these systems the system temperatures do not reliably reflect AH or RH, only the temperature differential between the two sites monitored. If the humidifier is cooler than the gas in the inspiratory limb, AH remains the same whereas RH is decreased. Under these circumstances, the circuit will have no condensate, so the practitioner cannot be certain that the gas is being humidified. Similarly, when the humidifier is minimally hotter than the gas in the circuit, RH increases or stays the same with minimal reduction in AH; little or no condensate forms in the circuit. To ensure that the inspired gas is being humidified, the temperature differential should be adjusted to the point that a few drops of condensation form near the patient's airway connector. This minimal condensate is the most reliable indicator that gas is fully saturated. If no condensate is visible, the gas RH could be anywhere between 99% and 0%, and clinicians have no way to know without access to a reliable hygrometer.

When heated wire circuits are used for infants who are in an isolette or other thermal-neutral environment, care must be taken regarding placement of the thermistor in the circuit. Fig 3–21 illustrates what happens if the sensor measuring the patient's airway temperature is within the thermal neutral environment: the probe will sense the warm ambient temperature and reduce or shut down power to the heated wires. This will result in increased rainout in the circuit and a significant reduction in humidity delivered to the patient. When heated wire circuits are used under these circumstances, the sensor probe in the inspiratory limb must be located outside of the heated environment to allow the heated wire controller to maintain the desired temperature and water content of inspired gases.

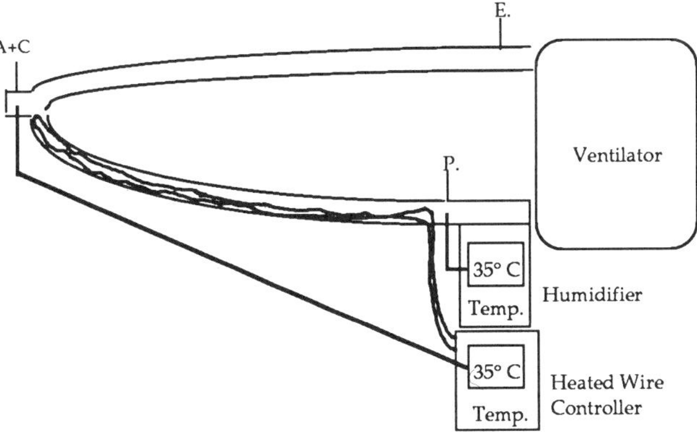

P. Proximal to heater outlet 35°C:AH 36:RH 90%
A. Patient Airway 35°C:AH 36:RH 90%
E. Exhaled Gas 28°C:AH 27 mg/L

Rainout from P to E = 9 mg/L

Heated wire on inspiratory side, with ambient cooling of expiratory limb of circuit means a lot of rainout between patient and exhalation valve of ventilator.

FIG 3–19
Standard configuration of a heated wire circuit on the inspiratory limb of the ventilator circuit. Ambient cooling on the expiratory limb of circuit creates condensate.

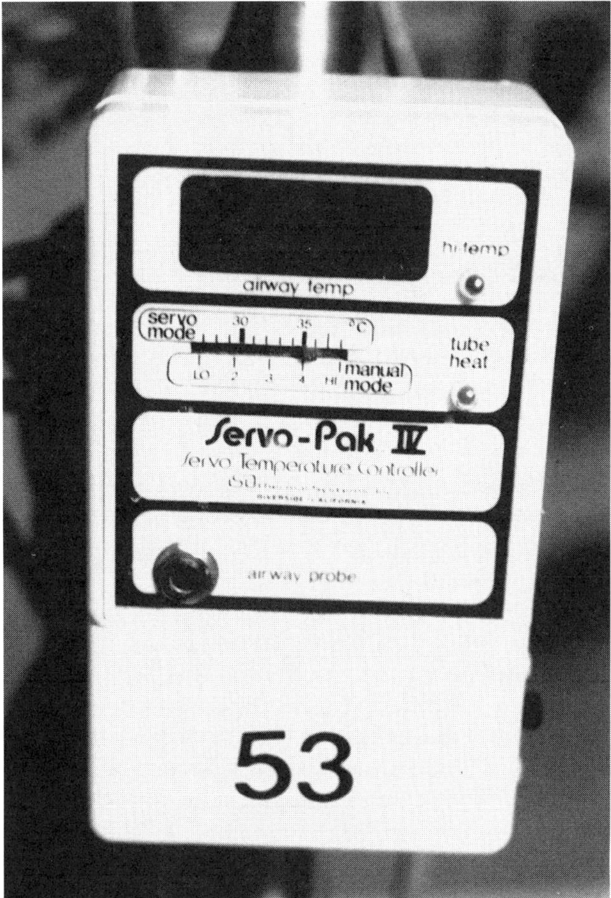

FIG 3–20
Isothermal Servo-Pak heated wire controller for use with nonheated wire–ready humidifiers.

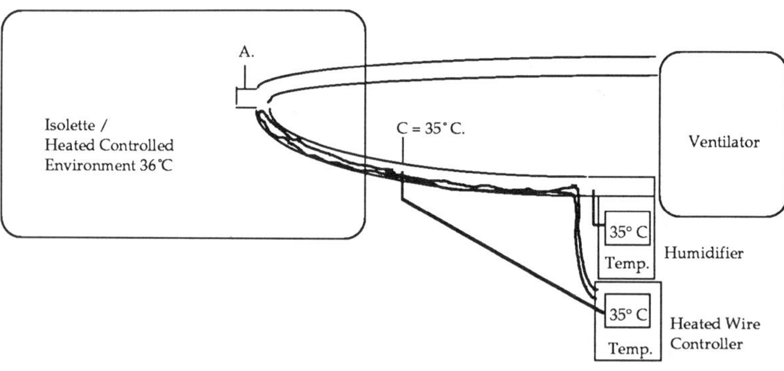

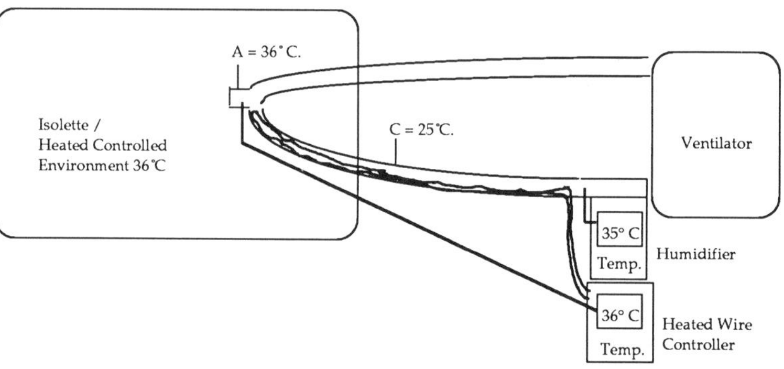

FIG 3–21
Effects of temperature probe placement in heated environments. Proper placement is in the circuit before entering the heated field. A probe placed in the heated area senses ambient heat, and the controller reduces the heat to the humidifier with a severe reduction in humidity to the patient.

Aerosol Generator

General Principles

Aerosol generators are commonly used by respiratory care practitioners to deliver humidity and medications. A variety of methods are used to generate aerosols for therapeutic use. The most common methods include jet nebulizers, MDIs, DPIs, powder inhalers (DPI), and ultrasonic nebulizers. Spinning disk nebulizers are rarely used in clinical respiratory care; they are more frequently used as room humidifiers.

Types of Aerosol Generators

Jet nebulizer. Jet nebulizers (Fig 3–22) use the Bernoulli principle; a high-pressure gas is driven through a restricted orifice (jet) positioned to intersect the top of a tube whose base is immersed in solution. The resulting venturi effect produces an area of low pressure that draws the solution up a capillary tube into the direct gas jet stream, which shatters the fluid stream into droplets. If properly designed, the stream of gas directs the droplets to impact against a baffle, the internal walls of the nebulizer, and/or the surface of the solution. Impaction removes the large particles from suspension and allows them to return to the reservoir, whereas smaller particles remain suspended in the gas and exit from the nebulizer. Droplet size and nebulization time are inversely proportional to gas flow through the jet. The higher the flow rate to the nebulizer, the smaller the particle size generated

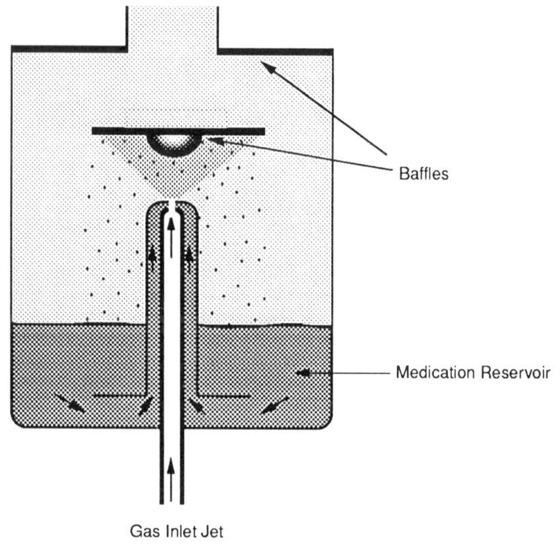

FIG 3–22
Jet nebulizer.

and the greater the time required to nebulize the contents of the nebulizer.

Metered dose inhaler. MDIs are Freon-powered nebulizers that provide multidose convenience through the use of a metering device (Fig 3–23). They are pressurized canisters containing a drug in the form of a micronized powder suspended with a mixture of two or more chlorofluorocarbon (CFC) propellants (Freons) along with a dispersal agent. MDIs are the most widely used form of aerosol device for the administration of bronchodilators, anticholinergics, and steroids; more formulations of these drugs are now available for use by MDI than for use with other types of nebulizers.

A variety of dispersal agents are used to improve drug delivery by keeping the drug in suspension. The most common dispersal agent is surfactant. The surfactants, commonly soya lecithin, sorbitan trioleate, and oleic acid, help to both keep the drug suspended in the Freon and lubricate the valve mechanism. The dispersal agents are usually present in amounts at least equal to or greater than the quantity of drug to be administered. The high concentration of the dispersal agent has clinical significance. Severe cough or wheezing caused by the propellant or surfactant develops in some patients, so care must be exercised when initiating therapy by MDI.[47]

The majority of the spray from most MDIs, up to 60% to 80% by weight, consists of CFCs with only 1% active drug. The large quantity of CFCs is also of clinical importance. Adverse reactions to CFC have also been reported, particularly in children.[48–50]

The output volume of MDIs varies from 30 to 100 μL, which contains 50 μg to 5 mg of drug, depending on the drug administered.[51, 52] Most MDIs use a 50-μL metering chamber to control drug delivery. Increasing the volume of the chamber does not improve drug delivery. More of the additional drug is lost at the actuator mouthpiece because of the lower rate of evaporation of the greater amount of propellant released and is therefore not available to the patient.[53]

Aerosol production from an MDI takes approximately 20 ms. Aerosolization of the liquid released from the metered dose canister begins as the propellants vaporize or "flash" and continues as the propellant evaporates. The velocity of the liquid spray leaving the MDI is about 15 m/sec. The speed falls to less than half the maximum velocity within 0.1 seconds as a cloud develops and moves away from the actuator orifice.[54] The particles produced from the "flashing" of propellants are initially 35 μm and rapidly decrease in size because of evaporation as the particle moves away from the nozzle.[55]

The particle size has an influence on the delivery of drug by MDI. Because of the velocity of the jet fired from the MDI, approximately 80% of the dose impacts and is deposited in the oropharynx, especially when the canister is fired from inside the mouth.[52, 55] Manufacturers of MDIs can adjust the particle size delivered by the device to influence drug targeting and subsequent absorption. The particle size and spray pattern produced by MDIs are determined by a variety of factors. A primary determinant is the vapor pressure of the canister. For most MDIs, the propellant vapor pressure varies from about 300 to 500 kPa at 20°C and creates a heterodisperse aerosol with MMADs of 3 to 6 μm and a GSD of 2.[8] The higher the vapor pressure, the smaller the particle size. The major determinant of the vapor pressure is the composition of the CFC. The rate of evaporation of the CFC determines the coarseness of the spray. The slower the rate of evaporation, the coarser the spray. Finer sprays can be produced by using greater quantities of CFC 12 or more volatile compounds. Raising the temperature also increases the pressure and reduces the particle size. As a practical note, skiers and others who are exposed to cold

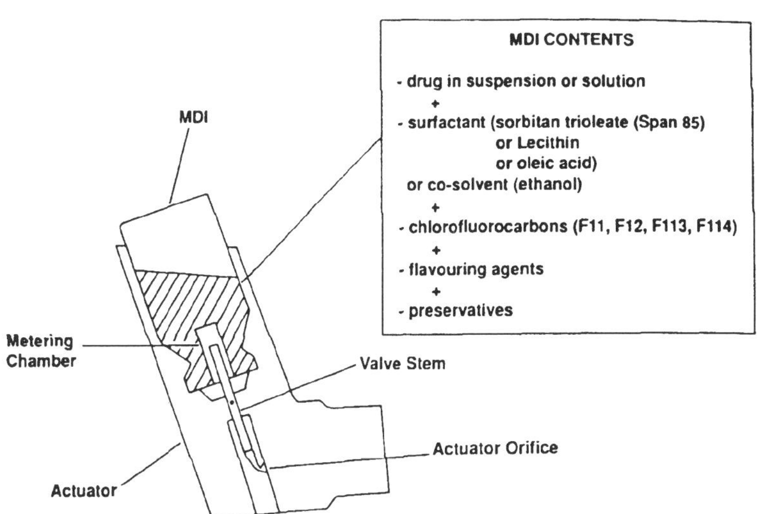

FIG 3–23
Metered dose inhaler *(MDI)* with contents. (Adapted from Newhouse MT, Dolovich M: Aerosol therapy in children, in *Basic Mechanisms of Pediatric Respiratory Disease: Cellular and Integrative.* Toronto, BC Decker, 1991.)

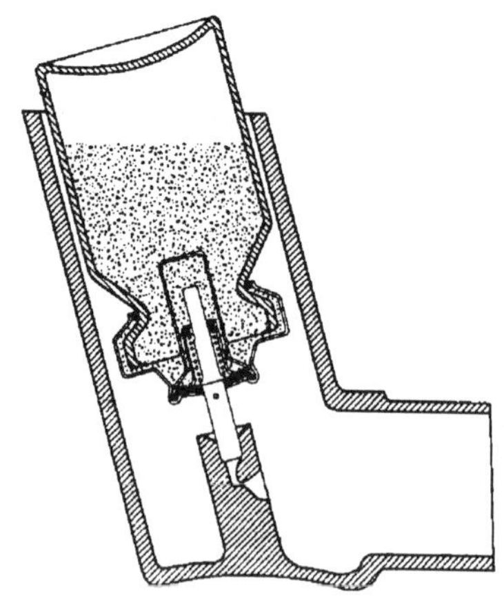

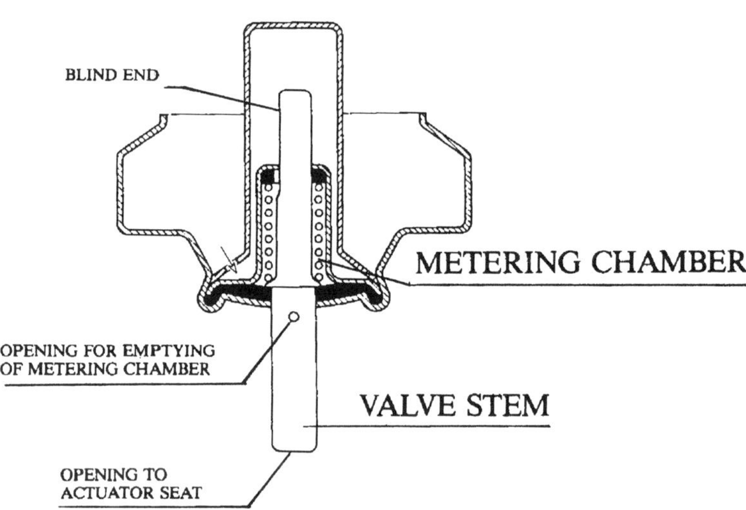

FIG 3–24
Metered dose inhaler with a valve assembly developed by Riker/3M. (Courtesy of 3M Pharmaceuticals.)

for a long period should keep their MDIs in an inside pocket so that body heat will maintain the temperature within a normal operating range.

Other variables that can be adjusted to change the particle size include the size of the valve stem and the actuator orifice (Fig 3–24), the drug concentration, and the addition of cosolvents. The smaller the valve stem size and the actuator orifice size, the finer the spray. Higher drug concentrations produce coarser aerosols. Ethanol has also been used as a cosolvent for drug delivery.[8] Its use results in a coarser spray, which may facilitate delivery of some drugs. The CFCs evaporate more slowly in the presence of alcohol. The alcohol concentration must be taken into account when selecting an MDI for drug delivery. Concentrations of alcohol can be over 35% in some products and can be a respiratory irritant.

The MMAD of most MDIs is between 3 and 6 μm[57] with a deposition in the lung of about 10%.[58, 59] As much as 80% of the dose is deposited in the mouth and may be a factor in systemic absorption as opposed to direct aerosol delivery to the lung since the MDI delivers a significant amount of drug to the mucous membranes of the mouth and stomach. Unfortunately, the actual amount of drug delivered to an individual patient is unpredictable because of significant interpatient variability.[56]

A number of studies have documented the clinical efficacy of MDIs.[60–63] MDIs have been demonstrated to be at least as effective as other nebulizers used for drug delivery. As a result they are often the preferred method for delivering bronchodilators to spontaneously breathing as well as intubated, ventilated patients.[64, 65] Many MDIs incorporate spacers and chambers to hold aerosolized medications for patients who have difficulty in coordinating inspiration with operation of a standard MDI unit.

Dry powder inhaler. The DPI is another form of MDI. Inhalation of drug in a crystalline or powder form has become increasingly popular because this delivery system is relatively inexpensive, does not depend on the use of CFCs, and does not require the hand-breath coordination required of MDIs. Aerosols of dry powder are created by drawing air through an aliquot of the powder. The high inspiratory flow rates required for optimal performance result in pharyngeal impaction of drug in a manner similar to MDIs. The clinical efficacy of drugs delivered by DPI appears to be similar to the results with MDIs, particularly when the MDI is used without an accessory chamber.[56]

A variety of factors have an influence on drug delivery by DPI.[66] DPIs are breath actuated. Relatively high inspiratory flow rates are required to release the powder as respirable particles.[67–69] The required high inspiratory flow rates make DPIs ineffective in small children or any patients who are so compromised that they cannot achieve flow rates of 0.5 to 1 L/sec or greater. DPIs are usually restricted to use for prophylactic and maintenance therapy. They are not acceptable for use during an acute bronchospastic episode and are generally not recommended for infants or children less than 6 years of age.[69] For maintenance therapy, however, DPI is preferred by many patients, both adults and older children.[56]

Although hand-breath coordination is not as important an issue with DPI vs. MDI, coordination in use of the device can have an influence on drug delivery. Exhalation into the device can result in loss of drug delivered to the lung. Some devices also require assembly, which can be cumbersome or difficult for some patients.

High humidity can also affect drug availability from DPIs.[56] The hygroscopic powder will clump if exposed to high humidity, and larger particles will be created that are not as effectively inhaled. Drugs delivered by DPI are carried in lactose or glucose. The drug particle size is from 1 to 2 μm, and the carrier has a particle size of approximately 20 to 25 μm. Most of the carrier impacts in the oropharynx, where it can cause irritation. DPIs may not reliably be used for patients with artificial airways, either endotracheal or tracheotomy tubes.

Several DPIs use individual doses administered as gelatin capsules that are punctured before inhalation (Spinhaler, Rotohaler) or use individual blister packets of drug (Diskhaler). The Turbohaler is a multidose preloaded powder system with 200 doses of drug, terbutaline sulfate or budesonide.

Ultrasonic nebulizer. An ultrasonic nebulizer uses a piezoelectric crystal vibrated at a high frequency, greater than 1 MHz, to create an aerosol. The crystal transducer, composed of substances such as quartz-barium titanate, converts electricity into sound. The beam of sound is focused in the liquid above the transducer to create waves in the liquid immediately above the transducer. If the frequency is high enough and the amplitude of the signal strong enough, the oscillation waves crest, disrupt the surface of the liquid, and create a "geyser" of droplets.

Large-volume ultrasonic nebulizers usually have the transducer built into an apparatus that includes multiple electronic components as shown in Figs 3–25 and 3–26. The devices utilize relatively inexpensive medication cups for individual patient use, thus eliminating the need to sterilize the entire apparatus between patients. They use water as a couplant between the transducer and the medication being nebulized. The medication cup, with a flexible diaphragm on the bottom, is seated into a couplant chamber filled with enough water to allow a firm water seal between the transducer and cup. This water conducts the sound energy to the diaphragm or cup bottom, which in turn vibrates the medication to produce an aerosol. The water used as couplant must be changed regularly and the unit cleaned to minimize contamination from direct physical contact with the nebulizer and medication cups between treatments.

Ultrasonic nebulizers tend to have a higher output

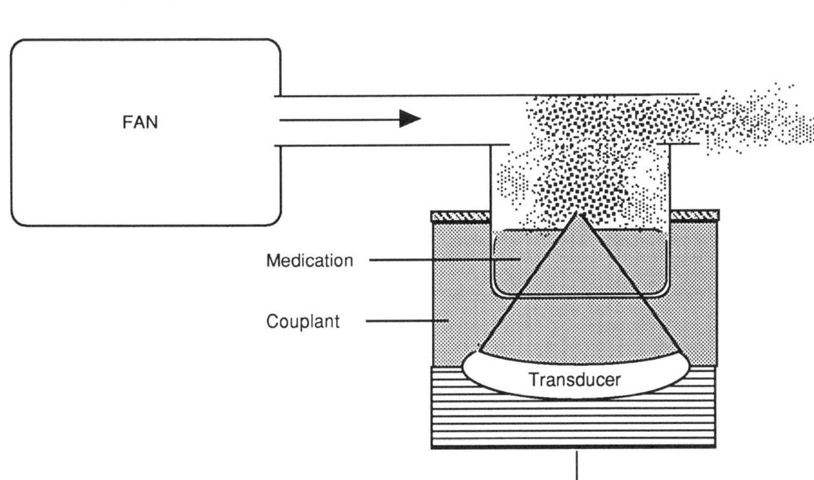

FIG 3–25
Ultrasonic nebulizers with medication cups that are exchanged between patients use a liquid couplant between the transducer and the medication. The fan is used to drive aerosol to the patient.

rate (0.5 to 7 mL/min) and higher mist density than conventional jet nebulizers. The particle or droplet size (MMAD) delivered by an ultrasonic nebulizer is related to the frequency at which the crystals vibrate. The frequency is usually specific to the device selected and is rarely adjustable by the user. The particle size is inversely proportional to frequency. For example, the DeVilbiss Portasonic operates at a frequency of 2.25 MHz and produces an MMAD of 2.5 μm, whereas the DeVilbiss Pulmosonic operates at 1.25 MHz and produces a much less respirable particle range of 4 to 6 μm MMAD. The amplitude of the signal affects the output from the nebulizer. The greater the amplitude, the greater the output from the nebulizer, up to the limit of the device design. Increases beyond that specific upper limit will not improve the device output.

Particle size and aerosol density are also affected by the source and flow of gas that conducts the aerosols from the nebulizer to the patient. If the nebulizer is producing a steady output of particles, the greater the flow of gas through the chamber, the more dilute the same number of particles will be in the larger volume of gas. The faster the flow of gas, the greater chance that large particles will be driven out of the nebulizer before they can coalesce with other particles and settle out. Low flow rates are associated with smaller particles and a higher density of mist. High flow rates yield larger particles and less density. Unlike jet nebulizers, the temperature of the solution placed in the ultrasonic nebulizer increases during use. As the temperature increases, the drug concentration will also rise, thereby increasing the likelihood of undesired side effects.

The larger commercial units like the Medisonic Compact NF-31 (shown in Fig 3–27) use low-flow blowers that can deliver either air or other compressed gases via a flowmeter. A blender can be added to the delivery system to more precisely control the delivered gas concentration. Aerosol tubing, a mask, or a mouthpiece can be used to administered the ultrasonically nebulized solution.

Smaller ultrasonic nebulizers such as the Medismil have been designed primarily for individual use (an example is shown in Fig 3–28). They do not use water-filled couplants. Medication is placed directly into the manifold in direct contact with the transducer. The transducers are connected by cable or connector to a power source, often battery powered to increase portability. The small nebulizers that incorporate the transducer manifold at the patient airway rely upon the patient's inspiratory flow rate to evacuate the aerosol from the nebulizer to the lung.

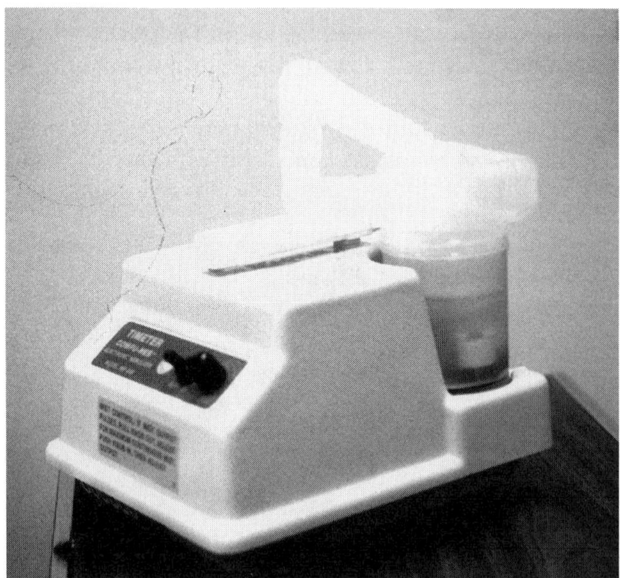

FIG 3–26
The Timeter Compu-Neb ultrasonic nebulizer uses liquid couplant and an internal fan/blower.

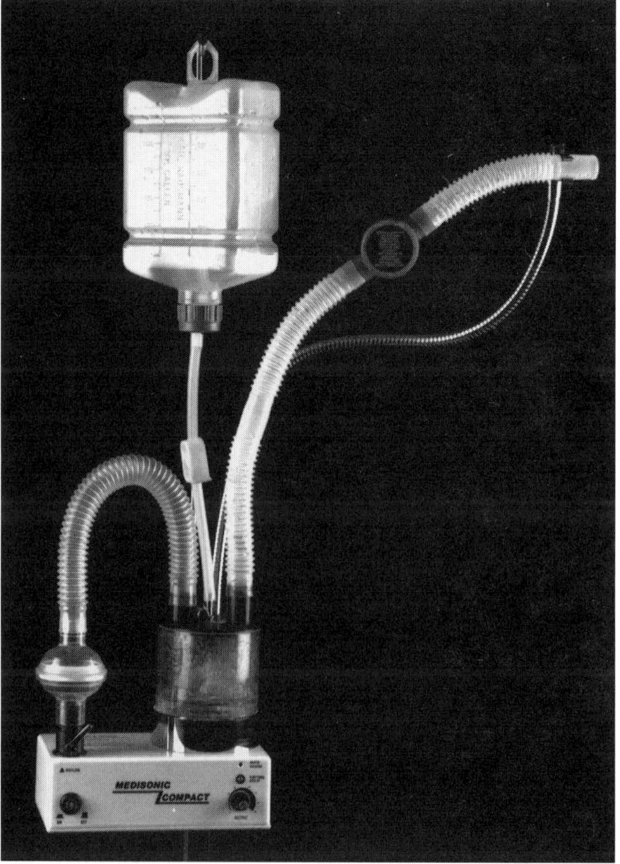

FIG 3–27
Medisonic Compact NF-31 Humidifier/Inhaler shown with bacteria filter and heater. (Courtesy of Medisonic USA, Inc.)

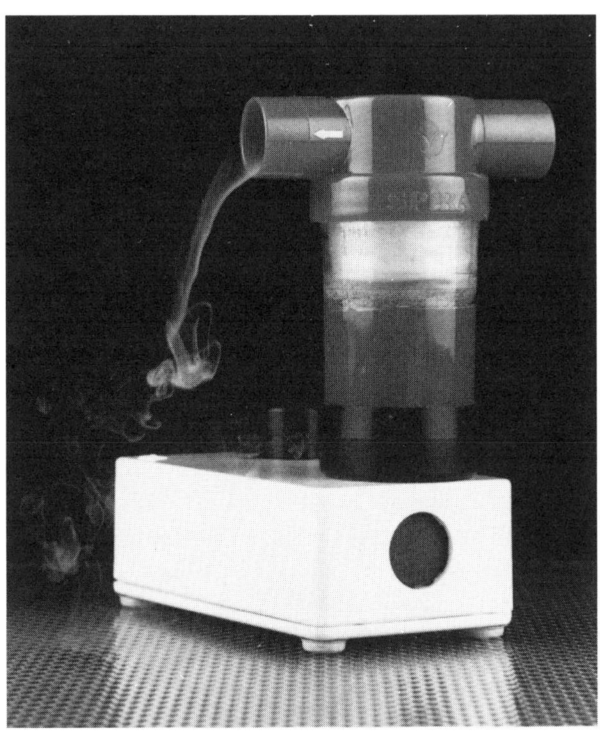

FIG 3–28
The Medisonic Microsonic ultrasonic nebulizer is a portable and lightweight and will operate on 12 V dc or with a 110-V adaptor. (Courtesy of Medisonic USA, Inc.)

EQUIPMENT SELECTION

Matching the needs of the patient to the appropriate tool in order to effectively meet clinical goals is key to providing appropriate therapy.

Humidifiers

The majority of patients who receive supplemental oxygen therapy should have the inspired gases humidified. Some of the key factors associated with different types of humidification devices are itemized in Table 3–3. Some practitioners have not used humidifiers for patients requiring supplemental oxygen at low flow rates or for short periods of time. Recently, the American College of Chest Physicians (ACCP) has suggested that simple bubble humidifiers are not necessary when delivering fresh gas flows of 4 L/min or less.[70] Their recommendation is based on the absence of data demonstrating the clinical value of added humidification when low flows of gas are administered. On the basis of their recommendations, humidifiers are often not added to low-flow oxygen delivery systems in such settings as recovery rooms, where the oxygen administration time is usually short. Eliminating the use of humidifiers for low-flow oxygen reduces costs for routine administration. The cost savings, however, are not so great that they should not be provided for patients who experience nasal dryness or irritation associated with unhumidified inspired gases. However, all patients receiving low-flow gas should be monitored for complaints of dryness or irritation, and when either exists, a humidifier should be added to the inspired delivery system.[71]

Humidifiers are added to the oxygen delivery system for most nonintubated and all intubated patients. Commercially available humidifiers are either unheated or add heat to increase the humidity output. Unheated BTHs are capable of humidifying dry medical gas to an AH between 10 and 13 mg/L when used at flow rates between 2 and 10 L/min.[71] Unheated bubble humidifiers are less efficient at flow rates above 5 L/min and are of limited effectiveness at flow rates above 10 L/min. When flows greater than 10 L/min are required, another type of humidifying device should be selected. Table 3–4 describes the AH achieved when oxygen is bubbled through four commercially available disposable BTHs. Note that the AH increases as the flow rate is reduced.

TABLE 3–3
Key Factors in Humidification Strategies

Factor	Unheated Humidifier	Heated Humidifier	Passover Humidifier	Gas-Driven Nebulizer	Mechanical Nebulizer	HME*
Output	15–20	35–50	35–50	20–40	40–1,000	20–35
Temperature	15–20	34–40	34–40	15–20	15–25	22–28
Maintain body temperature	–	+ + +	+ + +	–	– – –	+
Electric hazards(potential)	–	+	+	–	+	–
Infection	+	+	+	+ + +	+ + +	–
Overheating	–	+	+	+ +	+	–
Hypothermia	+	– –	– –	+	+	–
Overhydrate	–	+	+	+ +	+ + +	–
Underhydrate	+	–	–	+ +	+	+ +
Increase inspiratory resistance	+	+	–	–	–	+ +

* HME = heat and moisture exchanger.

TABLE 3–4

Absolute Humidity Provided by Four Commercially Available Bubble-Type Humidifiers*†

Liters per Minute	Aerwey 300	Aquapak 301	McGaw 250	Travenol 500
2	17.2	17.6	20.4	20.4
4	16	17.7	18.4	19.5
6	15.6	16.9	16.9	16.2
8	14.6	14.9	14.9	15.7

* Data from Darin J, Broadwell J, MacDonnell R. *Respir Care* 1981; 27:41.
† Absolute humidity is in milligrams per liter for four unheated bubble humidifiers at increasing liter flow rates.

Unheated Humidifiers

Unheated humidifiers should meet the recommendations contained in ANSI Z-79.9, section 3.1.1.1.[21] The recommendation is that a fluid output of 10 mg/L should be provided by the humidifier. The minimum level of 10 mg/L is felt to be the lowest acceptable humidity level necessary to minimize mucosal damage to the upper airway under a variety of use environments. In addition, 10 mg/L of water will provide approximately 50% RH at 72°F ambient conditions and enhance the dissipation of static electricity in order to prevent fires in areas that may contain flammable gases or materials.

Heated Humidifiers

Most often when supplemental oxygen is provided to either intubated or nonintubated patients, supplemental humidity should be provided with a heated humidifier. A variety of devices are commercially available to provide heated humidity. Selection of a heated humidifier should be based on a variety of criteria based on ANSI standards,[21] American Association of Respiratory Care (AARC) Clinical Practice Guidelines[73] (see Appendixes 3–1 and 3–2) and reports from the ECRI:

1. The gas temperature at the patient should not be able to be set above 40°C. When temperatures of 40°C or above are reached, audible and visual alarms should indicate an overtemperature condition and interrupt power to the heater.

2. Audible and visual alarms should indicate when remote temperature sensors are disconnected, absent, or defective. In these situations, power to the heater should be interrupted to protect from overheating.

3. Temperature overshoot can occur with any humidifier and produce gas hotter than 40°C. Short-term overshoot is common with improper operation. Servo-controlled units can overshoot when the unit is allowed to warm up without flow through the circuit, when the patient airway temperature probe is not inserted in the circuit (or becomes dislodged during operation), or when flow is increased, decreased, or interrupted during normal operation. Non–servo-controlled units can overheat gas when the temperature controls are set too high or gas flow is abruptly reduced.

4. Controls and indicators for delivered gas temperature should be accurate to within 3°C of the indicated value.

5. During normal operation humidifier temperature output should not vary more than 2°C from the set value (at the patient).

6. Warm-up time should not take more than 10 to 15 minutes.

7. The water level should be readily visible in either the humidifier or remote reservoir.

8. Humidifiers should be able to withstand ventilation pressures of 100 cm H_2O or greater.

9. Internal compliance should be relatively stable so that changes in water level do not make significant changes in the delivered tidal volume. ECRI recommends that the compliance be less than that of the intended patient (<1 mL/cm H_2O for neonates) and vary less than 0.3 mL/cm H_2O from high to low water levels.

10. During operation the humidifier should not be too hot to touch. Readily accessible surfaces should not be hotter than 37.5°C. A warning label should warn if the metal surface of the heat source can reach 50°C and is accessible when changing the humidification chamber or during disassembly.

11. Humidifiers should not be damaged by spilled fluids. The operator or feed system must not be able to overfill the humidifier to the point that water can block gas flow through the humidifier or ventilator circuit.

12. Electromagnetic interference (EMI) from other devices should not affect humidifier performance. The unit should not be damaged between 95 and 135 V rms.

13. The unit should have adequate overcurrent protection to prevent ventilator shutdown or loss of power to other equipment on the same branch circuit because of internal equipment failures. Fuses or circuit breakers should be clearly labeled and easy to reset or replace.

14. Misassembling the unit in a way that would be hazardous to the patient should not be possible. The direction of gas flow should be indicated on components for which proper direction is essential.

15. The humidifier should be assembled and filled in a manner that minimizes the introduction of infection or other materials.

16. Operating and service manuals should be provided with the humidifier and should cover all aspects of use and service.

Table 3–5 provides a brief summary of a few critical factors such as the ability to maintain a fixed volume if used with neonates.

The following descriptions are based in large part on manufacturer specifications and product reports.[43, 44]

Bubble-type humidifiers.

Bourns humidifier. The Bourns humidifier is a heated BTH system. It is available in two sizes, adult and infant. The design of the humidifiers is identical, except that the infant humidifier has less air space above the water level, thereby minimizing compressible volume, and it operates as a passover humidifier. The water temperature is controlled at the humidifier; the system is not servo-controlled but has alarms to warn of low water, overheating, and inoperability.

Puritan Bennett Cascade humidifier. The Puritan Bennett Cascade humidifier is a BTH usually used as part of the ventilator circuit for intubated, mechanically ventilated patients. As seen in Fig 3–29, unhumidified gas enters the unit and is directed down a tower where it displaces water away from the distal portion of the tower and a grid that is attached to the tower. Gas then flows upward through the grid, which is covered by a thin film of water that constantly cascades through the orifice in the wall of the grid and spreads across the surface of the grid. This film of water, when exposed to the gas flow passing upward through the grid, creates a froth of bubbles that rapidly diffuses water vapor to the inspired gas. The cascade employs a thermostatically controlled electric heater. It can deliver 100% RH at body temperature. The control is set on the heater and drives a heating element that fits into a metal sleeve at the top of the humidifier; a thermoswitch controls current to the heater. A safety shutoff switch is included in the system and must fit properly between the cascade and the heater for the system to operate.

The cascade delivery system imposes a high–flow-resistive work load on the circuit. The gas must pass through the tower and heated water. The work of breathing imposed by the cascade-type design is greater than the work of breathing through passover humidifiers or HME humidifiers.[40] This resistance is significantly reduced with removal of the tower as shown in Fig 3–30, which converts the cascade to a passover humidifier.

In addition to the added work of breathing, there is also a large compressible volume in the cascade humidifier. These factors are of particular concern when a cascade humidifier is used as part of the breathing circuit for a pediatric patient or a critically ill adult who may not be able to overcome the increased work of breathing during weaning. The reservoir of the cascade humidifier requires intermittent manual filling, usually necessitating temporary discontinuation of operation to unscrew the canister, add water, and replace the canister into the system.

TABLE 3–5
Summary of Heated Humidifiers

Brand	Method Type of Heater	Chamber Volume	Auto-Feed	Servocontrolled
Bourns	BTH* Passover Plate	Medium, variable	No	No
Cascade II	BTH Immersion	Large, variable	No	Yes
Bird	Wick Wrap	Small, fixed	Yes	No
Fisher Paykel	Wick/passover Plate	Medium, variable	Limited	Yes
RCI Concha	Wick Wrap	Medium, fixed (pediatric)	Yes	Yes
Inspiron	Passover/filter Plate	Small, fixed	Yes	No
Marquest	Passover Plate	Medium, fixed	Yes	Yes
LDS	Wick Plate	Medium, variable	Yes	Yes
Mona Loa	Wick Immersion	Small, fixed	Yes	Yes
HPD Medical	Wick/passover Plate	Medium, variable	Limited	Yes

* BTH = bubble-type humidifier.

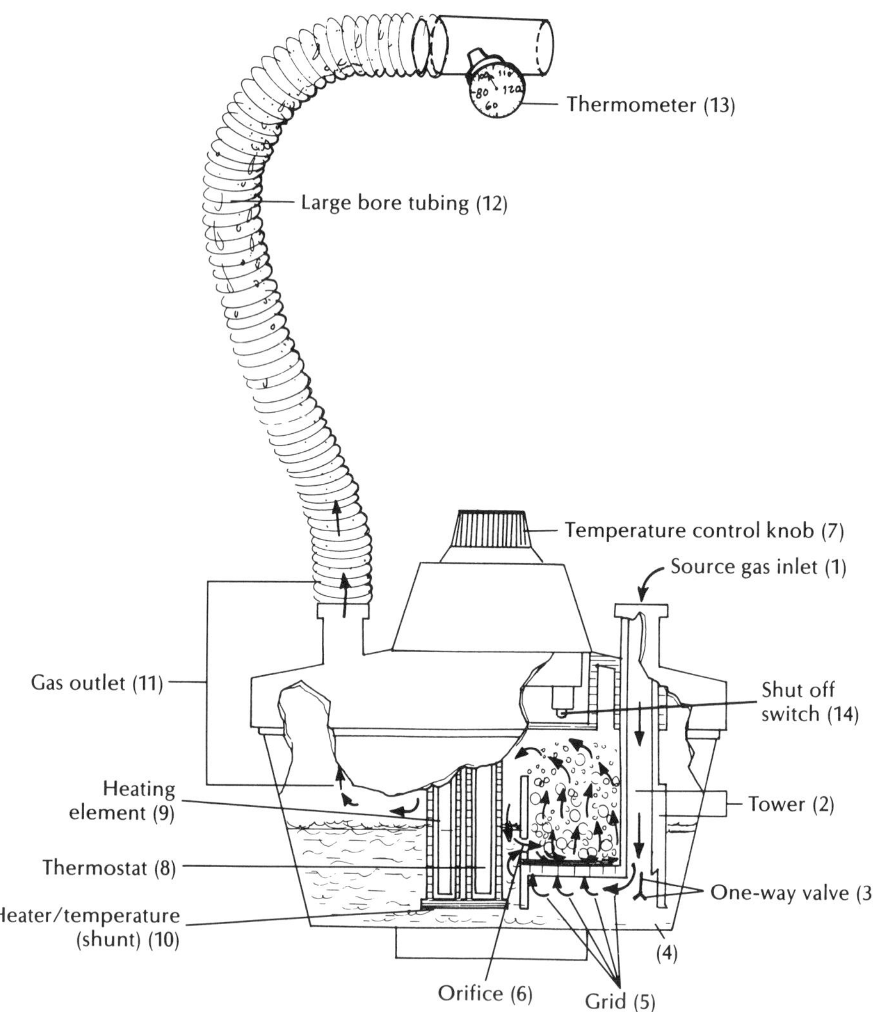

FIG 3–29
Schematic of the Bennet Cascade humidifier with components and function. (From Eubanks DH, Bone RC: Module II, Humidity Therapy, in *Comprehensive Respiratory Care,* ed 2. St Louis, Mosby, 1990. Used by permission.)

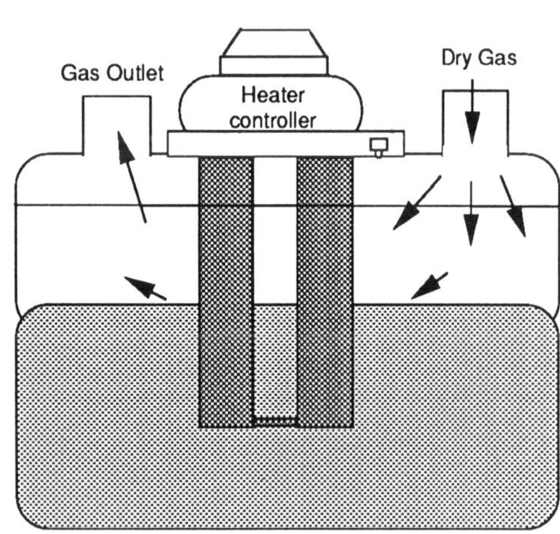

FIG 3–30
Removing the tower from the Cascade humidifier converts it to a passover humidifier with a significant reduction in airway resistance and aerosol production.

Puritan Bennett Cascade II humidifier. The Puritan Bennett Cascade II humidifier is a servo-controlled heated humidifier, similar to the Puritan Bennett Cascade humidifier. It has the added feature of a proportioning heater system incorporating a temperature sensing probe at or near the patient airway and a display at the control panel. An alarm system warns of probe disconnection, high gas temperature, low water level, and most controller malfunctions. Other features of this humidifier include the following:

- Water feed mechanism: None
- Humidification method: Bubble-through, reusable
- Chamber volume: 900 mL
- Temperature: Servo-controlled; range, 20 to 43°C
- Overtemperature alarm: User controlled; range, 0 to 43°C
- Alarms: Alarm test button, 42°C alarm, and water temperature alarm of over 88°C; does not have an alarm mute

Passover Humidifiers

Marquest SCT 2000 and Marquest SCT 3000 humidifiers. The Marquest SCT 2000 (not shown) is a microprocessor-controlled passover-type humidifier. It is a servo-controlled unit that adjusts for both airway temperature and relative humidity when included in a system with a heated wire circuit. The temperature control determines the temperature of the gas as it exits the patient circuit. The thermistor probes monitor gas at the outlet of the humidifying chamber and at the patient airway.

At start-up the temperature setting defaults to 37°C (with a range of 30 to 39°C), and the RH setting defaults to 6 (on a scale of 1 to 10). There is a diagnostic mode for indicating hardware and software failures. These humidifiers can be used with single or dual heated wire circuits.

The Marquest SCT 3000 humidifier is identical to the SCT 2000 except that it can be used without a heated wire circuit, has a maximum temperature of 37°C when used without the heated wire circuit, and does not incorporate an RH control.

The Marquest humidification chamber has a unique design (see Fig 3–16) that allows continuous feed from a large reservoir surrounding the chamber. Filling the reservoir is accomplished without interruption of ventilation by clamping of the feed tube from the reservoir before opening the fill port.

BEAR VH-820 humidifier. The BEAR VH-820 humidifier (not shown) is a microprocessor-controlled passover humidifier that channels gas through a labyrinth of vanes above the surface of water. Heated wire circuits are available in 4- and 6-ft inspiratory limb lengths but need not be included in the circuit. An adapter allows the use of other manufacturers' heated wire circuits. The unit has a continuous water feed mechanism with a solenoid-actuated tube clamp controlling the water flow to the humidification chamber by a feedback mechanism from a thermister located within the heater. An alarm recall button allows the operator to display error codes. The humidifier has a standby mode that interrupts power to the heater and shuts down the tube clamp for 2 minutes to prevent temperature overshoot when the patient is disconnected for clinical interventions.

- Water feed mechanism: Utilizes a tube clamp
- Humidification method: Passover, reusable
- Chamber volume: 5 to 10 mL
- Temperature: Dual servo-controlled with a range of 26 to 38°C
- Overtemperature alarm: 2.5°C above the set temperature
- Alarms: Water depletion, low temperature, overfill, heated wire disconnect, and circuit board malfunction; has a 1-minute alarm mute.

Fisher Paykel MR 600 humidifier. The Fisher Paykel MR 600 humidifier (not shown) is a microprocessor servo-controlled unit with reusable or disposable heated wire circuits available. Disposable and reusable humidification chambers are available in wick and passover style in sizes appropriate for adults and children. A heated wire is required in the inspiratory limb, and an optional heated wire can be used in the expiratory limb.

- Water feed mechanism: Manual for most chambers; limited autofeed available
- Humidification method: Passover and wick, reusable or disposable
- Chamber volume: Adult, 280 mL; pediatric, 230 mL
- Temperature: Dual servo-controlled; range, 30 to 39°C
- Overtemperature alarm: 2°C over the set temperature
- Alarms: low temperature, probe disconnect, and heated wire disconnect; 3-minute alarm mute.

Fisher Paykel MR 730 humidifier. The Fisher Paykel MR 700 microprocessor servo-controlled humidifier (Fig 3–31) is similar in design and function to the MR 600 humidifier. It is available with reusable or disposable heated wire circuits. The same disposable and reusable humidification chambers are available in wick and passover style in sizes appropriate for adult and children. A heated wire is optional in the inspiratory and expiratory limbs of this humidifier. Heated wire circuits from a variety of manufacturers can also be used.

- Water feed mechanism: Manual for most chambers, limited auto-feed available for select chambers
- Humidification method: Passover and wick, reusable or disposable
- Chamber volume: Adult, 280 mL; pediatric, 230 mL
- Temperature: Dual servo-controlled; range, 30 to 39°C
- Overtemperature alarm: 2°C above the set temperature
- Alarms: low temperature, probe disconnect, and heated wire disconnect; 3-minute alarm mute.

HPD Medical Incorporated Heater Base Model MI-500. The HPD model MI-500 is a microprocessor servo-controlled humidifier that can be used with or without permanent or disposable heated wires from any manufacturer. One in a line of three units (shown in Fig 3–32), the HPD heater bases fit Fisher Paykel humidifier chambers.

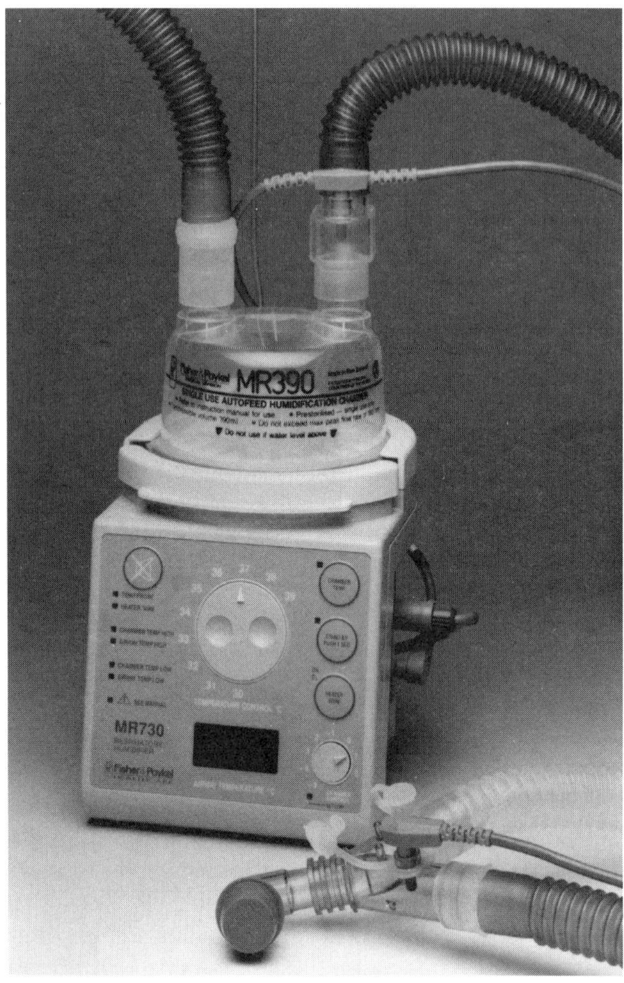

FIG 3–31
Fisher Paykel MR730 heated humidifier. (Courtesy of Fisher Paykel.)

- Humidification method: Passover/wick, reusable or disposable chambers with manual gravity feed
- Alarms: low water, low temperature, high temperature, and probe disconnect

Inspiron Vapor-Phase humidifier. The Inspiron Vapor-Phase humidifier is a non–servo-controlled humidifier that uses a disposable humidification chamber with a hydrophobic filter that acts as a barrier to microbial penetration and allows only molecular water to pass into gas en route to the breathing circuit. Continuous water feed to the heater plate is limited by the hydrophobic barrier, so a simple gravity feed suffices. This device offers the opportunity to use distilled or tap water as a cost-effective alternative to sterile packaged water.

- Water feed mechanism: Remote continuous gravity feed, hydrophobic barrier
- Humidification method: Passover, disposable

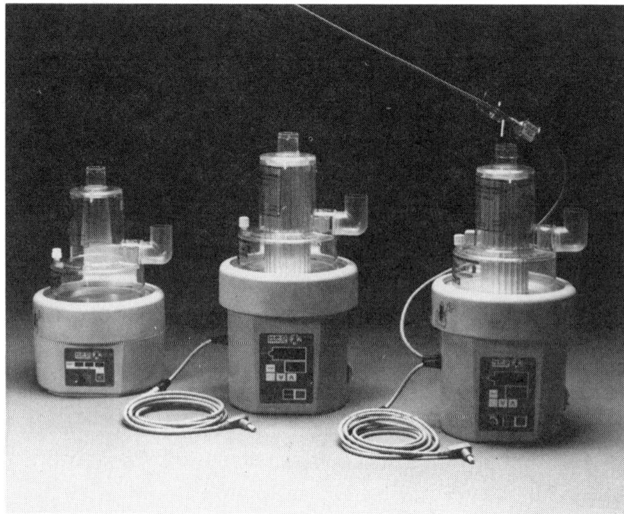

FIG 3–32
HPD series of heater bases. From *left to right:* model MI-100 with a model 3010 humidifying chamber and MI 200 and MI 500 heater bases with model 3000 humidifying chambers. (Courtesy of HPD.)

- Chamber volume: 10 mL
- Temperature: Non–servo-controlled, 30 to 39°C
- Alarms: Overtemperature (40°C), low temperature, and probe failure; 2-minute alarm mute.

Bird Humidifier Model 3000 humidifier. The Bird Humidifier Model 3000 humidifier (not shown) is a non–servo-controlled unit that uses an absorbent "blotting" paper (wick) to absorb water from the base of the unit. It is surrounded by the heater. Gas enters the chamber in which evaporation occurs. A constant water level is maintained by a reservoir feed system with a float within the humidifier chamber. Float failure can result in chamber overfilling. The temperature is adjusted by a calibrated control mechanism that carries with it a reference number. An external probe monitors the temperature distal to the humidifier, which is displayed at the controller. It will detect a gas temperature over 40°C, trigger an alarm, and turn the heater off. It does not otherwise adjust the power to regulate temperature. This device has low resistance to airflow. The humidifier chamber is nondisposable but requires replacement of the disposable wick.

- Water feed mechanism: Remote continuous feed, float mechanism
- Humidification method: Passover wick, reusable with a disposable wick
- Chamber water volume: 20 mL
- Temperature: Non–servo-controlled
- Alarms: overtemperature (40°C), probe disconnect, and humidification module disconnect; no alarm mute

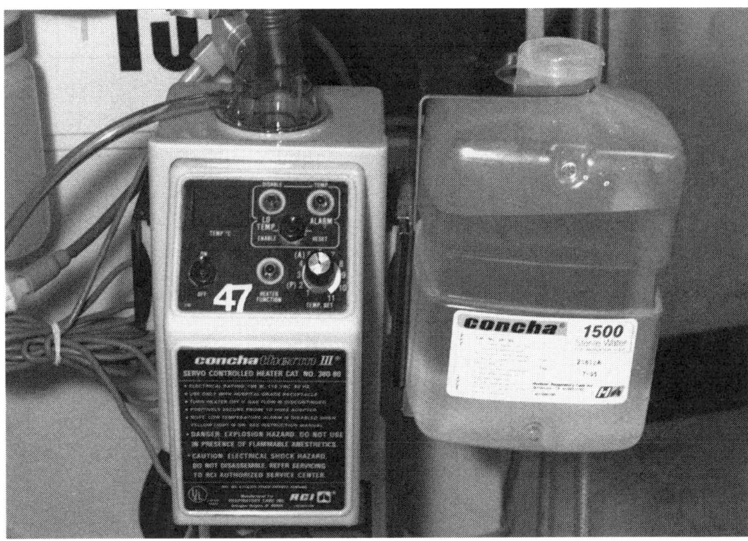

FIG 3–33
Hudson RCI ConchaTherm III with a 1,500-mL water reservoir.

Conchatherm III (Hudson/RCI) humidifier. The Conchatherm III (Hudson/RCI) humidifier (Fig 3–33) is a servo-controlled heated humidifier that utilizes a paper wick in a disposable humidifier canister inserted into a controller. The canister is surrounded by the heating element and thus shielded by the body of the unit. An external gravity-fed reservoir provides a good view of the water level and cannot be overfilled. Fig 3–34 illustrates how the pediatric chamber with an automated, "chicken feeder" filling system maintains a constant water level and gas volume in the column. A low-temperature alarm is disabled for the first 20 minutes after turning on the heater. If a temperature of 28°C has not been reached after the alarm is activated, the low-temperature alarm sounds.

- Water feed mechanism: Remote continuous feed, gravity
- Humidification method: Passover wick, disposable
- Chamber volume: Adult, 182 mL; pediatric, 75 mL
- Temperature: Servo-controlled
- Alarms: Overtemperature (40°C), low temperature, and probe disconnect; no alarm mute

ALP Opti-Mol molecular humidification system. The Opti-Mol system (not shown) is a chamber option for use with the Hudson/RCI Conchatherm III humidifier heater. A wick humidifier chamber, it uses a built-in automatic float system to maintain a constant water level in the column and is used with a gravity feed system.

Mauna Loa Lavapak-3. The Lavapak-3 (Fig 3–35) is a servo-controlled humidifier developed for use with infants and pediatric patients. It is designed for ready use in transports. The disposable humidification chamber has a small fixed volume with an internal float that

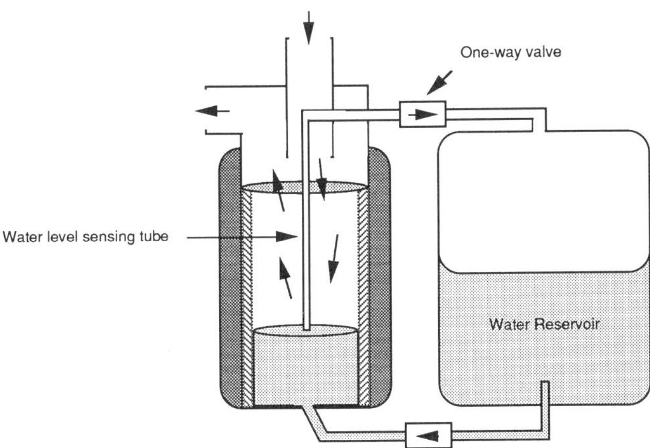

FIG 3–34
Schematic of the Pediatric Low Compliance Concha Column.

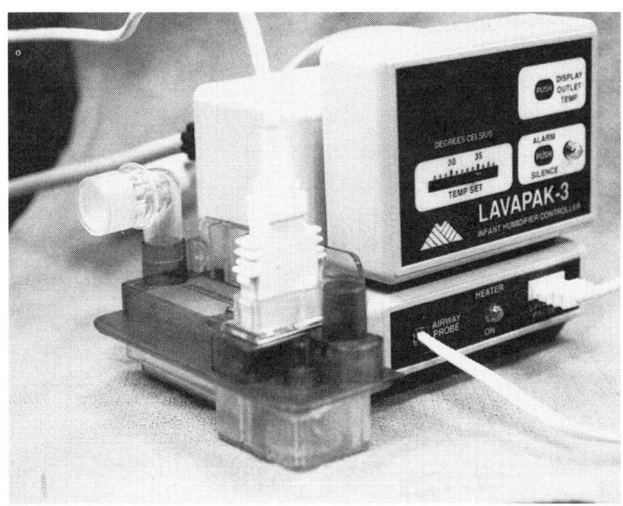

FIG 3–35
Mauna Loa Lavapak-3 infant humidifier.

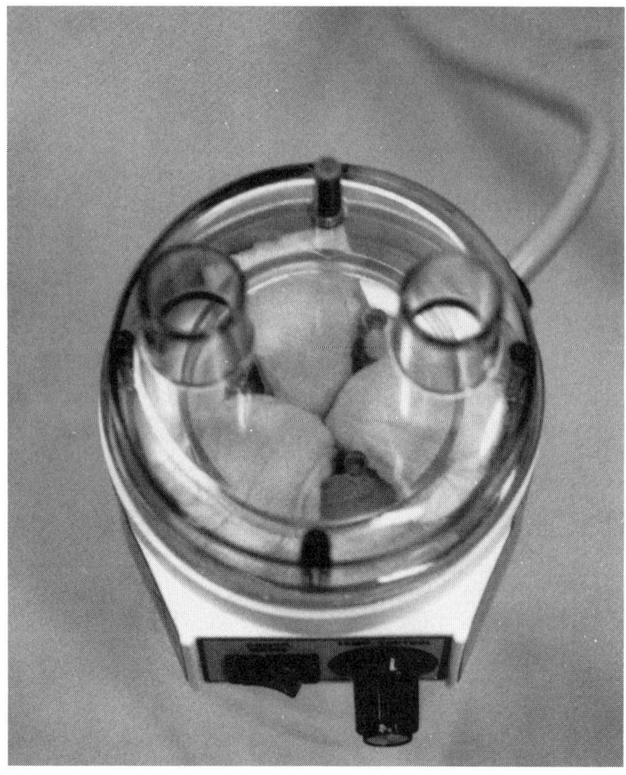

FIG 3–36
Thera-Mist P3500 humidifier.

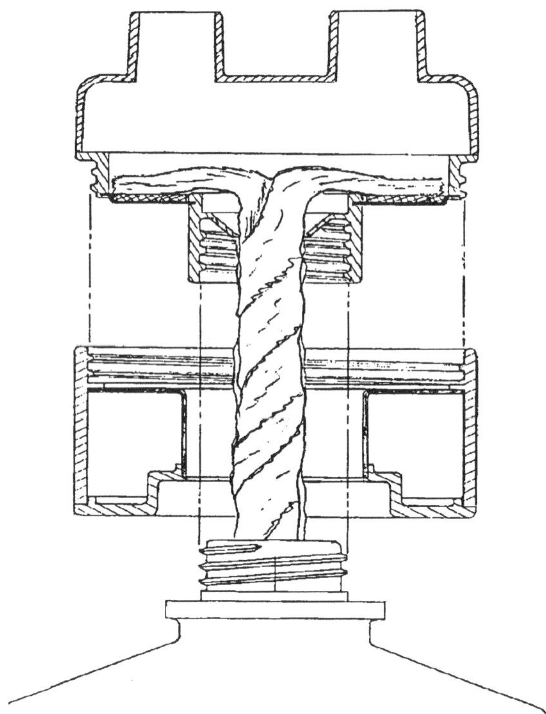

FIG 3–37
Cross-sectional assembly diagram of the reusable Thera-Mist humidifier. (Adapted from Pegasus Research Corp. sales literature.)

keeps water levels constant. The core of the Lavapak is a honeycomb of heated wires wrapped around several layers of plastic wafer that are also wrapped with layers of absorbent paper. This combination of heater element and wick is partially immersed in water. Dry gas enters the humidifier and passes through the layers of heated wires and wet paper.

Pegasus Thera-Mist humidifier. The Thera-Mist humidifier (Fig 3–36) is a non–servo-controlled wick humidifier designed to provide temperatures of 35°C or less at flows up to 20 L/min with 6-ft standard aerosol tubing. The humidifier chamber (disposable or reusable) sits on a heater base that attaches to a Baxter 1-L water bottle. The cotton wick draws water from the bottle up to the chamber, where it sits on a Goretex wick disk placed above the heater plate. The humidifier chamber is aseptically isolated from the heater. The humidifier chamber (Figs 3–37 and 3–38) comes in reusable form with disposable wick tops (that fold up and in the wick disk). This system also interfaces with nebulizer options.

Jet Nebulizers

Jet nebulizers, when used as humidifiers, are identical to the large-volume nebulizers described below. No data support the use of a jet nebulizer as opposed to any other type of heated humidifier.

Heat and Moisture Exchangers

HMEs provide an inexpensive alternative to humidifiers when used for the short-term ventilation of adult patients who do not have complex humidification needs such as might be required for a brief period of time in a recovery room, in the emergency department, during transport, or to complete a radiologic procedure. The HME does not provide sufficient heat or humidification

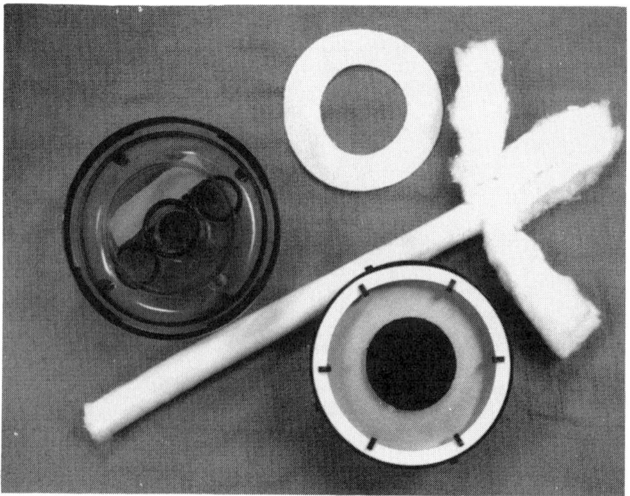

FIG 3–38
Components of the Thera-Mist humidifier assembly.

TABLE 3–6

Commercially Available Heat and Moisture Exchangers*

Brand	Dead Space (mL)	Output (mg/L)	Material
Pall conserve	98	23	Hydrophobic ceramic fiber
Siemens Servo 150	92	25	Cellulose sponge and felt
Engstrom Edith	89	26	Hygroscopic polypropylene fiber
Mallinckrodt Nose	61	21	Hygroscopic plastic foam
Airlife HumidAir	41	24	Hygroscopic synthetic felt
Terumo Breathaid	11.5	14	Alternating aluminum/cellulose fiber
Portex Humid Vent-1	10	23	Hygroscopic paper roll

* Data from ECRI: *Health Devices* 1983; 12:133; and Branson RD, Hurst JM: *Respir Care* 1987; 32:741–747.

for long-term management. When an HME is to be used, a device appropriate for the individual patient, based on size and tidal volume, should be selected. Table 3–6 itemizes dead space, measured output, and materials used in several available HMEs. HMEs come in a wide variety of shapes and sizes, as demonstrated in Fig 3–39. Pall (Fig 3–40) has recently introduced an HME with a port to attach to a sidestream capnograph. Several HME devices have been designed for the application of low-flow oxygen to patients with bypassed upper airways (Figs 3–41 and 3–42).

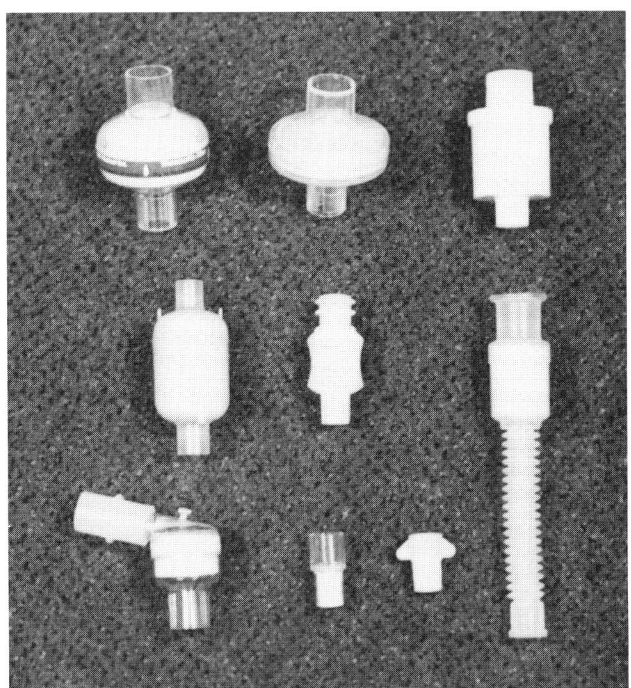

FIG 3–39
Heat and moisture exchangers come in a wide variety of shapes and sizes *(left to right, top to bottom):* ARC Medical Inc. ThermoFlo Filter, Intertech Filtered HMC, Siemens-Elema Servo Humidifier 152, Mallinkrodt, Vital signs HCH 5701, Hudson RCI AQUA+ Flex, Gibeck Respiration Humid-Vent 2, Hudson RCI AQUA+ N, and Vital Signs HCH 5704.

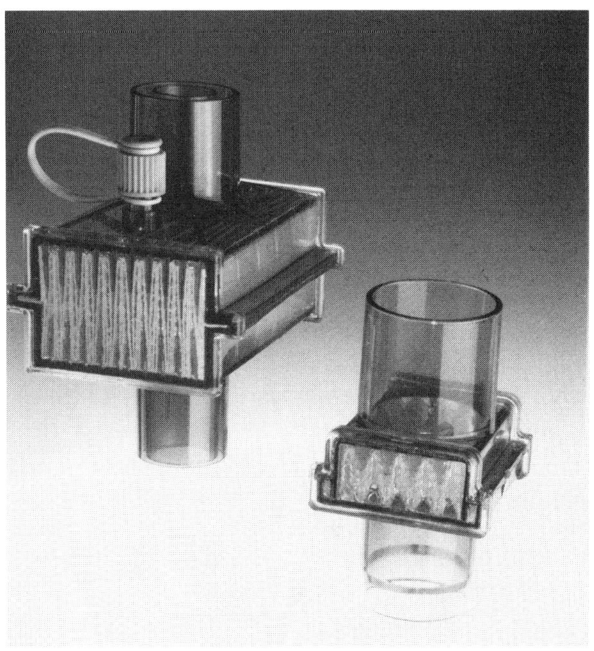

FIG 3–40
Pall's HME 15–22M with a CO_2 monitoring port *(left)* and PS-30S *(right)* (Courtesy of Pall Corp.)

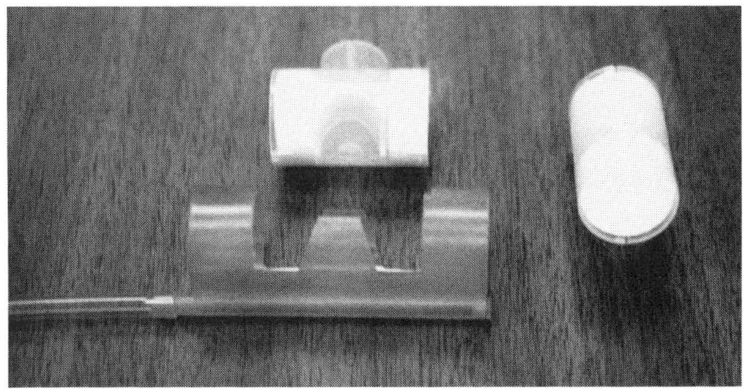

FIG 3–41
The Portex ThermoVent T is a heat and moisture exchanger for providing low-flow oxygen to the tracheostomized or intubated patient.

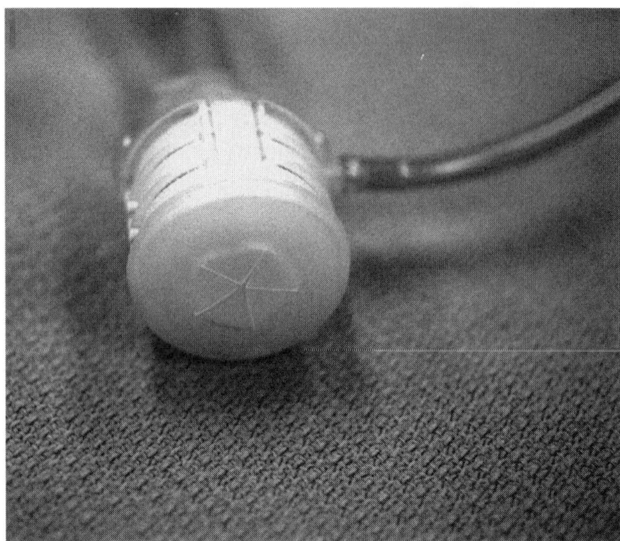

FIG 3–42
Hudson RCI AQUA T+ hygroscopic condensor humidifier is designed for the intubated or tracheostomized patient.

HMEs are contraindicated for a variety of clinical situations.[73] They should not be used as part of the ventilator circuit for patients with thick, copious, or bloody secretions or for patients with a large leak around an endotracheal tube, such as might occur with a large bronchopleurocutaneous fistula or leaking endotracheal tube cuff. In this situation, if the exhaled tidal volume is less than 70% of the delivered tidal volume, incomplete rebreathing will minimize the humidification that can be accomplished with the HME. HMEs are also contraindicated for patients whose body temperature is less than 32°C and patients with a minute ventilation greater than 10 L/min. Hazards associated with use of the HME include hypothermia, underhydration and impaction of pulmonary secretions, potential increase in the resistive work of breathing through the HME or as a result of mucus plugging the airways, hypoventilation resulting from increased added dead space, and an inaccurate low-pressure alarm upon ventilator disconnection because of the high resistance when ventilating through the HME. In addition, HMEs must be removed from the patient circuit during aerosol administration.

Aerosol Therapy

Bland Aerosol Therapy

Aerosol therapy is used to provide humidification, to obtain samples of pulmonary secretions for diagnosis, and to provide pharmacologic therapy, including bronchodilators, steroids, and antibiotics, directly to the airways. Aerosol therapy with bland solutions such as saline is used for therapeutic and diagnostic purposes. Large-volume ultrasonic nebulizers, Babbington nebulizers, and mist tents are commonly used for these purposes.

Large-volume nebulizers. Large-volume pneumatic nebulizers with reservoir volumes greater than 100 mL are commonly used to aerosolize solutions such as saline for prolonged periods of time. These devices have also been used to provide continuous administration of active medications such as bronchodilators.

Large-volume nebulizers with bland solutions are primarily indicated to provide humidification of medical gases for patients with bypassed upper airways, to treat upper airway inflammation with cold mist for local vasoconstriction, and to induce sputum production, most often for diagnostic purposes.

Although bland aerosol therapy with large-volume nebulizers has been advocated as a method to hydrate dehydrated patients, few data document the benefit of this method of fluid delivery. Most often parenteral fluid administration by the oral or intravenous route is superior and is associated with less risk, particularly for infection, and has a lower cost. For delivery of humidified inspired gases, large-volume nebulizers offer little advantage over alternative methods.

Most large-volume nebulizers operate by using the 50-psig gas source regulated by a flowmeter. The total gas flow delivered through large-volume nebulizers depends on the design of the delivery system. Venturi entrainment is used with most of these units to provide the desired F_{IO_2}; oxygen is the gas source, and air is used for entrainment. Oxygen flow through the flowmeter is generally limited to between 10 and 15 L/min. The total flow depends on the flow rate of the driving gas and the selected F_{IO_2} (the aperture size through which air is entrained). Any backpressure in this venturi system (e.g., mask continuous positive airway pressure [CPAP]) will reduce the total flow and hence increase the F_{IO_2}.

In general, large-volume pneumatic nebulizers are high-flow devices intended to provide enough flow to meet and exceed patient inspiratory flow rates. The high flows are generated because of the entrainment of room air superimposed on the high flow from the wall oxygen source. Table 3–7 shows the total gas flow developed at various F_{IO_2} concentrations and oxygen flows of 10 and 15 L/min with no backpressure. However, when the patient's inspiratory flow becomes exceedingly high, as can occur with a severe infiltrative pneumonia, the nebulizer may not be able to provide sufficient flow to guarantee a desired inspired oxygen concentration. For example, if a patient has an inspiratory flow rate of 50 L/min and the patient requires an F_{IO_2} of 0.60, the nebulizer will not provide sufficient flow to the patient. The maximum flow that will be provided is 20 to 30 L/min. If the patient is not to entrain more room air from around a mask, additional flow would have to be provided by adding additional nebulizers. As the required F_{IO_2} increases, the flow provided from each nebulizer falls because of less air entrainment. In order to ensure the desired F_{IO_2}, the number of nebulizers that must be added becomes unwieldy. In these clinical situations, high-flow nebulizers such as the Misty Ox Gas Injector Nebulizer or a heated humidifier with a blender should be used.

Although there are a variety of large-volume nebulizer designs, the nebulizers all provide similar humidification.[35, 36] When large-volume nebulizers are used to provide drug solutions such as bronchodilators, the concentration of the drug will increase with continued delivery because of the preferential evaporation of diluent.

One problem with large-volume nebulizers when used for continuous therapy is the noise generated by the high flows. As was pointed out earlier, the American Academy of Pediatrics recommends that sound levels remain below 58 dB to avoid hearing loss for patients in incubators and hoods. This level is exceeded by a number of nebulizers on the market. Environmental sound pollution is also an issue in nursing units with a large volume of patients in close proximity such as anesthesia recovery units.

Another potential concern with the use of large-volume nebulizers is the potential for overhydration when they are used for prolonged periods of time. This is particularly a problem when these devices are used for infants and small children. When large-volume nebulizers are used in these clinical situations, the patients must be closely monitored for clinical signs of fluid overload. Large-volume nebulizers can precipitate airway irritability and increase airway resistance, particularly if the nebulizers deliver cold aerosols. Finally, as is true of any delivery system that contains water, the risk of nosocomial infection must be considered. When disposable nebulizers are used, the risk is minimal as long as the disposable devices are not refilled. Reusable devices should be sterilized between patients.[33]

TABLE 3–7
Total Gas Flow With Air Entrainment at Various F_{IO_2} Values

F_{IO_2}	Air/Oxygen	Total Flow* 10 L/min	15 L/min
0.24	25.0/1	260	390
0.30	8.0/1	90	135
0.35	4.6/1	46	69
0.40	32/1	32	48
0.60	1.0/1	20	30
0.70	0.6/1	16	24
0.80	0.34/1	13.4	20
0.9	0.14/1	11	16
1.0	0/1	10	15

* Liters of air per liter of oxygen $= \frac{1.0 - F_{IO_2}}{F_{IO_2} - 0.21}$.

Nondisposable large-volume nebulizers. The following are the features of some of the commercially available large-volume nebulizers:

Ohmeda Ohio Deluxe Nebulizer

- Reservoir volume: 800 mL
- Relative humidity: 80% (cold), 125% (heated)
- F_{IO_2} capability: 0.4, 0.6, 1.0
- Heater: Nonimmersible base

Puritan-Bennett All Purpose Nebulizer

- Reservoir volume: 375 mL
- Relative humidity: 70% (cold), 87% (heated)
- Heater: Immersion

Bird Inline Micronebulizer

- Reservoir volume: 500 mL
- Relative humidity: 70% (cold), 105% (heated)
- Heater: Immersion

Pegasus Thera-Mist Nebulizer

- Reservoir volume: 1,000 mL
- Relative humidity: 80% (cold), 110% heated
- Heater: Plate

Disposable large-volume nebulizers. Disposable large-volume nebulizers are manufactured by a number of companies; each offers slight modifications in reservoir size, air entrainment options, and heater design and availability. The RH provided at body temperature ranges from 58% to 74% for disposable units when cold and 75% to 96% when heated.

The disposable devices utilize either immersion, bottom plate, wraparound, or yolk collar heaters (Fig 3–43); they rarely have sophisticated servocontrol systems to monitor and control the temperature of the aerosol delivered to the patient. Most systems do not shut down with low water levels and can overheat when empty. Disposable large-volume nebulizers heaters can malfunction; for example, they can operate cold without warning the practitioner when the heating element malfunctions or heat to the point of inflicting thermal injury, again without sounding an alarm.

RCI Aquapak Nebulizer. The RCI Aquapak nebulizer (Fig 3–44) uses a heater positioned between the reservoir and the nebulizer. Water is heated as it passes through the heater. This type of heater is thought to be self-sterilizing in that it creates enough heat to kill pathogens or at least does not contribute to the pathogen

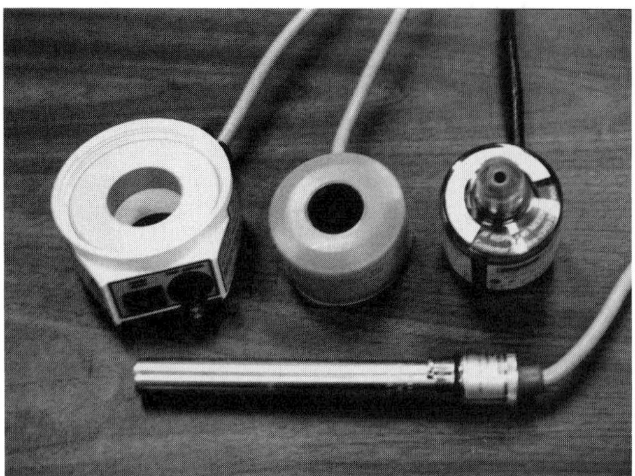

FIG 3–43
Types of heaters used with nebulizers and humidification systems. The TheraMist Heater (Pegasus) *(left)* sits at the base of the humidification chamber above the water bottle. The Travenol 2M8021 Nebulizer heater *(center)* fits around a metal collar on the neck of the nebulizer. The AquaTherm (Hudson/RCI) *(right)* heats water en route to the nebulizer. The Puritan Immersion Heater *(bottom)* extends directly into the reservoir.

load of the patient. The sterility of this device, however, is not well documented. It is unclear whether sterility can be guaranteed in situations where the heater is used with high flows that might overwhelm the heater's capabilities.

Professional Medical Products Prefil Nebulizer. This servo-controlled heater (Fig 3–45) uses a continuous temperature feedback to control an automatic safety shutoff to safeguard against the possibility of tracheal burns. Light-emitting diodes (LEDs) display the delivered aerosol temperature. It is used with the Prefil large-volume disposable nebulizer.

Misty Ox High F_{IO_2} High Flow Nebulizer. The Misty Ox nebulizer (Fig 3–46) uses a turboheater that sits with a detachable, easy-to-clean chamber between the reservoir bottle and the nebulizer manifold. Gas leaves the nebulizer and is routed into the heater chamber where it contacts the heater plate and exits to the patient. This unit can produce up to 60 L/min total flow at an F_{IO_2} of 0.6 by using high-flow flowmeters.

Inspiron. The Inspiron nebulizer utilizes an immersion heater that enters through the top of the nebulizer and directly contacts the solution in the reservoir.

Baxter/Travenol. The Baxter/Travenol nebulizer incorporates a collar heater that rests around the metal neck of the nebulizer body between the manifold and the reservoir. There is no contact between the heater and the aerosol.

Misty Ox Gas Injector Nebulizer. The Misty Ox Gas Injector Nebulizer (GIN) (Fig 3–47) is a high-flow nebulizer that does not depend upon entrainment ports to increase the total flow or mix oxygen. To develop high flows, the GIN uses two flowmeters, one source of gas operates the nebulizer, while the other source is injected past the nebulizer, blending oxygen and air to provide desired F_{IO_2}. The GIN can produce total flows of 80-110 lpm., with F_{IO_2} not affected by back pressure.

This system is suitable for patients with high minute volumes or CPAP, allowing a "flush" from gas sources. The GIN uses the same turboheater as the High Flow Nebulizer. A disadvantage is the relatively high sound levels generated by the high flows.

ALP High Efficiency Nebulizer System. The ALP High Efficiency Nebulizer has a unique design (Fig 3–48): a lightweight probe heater element extends from the electronic heat controller at the wall plug to reduce weight and bulk at the nebulizer. The probe element

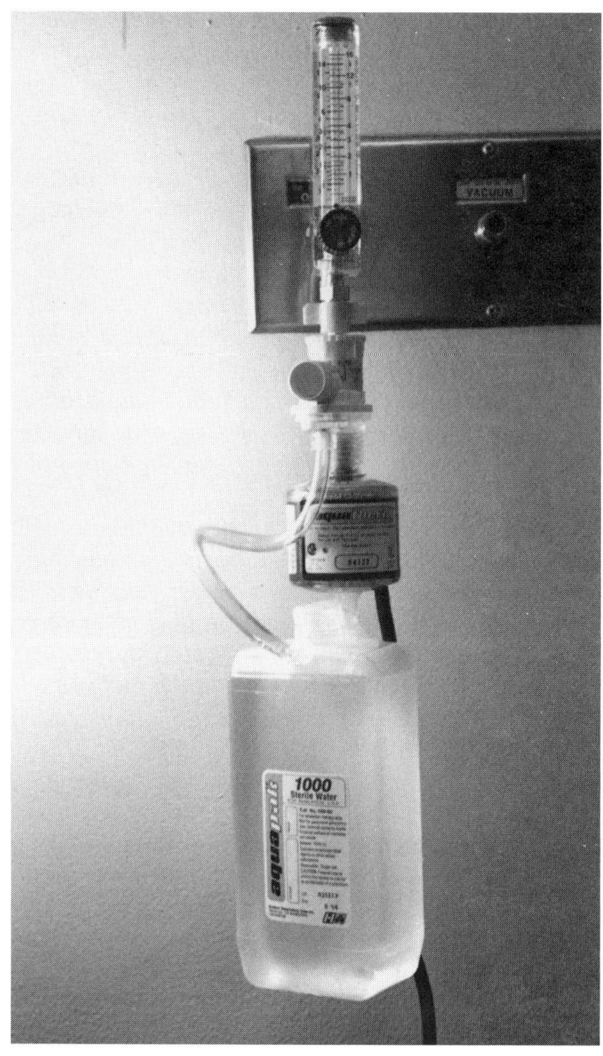

FIG 3–44
Hudson RCI Aqua Pak Nebulizer with heater.

inserts into a sleeve at the nebulizer. Water is drawn from the reservoir, around the outside of the heater sleeve, and onto the jet interface and makes no direct contact with the heater. Large particles that coalesce in the nebulizer can drain back into the reservoir.

Ultrasonic nebulizers. A variety of ultrasonic nebulizers are available. The particle size and output from the nebulizers vary considerably from one device to another. Some are capable of producing particle sizes up to 12 μm.

The primary use for the ultrasonic nebulizer is to induce sputum for diagnostic purposes. Small-volume ultrasonic nebulizers have also been promoted for bronchodilator therapy in nursing homes or other extended care facilities as an alternative to pneumatically driven small-volume nebulizers. The small-volume ultrasonic nebulizer may offer some advantage since most have less dead space than small-volume nebulizers do, thereby reducing the need for a large quantity of diluent to ensure delivery of drugs. The contained portable power source adds a great deal of convenience in mobility. Both theoretical advantages of the ultrasonic devices are outweighed by the high cost of the device, which may be up to 10 times the cost of a pneumatic nebulizer and 100 times the cost of treatment administered by MDI or DPI.

Ultrasonic nebulizers have also been used to administer undiluted bronchodilators to patients with severe bronchospasm.[74] Since the nebulizers have minimal dead space, the treatment time is shortened. Use of undiluted

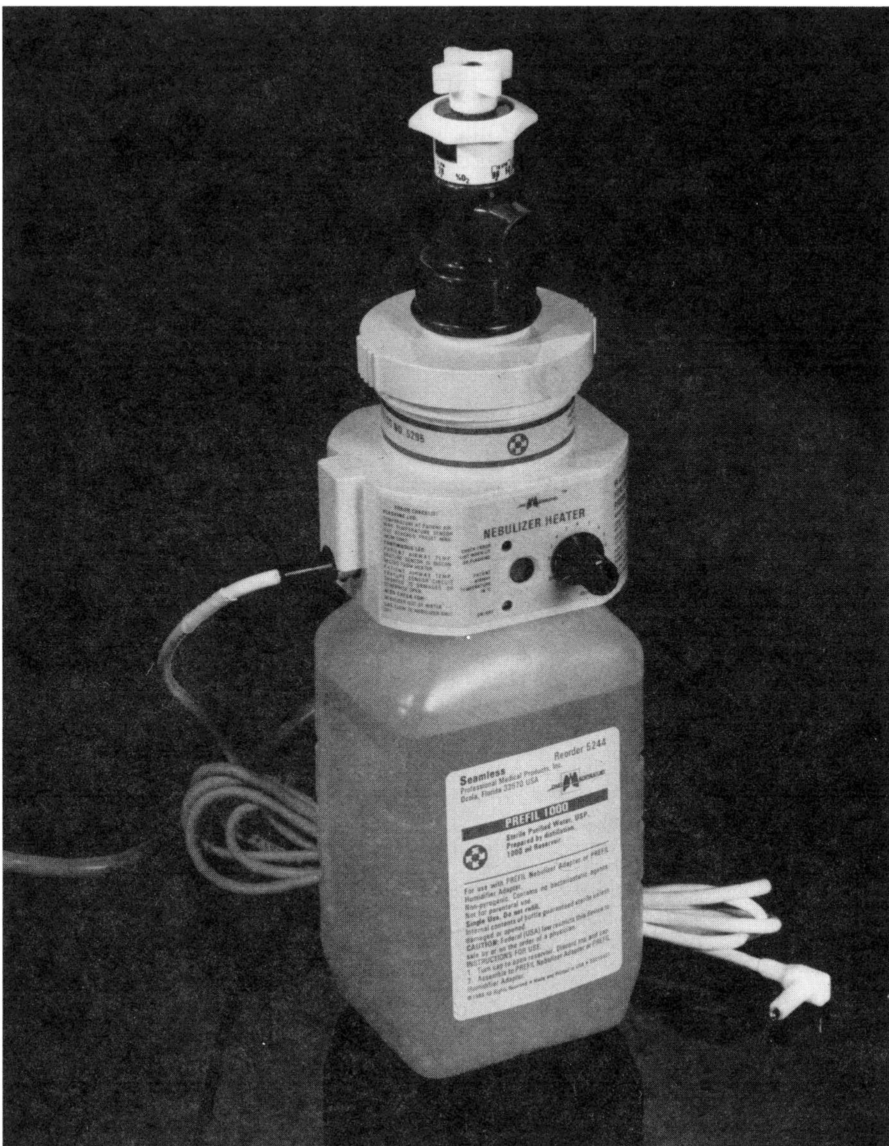

FIG 3–45
Seamless (Dart) Prefil adjustable electronic aerosol heater with a patient airway temperature sensor. (Courtesy of Professional Medical Products, Inc.)

bronchodilator is not new and is typically included in manufacturers' product dosing information found in the *Physician's Desk Reference.* Because the ultrasonic nebulizer manifold is prohibitively expensive, however, some practitioners have suggested a technique with the use of a one-way valve between the medication chamber and mouthpiece so that multiple patients can be treated consecutively without concern about infection (Fig 3–49). It is yet to be confirmed that a simple one-way valve manifold is adequate protection against contamination of the medication chamber; in addition, contact with infectious secretions on the outside of the nebulizer manifold could result in the transmission of pathogens from one patient to another.

Ultrasonic nebulizers have also found a place as room humidifiers and are often used as an alternative to steam vaporizers and centrifugal nebulizers in the home setting. When used for this purpose, it is important to remember that any ultrasonic nebulizer with an open water reservoir can become contaminated and transmit airborne pathogens. Care should be taken to ensure that these units are cleaned on a regular basis and that water is discarded from the reservoir periodically between cleanings. The recommended cleaning cycle is about once every 6 days.[75]

As suggested, the primary limitation to the use of ultrasonic nebulizers is the cost of the devices. The cost varies from $150 to over $1,000, considerably greater than the cost of acquisition and operation of other available nebulizers.

The use of ultrasonic nebulizers is associated with a number of potential complications, including overhydration, bronchospasm, infection, and disruption of the drug structure when used to administer medications.[76, 77]

Overhydration can occur as a result of the large fluid output from the nebulizers and their potential to deliver small particles to the lung parenchyma directly. Overhydration is of greatest risk after prolonged treatment of newborns, small children, and other patients with fluid and electrolyte imbalances. In addition to overhydration of the patient, pulmonary secretions can also swell after treatment with an ultrasonic nebulizer.

Bronchospasm can also occur after treatment with an ultrasonic nebulizer. The delivery of cold, high-density aerosols has been associated with increased airway resistance and irritability in a number of patients. In addition, sterile water administered through an ultrasonic nebulizer is known to be more irritating than normal saline.[78]

All nebulizers share the inherent hazard of transmitting pathogens via droplet nuclei. Contamination of the reservoirs of the ultrasonic nebulizers has been shown to cause airborne transmission of infection.[27–33]

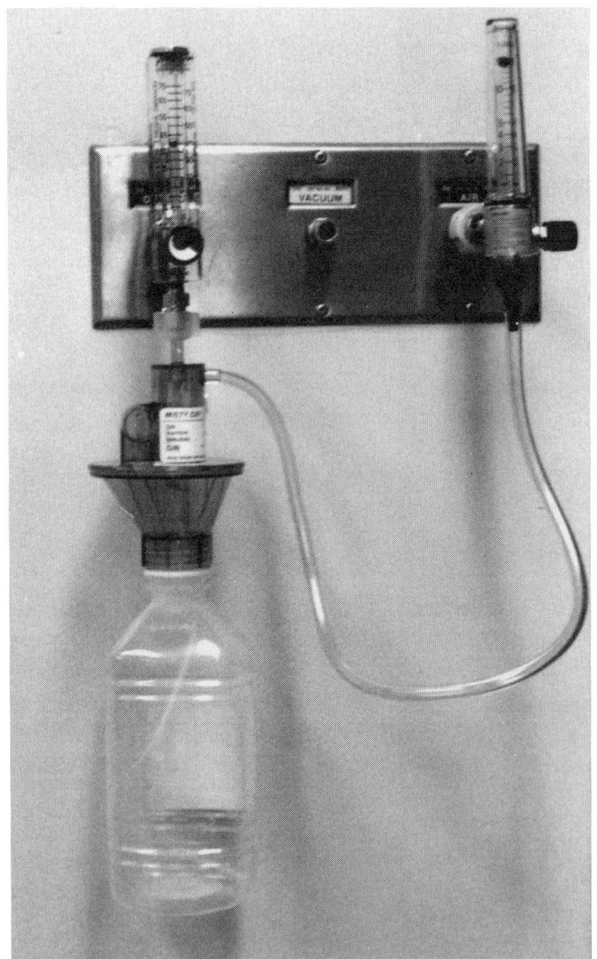

FIG 3–46
Misty Ox GIN.

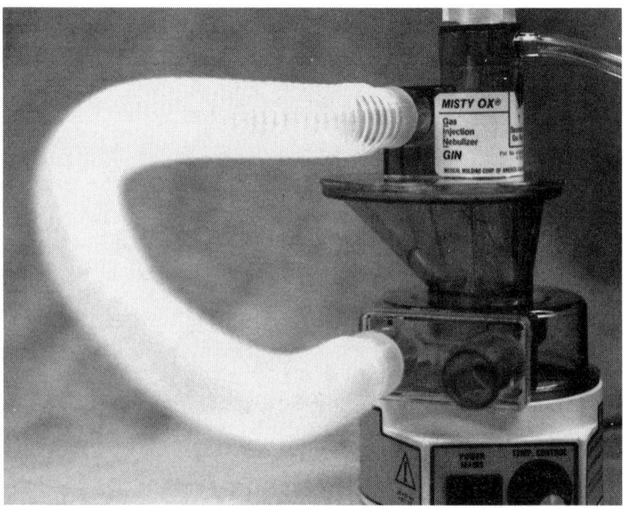

FIG 3–47
Misty Ox GIN with a turboheater.

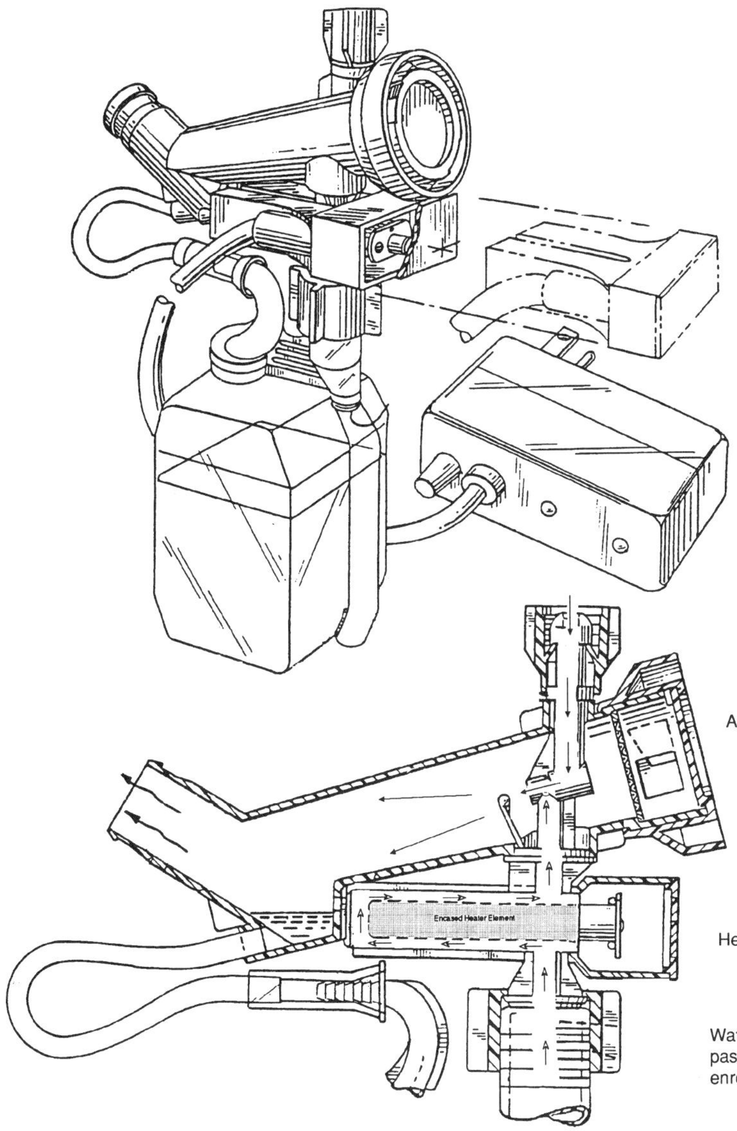

FIG 3–48
ALP High Efficiency Nebulizer System.

Heater element inserts into sleeve.
Heater base plugs into outlet away from neb.
Air Entrainment Port
Encased Heater Element
Heater inserts into sleeve
Water drawn up from bottle passes around heater sleeve enroute to jet.

Medications administered by ultrasonic nebulizer can become more concentrated during the treatment. This occurs because the solvent evaporates at a rate faster than the drug. Ultrasonic nebulizers have also been known to disrupt the structure of medications. Those nebulizers with an acoustic output of greater than 50 W/cm^2 cause changes in the structure of aerosolized medications. If the power output of the nebulizer is 50 W/cm^2 or less and the aerosol output is less than 2 mL/min, the nebulizers are reported to be safe when used to deliver medications.[77]

Babbington nebulizer. The Babbington nebulizer is a high-pressure gas source directed into a glass sphere with a slit from which the gas exits. The outside of the sphere is continuously bathed with a thin layer of liquid. As the gas leaves the sphere, it ruptures the film of water and sends particles toward an impactor baffle. A small stream of gas is directed up a siphon tube, which pumps solution from the reservoir to a holding chamber from which liquid drips onto the sphere. Three models have been produced in the United States: Solosphere, Hydrosphere, and Maxicool. They are no longer commercially available.

Solosphere, as its name implies, has a single sphere and can be used with a heater base. Hydrosphere and Maxicool both have two spheres and produce considerably higher output. They have been commonly used for tent applications. All have air entrainment capabilities, a high-density output, and an MMAD of about 4 μm.

The Solosphere provides a high-density mist of consistent particle size. It can deliver 15 to 63 L/min by face mask or tracheotomy collar and can be used as an alternative to standard pneumatic large-volume nebulizers.

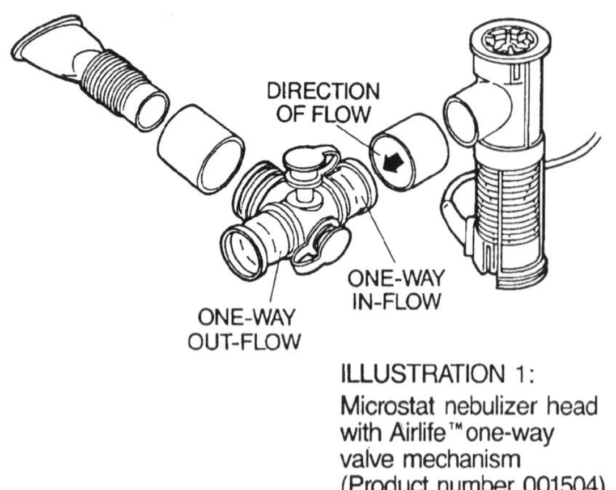

FIG 3–49
One-way valve assembly for use with the Mountain Medical Microstat nebulizer.

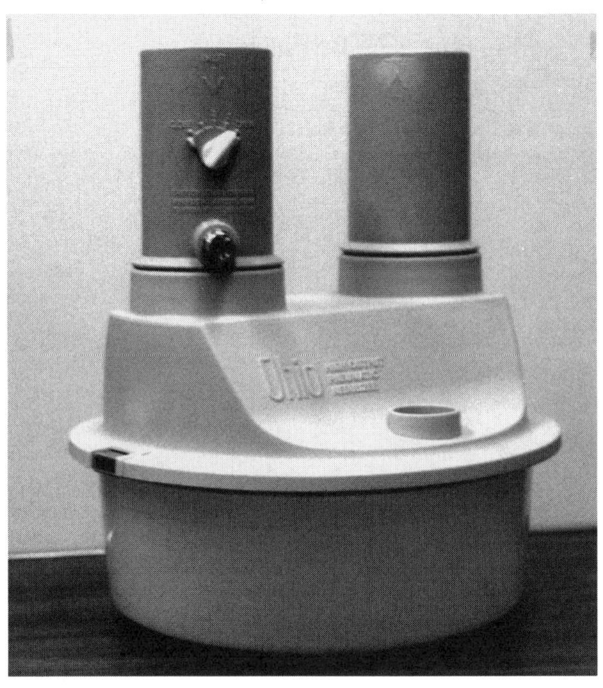

FIG 3–50
Ohio High Output Pneumatic Nebulizer.

The Hydrosphere provides 15- to 135-L/min flows, as compared with the Maxicool, which can generate flows of 30 to 257 L/min when the source gas is provided at 50 psig. These units are most commonly used with closed or open-top mist tents, where their high flow output flushes heat and carbon dioxide from the enclosed environment. They typically run cool enough so that they do not need ice or refrigeration for tent applications.

Mist tent. Mist tents have been used for the last 40 years for a variety of applications. They have been commonly used for the treatment of croup and have adopted the label "croup" tent. The cool aerosol is purported to promote peripheral vasoconstriction of the airway and reduce airway resistance.

Two potential areas of concern when a mist tent is used include increasing CO_2 concentrations within the tent and the tendency of the tents to retain heat from the body and raise the temperature within the tent. The CO_2 within the tent can be minimized by ensuring adequate fresh gas flow to the tent. The temperature problem is handled differently by each manufacturer. Most systems provide some mechanism to reduce the temperature in the tent to below room temperature. Some, like the Maxicool, utilize high fresh gas flows to cool the tent. Others, like the jet-type nebulizers used in some tents, have lower flows and must incorporate a cooling device. Air-Shields Croupette uses ice to cool the aerosol delivered to the patient. The Ohmeda Ohio Pediatric Aerosol Tent uses a large reservoir jet nebulizer with a "damper" (Fig 3–50) to effect circulation to the tent, and a refrigeration unit communicates directly with the inside of the tent to cool the air. The cooling effect of the unit causes considerable rainout, which is drained to a collection bottle outside of the tent. The Mistogen CAM-2 tent uses a Freon refrigeration device to cool water which circulates through a cooling panel. The Mistogen CAM-3 uses a Peltier effect–based thermoelectric system in which electric current passes through a semiconductor to augment heat absorption and release. As warm air is taken from the tent, heat is transferred and released in the room while cool air is returned to the tent.

Aerosol Drug Therapy

Aerosols are not only used for diagnostic purposes but are also frequently used to provide delivery of medications to the lung. The airways of the respiratory tract provide an ideal route for the administration of therapeutic agents. In many cases aerosols are superior, in terms of efficacy and safety, to the same systemically administered drugs used to treat pulmonary disorders.[79] Aerosols deliver a high drug concentration to the airway directly while providing very low systemic doses and minimizing systemic side effects. As a result, aerosol drug delivery has a high therapeutic index. Drugs can be delivered by aerosol from small-volume nebulizers, large-volume nebulizers, or MDIs. Ribavirin has been delivered by a specially manufactured device, the small-particle aerosol generator.

Small-volume nebulizer. Small-volume nebulizers are frequently used to deliver medication, particularly bronchodilators. A variety of different small-volume nebulizers are available. Each has specific characteristics, particularly with respect to output, that result in differences in delivery of drug to the lung (Table 3–8). Despite these differences, no studies have been done to date that demonstrate significant differences in clinical response based on small-volume nebulizer design. Similarly, no studies have been reported that suggest that the clinical response differs depending on the flow rates provided during the treatment.[80, 81] The lack of difference may be real or may represent how studies of nebulizer efficiency are performed. Each of the studies used high doses of drug, which may have masked any inefficiencies of the nebulizers themselves. One study did demonstrate that the dose delivered to stable asthmatics did make a difference.[82]

Device selection may be of greater importance for the administration of drugs other than bronchodilators, particularly to ensure efficient delivery of expensive drugs. Such substances include antiviral agents, α_1-antitrypsin, artificial surfactants, and pentamidine. Nebulizers with an MMAD less than 2 μm should be used for targeting delivery to the lung parenchyma. Small-volume nebulizers such as the Respirgard II (Fig 3–51) use auxillary baffles to create the desired particle size. Other specialty nebulizers such as the Vortran HEART and ICN SPAG-2 are described later in the chapter. The following factors affect the efficacy of small-volume nebulizers:

- Solution volume
- Nebulizer flow rate
- Intermittent vs. continuous nebulization
- Nebulizer design
- Temperature and humidity of the driving and entrained gas
- Output capabilities
- Amount aerosolized per unit time
- Particle size distribution

TABLE 3–8

Characteristics of a Variety of Nebulizers*

Nebulizer	MMAD†	GSD†
Jet nebulizers		
Respirgard II	0.93	±1.8
Centimist	1.1	±2.2
Aerotech II	2.0	±2.5
Fan JET	4.3	±2.5
Vortran HEART	3.5–2.2	±1.8–2.1
MedicAid Side-stream	2.75–3	
Ultrasonic Nebulizers		
FISO Neb	5.0	±2.0
Green Machine	>12.0	
Portasonic	1.6	±2.2
Pulmonsonic	4.2	±2.3

* Adapted from Fallat RI, Kandal K: *Respir Care* 1991; 36:1008–1016.

† MMAD = mean mass aerodynamic diameter; GSO = geometric standard deviation.

The amount of drug nebulized by a small-volume nebulizer increases as diluent is increased. Typical small-volume nebulizers will deliver more drug as an aerosol when the volume in the nebulizer is 4 mL as opposed to 2 mL with a constant nebulizer flow of 6 to 8 L/min. Particle size decreases as the flow rate increase. This has not been shown to correlate with difference in clinical response at varying diluent volumes and flow rates.[83] Another characteristic of small-volume nebulizers that is important to consider is the dead space volume. Dead space volume is the residual volume of medication that remains in the nebulizer after the nebulizer runs dry. It varies from 0.5 to 1.0 mL. The greater the dead space volume, the more drug wasted and the less efficient the delivery system.

Many of the commercially available small-volume nebulizers function only when kept in an upright position. Others are designed to operate in a variety of positions (Fig 3–52). This can be accomplished by directing a jet across the opening of multiple capillary tubes extending from a variety of points across the medication chamber. With this design, at least one capillary tube will be submerged in the medication no matter what the position of the nebulizer. The jet draws medication from the reservoir and directs the spray into an opposing baffle.

Humidity and temperature affect the performance of small-volume nebulizers. They each affect particle size and the concentration of drug remaining in the nebulizer. Evaporation of water and adiabatic expansion of gas can reduce the temperature of the aerosol to as much as 5°C

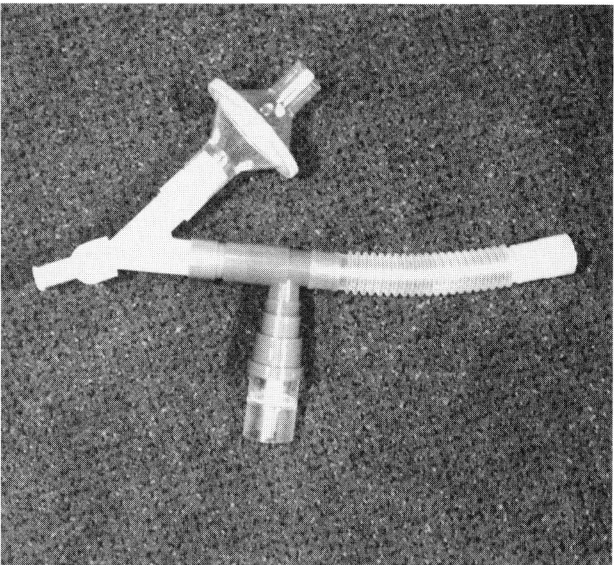

FIG 3–51
Respirgard II small-volume nebulizer.

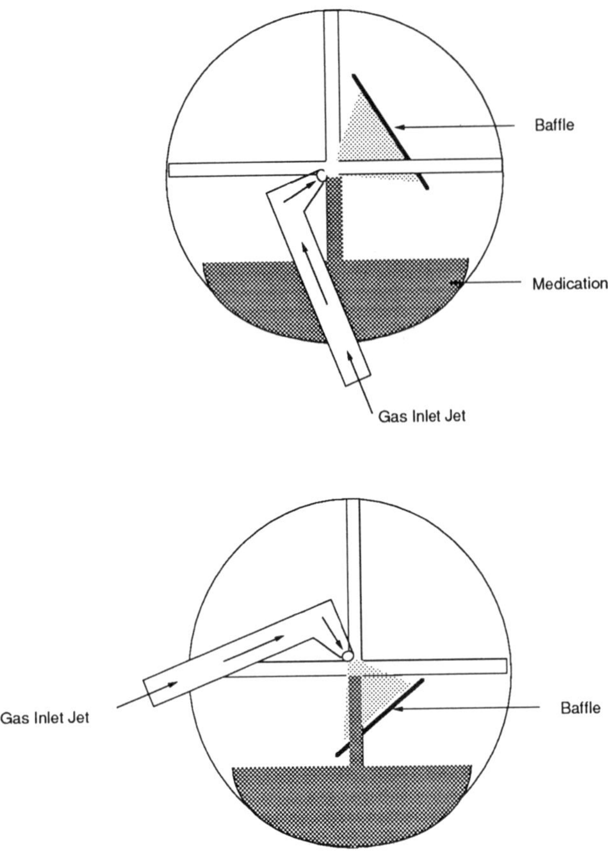

FIG 3–52
Diagram of a multipositional nebulizer.

below ambient temperature. As gas warms to room temperature, the particle size will be reduced. Aerosol particles entrained into a warm, fully saturated gas stream such as a ventilator circuit may increase in size.

Small-volume nebulizers will deliver the medication effectively only when used properly. Because the nose is such an efficient filter of particles over 5 μm, clinicians have long recommended that aerosol be inhaled through the mouth. Nose breathing filters out large particles and deposits more medication in the upper airway. Despite these theoretical differences, there appears to be no difference in clinical response between treatments given by mouthpiece or by mask when the patient is mouth breathing. Determination of the method of delivery, whether mask or mouthpiece, should be based on patient preference and comfort.

The ventilatory pattern does have an influence on the deposition of aerosols into the lower respiratory tract from small-volume nebulizers; in most situations, however, normal tidal breathing is encouraged during treatment. Slow inspiratory flow rates seem to be the most valuable maneuver to improve deposition. Deep breathing and breath holding during nebulizer therapy do not appear to augment the deposition of drug as compared with tidal breathing alone.[84]

Continuous nebulization during the entire respiratory cycle results in a considerable waste of drug. In between inspirations, the drug is lost to the environment. With a normal inspiratory:expiratory (I:E) ratio of 1:3, only 25% of the nebulized drug delivered to the face will get into the airway. Techniques to minimize drug loss have been used. Intermittent nebulization in which a patient-controlled finger port directs gas to the nebulizer only during inspiration provides greater opportunity to deposit more drug in the lung. It does, however, increase the duration of treatment by as much as three to five times the normal continuous administration time and requires considerably more patient hand-breath coordination than continuous nebulization does. Drug delivery can be significantly enhanced by the use of a valved storage chamber, such as the Mizer, that holds the aerosol generated during exhalation. The simple addition of a 50-mL tube as an expiratory reservoir to a nebulizer also improves drug delivery with small-volume nebulizers.

With the large number of small-volume nebulizers available on the market, it is clear that not all nebulizers are created equal. In fact, not all small-volume nebulizers work at all.[85] Care should be taken to evaluate the small-volume nebulizer that you use in same way that you would comparatively evaluate ventilator performance.

Aerosol administered by small-volume nebulizer to intubated and ventilated patients tends to be deposited in the tubing of the ventilator circuit; less medication is delivered to the patient. Deposition in the lung of ventilated patients has been measured in the range of 1.5% to 3.0%.[86, 87] McIntyre and associates estimated the deposition by this route to be only about 3% of the delivered dose,[87] whereas Fuller et al. found that the deposition of drug by small-volume nebulizer is 1.5%.[88]

When delivering medications by small-volume nebulizer to intubated, mechanically ventilated patients, the clinician must identify the most appropriate location for the nebulizer. Hughes and Saez[89] found that optimal placement of the nebulizer is in the inspiratory limb at the manifold of the ventilator circuit, about 18 in. from the patient wye. They demonstrated that the worst position for the nebulizer was between the patient and the wye connector of the circuit, particularly when using continuously nebulized medication; the drug that is nebulized after inspiration is complete is driven down the expiratory limb of the ventilator circuit and lost to the patient.

Large-volume nebulizer. Large-volume nebulizers can also be used to administer bronchodilators. Large-volume nebulizers are particularly useful when traditional dosing strategies are ineffective in treating severe bronchospasm. In the treatment of acute exacerbations of asthma with bronchodilators, a variety of methods are used to optimize treatment. When the patient does not respond, the frequency of administration of the bronchodilators is increased and may become as frequent as every 15 minutes. An alternative method of therapy to frequent small-volume nebulizer treatments is to provide continuous nebulization in a nebulizer with adequate solution to operate continuously and deliver a controlled rate of medication. Large-volume nebulizers can be used to provide continuous therapy. The continuous therapy ensures that the drug is not only delivered frequently enough to optimize bronchodilation but can also be delivered without patient interruption. The bronchodilator can be delivered while the patient sleeps.

Vortran's High Output Extended Aerosol Respiratory Therapy (HEART) nebulizer (Fig 3–53) has been used for providing continuous aerosol therapy with bronchodilators and other medications. This nebulizer has a 240-mL reservoir and produces particles between 3.5 and 2.2 μm in MMAD. The actual output and particle size vary based on the pressure at which the nebulizer operates and the flow rate.[90] The one problem with the use of a large-volume nebulizer for continuous treatment is that the concentration of drug increases over time as evaporation occurs. Patients receiving continuous bronchodilator therapy must be closely monitored for signs of drug toxicity.

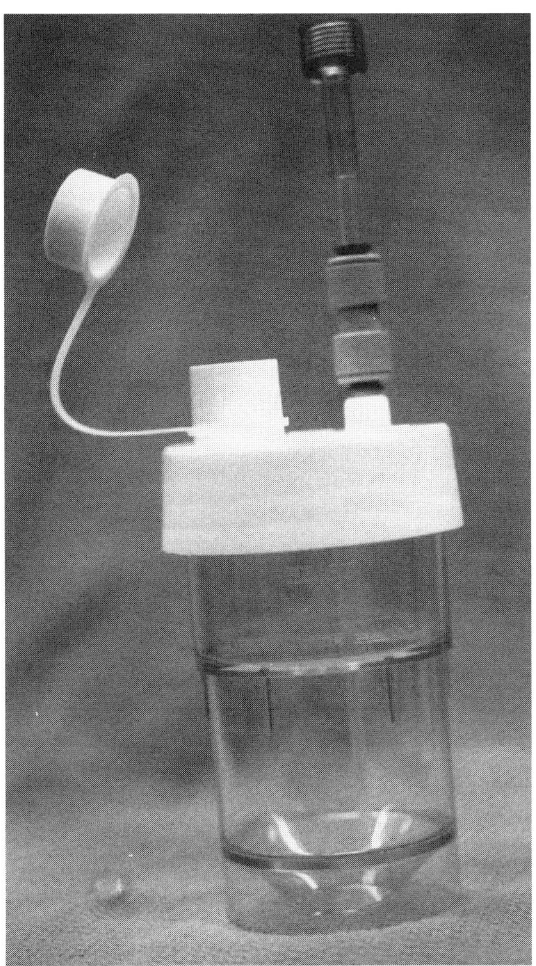

FIG 3–53
Vortan HEART nebulizer used for continuous nebulization of medication for patients requiring frequent treatment.

The HEART nebulizer can also be used with the Vortran Signal Actuated Nebulizer (VISAN) for mechanically ventilated patients to provide a high output of respirable particles on demand. The VISAN provides synchronous operation with aerosol produced at high flows during inspiration; it is actuated by an electronic signal from the ventilator so that timing is synchronized with inspiration. The device has a temperature bath to provide thermal control and a built-in air-controlled magnetic stirrer under the nebulizer reservoir to provide for uniform nebulization of suspension, colloids, and liposomes over extended periods.[90]

Another method for continuous delivery of bronchodilator by large-volume nebulizer is to use an intravenous infusion pump to drip premixed bronchodilator solution into a standard small-volume nebulizer. The cost and availability of infusion pumps make this an expensive device, but it appears to be capable of providing a dose each hour that is equivalent to treatments every 15 minutes by small-volume nebulizer with standard dosing.[91–101]

Metered dose inhalers. The MDI has become a common method to deliver drugs to the lung. The technique can now be used to administer all commonly used bronchodilators and steroids.

The successful administration of medications by MDI is very technique dependent. The patient must coordinate actuation of the MDI with early inspiration. The usual recommended method of delivery is to have the patient exhale to residual volume before inspiration and to close his lips tightly around the MDI actuator. Slow inspiratory flows of less than 0.75 L/sec with a breath hold of 10 seconds is reported to optimize lung deposition.[101–104]

Dolovich and others have shown increased deposition in the lung when the MDI is placed 4 cm from an open mouth position.[58] This technique improves lung deposition while decreasing oral deposition. The lung volume at which the aerosol is inhaled, beginning at residual volume, functional residual capacity, or 80% of total lung capacity, apparently does not significantly affect the amount of aerosol deposited in the lung or the clinical response to the bronchodilator.[105] It is possible that for patients with unstable airways, exhaling down to residual volume could result in closure of airways with a reduction in distribution of the next inhaled breath of aerosol to the lung. If true, the preferred technique might be for normal exhalation to functional residual capacity before inspiration and actuation of the MDI. The optimal technique for use of MDIs without accessory devices is as follows:

1. Warm the MDI to body temperature.
2. Assemble the apparatus (make sure that there are no objects or coins in the device that could be aspirated or obstruct outflow).
3. Shake the cannister vigorously, hold it upright, and place the actuator 4 cm (two fingers) away from the open mouth (aimed directly into the mouth).
4. After a normal exhalation, begin to inspire slowly (0.5 L/min) while actuating MDI. Continue inspiration to total lung capacity.
5. Hold the breath for 10 seconds.
6. Wait 1 minute between actuations.

Oral deposition of drug delivered by MDI can account for as much as 80% of the dose. The medication may be swallowed or absorbed by the mucous membranes and produce greater systemic side effects. The worst reported side effect of oral deposition with an MDI is increased oral thrush or opportunistic yeast infections associated with the use of inhaled steroids. Rinsing the mouth after steroid administration is essential to reduce the effects of oral deposition.

Improper MDI inhalation technique has been reported to range from 24% to 67% of previously instructed patients. This seems to correlate with findings that only 57% to 65% of physicians and nurses involved in outpatient instruction of patients in MDI technique performed at least four of seven steps properly.[106] Proper patient instruction is essential and rather time-consuming—requiring 10 to 28 minutes for initial instruction. Repeated instruction improves performance but must occur several times.[107–109] Even with the best instruction, some patients, especially infants, young children, and patients in acute distress, may be unable to coordinate proper administration; under these circumstances, accessory spacers or holding chambers should be considered.

Vitalograph has developed the Aerosol Inhalation Monitor (AIM) (Fig 3–54) to help teach pediatric patients the closed-mouth MDI administration technique. By using placebo aerosols, AIM monitors and provides visual feedback on coordinated inspiration with firing (depth charges are dropped and descend), appropriate inspiratory flow rates and duration of inspiration (depth charges blow up submarines), and breath holding (diver rises to the surface.) The proper sequence results in a merry tune.

Accessory devices. Because of the high deposition of drug in the mouth and the variability associated with coordination of breath control, techniques have been tried to improve drug delivery by MDI. Accessory devices have been used in conjunction with the MDI to reduce

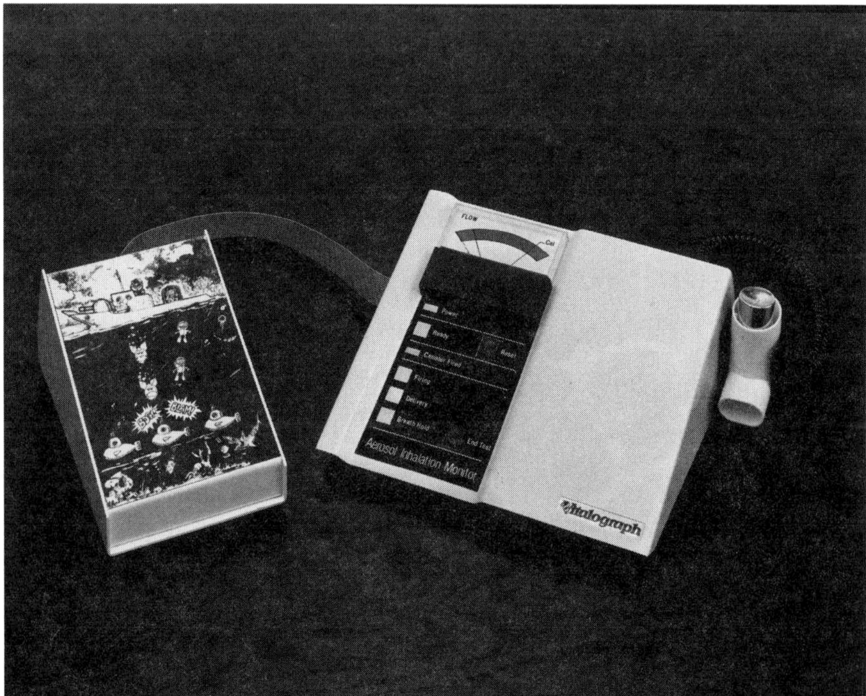

FIG 3–54
Vitalograph Aerosol Inhalation Monitor used to teach children and adults the closed-mouth technique of MDI administration.

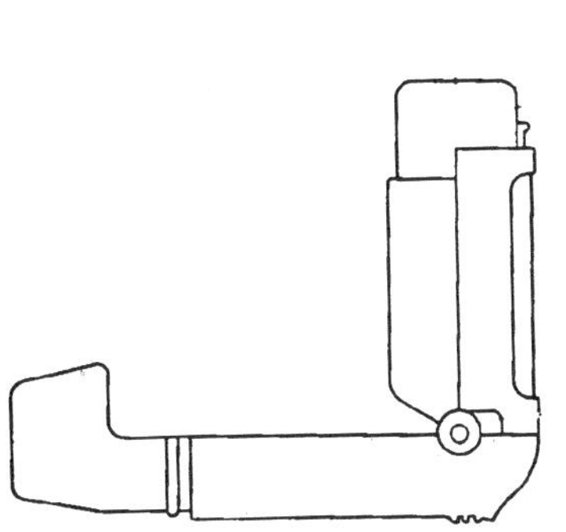
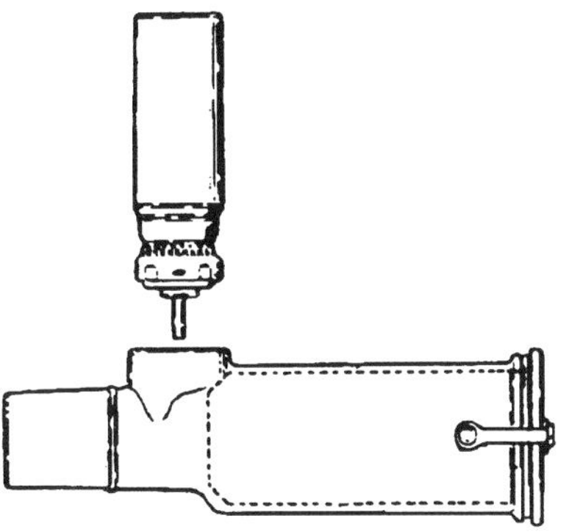

FIG 3–55
Diagram of the Open Spacer Synchroner and the closed spacer Optihaler. With no one-way valve or chamber capable of holding aerosol, the coordination of inspiration with firing of the MDI is critical for the patient to receive the dose.

oropharyngeal deposition and eliminate the need for hand-breath coordination. These devices have markedly improved the therapeutic efficacy of MDIs and made them consistently equivalent to treatment with small-volume nebulizers.

The accessories that appear to be most effective include spacers and holding chambers. Spacers, such as an open-ended straight tube, baggie, polyvinylchloride (PVC) tube, Open Spacer Synchroner, or Optihaler (Fig 3–55), provide space for the aerosolized medication or "plume" to expand and the CFCs to evaporate; this allows larger particles to impact on the walls of the device and reduces oropharyngeal deposition.[110] The spacer devices still require considerable coordination of actuation with breathing pattern. Exhalation immediately following actuation will clear the aerosol from the device and waste the dose. The open air–type spacer by design does not contain aerosol at all; it depends entirely on coordinated patient technique.

A holding chamber (Nebuhaler, Aerochamber, DHD Ace, shown in Fig 3–56) is similar to a spacer but incorporates a valve that permits the aerosol to be drawn from the chamber on inspiration but diverts exhaled gas on exhalation so that the remaining aerosol is not cleared. Use of the chamber allows patients with small tidal volumes to empty aerosol from the chamber with successive breaths. With the holding chamber in use, the patient can exhale into the mouthpiece or mask as the MDI is actuated without blowing away any of the medication. The InspirEase (Fig 3–56) is an example of a holding chamber without a one-way valve.

The DHD ACE (Fig 3–57) uses a mouthpiece with a one-way valve and inspiratory orifice at one end and a flow indicator attached to the other end of the chamber; this allows the device to do double duty as an accessory device for nonintubated as well as ventilated patients. Although the chamber works well in ventilated patients, the configuration has not been studied and reported in the literature.

The use of spacers and holding chambers has improved utilization of MDIs for delivery of bronchodilators. Larger doses of the medication are delivered to the

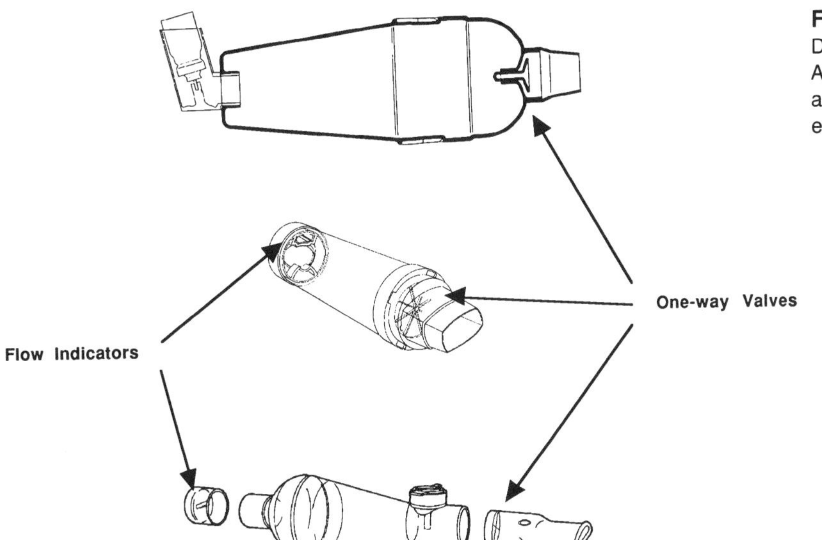

FIG 3–56
Diagram of three holding chambers (Nebuhaler, Aerochamber, and Ace). The one-way valve allows aerosol to remain in the chamber even if the patient exhales into the device.

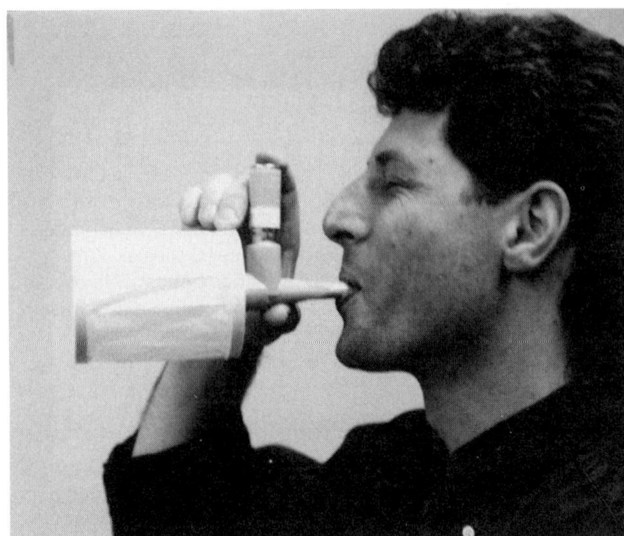

FIG 3–57
InspirEase device from Key Pharmaceuticals, Inc.

lower respiratory tract, with a greatly improved therapeutic ratio. Spacers and holding chambers tend to reduce oral deposition, reduce the bad taste of medication, and reduce the "cold Freon" effect that causes many children to stop inhalation with MDI actuation. Both accessory devices provide comparable advantages for patients who can coordinate MDI discharge with optimal breath control.[111] A holding chamber that incorporates an appropriately sized mask is available for use with infants, children, and adults (Fig 3–58). These units allow effective administration to patients who are unable to use a mouthpiece device because of size, age, coordination, or mentation (Fig 3–59).[112–120] Use of the MDI with a holding chamber may be as effective a method of delivering drugs as small-volume nebulizers.[121–131] Additional comparative studies will be helpful to more clearly define the clinical situations where one technique may be superior to the other.

The accessory devices used with the MDIs do cause a reduction in the MMAD[132] of the original spray through evaporation and impaction of the larger particles on the wall or valves of the device. The smaller particle size results in a 10- to 15-fold decrease in the dose of drug delivered to the pharynx.[110] Use of the holding chamber is particularly helpful when administering steroids since the total dose required will be less and systemic side effects can be minimized.[133] Even with a holding chamber in use, however, respirable particles do settle out and are deposited within the device.

Spacers are also used to optimize drug delivery by MDI to intubated, mechanically ventilated patients.[134] Three basic styles of adapter are available, including elbow, in-line, and chamber devices.

The elbow-style device (Fig 3–60) allows the MDI to be actuated directly into the airway by either an endotracheal or tracheostomy tube. The actuation is directed

FIG 3–58
Two mask Aerochamber designs from Monaghan for infants and children.

A

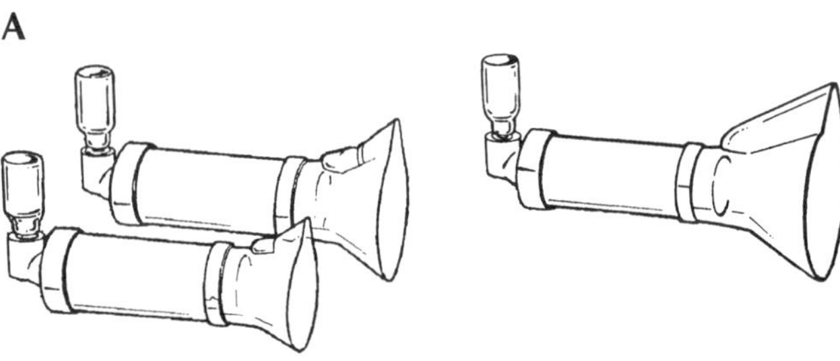

B

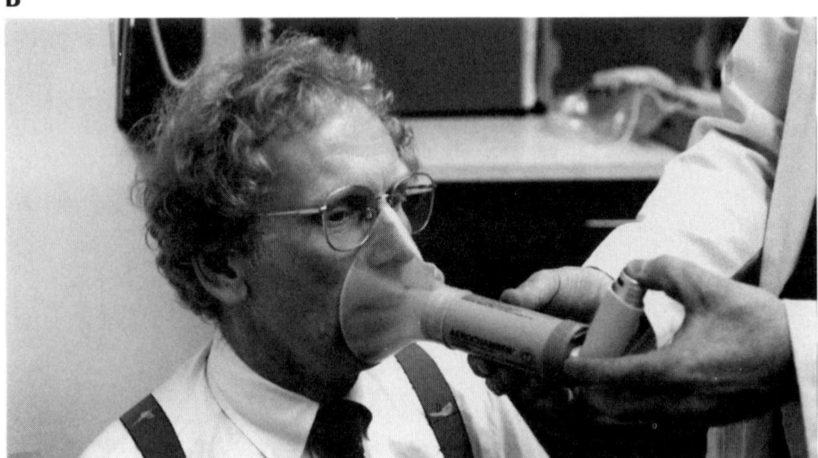

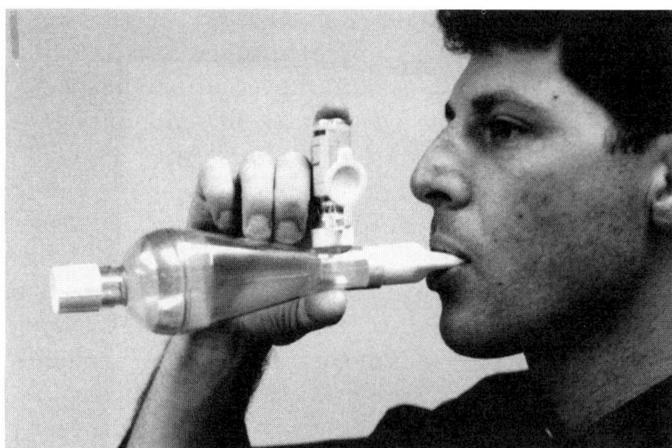

FIG 3–59
Adult being administered bronchodilator from an Aerochamber with a mask.

into a very constricted space; the majority of the CFCs and medication impact onto the walls of the artificial airway before evaporation and "aerosolization" of the medication. The result is a small percentage of respirable particles delivered beyond the tip of the airway into the lung.[135]

In-line devices (Fig 3–61) allow the MDI to be actuated in line with the ventilator circuit tubing. The in-line device and MDI are usually placed on the inspiratory limb of the ventilator circuit. Although the tubing is generally wider than the endotracheal tube, there is still a large percentage of medication trapped in the tubing; the delivered dose of respirable particles is low.

Chamber-style devices (Fig 3–62) are designed to allow an aerosol "plume" to develop. Within this cloud the CFCs evaporate before the bulk of the medication contacts the surface of the chamber or ventilator tubing. Use of the chamber device may result in less impaction of the medication on the walls of circuit tubing or airway as compared with the other devices used with ventilated patients.

One question that frequently arises when using drugs delivered by metered dose to ventilated patients is the dose of drug required. Many studies have suggested that the dose of drug delivered per puff from an MDI is less when administered to a ventilated patient as compared with the dose delivered to a nonintubated, spontaneously breathing patient. Bishop et al. utilized a bench model and determined that application of drug by MDI to an endotracheal tube by using the Monaghan AeroVent chamber, Instrumentation Industries RTC-22 spacer, or the Intermedical Intec 172275 spacer resulted in less drug being delivered vs. the drug delivered to a "normal airway." They estimated that if deposition of drug delivered by MDI to the normal airway is 10%, then these adapters might be expected to deposit only 1% of the

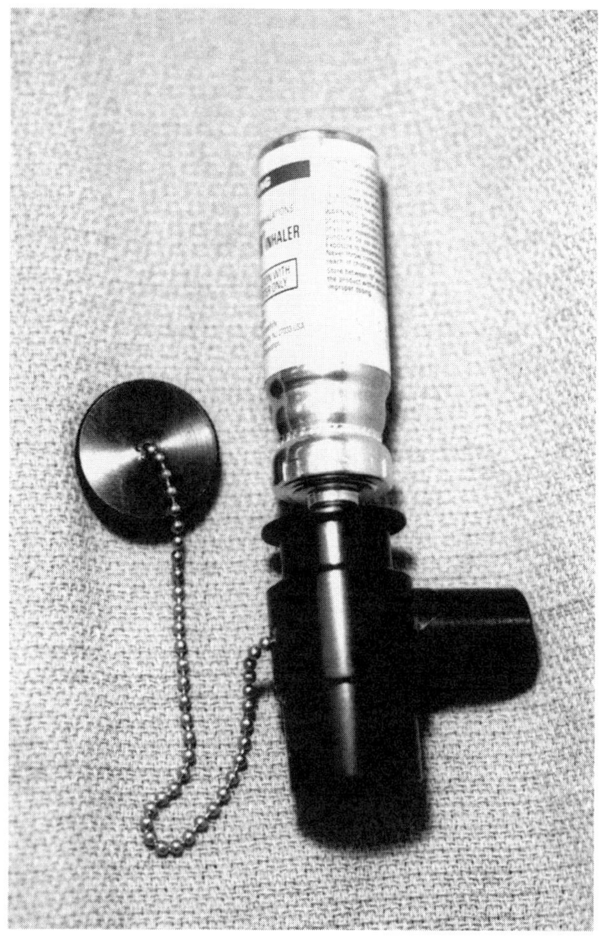

FIG 3–60
Elbow adapter for MDI administration to ventilated patients.

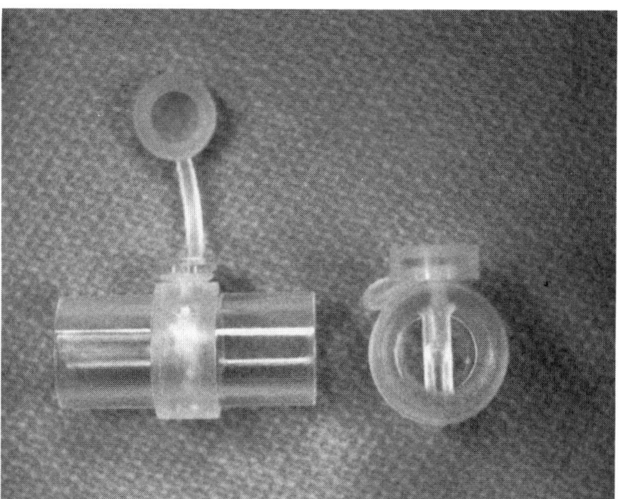

FIG 3–61
In-line adapter for MDI.

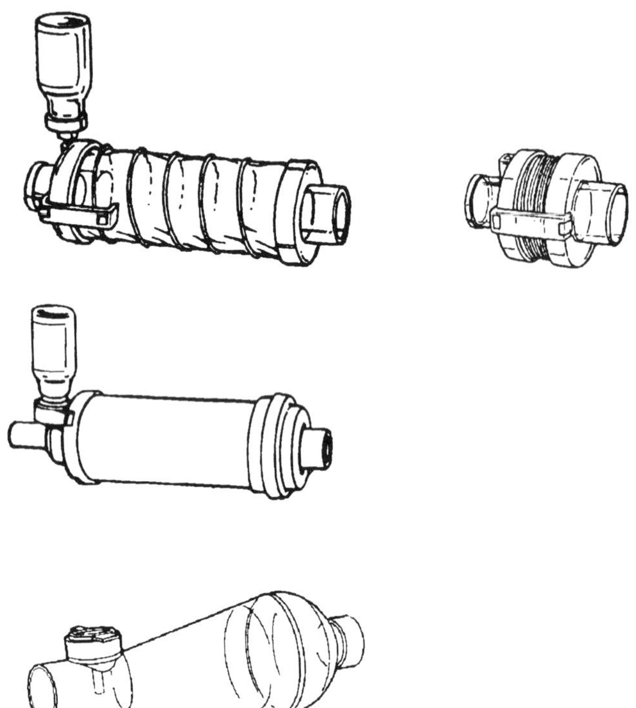

FIG 3–62
Chamber-style accessory devices studied by Ebert et al.: Monaghan Aerovent (extended for administration and compressed), Monaghan Aerochamber with a 15-mm connection for ventilated patients, and DHD Ace.

dose in the lung with the Intec chamber, 3% with the RTC-22 chamber, and 6% with the AeroVent chamber.[136] Using a similar bench model, Ebert et al. confirmed that chamber-style MDI devices produced a greater volume of respirable particles than the in-line or elbow-style devices (Fig 3–63).[137] Fuller et al., using the AeroVent chamber to deliver medication by MDI to intubated, ventilated patients, demonstrated a 5.5% deposition of drug delivered by MDI as compared with 1.5% deposition when delivered by small-volume nebulizer.[88]

It may be reasonable to assume that all intubated or ventilated patients receive a significantly smaller percentage of medication in the lung than nonintubated patients and that to deliver comparable amounts of medication to the lung larger doses (up to tenfold) may be required. A number of studies have demonstrated that the dose required is larger to achieve the same therapeutic end point for medications delivered by MDI to intubated vs. nonintubated patients. Since the specific dose required is unpredictable, our practice is to titrate the dose of bronchodilator delivered to ventilated patients using a MDI, usually with albuterol, and to incorporate an AeroVent adapter. Doses are administered in groups of 10 puffs administered twice, followed by 5 puffs administered up to four times at intervals of at least 5 minutes. Individual puffs are given at 1-minute intervals. The patient's response is monitored to determine the clinical response and the onset of side effects. If the patient demonstrates no side effects but continued clinical signs of increased airway resistance, repeated doses are administered by the protocol until the desired clinical response is achieved or toxicity develops. With this technique, only 60% of adult patients demonstrated any significant response to the bronchodilator when given up to 40 puffs. The patients had an optimal clinical response at approximately 24 puffs as shown in Fig 3–64. Adverse reactions (tachycardia or premature ventricular contractions) occurred in only 4 of 120 patients; all were minor and required no treatment. This evaluation suggests that more medication is required for clinical improvement in ventilated patients but that the higher doses are tolerated with minimal adverse reaction.[138]

Small-particle aerosol generator. The small-particle aerosol generator (SPAG) is a jet-type aerosol generator manufactured by ICN Pharmaceuticals specifically for the administration of ribavirin (Virazole). Ribavirin is an antiviral that has been recommended for the treatment of high-risk infants and children with respiratory syncytial virus (RSV) infections.[139] The effectiveness of this drug has been questionable. Few studies have demonstrated that ribavirin is useful therapy,[140] although recent data suggest that it is useful for ventilated infants with RSV.[141] The reason that the drug has recently been administered more commonly via the lung is that when administered by other routes, the systemic toxicity is very high.[141] The systemic toxicity is minimized and the

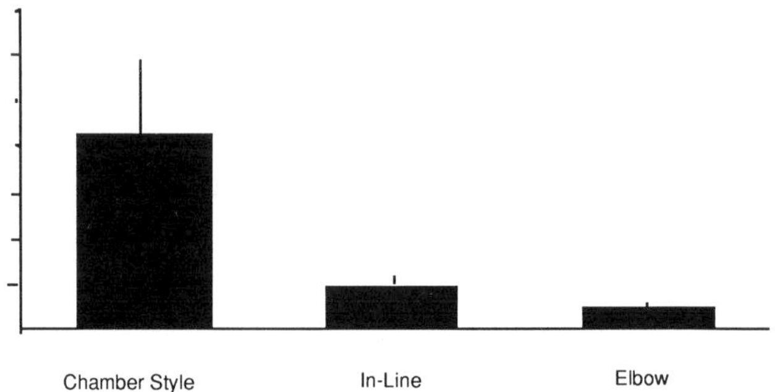

FIG 3–63
Comparison of available respirable particles delivered to an intubated, ventilated bench model with chamber, in-line, and elbow MDI adapters. (Adapted from Ebert J, Adams AB, Green-Eide B: An evaluation of MDI spacers and adapters: Their effect on the respirable volume of medication. *Respir Care* 1992; 37:862-868.)

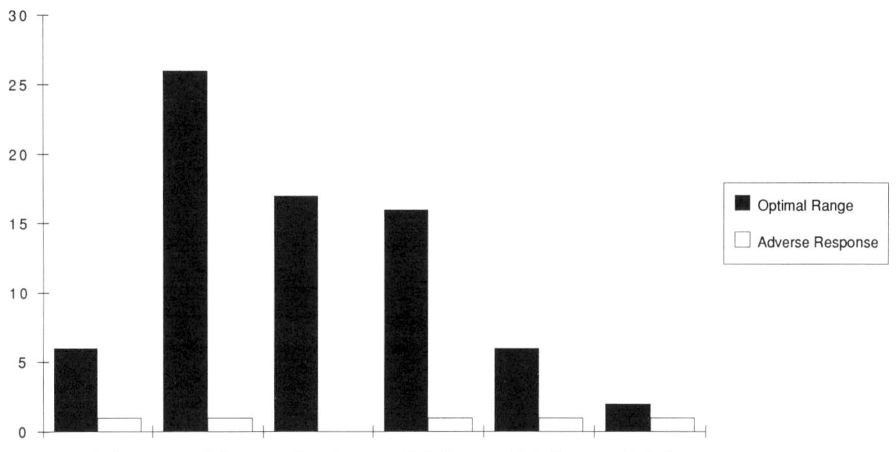

FIG 3–64
Optimal response and adverse effects of dose titration in 120 ventilated patients.

direct effect theoretically maximized when the drug is administered via the respiratory tract.[142]

The SPAG (Fig 3–65) was specifically designed to facilitate the administration of ribavirin. The device is unique in clinical respiratory care practice in that it incorporates a drying chamber with its own flow control to produce a stable aerosol. The SPAG reduces the medical gas source from the normal line pressure of 50 psig to as low as 26 psig; it has a variable regulator that is adjustable by the clinician. The regulator is connected to two flowmeters controlling flow to the nebulizer and drying chamber respectively. The nebulizer is located within the reservoir jar containing the medication and directs the aerosol output directly into the wall of the reservoir. As the aerosol leaves the medication reservoir/nebulizer and enters the long cylindrical drying chamber, a flow of dry gas is added to the aerosol. The dry gas serves to reduce particle size through evaporation and to transport the particles to the patient. Nebulizer flow should be maintained at about 7 L/min with total flow from both flowmeters not less than 15 L/min. The drying chamber helps to make the output almost monodisperse, with aerosol particles mostly between 1.2 and 1.4 μm. The SPAG II nebulizer tends to operate consistently even with backpressure and may be used with masks, hoods, tents, or ventilator circuits.

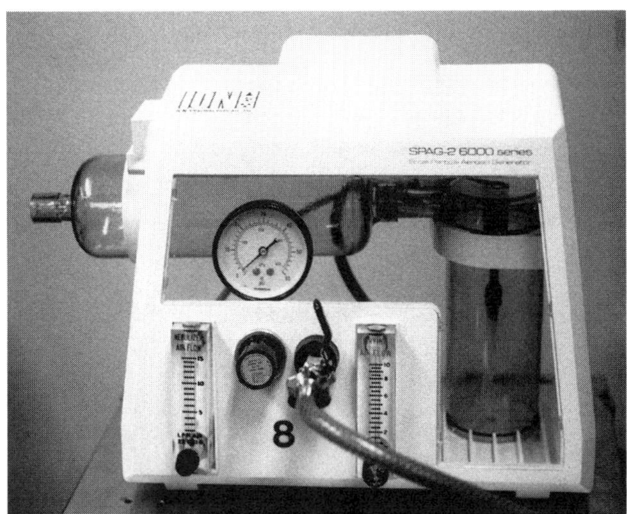

FIG 3–65
ICN SPAG-2 6000 series nebulizer.

A variety of toxicities have been reported by health care workers exposed to ribavirin. The most commonly reported include conjunctivitis, rash, and wheezing.[143–148] The possible risk of teratogenicity has also been considered, although no studies have confirmed that ribavirin is a risk to the fetus.[149] Because of the risks associated with administration of the drug, a number of environmental protective techniques are recommended[150]:

1. Ribavirin should be administered in a private room with negative-pressure ventilation and at least six air exchanges per hour. The room should be ventilated to the outside or have local exhaust filtered through a HEPA filter (Fig 3–66).

2. Canopies and scavenging systems should be used when ribavirin is administered to spontaneously ventilated patients. The expiratory limb of the ventilator circuit should be appropriately scavenged when ribavirin is administered through the ventilator circuit.

3. Whenever the patient requires other types of care, the aerosol should be interrupted. When discontinuing the treatment, the nebulizer should be turned off 5 minutes before opening a tent or 1 minute before disconnecting the ventilator circuit to reduce environmental exposure.

4. Personal protective equipment including goggles, respirator, gown, and gloves should be worn whenever the health care worker has direct contact with the drug.

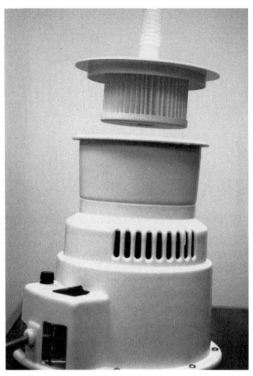

FIG 3–66
ICN HEPA filter scavenging unit shown with a disposable filter that is discarded after each 12- to 18-hour administration of ribavirin (Virazole).

5. Pregnant or lactating women should avoid contact with the drug. Health care workers who have had adverse reactions to ribavirin should also avoid further contact with the drug.[144]

When ribavirin is used to treat nonintubated, spontaneously breathing patients, techniques must be developed to minimize environmental contamination. Charney et al.[151] demonstrated the effectiveness of a two-tent containment system using two HEPA-filtered vacuum pumps to evacuate the space between the two tents. This system includes a shutoff valve that diverts the output from the SPAG to an aerosol device and allows easy diversion of blended oxygen to the patient when aerosol administration is interrupted. Kacmarek and Kratohvil[152] used a similar double-containment system with a hood (Fig 3–67) for three patients and confirmed that this level of scavenging is sufficient to reduce exposure levels. Cefaratt and Steinberg added a high-density aerosol to the space between the primary and secondary tent on the assumption that water-soluble ribavirin would increase the particle size and settle out more quickly, thereby reducing airborne exposure risk during tent opening.[153]

Ribavirin has been used most successfully to treat patients who require intubation and mechanical ventilatory support.[148] Unfortunately, the manufacturer of the drug suggests that it not be given through a ventilator circuit because of concern about drug accumulation and occlusion of the circuit. Demers et al. described a system for use with ventilator circuits that uses filters on the expiratory limb of the circuit and incorporates a water seal pop-off device and a one-way valve between the SPAG and humidifier outlet.[154] Kacmarek and Kratohvil[152] describe a system that incorporates a one-way valve connecting the SPAG to the inspiratory limb of the circuit of a Sechrist ventilator. The connection is made distal to the humidifier to prevent backflow of the aerosol during positive-pressure breaths. They also reduce the inspiratory flow by 7.5 L/min. A Pall filter was placed in the expiratory limb proximal to the exhalation valve. When either of these techniques is used to deliver ribavirin to mechanically ventilated patients, care should be taken to ensure that there is no leak around the cuff of the endotracheal tube. Gas leaking around the cuff will

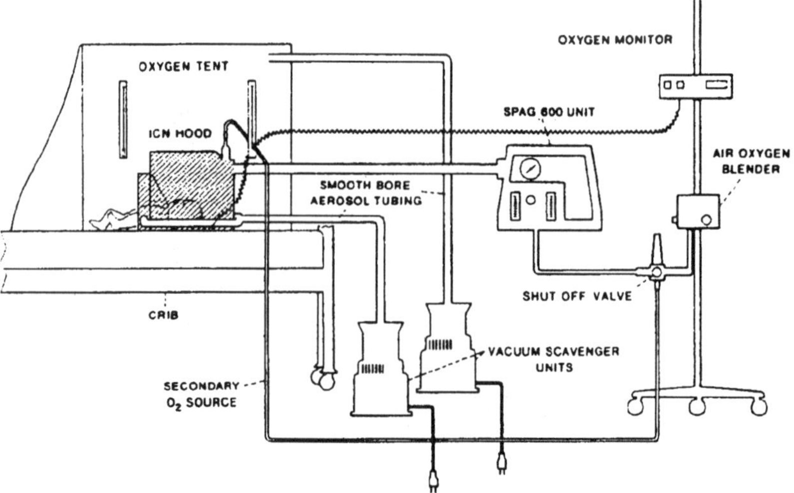

FIG 3–67
Double containment system for administering ribavirin to nonintubated patients. (Adapted from Kacmarek RM, Kratohvil J: *Respir Care* 1992; 37:37–45. Used by permission.)

contaminate the environment during positive-pressure breaths.

The benefits of ribavirin have only been demonstrated for intubated ventilated patients.[141] Additional studies will be needed to determine whether other patient populations will benefit from its use. In the meantime, in view of the high cost of the drug, approximately $450 per day, and the potential risk to health care workers, ribavirin should be restricted to use for ventilated patients presumed to be infected with RSV. Other patients should be only be treated as part of a well-designed study.

Infection Control Implications of Equipment Selection

Aerosol and condensate from ventilator circuits are known sources of patient contamination. Advances in circuit and humidifier technology have reduced the risk of contamination and nosocomial infection. Use of the wick or passover humidifier minimizes aerosolization of water from the heated reservoir. Heated wire circuits reduce the production and pooling of condensate within the circuit. Rhames et al. demonstrated that BTHs such as the Puritan Bennett Cascade humidifier produce aerosols that can carry bacteria.[32] Wick humidifiers do not. In addition, Gilmour et al. demonstrated that temperatures at which wick humidifiers operate can kill bacteria within the chamber.[155] In a study evaluating contamination of ventilator circuits that incorporate wick humidifiers with heated wire circuits, Fink et al. demonstrated that contamination of ventilator circuits occurs from the patient to the circuit rather than vice versa.[156] In no case did they find the reservoir infected with any organism that was not previously identified in patient sputum. The probable explanation for these findings is that since no aerosols are generated, there is no apparent route of transmission for bacteria from the humidifier to the patient.

The current Centers for Disease Control (CDC) guidelines regarding ventilator circuit changes, which suggest that circuits be changed every 48 hours, are based on the risk of nosocomial infection in critically ill patients. The frequent changes recommended by the CDC were the result of data using nonheated circuits and heated BTHs or large-reservoir nebulizers.[33]

Dreyfuss and coworkers compared 48-hour ventilator circuit changes with no circuit changes in patients who required over 96 hours of ventilation. They used wick humidifiers and circuits that did not include heated wires. They were able to find no difference in the incidence of pneumonia or duration of ventilatory support between the two groups and concluded that the frequency of ventilator circuit change had no effect on the rate of nosocomial pneumonia.[157]

Boher et al. evaluated the impact of 7-day ventilator circuit changes on the incidence of nosocomial lower respiratory tract infection rates. They compared the incidence of infection after 7-day circuit changes with historical controls whose circuits were changed every 48 hours. The study used wick-type humidifiers without heated wire circuits. They noted that infection rates decreased from 18 per 1,000 ventilator days with 48-hour circuit changes to 13 per 1,000 ventilator days with 7-day changes.[158]

Frequent ventilator circuit changes have themselves been identified as a risk factor for nosocomial pneumonia and death. Craven et al. found that patients who had the circuit changed every 24 hours were at greater risk than those whose circuit was changed every 48 hours. They speculated that the increased manipulation of the airway or tubing may have resulted in flushing contaminated condensate into the airway or increased leakage of bacteria around the endotracheal tube into the trachea.[159]

As a result of these studies, many institutions are now decreasing the frequency of ventilator circuit changes. The policy at the University of California, San Francisco, is to change ventilator circuits weekly or when the circuit becomes grossly contaminated with secretions or blood. This change has resulted in significant savings in equipment and personnel time. The cost of changing the ventilator circuit every 7 days is about $1,350 per ventilator per year as compared with $9,500 per ventilator per year if the circuit were changed daily.

Methods to Control Environmental Contamination

A variety of techniques are available to protect the environment, staff, and other patients from contamination during respiratory therapy procedures. Nebulized medication that escapes into the atmosphere from the nebulizer or is exhaled by the patient becomes a form of second-hand exposure to health care providers and others in the vicinity of the treatment.

Much recent attention has been raised regarding the risk to health care workers by exposure to some of the aerosolized medications, particularly ribavirin and pentamidine. Concerns have also been expressed about the potential teratogenicity of these agents. The risk imposed by continuous exposure to aerosolized antibiotics, steroids, and bronchodilators has also been raised, although no studies have demonstrated any significant risk. Although the risk has not been demonstrated, practitioners should be careful when administering any aerosolized agents.

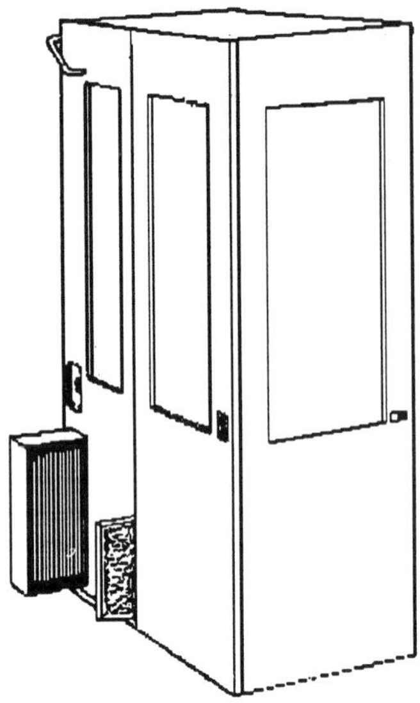

FIG 3–68
Emerson treatment booth to provide total containment of aerosol during therapy.

As previously stated, the greatest risk for health care workers at the present time is associated with the administration of ribavirin and pentamidine and from respiratory-transmitted diseases, particularly tuberculosis. Conjunctivitis, headaches, bronchospasm, shortness of breath, and rashes have been reported in health care workers administering ribavirin and pentamidine.[160] When treating patients with ribavirin or pentamidine, a number of protective measures should be utilized as outlined for ribavirin earlier. The treatment should be provided in a private room or booth, tent, or specially designed station to minimize environmental contamination. If the treatment is provided in a private room, the room should have negative-pressure ventilation with adequate air exchanges (at least six per hour) to clear the room of residual aerosol before the next treatment, or a tent should be used to minimize environmental exposure. HEPA filters should be used to filter room or tent exhaust, or the aerosol should be shunted to the outside.

Chambers and Booths

Booths or stalls should be used for sputum induction and aerosolized medication in any area in which multiple patients are treated. They should be designed to provide adequate airflow to draw aerosol and droplet nuclei from the patient to an appropriate filtration system or exhaust directly to the outside. Booths and stalls should be adequately cleaned between patients.

A variety of booths and specially designed stations are now available for delivery of pentamidine or ribavirin. The Emerson containment booth (Fig 3–68) is a

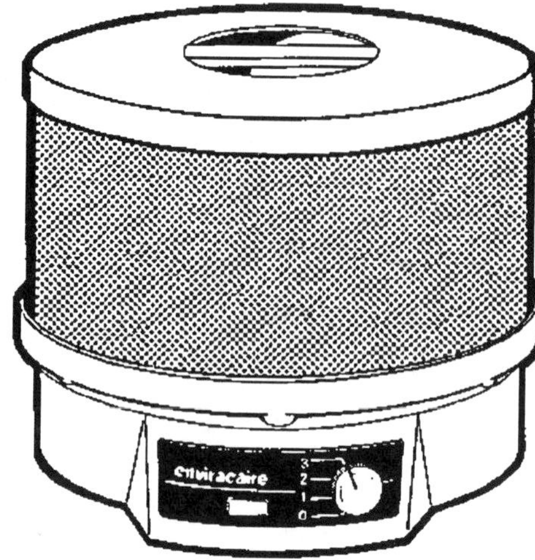

FIG 3–69
Enviracare room HEPA filter to provide local exhaust ventilation.

good example of a system that completely isolates the patient during aerosol administration; it draws all gas through a prefilter and a HEPA filter.

In areas where proper air exchanges do not exist, devices such as the Enviracare (Fig 3–69) have been used to provide local exhaust ventilation through a HEPA filter medium. Few data exist that support the efficacy of these

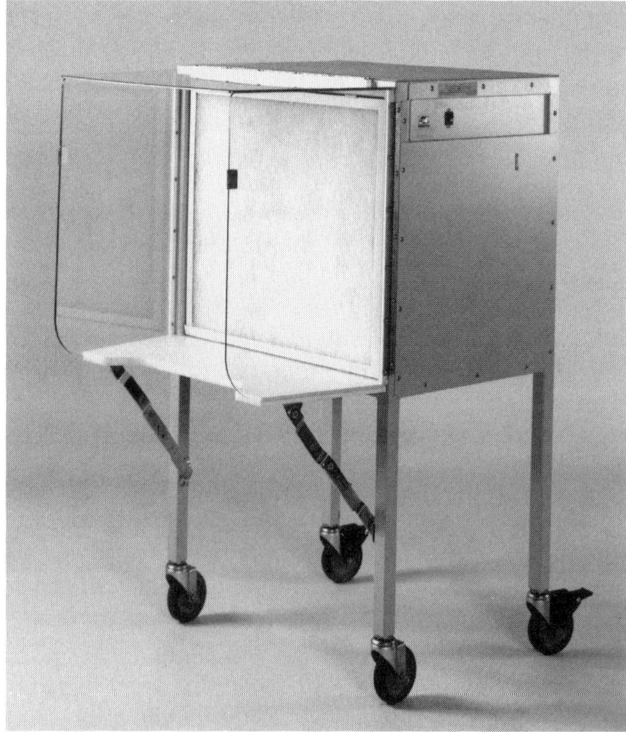

FIG 3–70
BioSafety Systems AeroStar aerosol protection cart. (Courtesy of BioSafety Systems, Inc.)

devices, although they are recently enjoying some popularity in use for the home.

The AeroStar Aerosol Protection Cart (Respiratory Safety Systems, San Diego) is one such portable patient isolation station for the administration of hazardous aerosolized medication (Fig 3–70). It has been used frequently during sputum induction and for pentamidine treatment. The patient compartment is collapsible with a swing-out counter and three polycarbonate walls. Captured aerosols are removed by a HEPA filter. A prefilter is used to retain larger dust particles and prevent early loading of the more expensive HEPA filter. A Minihelic pressure gauge is used to monitor HEPA filter performance.

The HR Aerosol Treatment Guard (Fig 3–71) is a similar product with different design. Selection should be made on unit specifications and performance.

Filters and nebulizers used in treatments with pentamidine and ribavirin should be treated as hazardous waste and disposed of accordingly. Goggles, gloves, and gowns should be used to serve as splatter shields and to reduce exposure to medication residues and body substances. The staff should be screened for adverse effects of exposure to the aerosol medication. The risks and safety procedures should be reviewed regularly.

In addition to the risks associated with aerosol medication administration, the risk of tuberculosis transmission has become of great concern recently because of an increase in case numbers and the development of multidrug-resistant strains of the organism.[161–163] Tuberculosis is transmitted in the form of droplet nuclei 0.3 to 0.6 μm in diameter that carry the tuberculosis bacilli. Consequently, protection from aerosols that can transmit tuberculosis requires the same protection that should be

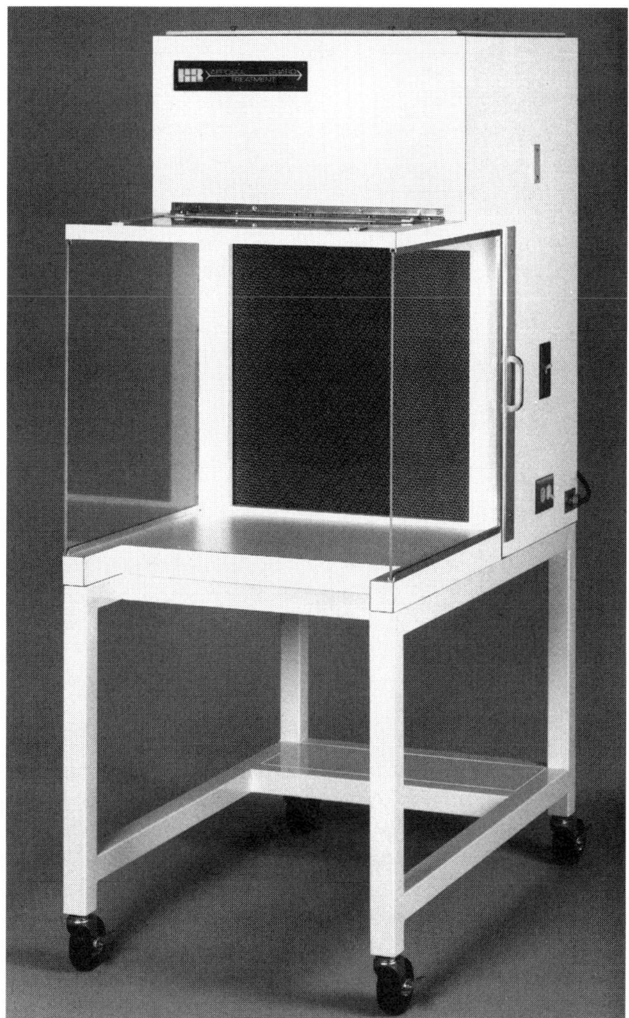

FIG 3–71
Aerosol Treatment Guard. (Courtesy of HR, Inc.)

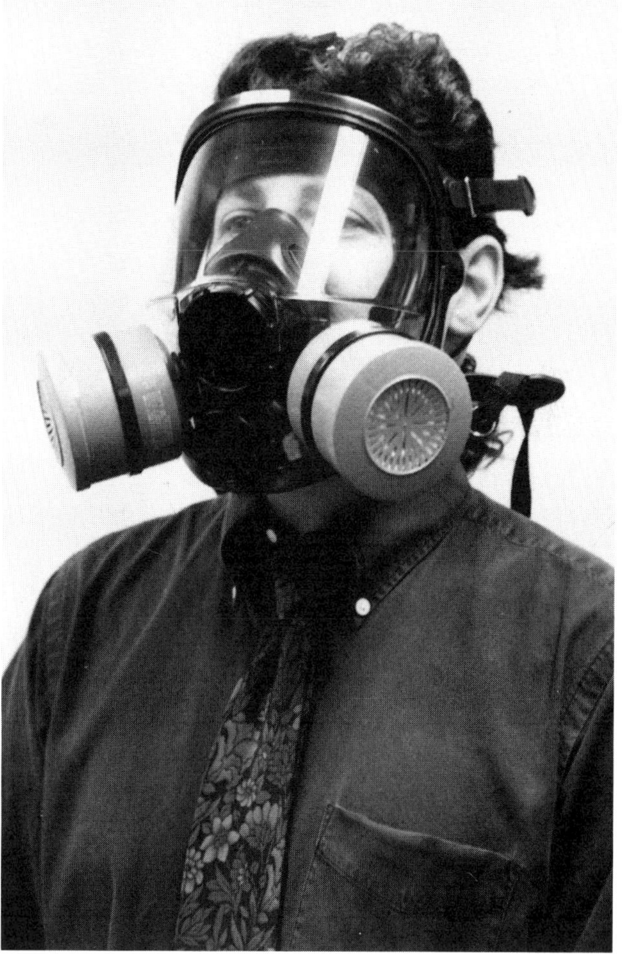

FIG 3–72
Respiratory care patient wearing a North 7600 Series Air Purifying Respirator with a full face piece.

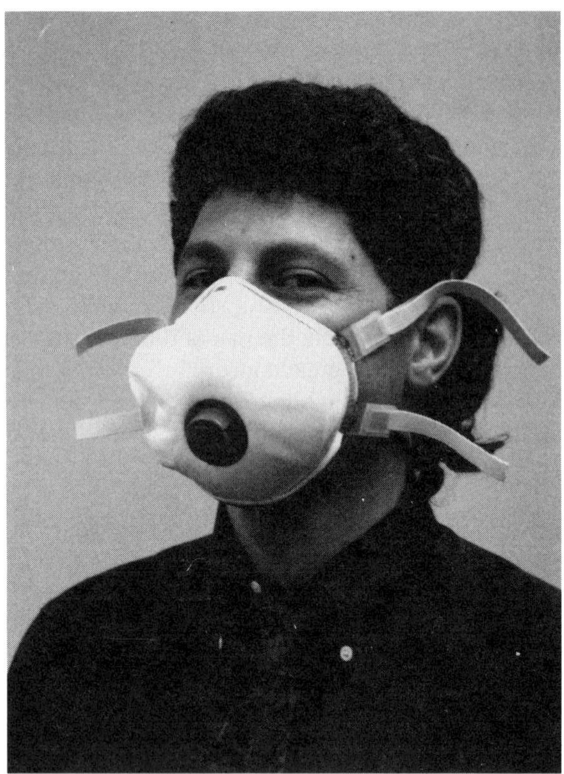

FIG 3–73
Respiratory care patient wearing a 3M 9970 High Efficiency Respirator.

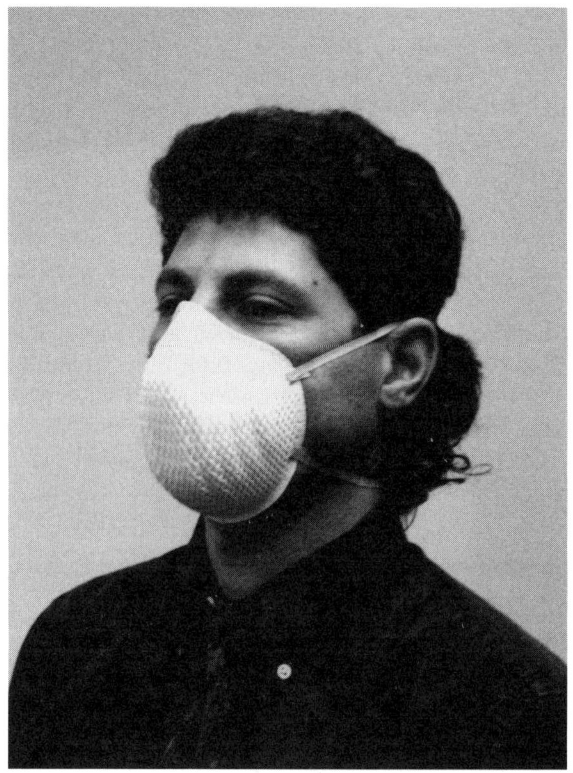

FIG 3–74
Respiratory care patient wearing a Moldex 2200 Dust and Mist Respirator.

exercised to reduce exposure to other aerosols in the 1- to 10-μm range. Known or suspected tuberculosis patients should be placed in private rooms with negative-pressure ventilation that has exhaust to the outside. If environmental isolation is not possible or the health care worker must enter the patient room, personal protective equipment should be used.

Personal Protective Equipment

Personal protective equipment is recommended when caring for any patient with a disease that can be spread by respiration. The greatest risk is for communication of tuberculosis or chicken pox. While environmental controls should be instituted when caring for these patients, universal precautions and respiratory isolation techniques should also be implemented.

A variety of masks and respirators (Figs 3–72 to 3–74) have been recommended for use when caring for a patient with tuberculosis or other respiratory-transmitted diseases. Traditional surgical masks, particulate respirators, disposable and reusable HEPA filters, and powered air-purifying respirators (PAPR) have all been used. Unfortunately, no data are available to determine the most effective and clinically most useful device to protect the health care worker or others.

REFERENCES

1. Shelley MP, Lloyd GM, Park GR: A review of the mechanisms and the methods of humidification of inspired gas. *Intensive Care Med* 1988; 14:1–9.
2. Walker JEC, Wells RE Jr, Merrill EW: Heat and water exchange in the respiratory tract. *Am J Med* 1961; 30:259–267.
3. McFadden ER Jr, Pichurke BB, Bowman HF, et al: Thermal mapping of the airways in humans. *J Appl Physiol* 1985; 2:564–570.
4. Sara C, Currie T: Humidification by nebulization. *Med J Aust* 1965; 1:174–179.
5. Primiano FP Jr, Montague FW Jr, Saidel GM: Measurement system for water vapor and temperature dynamics. *J Appl Physiol* 1984; 56:1679–1685.
6. Shapiro BA, Kacmarek RM, Cane RD, et al: *Clinical Application of Respiratory Care,* ed 4. St Louis, Mosby–Year Book, 1991, pp 57–73.
7. Kapadia FN, Shelley MP: Normal mechanisms of humidification. Recent advances in humidification. *Probl Respir Care* 1991; 4:395–402.
8. Dolovich M: Physical principles underlying aerosol therapy. *J Aerosol Med* 1989; 2:171–186.
9. Heyder J, Gebbart J, Rudolf G, et al: Physical factors determining particle deposition in the human respiratory tract. *J Aerosol Sci* 1980; 11:505–515.

10. Newman SP, Bateman JRM, Pavia D, et al: The importance of breath-holding following the inhalation of pressurized aerosol bronchodilators, in Baran D (ed): *Recent Advances in Aerosol Therapy: First Belgian Symposium on Aerosols in Medicine.* Brussels, 1979, pp 117–122.
11. Yu CP, Nicolaides P, Soong TT: Effect of random airway sizes on aerosol deposition. *Am Ind Hyg Assoc J* 1979; 40:999–1005.
12. Ingelstedt S: Studies on the conditioning of air in the respiratory tract. *Acta Otolaryngol Suppl (Stockh)* 1956; 131:1.
13. Chalon J, Loew DAY, Malbranche J: Effects of dry air and subsequent humidification on tracheobronchial ciliated epithelium. *Anesthesiology* 1972; 37:338.
14. Chatburn RL, Primiano FP: A rational basis for humidity therapy. *Respir Care* 1987; 32:249–253.
15. Ward JJ, Helmholtz HF: Applied humidity and aerosol therapy, in Burton GG, Hodgkin JE, Ward JJ (eds): *Respiratory Care: A Guide to Clinical Practice,* ed 3. Philadelphia, JB Lippincott, 1991, pp 355–396.
16. Scanlan C: Humidity and aerosol therapy, in Scanlan CL, Spearman CB, Sheldon RL (eds): *Egan's Fundamentals of Respiratory Care,* ed 5. St Louis, Mosby–Year Book, pp 557–583.
17. Anderson S, Herbring BG, Widman B: Accidental profound hypothermia. *Br J Anaesth* 1970; 42:653.
18. Wells RE, Walker JEC, Hickler RB: Effects of cold air on respiratory airflow resistance in patients with respiratory-tract disease. *N Engl J Med* 1960; 263:268.
19. Kacmarek RM: Humidity and aerosol therapy, in Pierson DJ, Kacmarek RM (eds): *Foundations of Respiratory Care.* New York, Churchill Livingstone, 1992, pp 793–824.
20. Gray HSJ: Humidifiers. *Probl Respir Care* 1991; 4: 423–434.
21. American National Standards Institute: *American National Standards for Nebulizer and Humidifiers.* American National Standards Institute Publication Z79.9, New York, 1979.
22. Seigel D, Romo B: Extended use of prefilled humidifier reservoirs and the likelihood of contamination. *Respir Care* 1990; 35:806–810.
23. Reinarz JA, Pierce AK, Mays BB, et al: The potential role of inhalation therapy equipment in nosocomial pulmonary infection. *J Clin Invest* 1965; 44:831–839.
24. Hoffman MA, Finberg L: *Pseudomonas* infections in infants associated with a high-humidity environment. *J Pediatr* 1955; 46:626–630.
25. Macpherson CR: Oxygen therapy—an unsuspected source of hospital infections? *JAMA* 1958; 167:1083–1086.
26. Sever JL: Possible role of humidifying equipment in spread of infections from the newborn nursery. *Pediatrics* 1959; 24:50–53.
27. Schulze T, Edmondson EB, Pierce AK, et al: Studies of a new humidifying device as a potential source of bacterial aerosols. *Am Rev Respir Dis* 1965; 96:517–519.
28. Phillips I: *Pseudomonas aeruginosa* respiratory tract infections in patients receiving mechanical ventilation. *J Hyg (Camb)* 1967; 65:229–235.
29. Pierce AK, Edmondson EB, McGee G, et al: An analysis of factors predisposing to gram-negative bacillary necrotizing pneumonia. *Am Rev Respir Dis* 1966; 94:309–315.
30. Pierce AK, Sanford JP, Thomas GD, et al: Long-term evaluation of inhalation therapy equipment and the occurrence of necrotizing pneumonia. *N Engl J Med* 1970; 282:528–531.
31. Pierce AK, Sanford JP: Bacterial contamination of aerosols. *Arch Intern Med* 1973; 131:156–159.
32. Rhame FS, Streifel A, McComb C, et al: Bubbling humidifiers produce microaerosols which can carry bacteria. *Infect Control* 1986; 7:403–406.
33. Centers for Disease Control: *Guideline for the Prevention of Nosocomial Pneumonia and Guideline Ranking Scheme. Guidelines for Prevention and Control of Nosocomial Infections.* Atlanta, Centers for Disease Control, July 1982.
34. Mercer TT, Goddard RF, Flores RL: Output characteristics of several commercial nebulizers. *Ann Allergy* 1965; 23:314–326.
35. Klein EF, Shah DA, Shah NJ, et al: Performance characteristics of conventional prototype humidifiers and nebulizers. *Chest* 1973; 64:690–696.
36. Hill TV, Sorbello JG: Humidity outputs of large-reservoir nebulizers. *Respir Care* 1987; 32:225–260.
37. Shelly MP: Inspired gas conditioning. *Respir Care* 1992; 37:1070–1080.
38. Branson RD, Hurst JM: Laboratory evaluation of moisture output of seven airway heat and moisture exchangers. *Respir Care* 1987; 32:741–747.
39. Ploysongsang Y, Branson D, Rashkin MC, et al: Effect of flowrate and duration of use on the pressure drop across six artificial noses. *Respir Care* 1989; 343:902–907.
40. Nishimura M, Nishijima MK, Okada T, et al: Comparison of flow-resistive work load due to humidifying devices. *Chest* 1990; 97:600–604.
41. Cadwallader HL, Bradley CR, Ayliffe GAJ: Bacterial contamination and frequency of changing ventilator circuitry. *J Hosp Infect* 1990; 15:65–72.
42. Hedley RM, Allt-Graham J: A comparison of the filtration properties of heat and moisture exchangers. *Anaesthesia* 1992; 47:414–420.
43. ECRI: Heated humidifiers. *Health Devices* 1987; 16: 223–250.
44. ECRI: Single product review: Marquest SCT 2000 heated humidifier. *Health Devices* 1991; 20:23–27.
45. Craven DE, Goularte TA, Make BJ: Contaminated condensate in mechanical ventilator circuits. A risk factor for nosocomial pneumonia. *Am Rev Respir Dis* 1984; 129:625–628.
46. Centers for Disease Control: Update: Universal precautions for prevention of transmission of human immunodeficiency virus, hepatitus B virus, and other blood

borne pathogens in health care settings. *MMWR* 1988; 37:377–388.
47. Boyce JM, White RL, Spruill EY, et al: Cost-effective application of the Centers for Disease Control guidelines for prevention of nosocomial pneumonia. *Am J Infect Control* 1985; 13:228–232.
48. Des Jardins T: Freon-propelled bronchodilator use as a potential hazard to asthmatic patients. *Respir Care* 1980; 21:50–57.
49. Breeden CC, Safirstein BH: Albuterol and spacer-induced atrial fibrillation. *Chest* 1990; 98:762–763.
50. Silverglade A: Cardiac toxicity of aerosol propellants. *JAMA* 1972; 222:827–828.
51. Moren F: Aerosol dosage forms and formulations, in Moren F, Newhouse MT, Dolovich MB (eds): *Aerosols in Medicine: Principles, Diagnosis and Therapy.* Amsterdam, Elsevier, 1985, pp 261–287.
52. Hallworth GW: The formulation and evaluation of pressurized metered dose inhalers, in Ganderton D, Jones T (eds): *Drug Delivery to the Respiratory Tract.* Chichester, England, Ellis Horwood, 1987, pp 87–118.
53. Newhouse MT, Dolovich M: Aerosol therapy in children, in *Basic Mechanisms of Pediatric Respiratory Disease: Cellular and Integrative.* Toronto, BC Decker, 1991.
54. Dhand R, Malik SK, Balakrishan M, et al: High speed photographic analysis of aerosols produced by metered dose inhalers. *J Pharm Pharmacol* 1988; 40:429–430.
55. Wiener MV: How to formulate aerosols to obtain the desired spray pattern. *Soc Cos Chem* 1958; 9:289–297.
56. Newman SP: Aerosol generators and delivery systems. *Respir Care* 1991; 36:939–951.
57. Kim CS, Trujillo D, Sackner MA: Size aspects of metered-dose inhaler aerosols. *Am Rev Respir Dis* 1985; 132:137–142.
58. Newman SP, Pvia D, Moren F, et al: Deposition of pressurized aerosols in the human respiratory tract. *Thorax* 1981; 36:52–55.
59. Dolovich M, Ruffin RE, Roberts R, et al: Optimal delivery of aerosols from metered dose inhalers. *Chest* 1981; 80(suppl):911–915.
60. Jenkins SC, Heaton RW, Fulton TJ, et al: Comparison of domicilliary nebulized salbutamol and salbutamol from a metered-dose inhaler in stable chronic airflow limitation. *Chest* 1987; 91:804–807.
61. Cissik JH, Bode FR, Smith JA: Double-blind crossover study of five bronchodilator medications and two delivery methods in stable asthma. Is there a best combination for use in the pulmonary laboratory? *Chest* 1990; 90:489–493.
62. Shim CS, Williams MH Jr: Effect of bronchodilator administered by canister versus jet nebulizer. *J Allergy Clin Immunol* 1984; 73:387–390.
63. Mestitz H, Coplan J, McDonald C: Comparison of outpatient nebulized vs metered dose inhaler terbutaline in chronic airflow obstruction. *Chest* 1989; 96:1237–1240.
64. AARC Clinical Practice Guidelines: Selection of aerosol delivery device. *Respir Care* 1992; 37:891–897.
65. Faculty and Working Group, American Association for Respiratory Care: Aerosol Consensus Conference Statement—1991. *Respir Care* 1991; 36:916–921.
66. Pederson S: How to use a Rotohaler. *Arch Dis Child* 1986; 61:11–14.
67. Pederson S, Hansen OR, Fuglsang G: Influence of inspiratory flowrate upon the effect of a Turbuhaler. *Arch Dis Child* 1990; 65:308–310.
68. Engel T, Heinig JH, Madsen F, et al: Peak inspiratory flowrate and inspiratory vital capacity of patients with asthma measured with and without a new dry powder inhaler device (Turbuhaler). *Eur Respir J* 1990; 3:1037–1041.
69. Hansen OR, Pederson S: Optimal inhalation technique with terbutaline Turbuhaler. *Eur Respir J* 1989; 2:637–639.
70. American College of Chest Physicians—NHLBI: National conference on oxygen therapy. *Respir Care* 1984; 29:922.
71. Darin J: The need for rational criteria for the use of unheated bubble humidifiers (editorial). *Respir Care* 1982; 27:945–947.
72. Darin J, Broadwell J, MacDonnell R: An evaluation of water-vapor output from four brands of unheated prefilled humidifiers. *Respir Care* 1981; 27:41.
73. AARC Clinical Practice Guidelines: Humidification during mechanical ventilation. *Respir Care* 1992; 37:887–890.
74. Ballard RD, Bogin RM, Pak J: Assessment of bronchodilator response to a β-adrenergic delivered from an ultrasonic nebulizer. *Chest* 1991; 100:410–415.
75. Chatburn RL, Lough MD, Klinger JD: An in-hospital evaluation of the sonic mist ultrasonic room humidifier. *Respir Care* 1984; 29:893–899.
76. Doershuk CF, Mathews LW, Gillespie CT, et al: Evaluation of jet type and ultrasonic nebulizers in mist tent therapy for cystic fibrosis. *Pediatrics* 1968; 41:723–732.
77. Boucher RGM, Kreuter J: Fundamentals of the ultrasonic atomization of medicated solutions. *Ann Allergy* 1968; 26:59.
78. Lewis RA, Ellis CJ, Fleming JS, et al: Ultrasonic and jet nebulizers: Differences in the physical properties and fractional deposition on the airway responses to nebulized water and saline aerosols (abstract). *Thorax* 1984; 39:712.
79. Svedmyr N: Clinical advantages of the aerosol route of drug administration. *Respir Care* 1991; 36:922–930.
80. Hadfield JW, Windebank WJ, Bateman JRM: Is driving gas flow clinically important for nebulizer therapy? *Br J Dis Chest* 1986; 80:550–554.
81. Douglas JG, Leslie MJ, Crompton GK, et al: A comparative study of two doses of salbutamol nebulized at 4 and 8 L/min in patients with chronic asthma. *Br J Dis Chest* 1986; 80:55–58.
82. Johnson MA, Newman SP, Bloom R, et al: Delivery of albuterol and ipratropium bromide from two nebulizer systems in chronic stable asthma: Efficacy and pulmonary deposition. *Chest* 1989; 96:1–10.
83. Hess D, Horney D, Snyder T: Medication-delivery performance of eight small-volume, hand-held nebulizers:

Effects of diluent volume, gas flowrate and nebulizer model. *Respir Care* 1989; 34:717–723.
84. Zainuddin BM, Tolfree SEJ, Short M, et al: Influence of breathing pattern on lung deposition and bronchodilator response to nebulized salbutamol in patients with stable asthma. *Thorax* 1988; 43:987–991.
85. Alvine GF, Rodgers P, Fitzsimmons KM, et al: Disposable jet nebulizers: How reliable are they? *Chest* 1992; 101: 316–319.
86. Dahlback M, Wollmer P, Drefeldt B, et al: Controlled aerosol delivery during mechanical ventilation. *J Aerosol Med* 1989; 4:339–347.
87. Malntyre NR, Silver RM, Miller CW, et al: Aerosol delivery in intubated, mechanically ventilated patients. *Crit Care Med* 1985; 13:81–84.
88. Fuller HD, Dolovich MB, Posmituck G, et al: Pressurized aerosol versus jet aerosol delivery to mechanically ventilated patients: Comparison of dose to the lungs. *Am Rev Respir Dis* 1990; 141:440–444.
89. Hughes JM, Saez J: Effects of nebulizer mode and position in a mechanical ventilator circuit on dose efficiency. *Respir Care* 1987; 32:111–1135.
90. Raabe OG, Lee JIC, Wong GA: A signal actuated nebulizer for use with breathing machines. *J Aerosol Med* 1989; 2:201–210.
91. Colacone A, Wolkove N, Stern E, et al: Continuous nebulization of albuterol (salbutamol) in acute asthma. *Chest* 1990; 97:693–697.
92. Moler FW, Hurwitz ME, Custer JR: Improvement in clinical asthma score and $Paco_2$ in children with severe asthma treated with continuously nebulized terbutaline. *J Allergy Clin Immunol* 1988; 81:1101–1109.
93. Portnoy J, Aggarwal J: Continuous terbutaline nebulization for the treatment of severe exacerbations of asthma in children. *Ann Allergy* 1988; 60:368–371.
94. Robertson C, Smith F, Beck R, et al: Response to frequent low doses of nebulized salbutamol in acute asthma. *J Pediatr* 1985; 106:672–674.
95. Schuh S, et al: High- versus low dose, frequently administered nebulized albuterol in children with severe acute asthma. *Pediatrics* 1989; 83:513–518.
96. Rebuck AS, Chapman KR, Abboud R, et al: Nebulized anticholinergic and sympathomimetic treatment of asthma and chronic obstructive airway disease in the emergency room. *Am J Med* 1987; 82:59–64.
97. Ba M, Thivierge RL, Lapierre JG, et al: Effects of continuous inhalation of salbutamol in acute asthma (abstract). *Am Rev Respir Dis* 1987; 135:326.
98. Amado M, Portnoy J, King K: Comparison of bolus and continuously nebulized terbutaline for treatment of severe exacerbations of asthma (abstract). *Ann Allergy Clin Immunol* 1988; 81:318.
99. Amado M, Portnoy J: A comparison of low and high doses of continuously nebulized terbutaline for treatment of severe exacerbations of asthma (abstract). *Ann Allergy* 1988; 60:165.
100. Heimer D, Shim C, Williams MH: The effect of sequential inhalations of metaproterenol aerosol in asthma. *J Allergy Clin Immunol* 1980; 66:75–77.
101. Newman SP, Pavia D, Clarke SW: Simple instructions for using pressurized aerosol bronchodilators. *J R Soc Med* 1980; 73:776–779.
102. Riley DJ, Liu RT, Edelman NH: Enhanced response to aerosolized bronchodilator therapy in asthma using respiratory maneuvers. *Chest* 1979; 76:501–507.
103. Grainger JR: Correct use of aerosol inhalers. *Can Med Assoc J* 1977; 116:584–585.
104. Woolf CR: Correct use of pressurized aerosol inhalers. *Can Med Assoc J* 1979; 121:710–711.
105. Riley DJ, Weitz BW, Edelman NH: The responses of asthmatic subjects to isoproterenol inhaled at differing lung volumes. *Am Rev Respir Dis* 1976; 114:509–515.
106. Guidry GG, Brown WD, Stogner SW, et al: Incorrect use of metered dose inhalers by medical personnel. *Chest* 1992; 101:31–33.
107. Crompton GK: Problems patients have using pressurized aerosol inhalers. *Eur J Respir Dis* 1982; 119(suppl):101–104.
108. De Blaquiere P, Christensen DB, Carter WB, et al: Use and misuse of metered-dose inhalers by patients with chronic lung disease: A controlled randomized trial of two instruction methods. *Am Rev Respir Dis* 1989; 140:910–916.
109. Allen SC, Prior A: What determines whether an elderly patient can use a metered dose inhaler correctly? *Br J Dis Chest* 1986; 80:45–49.
110. Kim CS, Eldridge MA, Sackner MA: Oropharyngeal deposition and delivery aspects of metered-dose inhaler aerosols. *Am Rev Respir Dis* 1987; 135:157–164.
111. Tschopp JM, Robinson S, Caloz JM, et al: Bronchodilating efficacy of an open-spacer device compared to three other spacers. *Respir Care* 1992; 37:61–64.
112. Lee N, Rachelefsky G, Kobayashi RH, et al: Efficacy and safety of albuterol administered by power driven nebulizer (PDN) versus metered dose inhaler (MDI) with Aerochamber and mask in infants and young children with acute asthma (abstract). Presented at a meeting of the American Academy of Pediatrics, November 1990.
113. Kraemer R, Frey U, Sommer CW, et al: Short-term effect of albuterol, delivered via a new auxiliary device, in wheezy infants. *Am Rev Respir Dis* 1991; 144:347–351.
114. Hodges IGC, Milner AD, Stokes GM: Assessment of a new device for delivering aerosol drugs to asthmatic children. *Arch Dis Child* 1981; 56:787–789.
115. Lee H, Evans HE: Evaluation of inhalation aids of metered dose inhalers in asthmatic children. *Chest* 1987; 91:366–369.
116. Gurwitz G, Levison H, Mindorf C, et al: Assessment of a new device (Aerochamber) for use with aerosol drugs in asthmatic children. *Ann Allergy* 1983; 50:166–170.
117. Barbera JM, Sly RM, Eby DM, et al: Responses to a bronchodilator aerosol delivered by Aerochamber to young children. *Ann Allergy* 1984; 52:224.
118. Katz R, Rachelefsky G, Rohr A, et al: Use of tube spacer, Aerochamber (A) to improve the efficacy of a metered

dose inhaler (MDI) in asthmatic children. *J Allergy Clin Immunol* 1986; 77:185.
119. Konig P, Gayer D, Kantak A, et al: A trial of metaproterenol by metered-dose inhaler and two spacers in preschool asthmatics. *Pediatr Pulmonol* 1988; 5:247–251.
120. Conner WT, Dolovich MB, Frame RA, et al: Reliable salbutamol administration in 6- to 36-month old children by means of a metered dose inhaler and Aerochamber with mask. *Pediatr Pulmonol* 1989; 6:263–267.
121. Madsden EB, Bundgaard A, Hidinger KG: Cumulative dose-response study comparing terbutaline pressurized aerosol administered via a pear shaped spacer and terbutaline in a nebulized solution. *Eur J Clin Pharmacol* 1982; 23:27–30.
122. Morgan MDL, Sing BV, Frame MH, et al: Terbutaline aerosol given through pear spacer in acute severe asthma. *BMJ* 1983; 285:849–850.
123. Berenberg MJ, Baigelman W, Cupples LA, et al: Comparison of metered-dose inhaler attached to an Aerochamber with an updraft nebulizer. *J Asthma* 1985; 22:87–92.
124. Newhouse MT, Dolovich MB: Control of asthma by aerosols. *N Engl J Med* 1986; 315:870–874.
125. Newman SP, Woodman G, Clarke SE, et al: Effect of InspirEase on the deposition of metered-dose aerosols in the human respiratory tract. *Chest* 1986; 89:551–556.
126. Newhouse MT, Dolovich MB: Aerosol therapy: Nebulizer vs metered dose inhaler. *Chest* 1987; 91:799–800.
127. Mestitz H, Copland JM, McDonald CF: Comparison of outpatient nebulized vs metered dose inhaler terbutaline in chronic airflow obstruction. *Chest* 1989; 96:1237–1240.
128. Berry RB, Shinto RA, Wong FH, et al: Nebulizer vs spacer for bronchodilator delivery in patient hospitalized for acute exacerbations of COPD. *Chest* 1989; 96:1241–1246.
129. Hodder RV: Metered dose inhaler with spacer is superior to wet nebulization for emergency room treatment of acute severe asthma. *Chest* 1988; 94(suppl):52.
130. Gervais A, Begin P: Bronchodilatation with a metered-dose inhaler plus an extension, using tidal breathing vs jet nebulization. *Chest* 1987; 92:822–824.
131. Summer W, et al: Aerosol bronchodilator delivery methods relative impact on pulmonary function and cost of respiratory care. *Arch Intern Med* 1989; 149:618–622.
132. Dolovich M, Chambers C, Mazza M, et al: Relative efficiency of four metered dose inhaler (MDI) holding chambers (HC) compared to albuterol MDI. Presented at American Lung Association American Thoracic Society 1992 International Conference at the Symposium on Aerosol Delivery Systems. 1992.
133. Salzman GA, Pyszczynski DR: Oropharyngeal candidiasis in patients treated with beclomethasone dipropionate delivered by metered-dose inhaler alone and with Aerochamber. *J Allergy Clin Immunol* 1988; 81:424–428.
134. Toogood JH, Baskerville J, Jennings B, et al: Use of spacer to facilitate inhaled corticosteroid treatment of asthma. *Am Rev Respir Dis* 1984; 129:723–729.
135. Crogan SJ, Bishop MJ: Delivery efficiency of metered dose aerosols given via endotracheal tube. *Anesthesiology* 1989; 70:1008–1010.
136. Bishop MJ, Larson RP, Buschman DL: Metered dose inhaler aerosol characteristics are affected by the endotracheal tube actuator/adapter used. *Anesthesiology* 1990; 71:1263–1265.
137. Ebert J, Adams AB, Green-Eide B: An evaluation of MDI spacers and adapters: Their effect on the respirable volume of medication. *Respir Care* 1992; 37:862–868.
138. Fink JB, Cohen N, Covington J, et al: Titration for optimal dose response to bronchodilators using MDI and spacer in 120 ventilated adults. In preparation.
139. Kacmarek RM: Ribavirin and pentamidine aerosols: Caregiver beware (editorial)! *Respir Care* 1990; 35: 1034–1036.
140. Herbert MF, Gugliemo BJ: What is the clinical role of aerosolized ribavirin? *Drug Intell Clin Pharmacol* 1990; 24:735–738.
141. Smith DW, Frankel LR, Mathers LH, et al: A controlled trial of aerosolized ribavirin in infants receiving mechanical ventilation for severe respiratory syncytial virus infections. *N Engl J Med* 1991; 325:24–29.
142. Committee on Infectious Diseases, American Academy of Pediatrics: Ribavirin therapy of respiratory syncytial virus. *Pediatrics* 1987; 79:475–478.
143. Harrison R: Assessing exposures of health care personnel to aerosols of ribavirin—California. *MMWR* 1988; 37:560–568.
144. Harrison R: Reproductive risk assessment with occupational exposure to ribavirin aerosol. *Pediatr Infect Dis J* 1990; 9(suppl):102–105.
145. Arnold SD, Buchan RM: Exposure to ribavirin aerosol. *Appl Occup Environ Hyg* 1991; 6:271–279.
146. Rodriguez WJ, Bui RH, Connor JD, et al: Environmental exposure of primary care personnel to ribavirin aerosol when supervising treatment of infants with respiratory syncytial virus infections. *Antimicrob Agents Chemother* 1987; 31:1143–1146.
147. Diamond SA, Dupuis LL: Contact lens damage due to ribavirin exposure (letter). *Drug Intell Clin Pharmacol* 1989; 23:428–429.
148. Adderley RJ: Safety of ribavirin with mechanical ventilation. *Pediatr Infect Dis J* 1990; 9(suppl):112–114.
149. Waskin H: Toxicology of antimicrobial aerosols: A review of aerosolized ribavirin and pentamidine. *Respir Care* 1991; 36:1026–1036.
150. Massachusetts Department of Labor and Industries, Division of Occupational Hygiene: *Ribavirin Alert.* DOH Publication No 1558, July 1989.
151. Charney W, Corkery KJ, Kraemer R: Engineering administration controls to contain the delivery of aerosolized ribavirin: Results of simulation and application to one patient. *Respir Care* 1990; 35:1042–1048.
152. Kacmarek RM, Kratohvil J: Evaluation of a double-enclosure double-vacuum unit scavenging system for ribavirin administration. *Respir Care* 1992; 37:37–45.

153. Cefaratt JL, Steinberg EA: An alternative method for delivery of ribavirin to nonventilated pediatric patients. *Respir Care* 1992; 37:877–881.
154. Demers RR, Parker J, Frankel LR, et al: Administration of ribavirin to neonatal and pediatric patients during mechanical ventilation. *Respir Care* 1986; 31:1188.
155. Gilmour IJ, Boyle MJ, Streifel A: Humidifiers kill bacteria (abstract). *Anesthesiology* 1991; 75:498.
156. Fink J, Mahlmeister M, York M, et al: Patterns of contamination of ventilator circuits: Implications for frequency of circuit changes in critically ill patients. Submitted for publication.
157. Dreyfuss D, Djedaini K, Weber P, et al: Prospective study of nosocomial pneumonia and of patient and circuit colonization during mechanical ventilation with circuit changes every 48 hours versus no change. *Am Rev Respir Dis* 1991; 143:738–743.
158. Boher M, Lohse S, Glasby C, et al: Impact of 7-day circuit changes on nosocomial lower respiratory tract infections. *Am J Infect Control* 1991; 20:103.
159. Craven DE, Kunches LM, Kilinsky V, et al: Risk factors for pneumonia and fatality in patients receiving continuous mechanical ventilation. *Am Rev Respir Dis* 1986; 133:792–796.
160. Fallat RJ, Kandal K: Aerosol exhaust: Escape of aerosolized medication into the patient and caregiver's environment. *Respir Care* 1991; 36:1008–1016.
161. Reykus JF: There's more to respirators than meets the eye. *Occup Health Safety* 1989; Oct:50–58.
162. ECRI: Tuberculosis, part II: Respirators and recommendations. *Technol Respir Ther* 1992; 13:1–4.
163. Dooley SW, Castro KG, Hutton MD, et al: Guidelines for preventing the transmission of tuberculosis in health-care setting, with special focus on HIV-related issues. *MMWR* 1190; 39.

SUGGESTED READING

Ballard K, Cheeseman T, Ripiner T, et al: Humidification of ventilated patients. *Intensive Crit Care Nurs* 1992; 8:2–9.

Barnes KL, et al: Bacterial contamination of home nebulizers. *BMJ* 1987; 295:812.

Baumgart S, Engle WD, Fox WW, et al: Effect of heat shielding on convective and evaporative heat losses and on radiant heat transfer in the premature infant. *J Pediatr* 1981; 99:948.

Bowton DL, Goldsmith WM, Haponik EF: Substitution of metered-dose inhalers for hand-held nebulizers: Success and cost savings in a large acute-care hospital. *Chest* 1992; 101: 305–308.

British Standards Institution: *Specifications for Humidifiers for Use With Breathing Machines BS 4494.* London, 1970.

Centers for Disease Control: Nosocomial transmission of multi-drug resistant TB to health-care workers and HIV infected patients in an urban hospital—Florida. *MMWR* 1990; 39:718–722.

Chatburn RL: Physiologic and methodologic issues regarding humidity therapy (editorial). *J Pediatr* 1989; 114:418–420.

Chernick V: Why intermittent positive pressure when normal inhalations will do (editorial)? *J Pediatr* 1977; 1:361–362.

Cohen IL, Weinberg PF, Fein IA, et al: Endotracheal tube occlusion associated with the use of heat and moisture exchangers in the intensive care unit. *Crit Care Med* 1988; 16:277–279.

Corr D, Dolovich M, McCormack D, et al: Design and characteristics of a portable breath actuated, particle size selective medical aerosol inhaler. *J Aerosol Sci* 1982; 13:1.

Cushing IE, Miller WF: Considerations in humidification by nebulization. *Dis Chest* 1958; 34:388–403.

Dolovich M: Clinical aspects of aerosol physics. *Respir Care* 1991; 36:931–938.

Dolovich MB, Killian D, Wolff RK, et al: Pulmonary aerosol deposition in chronic bronchitis: Intermittent positive pressure breathing versus quiet breathing. *Am Rev Respir Dis* 1977; 115:397–402.

Eckerbom B, Lindholm CE: Laboratory evaluation of heat and moisture exchangers. Assessment of the Draft International Standard (ISO/DIS 9360) in practice. *Acta Anaesthesiol Scand* 1990; 34:291–295.

Eckerbom B, Lindholm CE, Mannting F: Mucocilliary transport with and without the use of a heat and moisture exchanger. An animal study. *Acta Anaesthesiol Scand* 1991; 35:297–301.

Gelmont DM, Balmes JR, Yee A: Hypokalemia induced by inhaled bronchodilators. *Chest* 1988; 94:763–766.

Georgopoulos D, Wong D, Anthonisen NR: Tolerance to β_2-agonists in patients with chronic obstructive pulmonary disease (COPD) (abstract). *Am Rev Respir Dis* 1989; 139:12.

Intermittent Positive Pressure Breathing Trial Group: Intermittent positive pressure breathing therapy of chronic obstructive pulmonary disease: A clinical trial. *Ann Intern Med* 1983; 99:612–620.

Kahn RC: Humidification of the airways adequate for function and integrity? *Chest* 1983; 84:510–511.

Lomholdt N, Cooke R, Lundig M: A method of humidification in ventilator treatment of neonates. *Br J Anaesth* 1968; 40:335.

Mancebo J, Amaro P, Lorino H, et al: Effects of albuterol inhalation on the work of breathing during weaning from mechanical ventilation. *Am Rev Respir Dis* 1991; 144:95–100.

Martin C, Perrin G, Gevaudan MJ, et al: Heat and moisture exchangers and vaporizing humidifiers in the intensive care unit. *Chest* 1990; 97:144–149.

McPherson SP: *Respiratory Therapy Equipment,* ed 4. St Louis, Mosby–Year Book, 1990.

Misset B, Escudier B, Rivara D, et al: Heat and moisture exchanger vs heated humidifier during long-term mechanical ventilation. A prospective randomized study. *Chest* 1991; 100:160–163.

Montgomery AB, Debs RJ, Luce JM, et al: Aerosolized pentamidine as sole therapy for *Pneumocystis carinii* pneumonia in patients with acquired immunodeficiency syndrome. *Lancet* 1987; 2:480–483.

Murray JF: Review of the state of the art in intermittent positive pressure breathing therapy. *Am Rev Respir Dis* 1974; 110:193–199.

Nelson D, McDonald JS: Heated humidification temperature control and rainout in neonatal ventilation. *Perinatol Neonatol* 1977; 1:23–42.

Nelson MS, Hofstadter A, Parker J, et al: Frequency of inhaled metaproterenol in the treatment of acute asthma exacerbation. *Ann Emerg Med* 1990; 19:21–25.

Newman SP, Clarke SW: Aerosols in therapy, in Moren F, Newhouse MT, Dolovich MB (eds): *Aerosols in Medicine: Principles, Diagnosis and Therapy.* Amsterdam, Elsevier, 1985, pp 289–312.

O'Hagan M, Reid E, Tarnow-Mordi WO: Is neonatal inspired gas humidity accurately controlled by humidifier temperature? *Crit Care Med* 1991; 19:1370–1373.

Pierce AK, Salzman HA: Intermittent positive pressure breathing therapy. *Am Rev Respir Dis* 1974; 110:13–15.

Proctor D: Physiology of the upper airway, in Vischer MB, Hasting AB, Pappenhiemer JR, et al (eds): *Handbook of Physiology—Respiration 1.* Baltimore, Williams & Wilkins, 1985, pp 323–325.

Reisman J, Galdes-Sebalt M, Kazim F, et al: Frequent administration by inhalation of salbutamol and ipratropium bromide in the initial management of severe acute asthma in children. *J Allergy Clin Immunol* 1988; 81:16–20.

Repsher LH, Anderson JA, Bush RK, et al: Assessment of tachyphylaxis following prolonged therapy of asthma with inhaled albuterol aerosol. *Chest* 1984; 85:34–38.

Sears MR, et al: 75 deaths in asthmatics prescribed home nebulizers. *BMJ* 1987; 294:477–480.

Singer OP, Wilson WJ: Laryngotracheobronchitis: 2 years' experience with racemic epinephrine. *Can Med Assoc J* 1976; 115:132–134.

Suzukawa M, Usuda Y, Katsuo N: The effects on sputum characteristics of combining an unheated humidifier with a heat-moisture exchanging filter. *Respir Care* 1989; 34:976–984.

Tarnow-Mordi WO, Reid E, Griffiths P, et al: Low inspired gas humidity and respiratory complications in very low birth weight infants. *J Pediatr* 1989; 114:438.

Tarnow-Mordi WO, Sutton P, Wilkonson AR: Inadequate humidification of respiratory gases during artificial ventilation. *Arch Dis Child* 1986; 61:698.

Thomas P, Williams T, Reilly PA, et al: Modifying delivery techniques of fenoterol from a metered dose inhaler. *Ann Allergy* 1984; 52:279–281.

Thomas SHL, Langford JA, George RDG, et al: Improving the efficiency of drug administration with jet nebulizers (letter). *Lancet* 1988; 1:126.

Turner JR, Corkery KJ, Eckman D, et al: Equivalence of continuous flow nebulizer and metered-dose inhaler with reservoir bag for treatment of acute airflow obstruction. *Chest* 1988; 93:476–481.

Appendix 3–1.

AARC Clinical Practice Guideline
Humidification during Mechanical Ventilation

HMV 1.0 PROCEDURE:

The addition of heat and moisture to inspired gases delivered to the patient during mechanical ventilatory support via an artificial airway

HMV 2.0 DESCRIPTION/DEFINITION:

When the upper airway is bypassed, humidification during mechanical ventilation is necessary to prevent hypothermia, inspissation of airway secretions, destruction of airway epithelium, and atelectasis.[1–7] This may be accomplished using either a heated humidifier or a heat and moisture exchanger (HME). (HMEs are also known as hygroscopic condenser humidifiers, or artificial noses). The chosen device should provide a minimum of 30 mg H_2O/L of delivered gas at 30°C.[8–10] Heated humidifiers operate actively to increase the heat and water vapor content of inspired gas.[11–14] HMEs operate passively by storing heat and moisture from the patient's exhaled gas and releasing it to the inhaled gas.[15–25]

HMV 3.0 SETTINGS:

3.1 Critical care
3.2 Acute care inpatient
3.3 Extended care and skilled nursing facility
3.4 Home care
3.5 Prolonged transport

HMV 4.0 INDICATIONS:

Humidification of inspired gas during mechanical ventilation is mandatory when an endotracheal or tracheostomy tube is present.[1–7]

HMV 5.0 CONTRAINDICATIONS:

There are no contraindications to providing physiologic conditioning of inspired gas during mechanical ventilation. An HME is contraindicated under some circumstances.

5.1 Use of an HME is contraindicated for patients with thick, copious, or bloody secretions.[8, 26–28]
5.2 Use of an HME is contraindicated for patients with an expired tidal volume less than 70% of the delivered tidal volume (eg, those with large bronchopleurocutaneous fistulas or incompetent or absent endotracheal tube cuffs).[15–25]
5.3 Use of an HME is contraindicated for patients with body temperatures less than 32°C.[8, 29]
5.4 Use of an HME may be contraindicated for patients with high spontaneous minute volumes (> 10 L/min).[8, 26, 29]
5.5 An HME must be removed from the patient circuit during aerosol treatments when the nebulizer is placed in the patient circuit.[8, 29]

HMV 6.0 HAZARDS/COMPLICATIONS:

Hazards and complications associated with the use of humidification devices include

6.1 potential for electrical shock—heated humidifiers;[11–14]
6.2 hypothermia—HME or heated humidifiers; hyperthermia—heated humidifiers;[11–14]
6.3 thermal injury to the airway from heated humidifiers;[30] burns to the patient and tubing meltdown if heated-wire circuits are covered or circuits and humidifiers are incompatible;
6.4 underhydration and impaction of mucus secretions—HME or heated humidifiers;[1–7]
6.5 hypoventilation and/or alveolar gas trapping due to mucus plugging of airways—HME or heated humidifier;[1–7]

6.6 possible increased resistive work of breathing due to mucus plugging of airways—HME or heated humidifiers,[1–7]
6.7 possible increased resistive work of breathing through the humidifier—HME or heated humidifiers;[31–34]
6.8 possible hypoventilation due to increased dead space—HME;[8, 15–25, 26–30]
6.9 inadvertent overfilling resulting in unintentional tracheal lavage—heated reservoir humidifiers;[35]
6.10 the fact that when disconnected from the patient, some ventilators generate a high flow through the patient circuit that may aerosolize contaminated condensate, putting both the patient and clinician at risk for nosocomial infection—heated humidifiers;[35]
6.11 potential for burns to caregivers from hot metal—heated humidifiers;
6.12 inadvertent tracheal lavage from pooled condensate in patient circuit—heated humidifiers;[35]
6.13 elevated airway pressures due to pooled condensation—heated humidifiers;
6.14 patient-ventilator dysynchrony and improper ventilator performance due to pooled condensation in the circuit—heated humidifiers;
6.15 ineffective low-pressure alarm during disconnection due to resistance through HME.[36]

HMV 7.0 LIMITATIONS OF METHODS:

7.1 Insufficient heat and humidification can occur with some HME devices, resulting in complications noted in HMV 6.0.[8, 15–28]
7.2 Insufficient heat and humidification can occur with heated humidifiers and result in complications noted in HMV 6.0 when
7.2.1 improper temperature settings are selected.
7.2.2 water level in the humidifier falls below manufacturer's suggested level.[37]
7.3 The HME selected should be appropriate to the patient's size and tidal volume.

HMV 8.0 ASSESSMENT OF NEED:

Humidification is needed by all patients requiring mechanical ventilation via an artificial airway. Conditioning of inspired gases should be instituted using either an HME or a heated humidifier.

8.1 HMEs are better suited for short-term use ($\leq$96 hours) and during transport.[8, 29]
8.2 Heated humidifiers should be used for patients requiring long-term mechanical ventilation ($>$96 hours) or for patients who exhibit contraindications for HME use.[8, 29]

HMV 9.0 ASSESSMENT OF OUTCOME:

Humidification is assumed to be appropriate if, on regular careful inspection, the patient exhibits none of the hazards or complications listed in HMV 6.0.

HMV 10.0 RESOURCES:

10.1 **Equipment:** Appropriate equipment should be available to provide for adequate humidification of the inspired gas. Such equipment may include but is not limited to
10.1.1 humidification device;
10.1.2 a system to monitor inspired gas temperature and to alarm when the temperature falls outside a preset range (for heated humidifier);
10.1.3 sterile water for heated humidifiers;
10.1.4 equipment necessary to comply with Universal Precautions.
10.2 Humidifier performance specifications should be checked to assure adequate heating and humidification during expected peak inspiratory flowrate and minute ventilation delivered by the mechanical ventilator. Heated humidifiers selected for use should meet specifications of the American National Standards Institute.[9]
10.3 **Personnel:**
10.3.1 **Level-I** personnel should possess
10.3.1.1 a complete understanding of the operation, maintenance, and troubleshooting of the ventilator, circuit, and humidifying device;
10.3.1.2 knowledge of and ability to implement Universal Precautions.
10.3.2 **Level-II** personnel should possess the abilities described in 10.3.1.1 and 10.3.1.2 and should also have
10.3.2.1 the ability to assess patient response to humidification;
10.3.2.2 the ability to recognize an adverse response to humidification;
10.3.2.3 the ability to appropriately respond to adverse events;
10.3.2.4 the ability to recommend modifications in humidification techniques as appropriate.

HMV 11.0 MONITORING:

The humidification device should be inspected visually during the patient-ventilator system check and condensate should be removed from the patient circuit as necessary. HMEs should be inspected and replaced if secretions have contaminated the insert or filter. The following variables should be recorded during equipment inspection:

11.1 **Humidifier setting** (temperature setting or numeric dial setting or both). During routine use on an intubated patient, a heated humidifier should be set to deliver an inspired gas temperature of 33 ± 2°C and should provide a minimum of 30 mg/L of water vapor.[8–10]

11.2 **Inspired gas temperature.** Temperature should be monitored as near the patient's airway opening as possible, if a heated humidifier is used.

11.2.1 Specific temperatures may vary with patient condition, but the inspiratory gas should not exceed 37°C at the airway threshold.

11.2.2 When a heated-wire patient circuit is used (to prevent condensation) on an infant, the temperature probe should be located outside of the incubator or away from the direct heat of the radiant warmer.[12]

11.3 **Alarm settings** (if applicable). High temperature alarm should be set no higher than 37°C, and the low temperature alarm should be set no lower than 30°C.[8, 10]

11.4 **Water level and function of automatic feed system** (if applicable).

11.5 **Quantity and consistency of secretions.** Characteristics should be noted and recorded. When using an HME, if secretions become copious or appear increasingly tenacious, a heated humidifier should replace the HME.

HMV 12.0 FREQUENCY:

All patients with an artificial airway requiring mechanical ventilation should receive continuous humidification of inspired gases.

HMV 13.0 INFECTION CONTROL:

13.1 Reusable heated humidifiers should be subjected to high-level disinfection between patients.[35] Clean technique should be observed when manually filling the water reservoir. Sterile water should be used.

13.2 When using a closed, automatic feed system, the unused portion of water in the water feed reservoir remains sterile and need not be discarded when the patient circuit is changed. However, the water feed system should be designated for single patient use only.

13.3 Condensation from the patient circuit should be considered infectious waste and disposed of according to hospital policy using strict Universal Precautions.[35, 38, 39]

13.4 Because condensate is infectious waste, it should never be drained back into the humidifier reservoir.[35, 38, 39]

Mechanical Ventilation Guidelines Committee:

Richard D Branson RRT, Chairman, Cincinnati OH
Robert S Campbell RRT, Cincinnati OH
Robert L Chatburn RRT, Cleveland OH
Jack Covington RRT, San Francisco CA

REFERENCES

1. Mercke U. The influence of varying air humidity on mucociliary activity. *Acta Otolaryngol* 1975; 79:133–139.
2. Marfatia S, Donahue PK, Henren WH. Effect of dry and humidified gases on the respiratory epithelium in rabbits. *J Pediatr Surg* 1975; 40:583–585.
3. Chalon J, Loew DAY, Malebranche J. Effect of dry anaesthetic gases on the tracheobronchial epithelium. *Anaesthesiology* 1972; 37:338.
4. Proctor D. Physiology of the upper airway. In: Vischer MB, Hastings AB, Pappenhiemer JR, Rahn H, eds. *Handbook of physiology—respiration 1*. Baltimore: Williams & Wilkins, 1985:323–325.
5. Moritz AR, Weisiger JR. Effects of cold air on the air passages and lungs. *Arch Intern Med* 1945; 75:233–240.
6. Burton JDK. Effects of dry anaesthetic gases on the respiratory mucus membrane. *Lancet* 1962; 1:235.
7. Dahlby RW, Hogg JC. Effect of breathing dry air on structure and function of airways. *J Appl Physiol* 1980; 61(1):312–317.
8. Branson RD. *Humidification of inspired gases during mechanical ventilation.* 1991; 3:55–66.
9. American National Standards Institute. Standard for humidifiers and nebulizers for medical use. *ANSI* Z79; 9, 1979.
10. Chatburn RL, Primiano FP Jr. A rational basis for humidity therapy. *Respir Care* 1987; 32:249–253.
11. Chamney AR. Humidification requirements and techniques. *Anaesthesia* 1969; 24:602.
12. Chatburn RL. Physiologic and methodologic issues regarding humidity therapy. *J Pediatr* 1989; 114:416–420.

13. Department of Health and Social Security. Evaluation of heated humidifiers. *Health Equipment Information* 1987; 177.
14. Emergency Care Research Institute. Heated humidifiers. *Health Devices* 1987; 16(7):223.
15. Branson RD, Hurst JM. Laboratory evaluation of moisture output of seven airway heat and moisture exchangers. *Respir Care* 1987; 32:741–747.
16. Shelly MP, Bethune DW, Latimer RD. A comparison of five heat and moisture exchangers. *Anaesthesia* 1986; 41:527–532.
17. Revenas B, Lindholm CE. The foam nose—new disposable heat and moisture exchanger: a comparison with other similar devices. *Acta Anaesthesiol Scand* 1979; 23:34–39.
18. Ogino M, Kopotic R, Mannino FL. Moisture-conserving efficiency of condenser humidifiers. *Anaesthesia* 1985; 40:990–995.
19. Leigh JM, White MG. A new condenser humidifier (letter). *Anaesthesia* 1984; 39:492–493.
20. Mebius CL. A comparative evaluation of disposable humidifiers. *Acta Anaesthesiol Scand* 1983; 27:403–409.
21. Gedeon A, Mebius C. The hygroscopic condenser humidifier: a new device for general use in anaesthesia and intensive care. *Anaesthesia* 1979; 34:1043–1047.
22. Chalon J, Markham JP, Ali MM, Ramanathan S, Turndorf H. The Pall Ultipor breathing circuit filter: an efficient heat and moisture exchanger. *Anaesth Analg* 1984; 63:566–570.
23. Weeks DB, Ramsey FM. Laboratory investigation of six artificial noses for use during endotracheal anaesthesia. *Anesth Analg* 1983; 62:758–763.
24. Walker AK, Bethune DW. A comparative study of condenser humidifiers. *Anaesthesia* 1976; 31:1086–1093.
25. Turtle MJ, Ilsley AH, Rutten AJ, Runciman WB. An evaluation of six disposable heat and moisture exchangers. *Anaesth Intensive Care* 1987; 15:317–322.
26. Cohen IL, Weinberg PF, Fein IA, Rowiniski GS. Endotracheal tube occlusion associated with the use of heat moisture exchangers in the intensive care unit. *Crit Care Med* 1988; 16:277–279.
27. Perch SA, Realey AM. Effectiveness of the Servo SH150 artificial nose humidifier: a case report. *Respir Care 1984;* 29:1009–1012.
28. Martin C, Perrin G, Gevaudan MJ, Saux P, Gouin F. Heat and moisture exchangers and vaporizing humidifiers in the intensive care unit. *Chest* 1990; 97:144–149.
29. Shelly MP, Lloyd GM, Park GR. A review of the mechanisms and methods of humidification of inspired gas. *Intensive Care Med* 1988; 14:1–9.
30. Klein EF Jr, Graves SA. "Hot pot" tracheitis. *Chest* 1974; 65:225–226.
31. Ploysongsang Y, Branson RD, Rashkin MC, Hurst JM. Pressure flow characteristics of commonly used heat-moisture exchangers. *Am Rev Respir Dis* 1988; 138:675–678.
32. Ploysongsang Y, Branson RD, Rashkin MC, Hurst JM. Effect of flow rate and duration of use on the pressure drop across six artificial noses. *Respir Care* 1989; 34:902–907.
33. Nishimura M, Nishijima MK, Okada T, Taenaka N, Yoshiya I. Comparison of flow-resistive workload due to humidifying devices. *Chest* 1990; 97:600–604.
34. Marini JJ. Strategies to minimize breathing effort during mechanical ventilation. *Crit Care Clin* 1990; 6:635–661.
35. Craven DE, Steger KA. Pathogenesis and prevention of nosocomial pneumonia in the mechanically ventilated patient. *Respir Care* 1989; 34:85–97.
36. Slee TA, Paulin EG. Failure of low pressure alarm associated with the use of a humidifier. *Anesthesiology* 1988; 69:791–793.
37. O'Hagan M, Reid E, Tarnow-Mordi WO. Is neonatal inspired gas humidity accurately controlled by humidifier temperature? *Crit Care Med* 1991; 19:1370–1373.
38. Centers for Disease Control. Update: Universal Precautions for prevention of transmission of human immunodeficiency virus, hepatitis B virus, and other blood-borne pathogens in health care settings. *MMWR* 1988; 37:377–388.
39. Boyce JM, White RL, Spruill EY, Wall M. Cost-effective application of the Centers for Disease Control guidelines for prevention of nosocomial pneumonia. *Am J Infect Control* 1985; 13:228–232.

Appendix 3–2.

AARC Clinical Practice Guideline
Selection of Aerosol Delivery Device

AD 1.0 PROCEDURE:

Selection of a device for delivery of aerosol to the lower airways

AD 2.0 DESCRIPTION:

The selection of a device for administration of pharmacologically active aerosol to the lower airway. The device selected should produce particles with a mass median aerodynamic diameter (MMAD) of 2–5 microns.[1, 2]

These devices include

Metered dose inhalers (MDI)
MDIs with accessory device (eg, spacer)
Dry powder inhalers (DPI)
Small volume nebulizers (SVN)
Large volume nebulizers (LVN)
Ultrasonic nebulizers (USN)

This guideline does not address bland aerosol administration and sputum induction.

AD 3.0 SETTING:

Aerosol therapy can be administered in a number of settings including hospital, clinic, extended care facility, and home.

AD 4.0 INDICATIONS:

The need to deliver—as an aerosol to the lower airways—a medication from one of the following drug classifications:

Beta adrenergic agents
Anticholinergic agents (antimuscarinics)
Anti-inflammatory agents (eg, corticosteroids)
Mediator-modifying compounds (eg, cromolyn sodium)
Mucokinetics

The selection of a device for delivery of aerosol for parenchymal deposition (eg, antibiotics) will be addressed in another Guideline.

AD 5.0 CONTRAINDICATIONS:

5.1 No contraindications exist to the administration of aerosols by inhalation.
5.2 Contraindications related to the substances being delivered may exist. Consult the package insert for product-specific contraindications.

AD 6.0 HAZARDS/COMPLICATIONS:

6.1 Malfunction of device[3–5] and/or improper technique[6–12] may result in underdosing.
6.2 The potential exists for malfunction of device and/or improper technique (inappropriate patient use) to result in overdosing.
6.3 Complications of specific pharmacologic agent may occur.
6.4 Cardiotoxic effects of Freon have been reported as an idiosyncratic response that may be a problem with excessive use of MDI.[13–18]
6.5 Freon may affect the environment by its effect on the ozone layer.[19–21]
6.6 Repeated exposure to aerosols has been reported to produce asthmatic symptoms in some caregivers.[22]

AD 7.0 LIMITATIONS OF PROCEDURE OR DEVICE:

7.1 Only a small percent of output deposits in the airway ($\leq 10\%$).[23–27]
7.2 Efficacy of the device is technique dependent (eg, coordination, breathing pattern, inspira-

tory hold).[6–9, 28–32] The reader is referred to *Kacmarek RM, Hess D. The interface between patient and aerosol generator. Respir Care 1991; 36:952–976* for detailed descriptions of optimal technique.

7.3 Efficacy of the device is design dependent (ie, output and particle size).[4, 5, 33]

7.4 Reduced deposition of aerosol to the lower airways is associated with the following and may require consideration of increased dose:

7.4.1 mechanical ventilation;[26, 27, 34–36]

7.4.2 artificial airways;[34–39]

7.4.3 airway caliber (eg, infants and children);[22, 37–39]

7.4.4 severity of obstruction.[40–42]

7.5 Patient compliance[12]

7.6 Limitations of specific devices

7.6.1 Metered Dose Inhaler:

7.6.1.1 Environmental concerns(CFC)[20, 21]

7.6.1.2 Inadequate technique[6–8, 28–32, 43]

7.6.1.3 Inadequate instruction[9–12]

7.6.2 MDI accessory device (spacer or holding chamber):

7.6.2.1 Adds to cost over MDI alone

7.6.2.2 More bulky than MDI alone

7.6.3 Dry powder inhaler:

7.6.3.1 At the present time, patients must load each dose for most medications.

7.6.3.2 Reduced inspiratory flow (< 60 L/min) can lead to reduced deposition.[44–46]

7.6.3.3 Irritation to airway[33]

7.6.3.4 Humidity may cause clumping of particles.

7.6.4 Small Volume Nebulizer:

7.6.4.1 Time- and labor-intensive

7.6.4.2 Less portable

7.6.4.3 Requires compressed-gas source or electricity

7.6.4.4 Vulnerable to contamination[47–50]

7.6.4.5 Lack of convenience may affect patient compliance

7.6.5 Large Volume Nebulizer:

7.6.5.1 Limited to acute and critical care setting

7.6.5.2 Requires close monitoring

7.6.5.3 Time- and cost-intensive

7.6.5.4 Vulnerable to contamination[46–49]

7.6.5.5 Reconcentration of solution may occur over long period of time due to evaporation by dry gas.

7.6.6 Ultrasonic Nebulizer:

7.6.6.1 Cost of device

7.6.6.2 Mechanical reliability

7.6.6.3 Requires electrical power source

7.6.6.4 Vulnerable to contamination

AD 8.0 ASSESSMENT OF NEED:

8.1 Based on proven therapeutic efficacy,[25, 51–60] variety of available medications, and cost-effectiveness[51, 61–64] the MDI with accessory device should be the first method to consider for administration of aerosol to the airway.

8.2 Lack of availability of prescribed drug in MDI, dry powder, or solution form.

8.3 Inability of the patient to use device properly with coaching and instruction should lead to consideration of other devices.

8.4 Patient preference for a given device that meets therapeutic objectives should be honored.

8.5 When there is need for large doses, MDI, SVN, or LVN may be used. Clear superiority of any one method has not been established. Convenience and patient tolerance of procedure should be considered.

8.6 When spontaneous ventilation is inadequate (eg, as in kyphoscoliosis or neuromuscular disorders, exacerbation of severe bronchospasm with impending respiratory failure that does not respond to other forms of therapy), delivery by a positive pressure breathing device (IPPB) should be considered.[65–67]

AD 9.0 ASSESSMENT OF OUTCOME:

9.1 Proper technique applying device

9.2 Patient response to or compliance with procedure

9.3 Objectively measured improvement (eg, increased FEV_1 or peak flow)

AD 10.0 RESOURCES:

10.1 Equipment:

10.1.1 MDI—canister with actuator supplied by manufacturer; MDI accessory device that properly fits MDI mouthpiece or mask; adapters for specific circumstances (eg, tracheostomy)

10.1.2 Small volume nebulizer—gas source, tubing, flowmeter, and mouthpiece or mask

10.1.3 **Large volume nebulizer**—gas source, flowmeter, connecting tubing, and mouthpiece or mask

10.1.4 **Mechanical ventilator**—SVN or MDI, adapter in inspiratory line of circuit

10.1.5 **IPPB machine** (i.e., pressure-limited ventilator)—nebulizer, gas source, connecting tubing, and mouthpiece or mask

10.1.6 **Manual resuscitator**—for 'bagging in' aerosol from MDI or SVN

10.2 Personnel:

10.2.1 Knowledge and skills at several levels are required to fully utilize and apply these devices.

10.2.1.1 Level II personnel provide initial assessments and care of the unstable patient:

10.2.1.1.1 utilizing proper technique for administration of MDI, accessory device, dry powder inhaler, SVN, LVN, USN; and SVN via IPPB;

10.2.1.1.2 practicing proper use, maintenance, and cleaning of equipment;

10.2.1.1.3 encouraging effective breathing patterns and coughing techniques;

10.2.1.1.4 modifying technique in response to adverse reactions;

10.2.1.1.5 modifying dosages and/or frequency as prescribed in response to severity of symptoms;

10.2.1.1.6 assessing patient condition and response to therapy;

10.2.1.1.7 performing auscultation and inspection and taking vital signs;

10.2.1.1.8 performing peak expiratory flowrate, spirometry, or ventilatory mechanics;

10.2.1.1.9 recognizing and responding to therapeutic and adverse responses and complications of medication and/or procedure;

10.2.1.1.10 understanding and complying with Universal Precautions.

10.2.1.2 The patient, family, or home caregiver; Level-I hospital personnel provide routine care of the patient:

10.2.1.2.1 preparing, measuring, and mixing medication;

10.2.1.2.2 demonstrating proper technique for administration of medication;

10.2.1.2.3 using equipment properly;

10.2.1.2.4 cleaning equipment;

10.2.1.2.5 encouraging effective breathing patterns and coughing techniques;

10.2.1.2.6 modifying technique in response to adverse reactions as instructed, with appropriate communication with physician or Level-II care provider;

10.2.1.2.7 modifying dosages and/or frequency as prescribed, with appropriate communication with physician, in response to severity of symptoms;

10.2.1.2.8 using the peak flowmeter properly and documenting results.

AD 11.0 MONITORING:

11.1 Performance of the device

11.2 Technique of device application

11.3 Assessment of patient response including changes in vital signs

AD 12.0 FREQUENCY:

12.1 Initiation of therapy after careful assessment of need (as outlined above)

12.2 The change from one type of device to another is based on a change in patient's condition or ability to use the specific device.

AD 13.0 INFECTION CONTROL:

13.1 Universal Precautions must be exercised for body substance isolation.[67]

13.2 SVN and LVN are for single patient use or should be subjected to high-level disinfection between patients.

13.3 Published data establishing a safe use-period for SVN and LVN are lacking; however they probably should be changed or subjected to high-level disinfection at approximately 24-hour intervals.

13.4 Medications:

13.4.1 Medications should be handled aseptically.

13.4.2 Tap water should not be used as the diluent.[69]

13.4.3 Medications from multidose sources in acute care facilities must be handled aseptically and discarded after 24 hours, unless manufacturer's recommendations specifically state that medications may be stored longer than 24 hours.

13.5 MDI accessory devices are for single patient use only. Cleaning of accessory devices is based on aesthetic criteria.

13.6 There are no documented concerns with contamination of medication in MDI canisters.

Aerosol Guidelines Committee:

Jon Nilsestuen PhD RRT, Chairman, Houston TX
Jim Fink MBA RRT, San Francisco CA
Theodore Witek Jr DrPH RPFT RRT, Ridgefield CT
James Volpe III MEd RRT, San Diego CA

REFERENCES

1. Dolovich M. Clinical aspects of aerosol physics. *Respir Care* 1991; 36:931–938.
2. Dolovich M. Physical principles underlying aerosol therapy. *J Aerosol Med* 1989; 2:171–186.
3. Merkus PJFM, van Essen-Zandlilet EEM, Parievliet E, Borsboom G, Sterk PJ, Kerrebijn KF, et al. Changes of nebulizer output over the years. *Eur Respir J* 1992; 5:488–491.
4. Sterk PJ, Plomp A, van de Vate JF, Quanjer PH. Physical properties of aerosols produced by several jet and ultrasonic nebulisers. *Bull Eur Physiopathol Respir* 1984; 20:65–72.
5. Alvine GF, Rodgers P, Fitzsimmons KM, Ahrens RC. Disposable jet nebulizers: how reliable are they? *Chest* 1991; 101:316–319.
6. Allen SC, Prior A. What determines whether an elderly patient can use a metered dose inhaler correctly? *Br J Dis Chest* 1986; 80:45–49.
7. Lindgren S, Bake B, Larsson S. Clinical consequences of inadequate inhalation technique in asthma therapy. *Eur J Respir Dis* 1987; 70:93–98.
8. Orehek J, Gayrard P, Grimaud C, Charpin J. Patient error in use of bronchodilator metered aerosols. *Br Med J* 1976; 1:76.
9. Guidry GG, Brown WD, Stogner SW, George RB. Incorrect use of metered dose inhalers by medical personnel. *Chest* 1992; 101:31–33.
10. Brashear RE. Pressurized aerosol bronchodilator instruction. *Chest* 1983; 84:117.
11. Newman SP, Clarke SW. The proper use of metered dose inhalers. *Chest* 1984; 86:342–344.
12. DeBlaquiere P, Christensen DB, Carter WB, Martin TK. Use and misuse of metered-dose inhalers by patients with chronic lung disease. *Am Rev Respir Dis* 1989; 140:910–916.
13. Speizer FE, Doll R, Heaf P. Observations on recent increase in mortality from asthma. *Br Med J* 1968; 1: 339–343.
14. Bass M. Sudden sniffing deaths. *JAMA* 1970; 212:2075–2079.
15. Speizer FE, Wegman DH, Ramirez A. Palpitation rates associated with fluorocarbon exposure in a hospital setting. *N Engl J Med* 1975; 292:624–626.
16. Brooks SM, Mintz S, Weiss E. Changes occurring after Freon inhalation. *Am Rev Respir Dis* 1972; 105:640–643.
17. Dollery CT, Williams FM, Draffan GH, Wise G, Sahyoun H, Paterson JW, et al. Artificial blood levels of fluorocarbons in asthmatic patients following use of pressurized aerosols. *Clin Pharmacol Ther* 1974; 15:59–66.
18. Paterson JW, Sudlow MF, Walker SR. Blood levels of fluorinated hydrocarbons in asthmatic patients after inhalation of pressurized aerosols. *Lancet* 1971; 2:565.
19. Silverglade A. Cardiac toxicity of aerosol propellants (editorial). *JAMA* 1972; 222:827–828.
20. Newman SP. Metered dose pressurized aerosols and the ozone layer. *Eur Respir J* 1990; 3:395–397.
21. Balmes JR. Propellant gases in metered dose inhalers: their impact on the global environment. *Respir Care* 1991; 36:1037–1044.
22. Kern DG, Franklin H. Asthma in respiratory therapists. *Ann Intern Med* 1989; 110:767–773.
23. Davis DS. Pharmacokinetics of inhaled substances. *Postgrad Med J* 1975; 51(Suppl 7):69–75.
24. Newhouse MT, Dolovich MB. Current concepts—control of asthma by aerosols. *N Engl J Med* 1986; 315:870–874.
25. Ruffin RE, Kenworthy MC, Newhouse MT. Response of asthmatic patients to fenoterol inhalation: a method of quantifying the airway bronchodilator dose. *Clin Pharmacol Ther* 1978; 23:338–345.
26. Fuller HD, Dolovich MB, Posmituck G, Wong Pack W, Newhouse MT. Pressurized aerosol versus jet aerosol delivery to mechanically ventilated patients: comparison of dose to the lungs. *Am Rev Respir Dis* 1990; 141:440–444.
27. Fernandez A, Lazaro A, Garcia E, Aragon C, Cerda E. Bronchodilators in patients with chronic obstructive pulmonary disease on mechanical ventilation: utilization of metered-dose inhalers. *Am Rev Respir Dis* 1990; 141:164–168.
28. Crompton GK. Problems patients have using pressurized aerosol inhalers. *Eur J Respir Dis* 1982; 63(Suppl 119):101–104.
29. O'Connell MB, Hewitt JM, Lacker TE. Consistency of evaluators assessing inhaler technique. *Ann Allergy* 1991; 67:603–608.
30. DeTullio PL, Corson ME. Effect of pharmacist counseling on ambulatory patients: use of aerosolized bronchodilators. *Am J Hosp Pharm* 1987; 44:1802–1806.
31. Self TH, Brooks JB, Lieberman P, Ryan MR. The value of demonstration and role of the pharmacist in teaching the correct use of pressurized bronchodilators. *Can Med Assoc J* 1983; 128:129–131.
32. Woodcock A. Training aid for pressurized inhalers. *Br J Dis Chest* 1980; 74:395–397.

33. Newman SP. Aerosol generators and delivery systems. *Respir Care* 1991; 36:939–951.
34. Gay PC, Patel HG, Nelson SB, Gilles B, Hubmayr RD. Metered dose inhalers for bronchodilator delivery in intubated, mechanically ventilated patients. *Chest* 1991; 99:66–71.
35. Cameron D, Clay M, Silverman M. Evaluation of nebulizers for use in neonatal ventilatory circuits. *Crit Care Med* 1990; 18:886–870.
36. MacIntyre NR, Silver RM, Miller CW, Schuyler F, Coleman RE. Aerosol delivery in intubated, mechanically ventilated patients. *Crit Care Med* 1985; 13:81–85.
37. Ahrens RC, Ries RA, Popendorf W, Wiese JA. The delivery of therapeutic aerosols through endotracheal tubes. *Pediatr Pulmonol* 1986; 2:19–26.
38. Crogan SJ, Bishop MJ. Delivery efficiency of metered dose aerosols given via endotracheal tubes. *Anesthesiology* 1989; 68:964–966.
39. Yu CP, Nicolaides P, Soong TT. Effect of random airway sizes on aerosol deposition. *Am Ind Hyg Assoc J* 1979; 40:999–1005.
40. Kim CS, Lewars GA, Sackner MA. Measurement of total lung aerosol deposition as an index of lung abnormality. *J Appl Physiol* 1988; 64:1527–1536.
41. Dolovich MB, Sanchis J, Rossman C, Newhouse MT. Aerosol penetrance: a sensitive index of peripheral airway obstruction. *J Appl Physiol* 1976; 40:468–471.
42. Ilowite JS, Gorvoy JD, Smaldone GC. Quantitative deposition of aerosolized gentamicin in cystic fibrosis. *Am Rev Respir Dis* 1987; 136:1445–1449.
43. Lindgren S, Bake B, Larsson S. Clinical consequences of inadequate inhalation technique in asthma therapy. *Eur J Respir Dis* 1987; 70:93–98.
44. Pedersen S. Treatment of acute bronchoconstriction in children with a tube spacer aerosol and a dry powder inhaler. *Allergy* 1985; 40:300–303.
45. Assoufi BK, Hodson ME. High dose salbutamol in chronic airflow obstruction: comparison of nebulizer with Rotacaps. *Respir Med* 1989; 83:415–420.
46. van Lunteren E, Coreno A. Inhaled albuterol powder for pulmonary function testing. *Chest* 1992; 101:985–988.
47. Reinarz JA, Pierce AK, Mays BM, Sanford JP. The potential role of inhalation therapy equipment in nosocomial pulmonary infection. *J Clin Invest* 1965; 44:831–839.
48. Pierce AK, Sanford JP, Thomas GD, Leonard JS. Long term evaluation of decontamination of inhalation therapy equipment and the occurrence of necrotizing pneumonia. *N Engl J Med* 1970; 282:528–531.
49. Pierce AK, Sanford JP. Bacterial contamination of aerosols. *Arch Intern Med* 1973; 131:156–159.
50. Wexler MR, Rhame FR, Blumenthal MN, Cameron SB, Juni BA, Fish LA. Transmission of gram-negative bacilli to asthmatic children via home nebulizers. *Ann Allergy* 1991; 66:267–271.
51. Mestitz H, Copland J, McDonald C. Comparison of outpatient nebulized vs metered dose inhaler terbutaline in chronic airflow obstruction. *Chest* 1989; 96:1237–1240.
52. Jenkins SE, Heaton RW, Fulton TJ, Moxham J. Comparison of domiciliary nebulized salblutamol and salbutamol from a metered-dose inhaler in stable chronic airflow limitation. *Chest* 1987; 91:804–807.
53. Sackner M, Kim C. Auxiliary MDI aerosol delivery systems. *Chest* 1985; 88(Suppl 2):161–169.
54. O'Reilly JF, Gould G, Kendrick AH, Laszlo G. Domiciliary comparison of terbutaline treatment by metered dose inhaler with and without conical spacer in severe and moderately severe chronic asthma. *Thorax* 1986; 41:766–770.
55. Morgan MDL, Singh BV, Frame MH, Williams SJ. Terbutaline aerosol given through pear spacer in acute severe asthma. *Br Med J* 1982; 285:849–850.
56. Cissik JH, Bode FR, Smith JA. Double-blind crossover study of five bronchodilator medications and two delivery methods in stable asthma. *Chest* 1986; 90:489–493.
57. Melville C, Phalan PD, Landau LI. Nebulized fenoterol compared with metered aerosol. *Arch Dis Child* 1985; 660:257–259.
58. Levinson H, Reilly A, Worslely GII. Spacing devices and metered dose inhalers in childhood asthma. *J Pediatr* 1985; 107:662–668.
59. Turner TR, Corkery KJ, Ecleman D, Gelb AM, Lipavsky A, Sheppard D. Equivalence of inhaler with reservoir bag for treatment of acute airflow obstruction. *Chest* 1988; 93:476–481.
60. Berry R, Shinto R, Wong F, Despers J, Light R. Nebulizer vs spacer for bronchodilator delivery in patients hospitalized for acute exacerbations of COPD. *Chest* 1989; 96:1241–1246.
61. Bowton DL, Goldsmith WM, Haponik EF. Substitution of metered-dose inhalers for hand-held nebulizers: success and cost savings in a large acute-care hospital. *Chest* 1992; 101:305–308.
62. Tenholder MF, Bryson MJ, Whitlock WL. A model for conversion from small volume nebulizer to metered dose inhaler aerosol therapy. *Chest* 1992; 101:634–637.
63. Jasper AC, Mohsenifar Z, Kahan S, Goldberg HS, Koerner SK. Cost-benefit comparison of aerosol bronchodilator methods in hospitalized patients. *Chest* 1987; 91:614–618.
64. Summer W, Elston R, Tharpe L, Nelson S, Haponik EF. Aerosol bronchodilatordelivery methods: relative impact on pulmonary function and cost of respiratory care. *Arch Intern Med* 1989; 149:618–623.
65. Gonzalez ER, Burke TG. Review of the status of intermittent positive pressure breathing therapy. *Drug Intell Clin Pharm* 1984; 18:974–976.
66. AHCPR. *Intermittent positive pressure breathing (IPPB) therapy.* AHCPR Health Technology Assessment Reports 1991; 1. Washington DC: U.S. Department of Health and Human Services, 1991.
67. O'Donohue WJ Jr. IPPB past and present (point of view). *Respir Care* 1982; 27:588–590.
68. Centers for Disease Control. Update: Universal Precautions for prevention of transmission of human immunodeficiency virus, hepatitis B virus, and other blood-borne

pathogens in health care settings. *MMWR* 1988; 37:377–388.

69. Arnow PM, Chou T, Weil D, Shapiro EN, Kretzschmar C. Nosocomial Legionnaires' disease caused by aerosolized tap water from respiratory devices. *J Infect Dis* 1982; 146:460–467.

ADDITIONAL BIBLIOGRAPHY

Faculty and Working Group. American Association for Respiratory Care. Aerosol Consensus Conference Statement—1991. *Respir Care* 1991; 36:916–921.

Newman SP. Delivery of therapeutic aerosols. In: Witek TJ, Schachter EN, eds. *Advances in respiratory care pharmacology.* Philadelphia: JB Lippincott, 1988; 1:53–82.

Moren F, Newhouse MT, Dolovich MD, eds. *Aerosols in medicine: principles, diagnosis, and therapy.* Amsterdam: Elsevier Science Publishers, 1985.

Witek TJ, Schachter EN. Delivery of drugs by aerosol. In: *Respiratory care pharmacology and therapeutics.* Philadelphia: WB Saunders, 1993.

Kim C, Eldridge M, Sackner M. Oropharyngeal deposition and delivery aspects of metered-dose inhaler aerosols. *Am Rev Respir Dis* 1987; 135:157–164.

Volpe J, Kendall H, Gilbert D, Stowe B, Dundovich K. Metered dose inhalers. *Respir Ther* 1990; 3(3):18–23.

Blake KV, Hoppe M, Harman E, Hendeles L. Relative amount of albuterol delivered to lung receptors from a metered-dose inhaler and nebulizer solution: bioassay by histamine bronchoprovocation. *Chest* 1991; 101:309–315.

Newhouse M, Dolovich M. Aerosol therapy: nebulizer vs metered dose inhaler. *Chest* 1987; 91:799–800.

Morley TF, Marozsan E, Zappasodi SJ, Gordon R, Griesback RM, Giudice JC. Comparison of beta-adrenergic agents delivered by nebulizer vs metered dose inhaler with InspirEase in hospitalized asthmatic patients. *Chest* 1988; 94:1205–1210.

Newhouse MT. Principles of aerosol therapy. *Chest* 1982; (Suppl):39S-41S.

Newhouse MT, Dolovich M. Aerosol therapy of reversible obstruction: concepts and clinical applications. *Chest* 1987; 91(Suppl):58S–64S.

Bryson MJ, Tenholder MF. Metered dose inhaler compliance with cost analysis. *Chest* 1990; 98(2, Suppl):32S.

Olivenstein R, Wolkove N, Cohen C, Frank H, Kreisman H. A comparison of responses to albuterol delivered by two aerosol devices. *Chest* 1986; 90:392–395.

Gervais A, Begin P. Bronchodilation with a metered-dose inhaler plus an extension, using tidal breathing vs jet nebulization. *Chest* 1987; 92:822–824.

Clausen JL. Self-administration of bronchodilators: cost effective? (editorial). *Chest* 1987; 91:475.

Shim C, Williams MH. The adequacy of inhalation of aerosol from canister nebulizers. *Am J Med* 1980; 69:891–894.

Paterson IC, Crompton GK. Use of pressurized aerosols by asthmatic patients. *Br Med J* 1976; 1:76–77.

Epstein SW, Manning CPR, Ashley MJ, Corey PN. Survey of the clinical use of pressurized aerosol inhalers. *Can Med Assoc J* 1972; 120:813–816.

Williams TJ. The importance of aerosol technique: does speed of inhalation matter? *Br J Dis Chest* 1982; 76:223–228.

Pedersen S, Hansen OR, Fuglsang G. Influence of inspiratory flow rate upon the effect of a Turbuhaler. *Arch Dis Child* 1990; 65:308–319.

Engel T, Heinig JM, Medsen F, Nikander K. Peak inspiratory flowrate and inspiratory vital capacity of patients with asthma measured with and without a new dry powder inhaler device (Turbuhaler). *Eur Respir J* 1990; 3:1037–1041.

Newman SP. Aerosol inhalers. *Br Med J* 1990; 300:1286–1287.

Ziment I. Bronchospasm. In: *Respiratory pharmacology and therapeutics.* Philadelphia: WB Saunders Co. 1978:105–146.

Schuh S, Parkin P, Rajan A, Canny G, Healy R, Rieder M, et al. High- versus low-dose, frequently administered, nebulized albuterol in children with severe, acute asthma. *Pediatrics* 1989; 83:513–518.

Nelson HS, Raine D Jr, Doner HC, Posey WC. Subsensitivity to the bronchodilator action of albuterol produced by chronic administration. *Am Rev Respir Dis* 1977; 116:871–878.

Plummer AL. The development of drug tolerance to beta2 adrenergic agents. *Chest* 1978; 73(Suppl):949–957.

4

Artificial Airways and Tubes

PAMELA L. BORTNER, B.S., R.R.T.
ROBERT A. MAY, M.D., R.R.T.

OBJECTIVES

- Compare the different types of oropharyngeal and nasopharyngeal airways as to their structure and clinical application.
- Differentiate between the various types of endotracheal tubes on the basis of structure and function.
- Discuss potential complications of endotracheal intubation.
- Identify different types of tracheostomy tubes.
- Explain the clinical applications and potential complications of various types of tracheostomy tubes.
- Point out the various types of adjunctive devices used in airway management such as stylets, cuff pressure manometers, and endotracheal tube exchangers.
- Contrast the various types of laryngoscopy and intubation equipment by their clinical application.
- Describe the hazards and possible complications associated with the use of each type of intubation equipment.

A patent airway is the foundation for ensuring adequate ventilation. Quite frequently, a disease process, trauma, or general anesthesia results in a potentially compromised airway. Artificial airways and endotracheal tubes are lifesaving and life-sustaining devices. However, improper placement or use of these devices by unskilled personnel may prove to be life-threatening. This chapter identifies various types of artificial airway equipment, explains the usage of each item, and discusses potential hazards or complications associated with these devices. It is imperative that the operator not only be familiar with the functional aspects of each piece of equipment but also receive practical training to become skilled in its use.

OROPHARYNGEAL AIRWAYS

Oropharyngeal airways are designed to be inserted into the mouth; they extend from the lips to the pharynx, fit between the lips and teeth, and follow the curvature of the tongue (Fig 4–1, A). They are made of metal, plastic, or rubber-like materials. Generally the design consists of three portions: the flange, the bite portion (body), and the air channel (Fig 4–1, B and C). The flange at the mouth opening prevents the airway itself from falling back into the mouth and becoming a source of obstruction. It also provides a means of stabilizing the airway in place against the lips or the teeth. The bite portion is straight and firm enough so that the patient cannot close the air channel by biting down as it fits between the teeth or gums. The air channel, or curved portion of the airway, extends upward and backward over the curve of the tongue and pulls it and the epiglottis away from the posterior pharyngeal wall to provide a patent air passage.

NOTE: Oropharyngeal airways are primarily used to prevent upper airway obstruction from the hypopharynx and to provide a passageway for suctioning. They are not a substitute for a tracheostomy or endotracheal tube.

Types of Oropharyngeal Airways

The various types of oropharyngeal airways are presented below:

Berman Airway

The Berman airway (Fig 4–1, C) is a plastic airway constructed with a rigid support beam through the center and sides that are open. There is no hollow center air passage.[1]

The open sides allow for ease of suctioning, as well as functioning as air channels. There is a flange at the oral end as described above. The center may have openings in it for suctioning should the airway become lodged sideways in the mouth. The advantages of the Berman airway over the other types are the ease with which it can be cleaned and the fact that it is less likely to become obstructed with mucus or foreign bodies because of its dual side air channels.

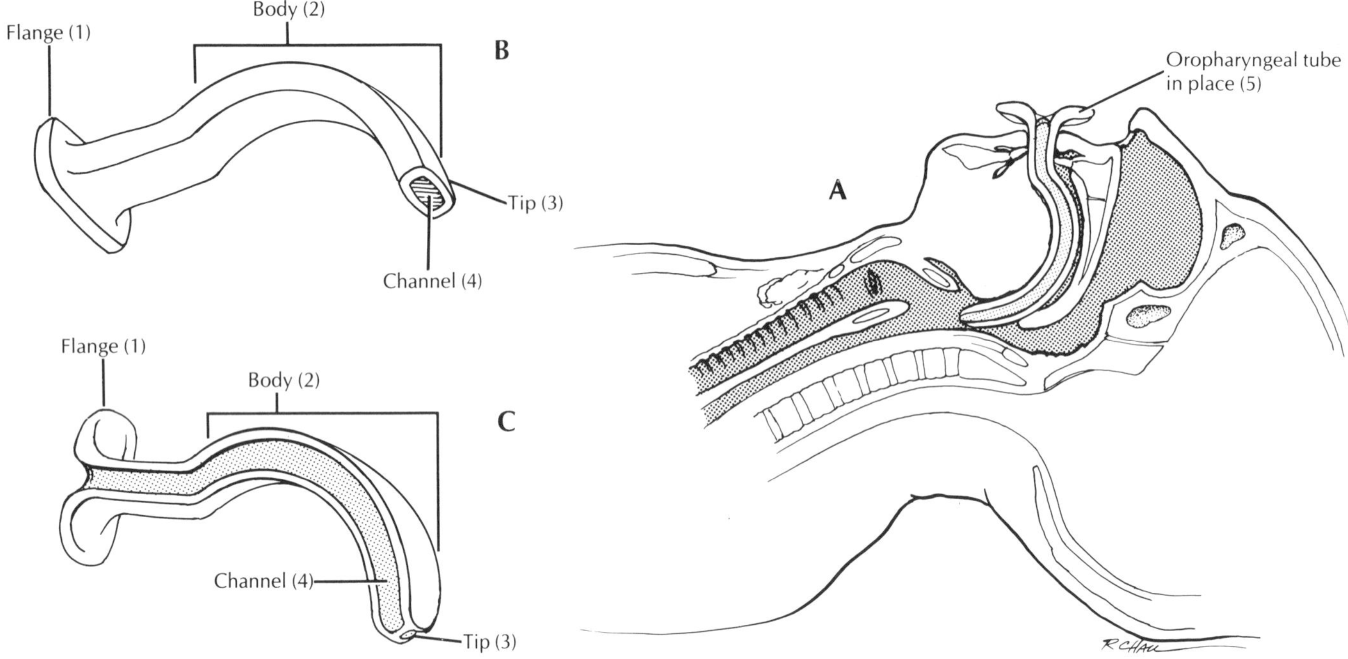

FIG 4–1
Oropharyngeal airways. **A,** airway in place. **B,** Guedel airway. **C,** Berman airway. (From Eubanks DH, Bone RC: *Comprehensive Respiratory Care,* ed 2. St Louis, Mosby–Year Book, p 548. Used by permission.)

Guedel Airway

The Guedel airway (Fig 4–1, B) may be constructed of several types of plastic and black rubber. It is perhaps the most frequently used type of oropharyngeal airway. The Guedel airway has a large flange at the oral end, a supportive bite area, and a less rigid material that forms the curved portion to follow the curve of the tongue. It differs from the Berman airway in that it has an enclosed tubular channel to facilitate air exchange and suction.

S-Tube Airways

Similar in construction to the Guedel-type airway is the S-tube oropharyngeal airway (Fig 4–2), except that it has a tube projected outward for mouth-to-airway ventilation. Its adequacy for this type of ventilation is questionable because of improper use by the rescuer. The central flange is reversible to facilitate use of either the short or the long end as the "airway" while the other end is used as a mouthpiece for the rescuer.

Use of Oropharyngeal Airways

An oropharyngeal airway is designed to prevent the patient's tongue from falling backward into the hypopharynx and causing partial or complete obstruction of the upper airway. Its use may be indicated during spontaneous, manual, or mouth-to-tube ventilation. It also permits ready access to the mouth and pharynx of the patient for suctioning. Oropharyngeal airways may be inserted in lieu of a bite block to prevent a patient from biting and occluding an oral endotracheal tube and also to change the shape of the patient's face, as in a patient who is edentulous or has facial trauma causing the cheeks to collapse and making an airtight mask seal impossible.[2]

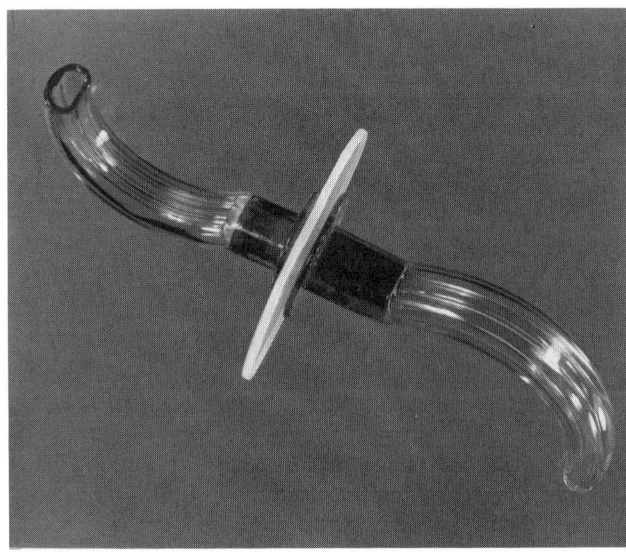

FIG 4–2
S-tube oropharyngeal airway. One airway is placed into the patient's mouth; the other airway is blown into by the rescuer to ventilate the patient.

It is important to note that the oropharyngeal airway, because of its position in the pharynx, may gag a semicomatose or alert patient, which could induce vomiting and increase the potential for aspiration.[3]

In most cases we recommend use of the Berman type of oral airway since it is more difficult for the patient to occlude the air channel by tissue or debris.

Insertion of Oral Airways

To insert an oral airway, stand at the patient's head, and use the cross-finger technique to open the mouth (Fig 4–3). One method of insertion is to turn the airway 180 degrees from its resting position as it is passed over the tongue in order to avoid pushing the tongue back into the pharynx. When the tip of the airway reaches the uvula, rotate the airway 180 degrees so that the tip is positioned behind the tongue and facing toward the larynx. The second method makes use of a tongue blade to hold the tongue in position. The airway can be inserted from the lateral aspect of the mouth and then rotated 90 degrees to the position in which it will rest (Fig 4–4). Once it is

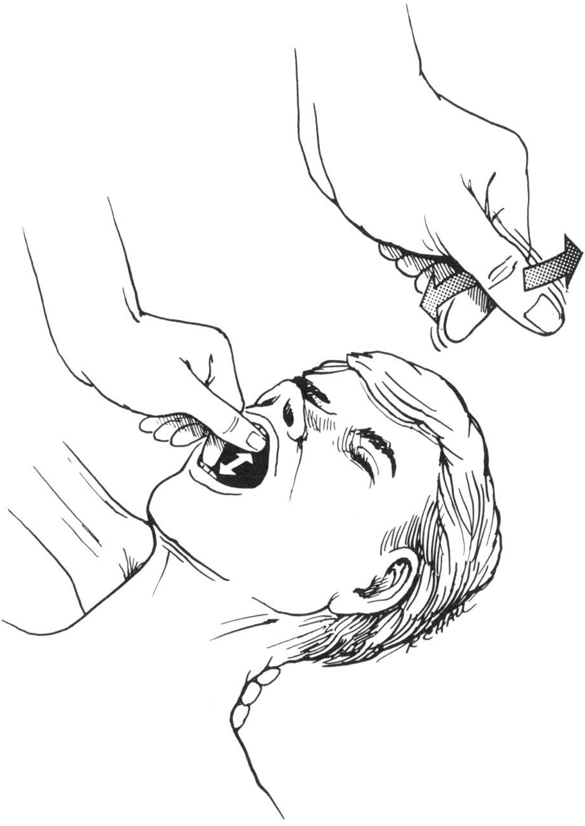

FIG 4–3
Opening the patient's mouth with the crossed-finger technique. (From Eubanks DH, Bone RC: *Comprehensive Respiratory Care,* ed 2. St Louis, Mosby–Year Book, 1990. Used by permission.)

A

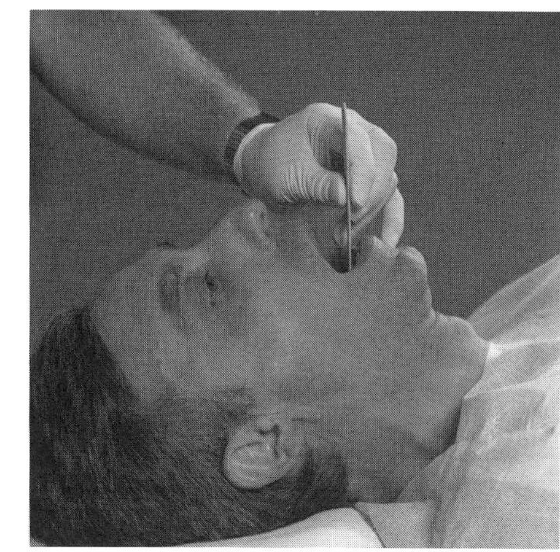

B

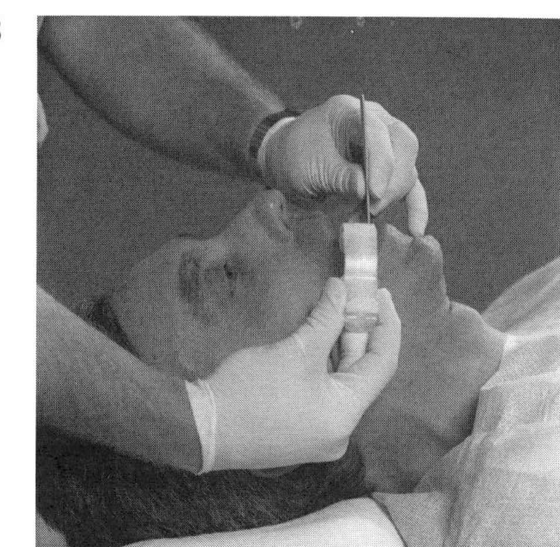

C

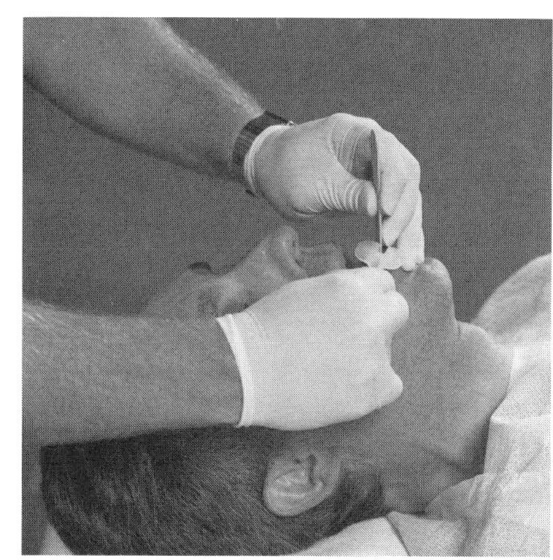

FIG 4–4
Insertion of an oropharyngeal airway. **A,** the tongue is displaced downward and anterior with the tongue blade. **B,** the oropharyngeal airway is inserted from the lateral aspect of the mouth along the tongue blade until the tip reaches the base of the tongue. **C,** the airway is rotated 90 degrees to its final resting position in the posterior of the pharynx.

in place, the airway should be assessed for proper size and position by determining whether or not it allows for unobstructed breathing.

NASOPHARYNGEAL AIRWAYS

The nasopharyngeal airway is available as an alternative to the oropharyngeal airway. Nasopharyngeal airways are inserted into the nose and directed along the floor of the nose parallel to the hard palate. They are curved to follow the anatomy of the nasopharynx, so the tip rests behind the tongue, just above the epiglottis.

These airways are made of plastic or rubber and resemble an endotracheal tube that has been shortened. All types have some degree of flange at the nasal end to facilitate the insertion and to help prevent accidental aspiration of the tube. The proper length of airway may be determined by measuring the distance from the tip of the nose to the meatus of the ear or from the tip of the nose to the tragus of the ear plus 1 in.[4]

Types of Nasopharyngeal Airways

The various types of nasopharyngeal airways are presented below.

Bardex Nasopharyngeal Airway

The Bardex nasopharyngeal airway (Fig 4–5, A) is made of soft rubber with a large flange at the nasal end and a bevel at the pharyngeal end.

Rusch Nasopharyngeal Airway

The Rusch nasopharyngeal airway (Fig 4–5, B) is made of rubber. It has a firm flange at the nasal end and a short bevel at the pharyngeal end.

Linder Nasopharyngeal Airway

The Linder airway is described in more detail because it is not as well known as the more popular models described above. The Linder airway is made of soft plastic and has a bubble-tip introducer that has a smooth rounded tip for easier insertion. The airway itself has a flat rather than beveled end. The Linder tube was designed to address the complications of bleeding encountered during introduction of a nasopharyngeal airway. A lower incidence of bleeding and mucosal damage may be expected because the Linder airway is made of soft plastic and has an introducer that provides a smooth round tip for insertion and the airway has no bevel. It was also found more often to be of the correct length when compared with red rubber airways. The Linder airway is supplied with a bubble-tip introducer consisting of a one-way valve, a hollow tube, and a distal balloon. With the introducer placed into the airway device, air is injected through the one-way valve to the dimensions of the outside wall of the airway. This complete assembly is placed through the nostril, and once in position, the air and the introducer are removed.[5]

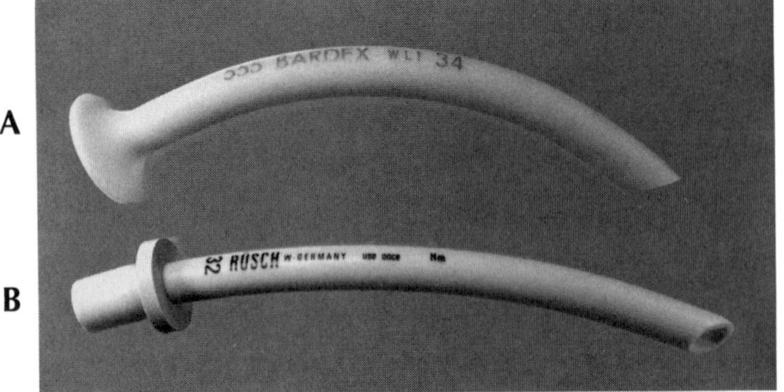

FIG 4–5
A, Bardex. **B,** Rusch, nasopharyngeal airways.

Use of Nasopharyngeal Airways

The nasopharyngeal airway is an alternative to the oropharyngeal airway in providing a patent airway. There are situations where the mouth cannot be opened or an oral airway does not relieve the obstruction. In this situation a nasopharyngeal airway is better tolerated and more comfortable in a semiawake patient than an oral airway. A nasopharyngeal airway also eliminates potential trauma and other problems involving the tongue and teeth that are caused by oral airways. Nasopharyngeal airways are used as aids to performing fiber-optic bronchoscopy, provide easy access to the trachea for nasotracheal suction, and protect the nasopharyngeal mucosa from the traumatic effects of repeated suctioning.[6] Nasopharyngeal airways have also been used in the management of airway problems found in Pierre Robin syndrome.[7]

For most uncomplicated situations we recommend either the Bardex or Rusch nasopharyngeal airway on the basis of the ease of insertion and low cost.

Insertion of Nasopharyngeal Airways

The nasopharyngeal airway should be lubricated with a water-soluble gel before insertion. To insert the airway, take a position at the head of the bed, introduce the airway into the naris, and point the end parallel to the hard palate. Advance it gently to avoid trauma and bleeding (Fig 4–6 A-C). If resistance is met, redirect the airway. If excessive resistance is met, attempt the other nostril, or choose a smaller airway. If the nasopharyngeal airway is too long, laryngospasm may occur. If it is too

A

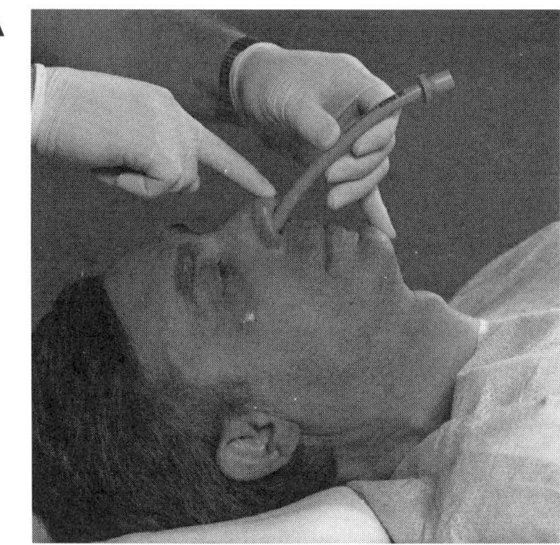

B

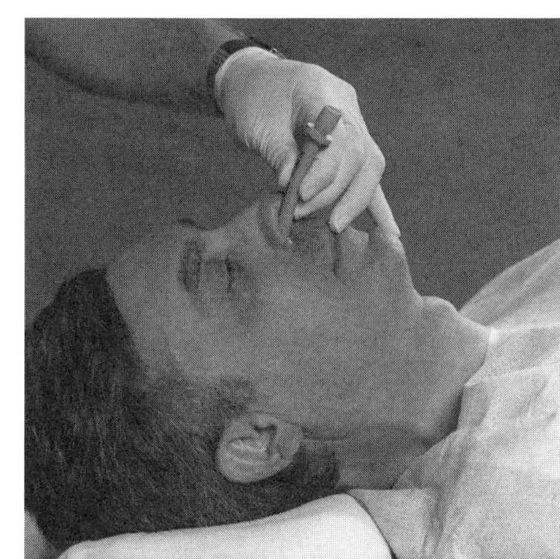

C

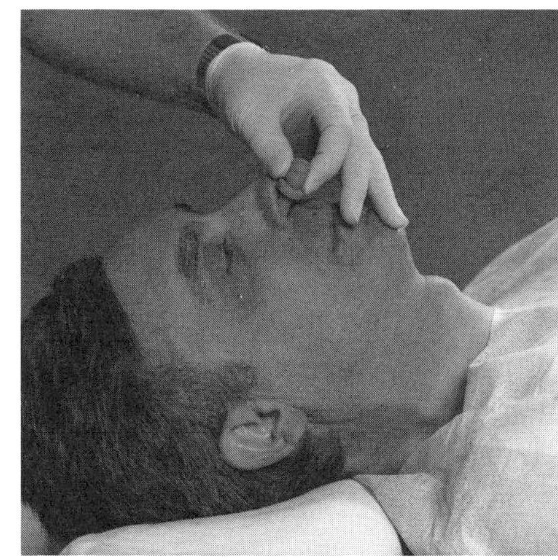

FIG 4–6
Insertion of a nasopharyngeal airway. **A,** the nasopharyngeal airway is initially directed through the naris in a slightly upward direction. **B,** after passing through the naris the airway should be advanced along a plane parallel to the floor of the nasal cavity. **C,** the airway should come to rest with the flange at the external naris.

short, complete airway patency will not be achieved. All oral and nasal airways should be clearly marked with their inside (ID) and outside (OD) diameters to facilitate the selection of a properly sized tube.

BITE BLOCKS

A bite block is placed between the teeth or the jaws in edentulous patients to prevent the patient from biting (occluding) an orotracheal airway or from biting his tongue or lips and causing bleeding and trauma to the mouth. The material should be tough but not rigid, and some have channels for air passage.

Types of Bite Blocks

A variety of materials and adaptations of other airways have been used as bite blocks. Oropharyngeal airways are sometimes used but may cause damage to the teeth.[3] As described earlier, the complications of using oropharyngeal airways when endotracheal tubes are in place for prolonged periods of time are not desirable. Some practical modifications of oral airways have been described where the pharyngeal portion has been removed.[8] Another airway gag was developed to address the needs of patients receiving electroconvulsive therapy (Fig 4–7). Made of wedge-shaped surgical rubber, it consists of a body with air channels, a flange, and a tongue depressor and retractor that holds the tongue in place but does not extend back into the pharynx deep enough to induce a gag reflex.[9] Still another commercially produced bite block is available with a special "C" shape and wing

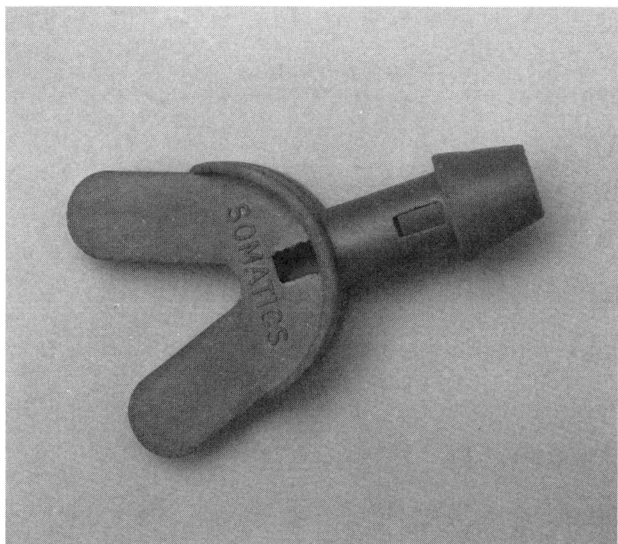

FIG 4–7
Bite block used for electroconvulsive therapy.

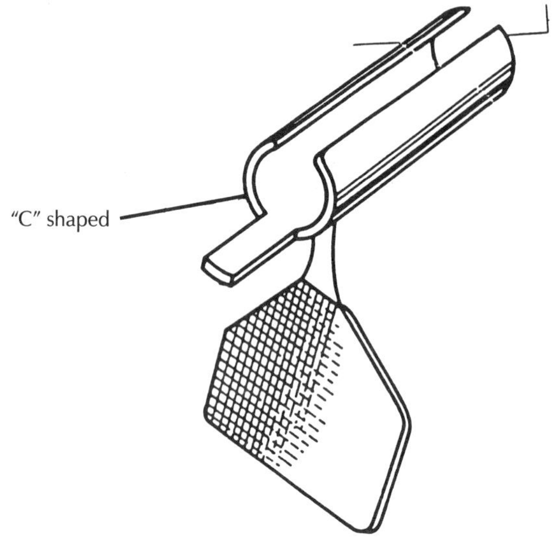

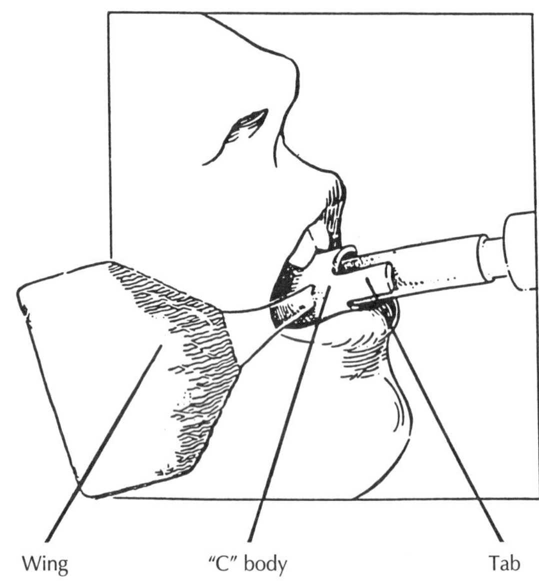

FIG 4–8
Bite-Blok. (Courtesy of Sontek Medical, Inc., Hingham, Mass.)

tab that makes it easy to use and prevents it from accidentally slipping out of position (Fig 4–8).

Use of Bite Blocks

As previously stated, bite blocks are used to prevent a patient from occluding an oral endotracheal tube by biting it during electroconvulsive therapy and in unconscious patients to prevent biting of the lips and/or tongue.

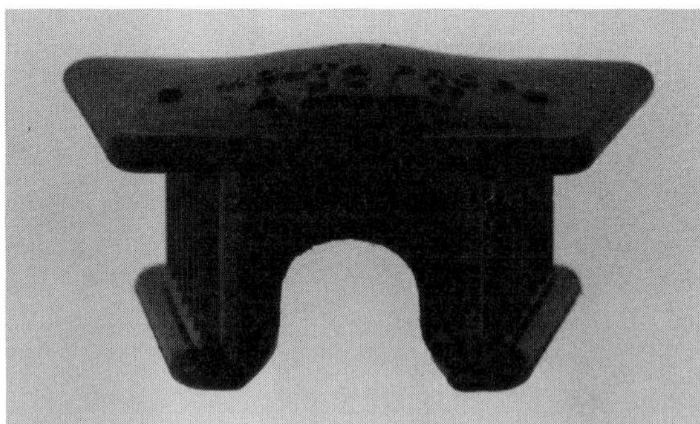

FIG 4–9
Dental bite block with guards placed between the molars.

A genuine bite block designed for dental surgery and placed between the molars rather than front teeth is the most easily tolerated device and of greater safety to the dentition[10] (Fig 4–9). As a safety feature, a long string is fixed to the block on one end and to the patient's gown or face on the other. In the event that the bite block becomes displaced into the patient's oropharynx or larynx, it can be easily removed by pulling the string rather than inadvertently wedging it further into the pharynx with your fingers.

Complications of Airways and Bite Blocks

Aspiration

As mentioned earlier, vomiting and aspiration are potential risks when using an oral airway. If the patient is biting the endotracheal tube, sedation or the use of neuromuscular blocking agents may be indicated, or a bite block as previously described may be inserted.

Airway Obstruction

If too large of an oropharyngeal airway is used, airway obstruction may occur by the tip of the airway pressing the epiglottis against the posterior pharyngeal wall or the larynx. If inserted improperly or if the airway is too small, airway obstruction may occur from pushing the tongue against the posterior of the pharynx. Therefore, selecting the proper size of oropharyngeal airway is extremely important. Obstruction can also occur should the central air channel become occluded by foreign bodies or other material such as vomitus or secretions.

Laryngospasm

Laryngospasm and coughing can be induced by insertion of a nasopharyngeal or oropharyngeal airway that is too long and consequently comes into contact with the epiglottis or vocal cords. This is more frequently found with use of oropharyngeal airways.

Dental Damage

Another frequently reported problem of oral airways is dental damage. Teeth can be broken or torn forcibly from the mouth as the patient bites down on the oral airway. Oral airways should be used judiciously if the patient has disease or decay of the teeth, if there are only isolated teeth remaining, and if caps, crowns, or other dental appliances are present. In these cases, the use of a nasopharyngeal airway or bite block may be indicated.[11]

Lip Injury

Damage to the lip may occur when an oral airway is in place and the lip is pinched between the teeth and the airway.

Tongue Injury

Continuous chewing motions in a comatose patient may cause damage to the tongue when an oropharyngeal airway is in place. Also, pressure necrosis of the tongue can occur should the airway be left in place for prolonged periods of time.

Epistaxis

Nose bleeds can occur from traumatic insertion or the use of too large of a nasopharyngeal airway. These airways should be used with caution in an anticoagulated patient. Improper insertion of nasopharyngeal airways may also cause damage to the turbinate.

Infection

Inserting a nasopharyngeal airway into a patient who is draining blood or cerebrospinal fluid may cause infection. Prolonged use of this airway may also be responsible for sinus infections.

Ulcers

Ulceration of the mucosa may be caused by the introduction of any foreign object, such as an endotracheal tube or a gastric tube, into the mouth and nose if the airway remains in place for long periods of time. Although ischemia is indeed a risk in this situation, if the goal is to maintain an airway and reduce the trauma from repeated insertion of a suction catheter, an oropharyngeal or nasopharyngeal airway may be associated with less trauma.[3]

Neurologic Complications

In patients with severe facial or head trauma, insertion of nasopharyngeal airways may, in rare instances, result in cranial vault intubation. Patients with basilar skull fractures are at greater risk for this occurrence.

ENDOTRACHEAL TUBES

Endotracheal tubes may be constructed from rubber, silicone, Teflon, polyethylene, or polyvinylchloride (PVC). In compliance with the American National Standard for Anesthetic Equipment, they must be made from nontoxic substances compatible with human tissue by implant testing. In addition to materials, other standard requirements include surface characteristics, dimensions, tolerances, cuff characteristics, and labeling of tubes and packages. Tubes that comply with all of the requirements of this standard should be marked "Z79."[12]

Endotracheal tubes may be transparent, translucent, or opaque, depending on the material used in construction. A standard radius of curvature is used to minimize kinking and more readily conform to anatomic structures. The machine (proximal) end is the end of the endotracheal tube projecting from the patient, whereas the patient (distal) end is the end inserted into the patient's trachea. Magill-type endotracheal tubes have a single, beveled opening at the patient end. The bevel faces left as the tube is inserted from the right side of the mouth to facilitate visualization of the larynx. Murphy-type endotracheal tubes have an additional opening in the sidewall of the tube at the patient end opposite the side of the bevel[12] (Fig 4–10). This extra opening is a safety feature to allow gas exchange to occur even if the beveled opening becomes obstructed and to enable the clinician to better direct gas flow toward a specific bronchus.

Standard Uncuffed Endotracheal Tubes

Standard, uncuffed endotracheal tubes have the basic design described in the general information section. Typically, a Murphy-type tube is used, and sizes are available from 2.5 to 10 mm ID. For sizes 6.0 mm and smaller, the OD will be marked, and the marking should be within 0.15 mm of the actual OD of the tube.[12] The

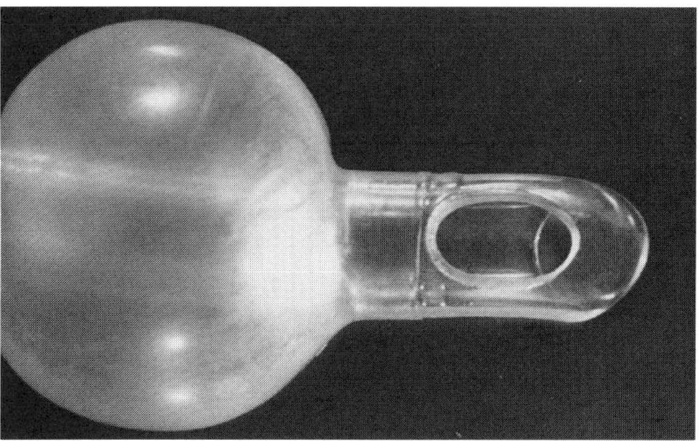

FIG 4–10
Murphy eye as seen on the distal end of a Murphy endotracheal tube (see Fig 4–13 also).

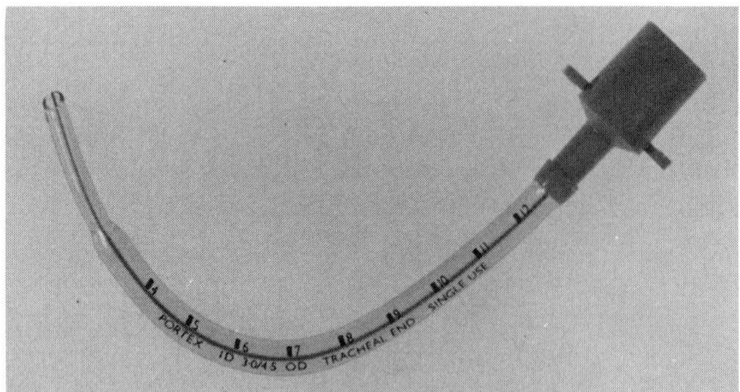

FIG 4–11
Cole endotracheal tube showing a tapered patient end.

Cole tube has a tapered patient end that fits through the vocal cords[13] (Fig 4–11).

The uncuffed tube is primarily for use in the pediatric population, where the cricoid ring is the narrowest point of the upper airway. In adults, the glottis is the narrowest point of the upper airway, so a cuff on the patient end of the tube is used to prevent excessive leak. An uncuffed tracheal tube may be used in adults during laryngeal surgery when the tube needs to be manipulated intraoperatively.

Since the narrowest point in the pediatric airway is the cricoid ring, it is difficult to determine the correct size of an uncuffed endotracheal tube on visualization of the larynx. Two formulas used in children for estimating the OD size in millimeters are based on age. In children over 6.5 years, use 4.5 plus age in years divided by 4, and for children under 6.5 years, use 3.5 plus age in years divided by 3 as an initial starting point.[14, 15] Keep in mind that these formulas only estimate the size needed and an experienced individual will also have tubes one-half size larger and smaller available. If age is unknown, a rule of thumb is to select a tube with an ID the size of the patient's small (pinky) finger. As the tube is inserted through the glottis, it should slide easily, and a small air leak should be heard when 10 to 30 cm H_2O positive pressure is gently applied during ventilation.

Uncuffed endotracheal tubes, with the exception of the Cole tube, have the advantage of maintaining a constant OD throughout. When used correctly in pediatric patients, minimal leak is present, which reduces trauma to the glottis at the cricoid ring. Endotracheal tube size, frequency of intubation, duration of intubation, and tube-related infections are thought to be contributing factors to the development of tracheal stenosis. Since uncuffed tubes do not seal the trachea, the possibility of aspiration of gastric contents exists. This is more of a concern in older children or adults, when the vocal cords become the narrowest portion of the upper airway. Other concerns associated with the use of endotracheal tubes include kinking, plugging, and the inability to remove tracheal secretions through a small tube. Since the use of an artificial airway bypasses natural nasal humidifying and warming systems, hypothermia and inspissation of secretions are potential complications and must be prevented. Uncuffed endotracheal tubes are intended to function with a small leak present. However, at times this leak can become so large that effective ventilation will not occur. In children, the leak may be too large if the tracheal tube is too small, if the Murphy eye is above the larynx, or if the glottis dilates as the edema resolves in epiglottitis or croup.[16] The use of Cole tubes has been associated with laryngeal dilation.[17]

NOTE: Uncuffed tubes tend to move up and down in the airway more easily than cuffed tubes and cause irritation, mucosal scarring, or tracheal erosion and possible hemorrhage.

Standard Cuffed Endotracheal Tubes

The addition of an inflatable cuff and pilot balloon assembly to the standard endotracheal tube enables sealing of the trachea. There is a maximum allowable distance from the tip of the tube to the machine end of the cuff that varies with the size of the endotracheal tube. Cuffs may be high residual volume, low pressure or may be low residual volume, high pressure by design (Fig 4–12, A and B). An inflation system includes a lumen in the endotracheal tube wall connecting the cuff to a pilot balloon and a spring-loaded valve assembly[12] (Fig 4–13). This enables inflation of the cuff with an air-filled syringe and retention of the air when the syringe is removed. The other features of this type of tube are similar to uncuffed tubes. Cuffed endotracheal tubes range in size from 5.0 through 10.0 mm, including half-sizes. Another type of cuffed endotracheal tube is the Bivona system (Fig 4–14—see the section on foam cuffed tracheostomy tubes).

Two primary reasons for using cuffed endotracheal tubes are (1) prevention of aspiration of foreign substances into the lungs and (2) creation of a closed system for ventilation of the lungs. Endotracheal tube movement is also minimized by the use of inflatable cuffs. Because of the increase in OD of cuffed endotracheal tubes and the short distance from the cricoid ring to the carina in smaller children, tubes below 5.0 mm are not available with inflatable cuffs.

When cuffed endotracheal tubes are used, many additional factors need to be considered. Before insertion of the tube, the cuff inflating assembly should be tested, including cuff integrity. Make certain that the cuff is then completely deflated to minimize cuff damage during the intubation procedure. Moistening the endotracheal tube

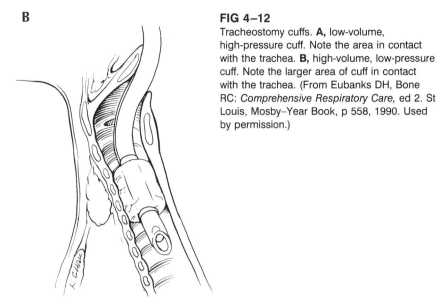

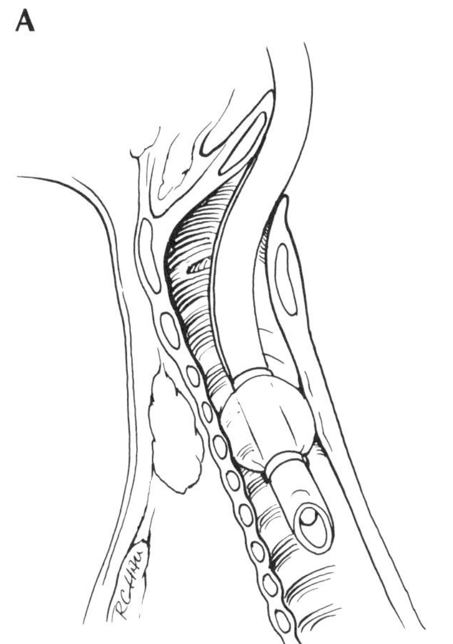

FIG 4–12
Tracheostomy cuffs. **A,** low-volume, high-pressure cuff. Note the area in contact with the trachea. **B,** high-volume, low-pressure cuff. Note the larger area of cuff in contact with the trachea. (From Eubanks DH, Bone RC: *Comprehensive Respiratory Care,* ed 2. St Louis, Mosby–Year Book, p 558, 1990. Used by permission.)

cuff with saline or a water-soluble gel may facilitate passage through the larynx. Lidocaine jelly for lubrication is not recommended because it has been reported to cause a higher incidence of sore throats following extubation.[18]

Proper inflation of the cuff once the endotracheal tube is in place is critical for safe and efficient performance of the endotracheal tube. A technique used to prevent excessive tracheal wall cuff pressures is the minimal leak technique. The cuff is inflated, and as positive pressure is applied, gradual deflation of the cuff occurs until a slight leak is heard from the mouth at 10 to 30 cm H_2O ventilating pressure. Alternately, a minimum-occlusion technique may be used in which air is inserted into the cuff until the leak stops at 30 cm H_2O ventilating pressure. With high-volume, low-pressure cuffs, the cuff pressures are generally less than 25 mm Hg, whereas with low-volume, high-pressure cuffs, the cuff pressures commonly exceed 50 mm Hg. Monitoring of cuff pressures should be performed intermittently to ensure safe levels as conditions change.[19]

Potential Problems

Endotracheal tube cuffs have been associated with many types of complications. Low-volume, high-pressure cuffs cause a more profound decrease in tracheal mucosal blood flow, which results in an increased chance of ulceration, hemorrhage, tracheal stenosis, tracheomalacia, tracheoesophageal fistula, and loss of mucosal cilia.[18–22] In addition to direct effects of the cuff on the trachea, other complications have been reported. Some ventilators that use a relative drop in airway pressure as

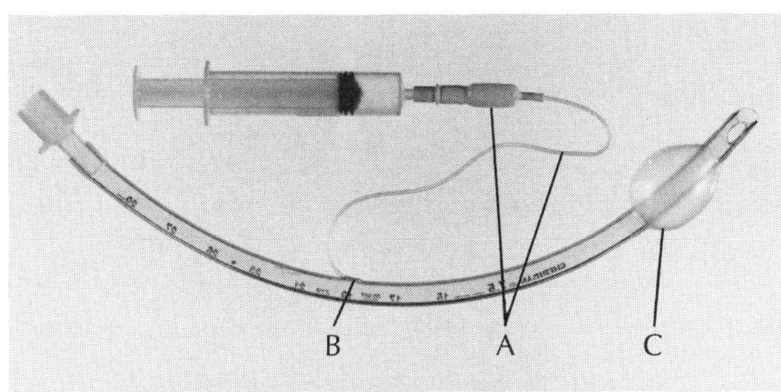

FIG 4–13
Endotracheal tube with an inflation system: Filling tube and spring-loaded valve *(A)* connecting a cuff *(C)* through a lumen in the tube wall *(B).*

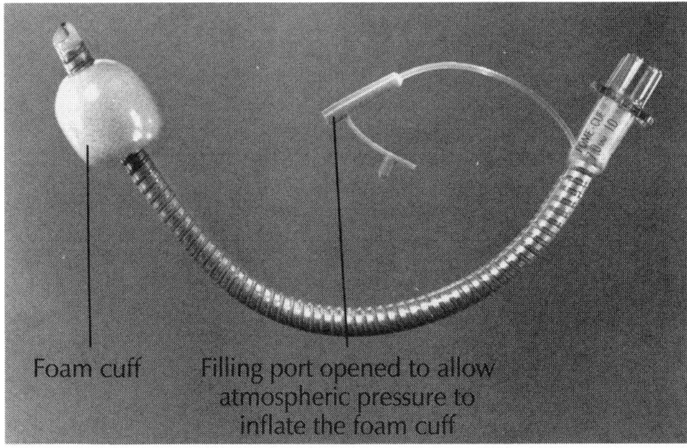

FIG 4–14
Bivona Fome-Cuf on a spiral-embedded laser-resistant endotracheal tube.

the signal to initiate inspiration may autocycle with a leaking endotracheal tube cuff.[23] The pilot balloon housing assembly can malfunction and cause either leaking or an inability to deflate the cuff.[24, 25] High-volume, low-pressure cuffs contain a larger volume of air and cover more surface area, so herniation over the end of the endotracheal tube can cause airway obstruction.[26] Because of the lower lateral wall pressure exerted on the trachea, gastric contents and even misplaced nasogastric tubes may more easily pass by a high-volume, low-pressure cuff into the trachea.[27]

As is the case with uncuffed endotracheal tubes, cuffed tubes also bypass the patient's humidification and warming systems, so drying of secretions, kinking and plugging of the tube, and hypothermia are potential problems. Bivona cuffs may convert to high pressure if an inexperienced operator adds air to eliminate a leak.

RAE Tubes

RAE tubes are preformed endotracheal tubes available in both oral and nasal types. Initially developed by Ring, Adair, and Elwyn for pediatric cases in 1971, the RAE tubes are currently used in adult and pediatric surgery of the head and neck.[28] The oral RAE tube (Fig 4–15) has a preformed bend to keep the machine end caudad to the site of surgery without kinking the tube. Nasal RAE tubes have a preformed bend that directs the machine end of the tube cephalad for use in oral and neck surgery (Fig 4–16). Both the oral and nasal RAE tubes have the preformed bend external to the patient. Cuffed, uncuffed, and half-sizes are available similar to standard endotracheal tubes. Other than the preformed bend as explained above, RAE tubes are structurally and functionally the same as standard endotracheal tubes.

During head and neck surgery, the operative field is in close proximity to the airway and endotracheal tube. In addition, the endotracheal tube is often draped out of view of the anesthesiologist. Under these circumstances, standard endotracheal tubes may become kinked if excessive angles of displacement are used. Preformed bends in RAE tubes keep the airway directed away from the surgical site and are much less prone to kinking.

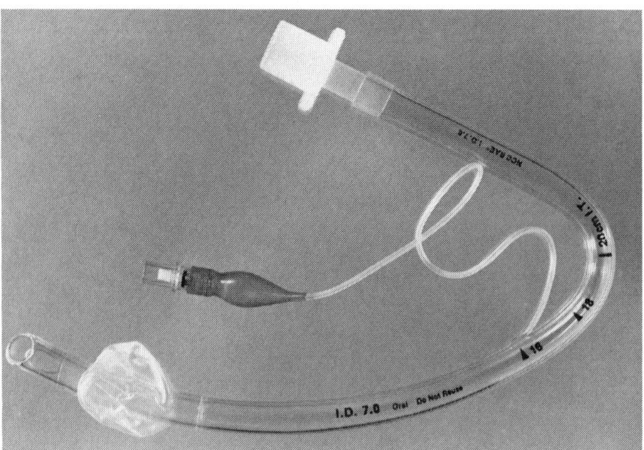

FIG 4–15
Oral RAE endotracheal tube.

Potential Problems

Since the bend is preformed at a fixed distance, it will correctly fit most patients; however, occasionally a RAE tube with a properly-sized ID may be too long or too short if placed to the depth of the bend. Uncuffed RAE tubes have two sideports, one on the long side of the bevel and one on the short side of the bevel, to provide bilateral ventilation if the tip of the RAE tube is inadvertently advanced into the mainstem bronchus.

Other potential problems with RAE tubes result from the preformed nature of the tube. Suctioning of the tube is more difficult because the catheter tends to get stuck at the bend. Small amounts of water-soluble lubricant or straightening of the bend temporarily will usually solve the problem. Placement of the RAE tube with a stylet, bronchoscopy through the tube, and endotracheal tube exchange are also difficult or not feasible with RAE tubes.

Spiral Embedded Tubes

Spiral embedded tubes contain metal wire completely encased in the rubber or PVC material (see Fig 4–14). The wire spirals through the entire length of the tube, with the exception of several millimeters at both the machine and patient ends. These tubes have the pilot tube placed near the machine end, so they cannot be shortened without damaging the cuff inflation tube. By design, spiral embedded endotracheal tubes are soft and pliable. Other features of this tube are similar to standard endotracheal tubes.

Spiral embedded tubes are useful in procedures where compression or kinking of the endotracheal tube

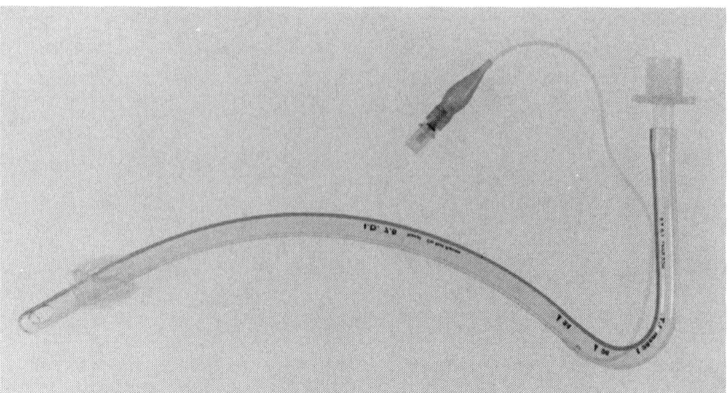

FIG 4–16
Nasal RAE endotracheal tube.

is likely. Surgery in the prone position, head and neck surgery, or placement into a tracheostomy stoma are potential uses for spiral embedded tubes.[29]

Spiral embedded tubes are intended to meet a specific need, namely, to prevent endotracheal tube occlusion when either patient position or surgical manipulation may cause the endotracheal tube to bend.

Potential Problems

In achieving its goal, several inherent potential problems exist. Not only does the pliability of the tube make insertion more difficult, but the ends of the tube without metal reinforcement are also more easily kinked. Another problem encountered with spiral embedded tubes, particularly when the tubes have been resterilized repeatedly, is the formation of intraluminal gas bubbles that expand when nitrous oxide is used. Expansion of the bubbles into the lumen of the endotracheal tube may cause obstruction or increased resistance to flow; this is most significant in pediatric patients.[30, 31]

Because of the pliable nature of the tube, a stylet may facilitate introduction into the trachea. A bite block or oral airway should be used to prevent permanent deformation of the tube with patient biting.[30]

Laser-Resistant Endotracheal Tubes

Laser-resistant endotracheal tubes (LRETTs) may be specifically made from laser-resistant material or may be standard tubes wrapped with laser-resistant material. Additionally, LRETTs may be designed specifically for CO_2, Nd-YAG, or KTP laser energy. It is important to note that currently no tube is completely safe from the risk of airway fire. The risk can be lowered by using LRETTs, but all tubes can burn in the right atmosphere if enough laser energy is applied.[32]

The Laser-Flex Mallinckrodt tube (Argyle, NY) is a flexible, stainless steel LRETT (Fig 4–17). It has a double-cuff design to protect the distal cuff from contact with the laser beam. Laser-Flex tubes are spiral wound, airtight, and flexible but maintain enough rigidity for intubation without the use of a stylet. The OD of the Laser-Flex is greater than that of standard tubes with equal ID.[33]

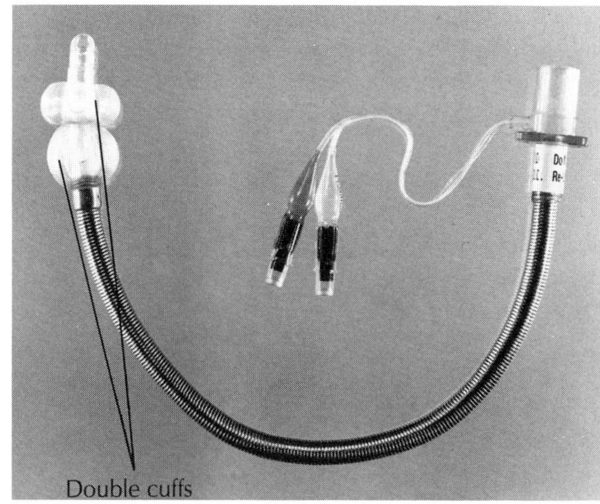

FIG 4–17
Laser Flex laser-resistant endotracheal tube showing a double-cuff design.

A silicone tube covered with an aluminum-filled silicone layer was marketed by Xomed (Jacksonville, Fla) and called Laser-Shield. This tube was involved in at least seven airway fires and was subsequently discontinued and replaced with the Laser-Shield II (Fig 4–18). *Health Devices* reported this tube to be acceptable for use with CO_2 and KTP lasers.[34]

Bivona's Fome-Cuf laser endotracheal tube consists of a flexible aluminum shaft encased in a silicone elastomer. This tube is designed for head and neck surgery use when a CO_2 laser is used in the pulsed mode. It utilizes a self-inflating Fome-Cuf that is filled with sterile water or saline after insertion of the tube into the trachea.

NOTE: "Normal" Fome-Cuf tubes *must not* be filled with *any* liquid.

LRETTs are used for all types of surgical procedures of the head and neck in which CO_2, Nd-YAG, and KTP lasers are employed. As indicated above, the different types of LRETTs are suitable only for specific laser types. Manufacturers' guidelines should be followed to prevent complications from these specialized tubes.

Preventing Complications With Laser Tubes

An airway fire is the most feared complication with the use of laser surgery in an intubated patient, although all of the previously mentioned complications of other endotracheal tubes can also apply to LRETTs. Prevention of airway fires requires meticulous planning and execution of safety procedures. Only use LRETTs designed for

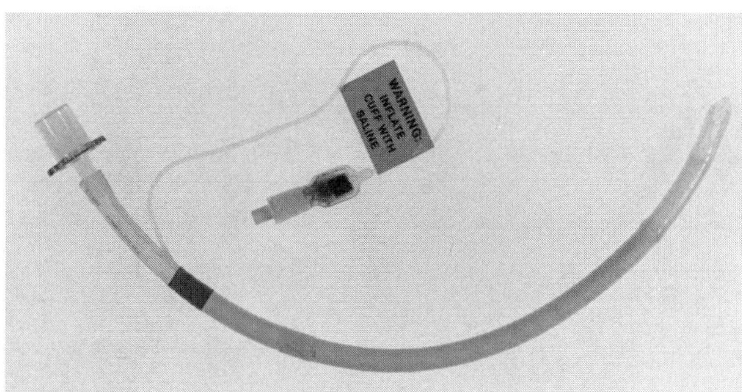

FIG 4–18
Laser-Shield II laser-resistant endotracheal tube.

a specific type of laser. Filling the cuff with liquid rather than gas that may support combustion is also important. Reducing the percentage of combustion-supporting gases such as oxygen and nitrous oxide can be done by using helium.[32]

At the first sign of airway fire, stop ventilation, and disconnect the breathing circuit. Cut the cuff pilot inflation tube and anchor devices, remove the tube, and douse it with water. Remove any burning ash or remnants of the tube from the airway, establish ventilation by mask or reintubation, and administer life support measures and other supportive treatment. Evaluate the extent of airway damage by laryngoscopy, bronchoscopy, or other required examinations, and then formulate a plan for continued ventilatory support.

If the injury is significant enough, postoperative intubation or mechanical ventilation may also be necessary. The use of steroids and antibiotics should be determined by evaluation of the airway and cultures of exudative material.[35] The use of laser-resistant wrappings over rubber silicone or PVC tubes may be less expensive; however, the chance for laser contact with flammable materials is higher. LRETTs may cost three to seven times the cost of wrapping a standard tube, but legal consequences may be difficult to avoid should an accident occur when wrapped tubes are used since specific LRETTs are now available.[32]

Endobronchial/Double-Lumen Tubes

Endobronchial or double-lumen endotracheal tubes (DLT) consist of a tube with two independent lumina of different lengths. The shorter tracheal lumen rests in the trachea above the carina, whereas the longer bronchial lumen is inserted into the right or left mainstem bronchus. Each lumen has a 15-mm connector at the machine end to enable separate modes of ventilation to each lung, or they can be connected to a wye piece and share a common source of ventilation (Fig 4–19). Two cuffs are employed. The proximal tracheal cuff is similar to standard high-volume, low-pressure cuffs, whereas the distal bronchial cuff is smaller and essentially a high-pressure, low-volume cuff. When this cuff is inflated in the bronchus, intracuff pressure may reach 200 mm Hg. To facilitate identification and confirmation of correct tube placement, the distal bronchial cuff is often colored radiopaque blue.

Current DLTs are composed of PVC, which becomes more flexible and malleable after warming to body temperature. Single-use DLTs are available in 41, 39, 37, and 35 F sizes, which correspond to each lumen having an ID of 6.5, 6.0, 5.5, and 5.0 mm, respectively.[36] Sizes 37 and 41 F can be used on most adults 68 in. in height or taller.[36] A pediatric 28 F DLT is also available. Table 4–1 presents endotracheal tube size equivalents for comparison.

A preformed stylet is supplied with the tube to enhance correct orientation of the bronchial lumen when inserted into the trachea. Because of the longer length and smaller diameter of the DLT when compared with standard endotracheal tubes, special suction catheters are needed for evacuation of tracheobronchial secretions.

Indications for DLT use fall into four major categories:

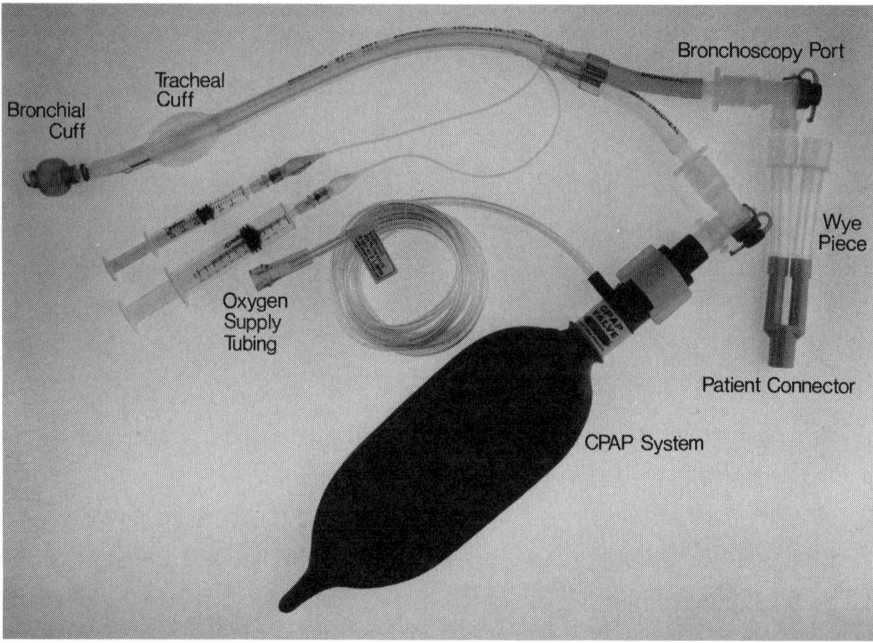

FIG 4–19
Double-lumen endotracheal tube shown with the optional continuous positive airway pressure *(CPAP)* system used with single-lung ventilation.

TABLE 4–1
Endotracheal Tube Size Equivalents*

Diameter Sizing			
Internal (mm)	External (mm)†	Magill†	French†
2.5	4.0		12
3.0	4.5	00	12–14
3.5	5.0		14–16
4.0	5.5	0–1	16–18
4.5	6.0	1–2	18–20
5.0	6.5		20–22
5.5	7.0	3–4	22
6.0	8.0		24
6.5	8.5	4–5	26
7.0	9.0	5–6	28
7.5	9.5	6–7	30
8.0	10.0	7–8	32
8.5	11.5	8	34
9.0	12.0	9–10	36
9.5	12.5		38
10.0	13.0	10–11	40
10.5	13.5		42
11.0	14.5	11–12	42–44
11.5	15.0		44–46

* From Eubanks DH, Bone RC: *Comprehensive Respiratory Care*, ed 2. St Louis, Mosby–Year Book, 1990. Used by permission.
† Since tube thicknesses vary from one style to another, the above is intended to serve as a guide only.

1. Intraoperatively in thoracic surgery, a DLT will provide a quiet operative field for pneumonectomy, lobectomy, esophageal resection, aortic aneurysm repair, and some thoracic spine procedures.

2. Selective airway protection may prevent spillage of pus or blood into the unaffected lung; in whole-lung lavage a DLT is used in the management of alveolar proteinosis.

3. In unilateral lung diseases, separation of therapy to each lung may improve overall oxygenation and ventilation.

4. The fourth general category is in selective management of the distribution of ventilation. Bronchopleural fistulas, tracheobronchial tree disruption, or surgical opening of a large conducting airway requires decreasing or stopping airflow through the opening in order to promote healing and effectively ventilate other regions of the lung.[37]

The DLTs in use today are much safer than the original DLTs. For example, the Carlen tube had a carinal hook that seated on the carina when appropriately positioned. This carinal hook could injure the larynx, trachea, or carina during insertion. In addition, the original DLTs were fitted with low-volume, high-pressure cuffs and were made of red rubber, which made them much stiffer than the current PVC tubes.

Potential Problems

Correct positioning of the DLT is the most important factor determining safe use.[38] Left-sided DLTs are relatively easy to place in the correct position because of the distal position of the left upper lobe bronchus as compared with the right. Since the right upper lobe bronchus is located near the origin of the right mainstem bronchus, placement of a right DLT may interfere with ventilation of the right upper lobe. With incorrect positioning or a change in tube position, hypoxemia and atelectasis may become significant problems. Mallinckrodt and Rusch right-sided DLTs have specially designed cuffs that facilitate ventilation of the right upper lobe through a sideport of the distal lumen. Positioning of this sideport at the level of the right upper lobe bronchus takeoff must be verified by fiber-optic bronchoscopy after the patient has been positioned.

During single-lung ventilation, oxygenation is usually adequate because of redistribution of pulmonary blood flow to the ventilated lung as a result of hypoxic pulmonary vasoconstriction (HPV). However, the HPV response may be altered by chronic obstructive pulmonary disease (COPD), hypothermia, sepsis, pulmonary hypertension, drugs, and other situations that may create a physiologic shunt and lead to profound hypoxemia. Mechanical dysfunction, endotracheal tube malposition, ventilation/perfusion abnormalities, and decreased cardiac output are additional factors associated with hypoxemia during single-lung ventilation. Under these circumstances, single-lung ventilation may not be tolerated without periods of reinflation or the application of continuous positive airway pressure to the deflated lung. Other complications of DLTs include laryngeal trauma, tracheobronchial rupture, displacement of tumors, and cuff inflation injuries. Relative contraindications to the use of DLTs are airway lesions or strictures, upper airway anatomy abnormalities, patients with a full stomach at risk for aspiration, and critically ill patients receiving mechanical ventilation and positive end-expiratory pressure (PEEP) who can not tolerate being off of the ventilator long enough for insertion and positioning of the DLT.[36]

TRACHEOSTOMY

Advantages and Disadvantages of Tracheostomy

The primary reason for performing a tracheostomy is to provide the patient with a secure artificial airway. Although tracheostomy is the preferred method for long-term airway management, much controversy still remains as to when the optimal time to perform a tracheostomy occurs. A tracheostomy should be performed only after the clinical benefits and risks to each individual patient are considered, not because a certain number of days of intubation have elapsed.

When compared with orotracheal or nasotracheal intubation, a tracheostomy has the advantages of (1) lowering airway resistance, (2) causing less movement of the tube within the trachea, (3) affording greater patient comfort, and (4) enabling the patient to swallow secretions and nourishment. The patient can communicate by moving his lips and even talk with the use of special tracheostomy tubes. If spontaneous decannulation occurs, the tube may be reinserted into the matured stoma easier than if an endotracheal tube is accidentally removed. Because the tracheostomy tube is shorter than an endotracheal tube, more of the airway below the cuff may be suctioned and more efficiently. Tracheostomy also avoids the oral, nasal, pharyngeal, and laryngeal complications of translaryngeal intubation.

Despite what seems like considerable advantages, a tracheostomy also has disadvantages. Performing a tracheostomy is a surgical procedure and has greater morbidity and mortality risks than endotracheal intubation does. Additional risks include incisional hemorrhage, subcutaneous emphysema, pneumothorax, and pneumomediastinum. Tracheal stenosis is common, and a permanent scar is unavoidable. Also, like endotracheal intubation, the tracheostomy tube bypasses normal defense mechanisms and impedes an effective cough since the glottis is also bypassed.

It is important to note that many complications experienced during conventional tracheostomy may be avoided when it is performed by a skilled surgeon as an elective procedure under optimal conditions when the patient's airway is already stabilized rather than at the bedside as an emergency effort.[39]

Methods of Performing Tracheostomy

Percutaneous Dilatational Tracheostomy

A relatively new advance has been described in which tracheostomy is performed by using a percutaneous procedure that is less traumatic than the conventional surgical method. This procedure may change prior opinions regarding acceptable locations and techniques for performing a tracheostomy.

The procedure is performed by making a small incision midway between the cricoid cartilage and the sternal notch. A 14-gauge cannula is inserted into the trachea between the first and second tracheal rings. A guidewire is introduced into the trachea and the tracheostomy dilated with increasing sizes of specially designed plastic dilators. Once the dilatation is complete, an appropriately sized tracheostomy tube is inserted over a small dilator and placed into position in the trachea.

The technique of percutaneous dilatational tracheostomy is advantageous in that it can be performed at the bedside in the intensive care unit, thereby reducing the risks that may be involved with moving an unstable high-risk patient to the operating room. With training, it can be performed by intensivists and not just exclusively by surgeons. Despite the relatively high cost of the disposable dilators, the estimated costs are reduced over conventional tracheostomy performed in the operating room by half. This technique also greatly reduces the risk of hemorrhage. One consideration when choosing the dilatation technique is that the dilatation creates an opening that fits tightly around the tracheostomy tube for several days rather than the large, secured opening created during conventional tracheostomy surgery. This could make reinsertion of the tracheostomy tube potentially difficult should early recannulation be necessary. Personnel skilled in airway care should be available. The incidence of longer-term problems associated with percutaneous dilatational tracheostomy, such as tracheal stenosis, is unknown.[40]

Emergency Tracheostomy Set

Although conventional tracheostomy is best performed in the operating room as an elective procedure, in certain circumstances an emergency tracheostomy must be performed at the bedside. For this reason, proper equipment must be checked routinely and be readily available on the unit should an emergency arise. The necessary equipment should include a light source, an appropriate selection of tracheostomy and endotracheal tubes, a suction system, assorted sizes of suction catheters, and an emergency tracheostomy tray. One type of sterile, single–patient use emergency tracheostomy set is NU-TRAKE, manufactured by International Medical Devices, Inc.[41]

The NU-TRAKE kit contains a bow-shaped needle for passage through the tissue. A tubular housing unit designed to rest on the cricoid cartilage is slanted to closely match the entrance angle of the needle. The blunt needle attached to the housing, which is divided lengthwise in order to open in a scissors-like fashion, can accommodate various-sized airways. Various-sized airways and their obturators are included in the set as well.

The procedure is performed by hyperextending the patient's head, identifying the cricothyroid membrane (between the thyroid cartilage and the cricoid cartilage), and using a knife blade to make a small incision in the skin. The stylet needle is placed through the tubular housing and the entire unit placed on the patient's neck at the incision site. The stylet is used to puncture the membrane and is removed from the housing. The blunt needle attached to the tubular housing is gently advanced into the trachea until the slanted housing rests on the patient's skin. The airway and obturator are inserted together through the distal end of the housing unit and pushed downward to divide the blunt needle lengthwise and spread it apart to accommodate the airway. The obturator is removed to leave a clear airway for ventilation.[41]

Still another way of managing an upper airway emergency is the insertion of a 12- to 14-gauge needle or intravenous catheter through the cricothyroid membrane. The distal end is then connected intermittently to a source of high-pressure oxygen, and the patient is moved immediately to the operating room where a tracheostomy is performed.

Tracheostomy Tubes

Historical Perspective—Metal Tracheostomy Tubes

Metal tracheostomy tubes of various types were used throughout the 19th century to relieve upper airway obstruction. In the early 1930s, Chevalier Jackson developed a systematic approach to the management of airway obstruction that became universally accepted. This approach made tracheostomy with double-lumen silver tubes the standard for treatment of airway obstruction.[40]

Silver has long been used in the manufacture of tracheostomy tubes because the metal walls can be kept very thin, which is an advantage when the inner cannula is used. Silver was selected for construction of the tracheostomy tubes because it is a completely nonreactive substance when in contact with human tissue. The disadvantage of using silver for tracheostomy tubes is that it is expensive and rigid and the curved shape does not conform well to the trachea, which can lead to compression damage along the tracheal wall and even erosion of major vessel walls.

The Jackson-type tracheostomy tube is constructed totally of silver. It has a rigid outer cannula with an attached fixed neck plate and a rigid inner cannula (Fig 4–20, A–C). These metal tracheostomy tubes are cuffless, but a rubber, reusable high-pressure cuff can be added to prevent leaks during mechanical ventilation. The size of the metal tubes is identified by the Jackson system,[42] which uses outer tube diameter. Disadvantages of metal tracheostomy tubes are their narrow ID, rigid structure of the neck plate, and the lack of a standard 15-mm adaptor for connection to most ventilatory devices. Problems associated with use of the reusable high-pressure cuffs were nonuniform expansion along the tracheal wall, lack of cuff strength, and danger of the cuff slipping over the end of tracheostomy tube and causing airway occlusion.[42, 43]

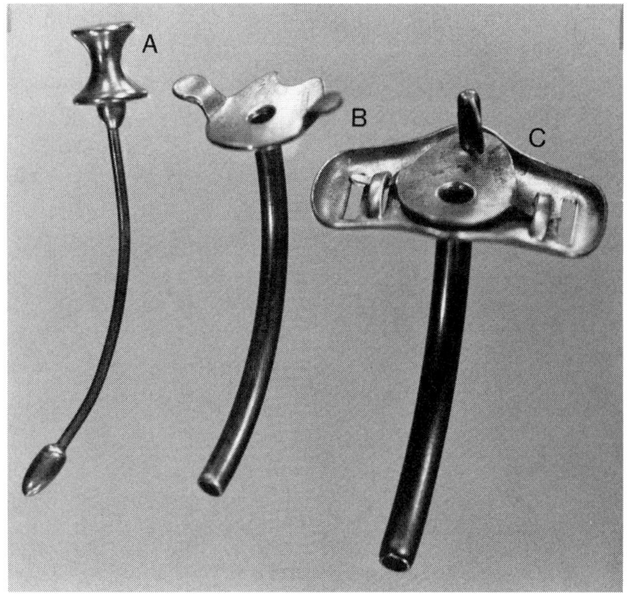

FIG 4–20
Jackson silver tracheostomy tube showing an obturator **(A)**, inner cannula **(B)**, and outer cannula **(C)**.

Metal tracheostomy tubes are available in pediatric and adult sizes; however, with the introduction of improvements in material design, the clinical use of these tracheostomy tubes today is almost nonexistent.

Current Construction

Tracheostomy tubes may be constructed of metal, rubber, silicone, Teflon, polyethylene, and PVC materials. Tracheostomy tubes, like endotracheal tubes, must satisfy American National Standards Equipment guidelines. Since they are in direct contact with body tissue, the ideal material will be nontoxic and determined by implant testing. In addition to materials, other standard requirements include surface characteristics, dimensions, tolerances, cuff characteristics, and labeling of tubes and packages. Tracheostomy tubes that comply with all of the requirements of these standards should have the "Z79" identifier stamped on the tube.[12]

The shape of the tracheostomy tube should conform as closely as possible to the anatomy of the airway. There are two main designs of tracheostomy tubes available: those that are curved and those that are angled to fit the trachea at one end and the area between the skin and the trachea at the other end.

Curved tracheostomy tubes usually have an inner cannula that can be removed for cleaning while the outer cannula remains in place. In addition, the outer cannula may have a window or fenestration to allow for speech when the inner cannula is removed. The disadvantages of the curved tube are that since the trachea is anatomically mostly straight, the curved tracheostomy tube often does not conform to the shape of the trachea, potentially allowing for compression of the membranous part of the trachea while the tip may traumatize the anterior portion. These tubes may also cause damage at the area of the stoma. Some examples of curved tracheostomy tubes are the Jackson tracheostomy tube and the Shiley cuffed (fenestrated and nonfenestrated) tracheostomy tube.[43]

Angled tracheostomy tubes have advantages because they enter the trachea at a less acute angle and cause less pressure damage at the stoma. In addition, because the tube portion that extends into the trachea is straight and conforms more closely to the anatomy of the airway, the angled tracheostomy tube is well centered in the trachea and causes less pressure necrosis along the tracheal wall. One disadvantage is that these types are generally difficult to fit with an inner cannula because the inner cannula must be flexible in order to conform to the angled tracheostomy tubes. Examples of angled tracheostomy tubes include the Portex uncuffed tracheostomy tube, the NCC tracheostomy tube, and the Rusch tracheostomy tube ULTRA Tracheoflex.[43]

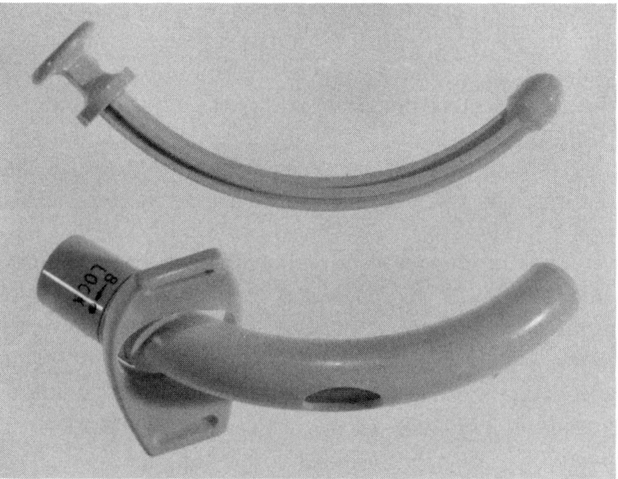

FIG 4–21
Shiley uncuffed tracheostomy tube with an obturator in place. (Courtesy of Sorin Biomedical, Inc., Irvine, Calif.)

Standard Uncuffed Tracheostomy Tubes

Standard, uncuffed tracheostomy tubes have the basic design described above. Modern plastic tracheostomy tubes are available in sizes 2.5 to 11.5 mm, according to their ID. Manufacturers delineate the various tracheostomy tube sizes according to the Jackson size of 0 to 12 mm. On most tracheostomy tubes the manufacturer should mark the ID as well as the OD as a guide to the user. On the flange attachment of some uncuffed adult tracheostomy tubes, such as those manufactured by Shiley (Fig 4–21), the letters *UNCUFFED* designate it as uncuffed, and the letters *FEN* designate the tracheostomy tube as fenestrated. If the tracheostomy tube chosen utilizes a removable inner cannula, the package in which it comes should have the size and make of the tube into which it is intended to fit.

The uncuffed tracheostomy tube is used primarily in the pediatric population, where the cricoid ring is narrower than the glottis. Because the tissues anterior to the trachea in the infant are thinner and the laryngeal and tracheal cartilages are softer, the use of cuffed tracheostomy tubes in infants and children up to 6 years old makes them susceptible to tracheal deformation. In children, especially infants, the shape of the neck plate of the tracheostomy tube is important. The usual straight neck plate does not fit well because of anatomic differences between infants and adults. Some of the anatomic discrepancies have been overcome with the development by Aberdeen of an anatomically shaped tracheostomy tube that easily conforms to the shape of the infant's neck, tracheostomy stoma, and trachea. This tube has served as the basis for design of pediatric tracheostomy tubes over the past several decades.[42]

One of the most critical factors in the production of pediatric tracheostomy tubes is to maintain an adequate ID even in the smallest sizes. Most pediatric tubes are made of PVC, a less-than-ideal substance from the standpoint of tissue reactivity but soft enough to conform to the trachea without kinking or collapsing. This property allows for a wall thickness that is malleable enough to provide an adequate ID for gas flow with minimal resistance. Both Shiley and Portex manufacture pediatric tracheostomy tubes of this type in various sizes. The most ideal substance is silicone rubber, which is the least irritating to human tissue; it has the added advantage of minimal adhesiveness, which reduces the likelihood of mucus sticking to the inner wall. This material also conforms to the trachea but requires thick walls to resist kinking or collapse. This loss of ID becomes critical in small infant or pediatric tracheostomy tubes. An example of this type of tracheostomy tube is produced by Dow Corning.[43]

Uncuffed tracheostomy tubes are intended to allow a small leak during ventilation. Unfortunately, there is a tendency to use a tube that fits rather snugly in order to decrease this leak. Also, a snugly fitting tube (one with the largest ID) is used when a thick-walled tube is employed in order to minimize airflow resistance through the tube. In either case, a large hole in the tracheal wall is required, and this increases the chance of stomal stenosis. These

Silastic tubes available for pediatric patients have a single lumen and do not require an inner cannula.

As previously discussed, in adults the glottis is the narrowest point of the upper airway, so a cuff on the patient end of the tube is used to prevent excessive leak during mechanical ventilation. Several studies indicate that adult tracheotomized patients can be safely and adequately ventilated with cuffless tracheostomy tubes.[44] The primary use of cuffless tracheostomy tubes is postlaryngectomy and in a patient with neuromuscular disease who needs frequent suctioning but not mechanical ventilation. Uncuffed tracheostomy tubes have also been used as a method of weaning; progressively smaller diameters of uncuffed tubes are used to allow suctioning and maintenance of the stoma while allowing patients to adapt to their normal airway. Since the absence of a cuff on tracheostomy tubes will not assist in the prevention of aspiration, this type of tube should not be used in an unconscious patient or someone who has lost the ability to protect his airway.

Standard Cuffed Tracheostomy Tubes

Like the uncuffed standard tracheostomy tube previously described, the typical cuffed tracheostomy tube is composed of outer and inner cannulas. The outer cannula forms the primary structure of the tube and also has the cuff assembly attached to its distal end (Fig 4–22, A and B). On several types of tracheostomy tubes, a removable inner cannula with a standard 15-mm adaptor tacks securely into place at the proximal end of the outer cannula to provide a point of attachment for humidification and ventilation systems. During normal use it is kept in place inside the outer cannula but can be removed for cleaning. Also placed at the proximal end is the inflation tube and pilot balloon with spring-loaded valve assembly for cuff inflation and deflation. An obturator with a rounded tip (not shown) is placed into the outer cannula before insertion of the tracheostomy tube. The rounded obturator tip extends beyond the distal end of the tube far enough to round the otherwise blunted end; this minimizes trauma to the mucosa of the tracheal wall during insertion of the tube. Finally, a radiopaque marker on the distal tip provides confirmation of tube position on radiographs.[45]

New, more modern tracheostomy tubes are similar in design to the metal Jackson tubes previously described. They differ primarily in that they are constructed of a lighter-weight plastic (PVC) or other synthetic materials instead of silver. These tubes are tissue compatible as determined by acceptable implant test methods and

A

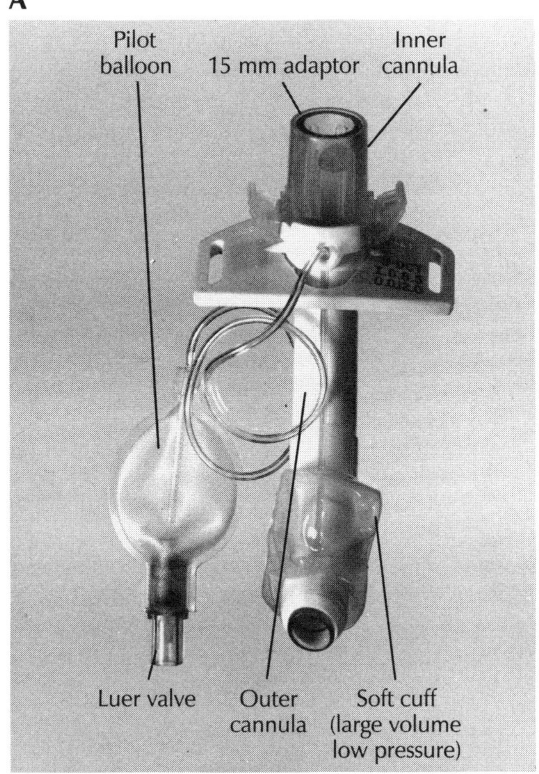

B

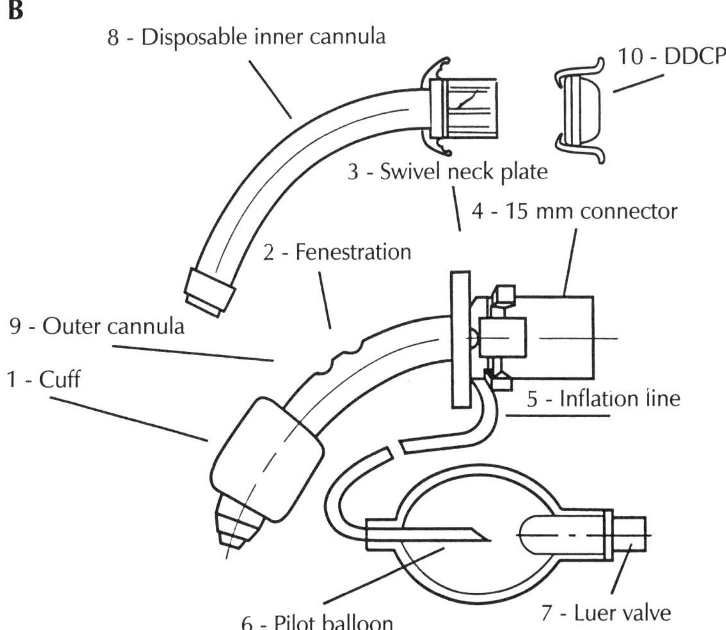

FIG 4–22
Shiley tracheostomy tubes. **A,** Shiley tracheostomy tube. **B,** double fenestrated tube with a snap-lock connector.

include more patient care options than the metal tubes do. The Shiley tracheostomy tube is one example of a modern tracheostomy tube system (Fig 4–22, A and B). This disposable tube system offers the practitioner a variety of tracheostomy tube models ranging from a standard system similar to the silver tracheostomy tube previously described to one with single and double fenestrations and pressure-limiting automatic relief valves that limit the internal cuff pressure to approximately 25 mm Hg (Fig 4–22, B). Like the endotracheal tube, some tracheostomy tubes include a radiopaque marker on the distal tip of the outer cannula to provide confirmation of tube positioning on radiographs.[45]

Complications With Cuffed Tracheostomy Tubes. As described in the section on standard cuffed endotracheal tubes, the use of cuffs has been associated with many types of complications. Efforts to limit these problems have resulted in numerous recent developments in the size and shape of tracheostomy tube cuffs. The design characteristics felt to be important are cuff volume and diameter of the cuff when fully expanded at atmospheric pressure.[46]

Another controversy in selection of the proper tracheostomy tube surrounds the use of a single-lumen tube vs. tubes with an inner cannula. As described above, Shiley is one such tracheostomy tube that provides a removable inner cannula for cleaning, as opposed to the single-lumen construction of Portex Soft Seal or Bivona. There remain many controversies with regard to selection of the proper cuffed tracheostomy tube, and careful consideration should be given to each clinical situation. Some considerations should be the cuff pressure necessary to achieve minimal leak, the transmission of pressure to the tracheal walls, the ability to monitor intracuff pressure, and finally the simplicity of design of the tube for optimum clinical use.

Specialized Tracheostomy Tubes

Foam Cuffed Tracheostomy Tubes

As previously stated in the section on endotracheal tubes, the foam cuff was designed by Kamen and Wilkinson and consists of a large-diameter, high–residual volume cuff composed of polyurethane foam covered by a silicone sheath.[47] This concept of the foam cuff was designed to address the issues of high lateral tracheal wall pressures that lead to complications such as tracheal necrosis and stenosis. Before insertion, air in the cuff must be evacuated by a syringe attached to the pilot port to make the foam contract (Fig 4–23, A). This allows insertion of the tracheostomy tube. Once the tracheostomy tube is in place, the syringe is removed to allow the cuff to reexpand until stopped by the tracheal wall (Fig 4–23, B). The pilot port remains open to the atmosphere, with the intracuff pressure kept at ambient levels. The open pilot port also permits compression and expansion of the cuff during the ventilatory cycle, which allows for intermittent perfusion of the tracheal tissue in contact with the tube without loss of volume during ventilation.

The degree of expansion of the foam is a determining factor of the degree of tracheal wall pressure that will be exerted. As the foam further expands, lateral tracheal wall

A

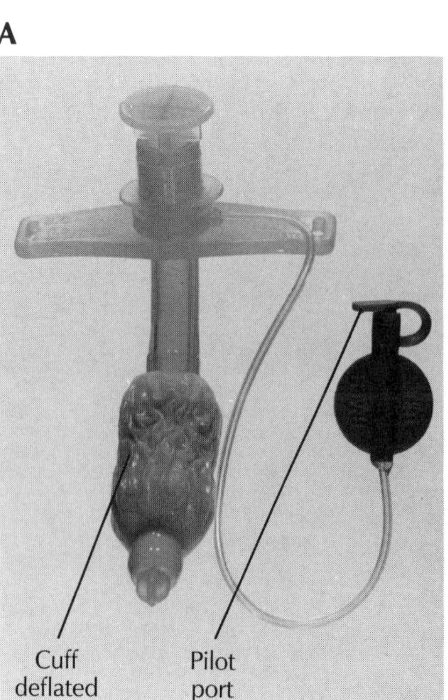

B

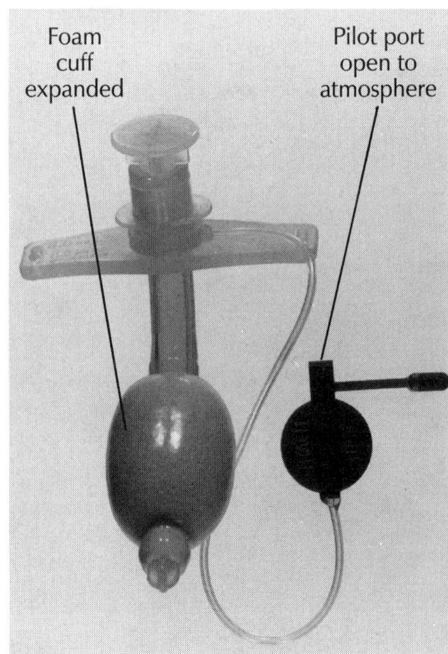

FIG 4–23
Tracheostomy tube with air removed from the foam cuff and the pilot port closed before insertion of the tube, **(A)** and with the foam cuff pilot port open to allow expansion of the cuff **(B)**.

pressure increases. When used properly, this pressure rarely exceeds 20 mm Hg.

When a foam cuff tracheostomy tube is selected, the proper size is important to maintain a seal and still benefit from the pressure-limiting advantages of the foam-filled cuff. If the tube is too small, the foam will inflate to its unrestricted size, and the cuff may leak and cause a loss of desired ventilation and protection against aspiration. If the tube is too large, the foam is unable to expand properly to provide the desired cushion, with resultant increased pressure against the tracheal wall. If air is injected into the cuff to increase the lateral wall pressure and provide a seal, the purpose and pressure-limiting benefits of the foam cuff will be defeated, and it may also cause the cuff to leak and create a loss of ventilator volume during inspiration.

The manufacturer recommends periodic cuff deflation to determine the integrity of the cuff and to prevent the silicone cuff from adhering to the tracheal mucosa. Bivona manufactures a tracheostomy tube that uses the foam cuff concept.[39, 43, 48]

Fenestrated Tracheostomy Tube

The fenestrated tracheostomy tube previously mentioned can be useful in assessing the patient's ability to be decannulated, and it allows the patient to talk when the tube is occluded and the cuff deflated. The fenestrated tracheostomy tube is similar in construction to regular tracheostomy tubes with the addition of an opening or "fenestration" in the posterior portion of the tube above the cuff (Figs 4–22, B and 4–24).

It is composed of a tracheostomy tube with a fenestration, a removable inner cannula, and a plastic plug. When the inner cannula is removed, the cuff deflated, and the normal air passage occluded with the plug, the patient can inhale and exhale through the fenestration and around the tube. This allows for assessment of the patient's ability to breathe through the normal oral/nasal route (preparing the patient for decannulation) and permits air to pass by the vocal cords (allowing phonation).

Personnel must be properly trained in use of the fenestrated tracheostomy tube. If the patient has been receiving humidified oxygen-enriched air via the tube, an alternate source must be provided such as a nasal cannula. Also critical to the process is the fact that the cuff must be completely deflated by evacuating all of the air before the proximal end is blocked. The tracheal cap is then put in place to allow the patient to breathe through the fenestrations and around the tube. If the cuff is left inflated during the capping procedure, the airway resistance will be excessive, and the patient will experience respiratory distress. The patient must be observed carefully for potential aspiration of secretions or oral fluids while the cuff is deflated. Obviously, because of the above-mentioned precautions, this type of tube should only be considered for alert, spontaneously breathing patients with normal upper airway reflexes.

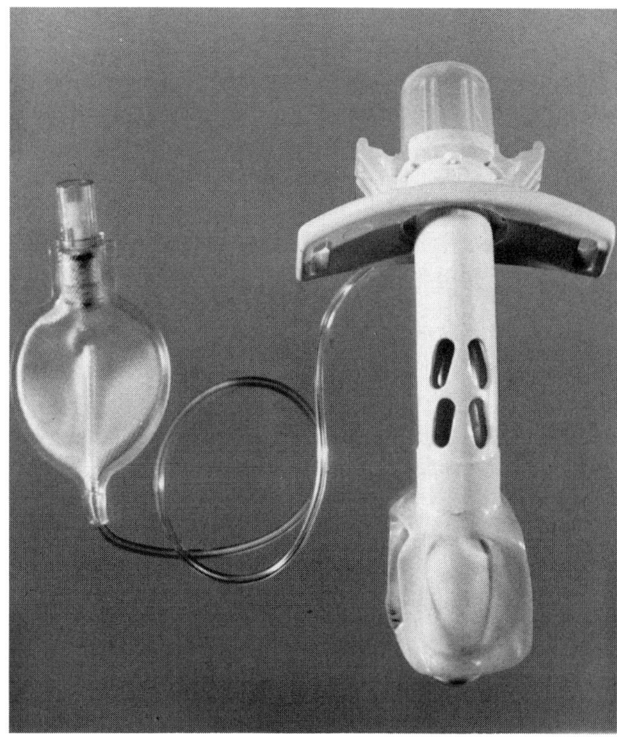

FIG 4–24
Shiley cuffed tracheostomy tube. Cuff, filling tube, and pilot balloon. Fenenestrations.

Talking Tracheostomy Tubes

The primary goal of a "talking" tracheostomy tube is to allow cognitively intact, ventilator-dependent patients the ability to communicate verbally. If a patient has normally functioning oral and laryngeal structures, the options available are an electrolarynx, a self-activated pneumatic system, or a "talking" tracheostomy tube.

The main problem with the electrolarynx is that the cost of the device is often beyond reasonable means. Patients are often frustrated by the unnatural vocal quality of the device, as well as the difficulty with some physically impaired patients in holding the device to the neck while speaking.

The pneumatic system is also limited by the dexterity required to operate the tone switch and the inability to speak clearly because of the intraoral catheter.[48, 49]

Several speaking tracheostomy tubes have been developed that provide intelligible verbal communication for ventilator-dependent patients with spinal cord injuries, neuromuscular diseases, and other causes of respiratory failure. The two most frequently used are the Communitrach I by Implant Techniques, Inc. (Fig 4–25), and the Portex "Talk" tracheostomy tube (not shown).

The Communitrach I is made of PVC, and is radiopaque except for the cuff. The tube has a low-pressure cuff and is designed for ventilator-dependent patients with a normal larynx. It is available in an adult size 7, and the machine end contains a 15-mm adaptor. There are fenestrations located on the posterior portion of the tube above the cuff. Independent channels, one for breathing and one for speech, are formed by seals between the inner and outer channels at both the distal and proximal ends of the Communitrach I. Air for breathing travels through the inner cannula only. The separate source of air for speech is via a speaking air supply connector. This air travels between the inner and outer cannulas, escapes through the fenestrations, is directed toward the vocal cords, and allows phonation while the cuff is inflated. Greater intensities in speech are produced by the additional flow of gas to the tracheostomy tube as compared with no additional flow. The Portex "Talk" (not shown) is similar in design, with the exception being that there is a single slot-type opening in the posterior portion above the cuff rather than several small fenestrations. It is supplied in sizes 7, 8, and 9 mm.

In comparative studies, there was no significant differences found in the degree of voice intensity produced by either tube. However, several design differences in posterior air openings and their incidence of plugging by secretions made the Portex "Talk" tracheostomy tube favorable for greater continuous communication.[50, 51] Two deficiencies cited with regard to the Portex "Talk" tube were that the air supply connector is too large, which causes the oxygen line to the tube to disconnect, and the inner cannula diameter is 2 mm smaller than the outer diameter, which creates increased airway resistance and difficulty in breathing with sizes less than 8 mm.[51]

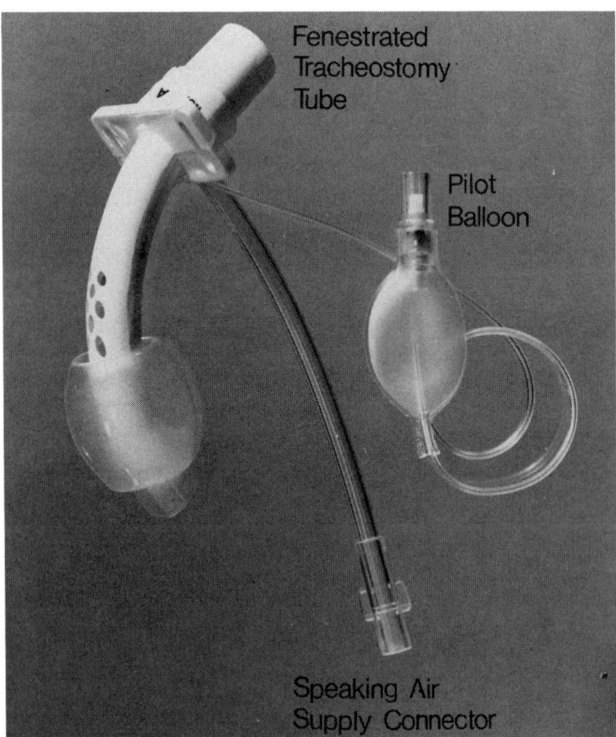

FIG 4–25
Communitrach I talking tracheostomy tube.

These talking tracheostomy tubes provide vital psychological support for tracheotomized patients—the ability to verbally communicate. With early speech rehabilitation, patients who are ventilator dependent or at risk of aspiration and require a cuffed tracheostomy tube will benefit from a speaking tracheostomy tube.

Passy-Muir Tracheostomy Speaking Valves

The Passy-Muir tracheostomy speaking valve (Fig 4–26, B and C) is designed to eliminate the need for finger occlusion in order to verbally communicate. It attaches to the 15-mm universal adaptor of all tracheostomy tubes and can be used in adult and pediatric patients. The valve opens on inspiration, air passing through to the lung, and closes on expiration, air directed into the trachea and up past the vocal cords to permit speech. This device can be used on a spontaneously breathing patient or one who is ventilator dependent (Fig. 4–26, A).

The Passy-Muir valve should be used with caution in patients who are at risk for aspiration because the cuff of the tracheostomy tube must be deflated to use this device. Increases in ventilatory volume may be needed to compensate for leaking around the tracheostomy tube during mechanical ventilation. Following removal of the Passy-Muir valve and reinflation of the tracheostomy cuff, the ventilator should be returned to previous settings to avoid overventilation of the patient. The Passy-Muir valve may also be used in the weaning process to reorient the patient to the use of the upper airway for breathing. Studies evaluating the Passy-Muir valve show that the valve provides natural PEEP, which may enhance the ability to be weaned.

Tracheal Buttons

Tracheal buttons (Fig 4–27) may be used to maintain tracheostomy stomas. These "trach buttons" are temporary appliances generally made of Teflon and consist of a hollow outer cannula and an inner solid cannula. This device fits from the skin to just inside the anterior wall of the trachea. The use of a tracheal button is indicated

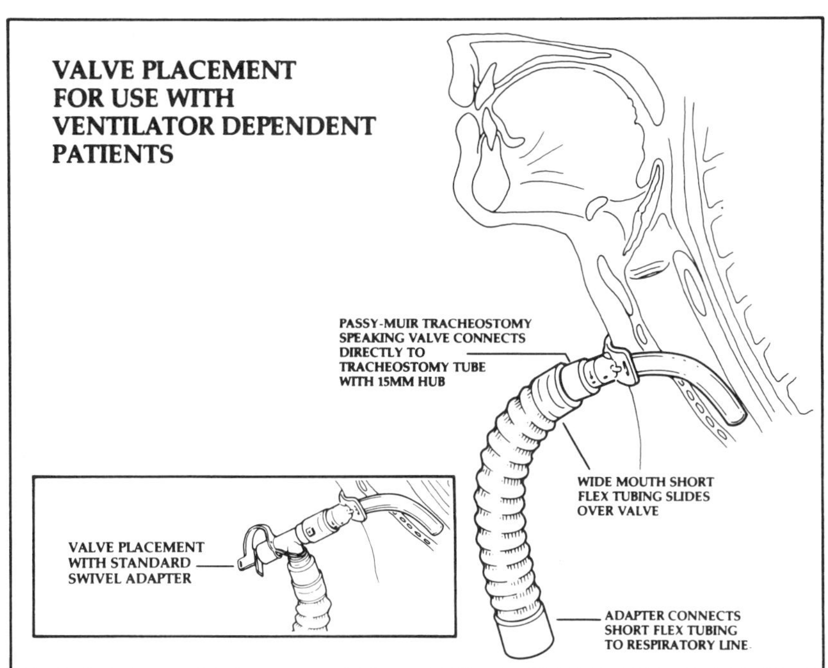

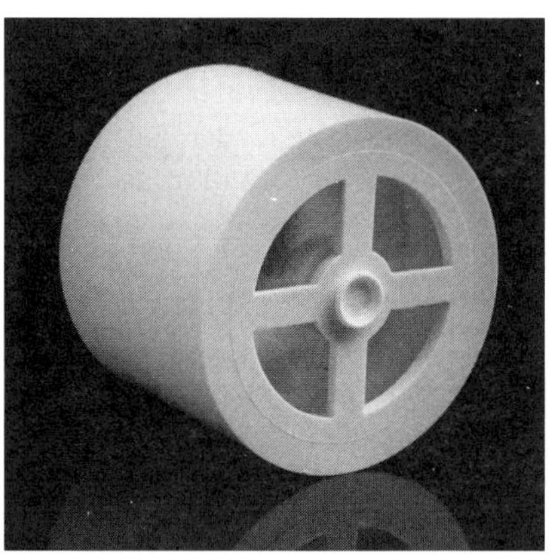

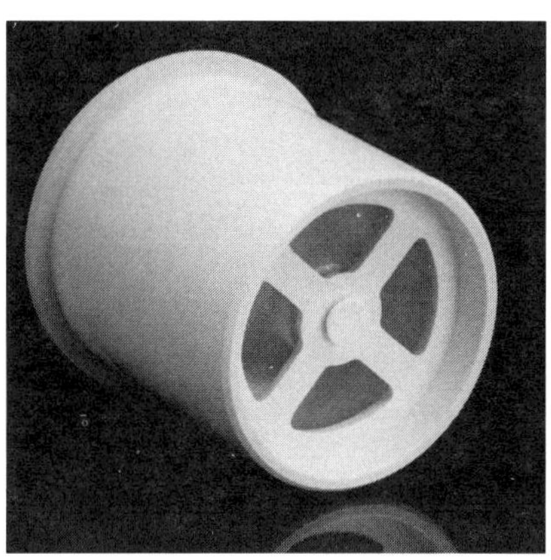

FIG 4–26
Passy-Muir Tracheostomy Speaking Valve. (Courtesy of Passy-Muir, Inc, Irvine, Calif.)

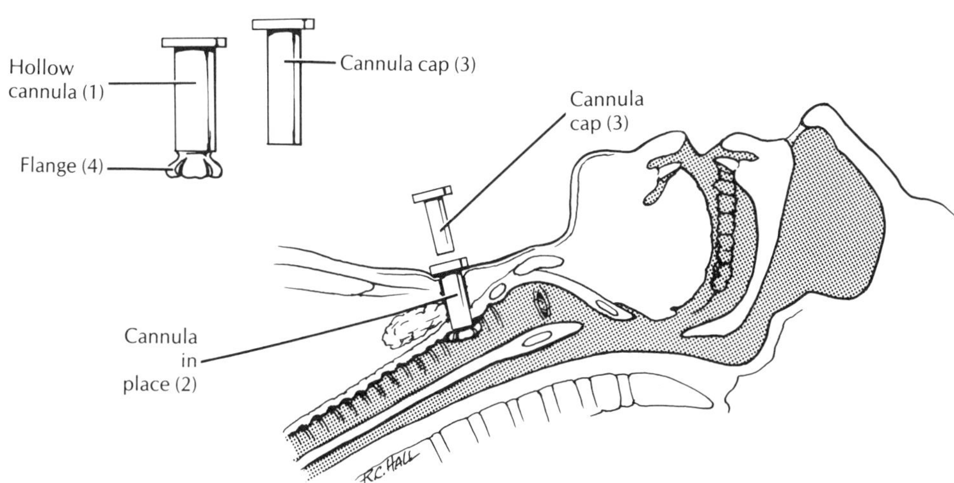

FIG 4–27
Tracheostomy button. (From Eubanks DH, Bone RC: *Comprehensive Respiratory Care,* ed 2. St Louis, Mosby–Year Book, 1990, p 571. Used by permission.)

when the tracheostomy stoma needs to be maintained for either replacement of a tracheostomy tube at a later date or to allow for suctioning. Since a tracheal button does not have a cuff, its use is limited when there is a risk of aspiration or during positive-pressure ventilation.[45]

SPECIAL AIRWAYS AND TUBES

Esophageal Obturator Airway

The esophageal obturator airway (EOA) is a hollow tube with an inflatable cuff near its end. Unlike an endotracheal tube, the EOA end is closed and is designed to be placed into the esophagus rather than the trachea. The tube, which passes through a mask, has several holes in its upper portion for ventilation (Fig 4–28).

The EOA is inserted blindly into the esophagus, where the inflated cuff seals off the lower part of the esophagus to prevent air passage and regurgitation of gastric contents. With the mask tightly sealed to the patient's face, air blown into the EOA is diverted out the pharyngeal holes in the upper portion of the tube and into the trachea and lungs. Since it is easier to place an EOA into the esophagus than an endotracheal tube into the trachea, many emergency medical technicians (EMTs) are trained to use an EOA in lieu of endotracheal intubation whenever an artificial airway is needed in the nonhospital setting. This type of airway may be used when head movement is contraindicated because of a cervical spine injury or after several attempts at endotracheal intubation have been unsuccessful.

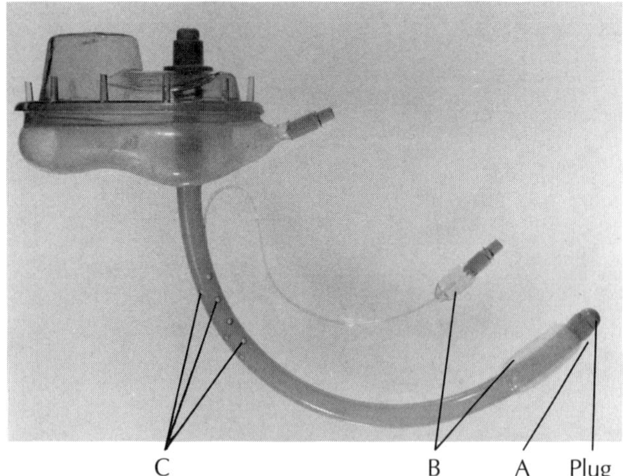

FIG 4–28
Esophageal obturator airway showing a plug blocking the distal end of the tube. **A,** inflatable cuff. **B,** filling tube. **C,** ventilation ports.

Potential Problems

The use of EOAs has several potentially life-threatening complications. The most common of these is inadvertent insertion into the trachea, which if not recognized immediately, results in asphyxia. If improperly positioned, pressure from the inflated EOA cuff expands the esophageal wall, which may compress the trachea and cause occlusion or constriction of the trachea. Esophageal rupture and laceration are other potential serious complications.

The EOA is contraindicated in conscious persons or those with spontaneous respirations. Because of the possibility of displacing the epiglottis in children and infants, it should not be used in persons under the age of 16 years. Its use should also be avoided in persons with known esophageal disease or those who have ingested caustic substances.

An EOA is not removed from an unconscious or semiconscious patient until after a cuffed endotracheal tube is in place. A modified version of an EOA, called an esophageal gastric tube airway (EGTA), includes a gastric tube that can be extended beyond the distal tip of the esophageal end to allow removal of stomach contents and reduce the risk of aspiration.

The continued use of EOAs is controversial. Even when used by trained personnel, an adequate seal is difficult to obtain, often making oxygenation and ventilation suboptimal.[52, 53]

Airway Adjuncts

Endotracheal Tube Exchangers

Occasionally an endotracheal tube needs to be replaced, either because of mechanical failure or because of anatomic changes (Fig 4–29). A leak in the cuff resulting from damage to the cuff or inflation system is the usual cause; however, tracheal dilation caused by prolonged cuff inflation may require placement of a larger tube.

Extubation and subsequent reintubation can be difficult in the presence of upper airway edema, coexisting nasogastric tubes, or cervical traction devices. Direct laryngoscopy in these situations is suboptimal and may even be impossible.

Numerous devices have been used as guides or stylets for endotracheal tube exchange, including nasogastric tubes, Fogarty catheters, central venous catheter conduits, flexible fiber-optic bronchoscopes, and endotracheal tube exchangers. The endotracheal tube exchanger is specifically designed for this purpose, with desirable features such as the proper length, a smooth blunt tip, and rigid but flexible integrity.

Following ventilation with 100% oxygen, the endotracheal tube exchanger is inserted into the existing

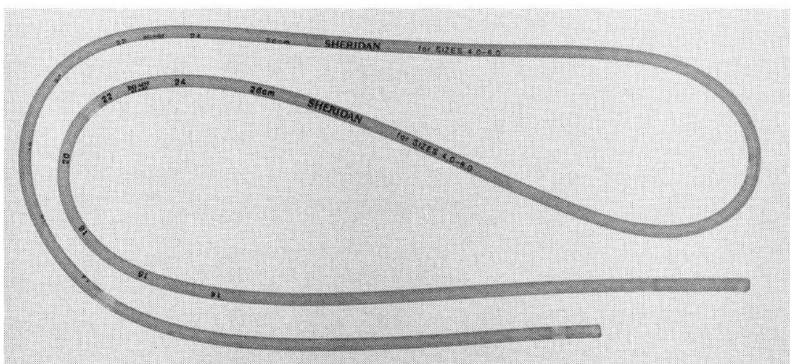

FIG 4–29
Endotracheal tube exchanger.

endotracheal tube beyond the distal end. The cuff is deflated and the endotracheal tube removed over the exchanger while holding the exchanger at its specified depth. Without retracting or advancing the exchanger, the new endotracheal tube is then advanced over the exchanger and into proper position in the trachea. Auscultation of breath sounds and chest radiography should be performed to verify correct positioning of the new endotracheal tube. Placement of the exchanger in the trachea does not ensure endotracheal tube passage, so other forms of emergency airway equipment must be at hand in case of difficulty. Since it is designed specifically for this purpose, it is recommended that the endotracheal tube exchanger be used for this procedure instead of the other devices mentioned.

Stylets

Several different types of stylets are available for use, both in adult and pediatric sizes (Fig 4–30). They are generally made of a malleable metal and are sometimes covered by a plastic material to soften the surface. A stylet is designed to be inserted into an endotracheal tube and then formed to the desired shape to ease insertion of the endotracheal tube. Lubrication of the surface of the stylet with a water-soluble material will facilitate removal of the stylet once the tip of the tube passes through the glottis. Stylets should not extend beyond the Murphy eye in the endotracheal tube, or inadvertent tracheal perforation may result. Laryngeal and pharyngeal trauma is often a potential hazard with the use of stylets because of the increased rigidity of the endotracheal tube. Shearing off pieces of the plastic covering upon withdrawal of the stylet has been reported but is not likely with modern endotracheal tubes.[4] It should also be noted that stylets should not be used when inserting an endotracheal tube nasally.

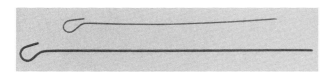

FIG 4–30
Stylets used for insertion of adult- and pediatric-sized tubes.

Cuff Pressure Manometers

Cuff inflation is required to provide a sealed airway for mechanical ventilation and to reduce or prevent the risks of aspiration. Some of the deleterious effects of cuff inflation are tracheal stenosis and tracheomalacia. These problems are related to the pressure exerted by the cuff against the tracheal wall. If this cuff pressure exceeds the perfusion pressure (18 to 20 mm Hg) along the mucosa, ischemia, ulceration and/or damage to the cartilage may result. As previously discussed, with the introduction of high–residual volume, low-pressure cuffs, damage to tracheal walls has lessened but has not been eliminated altogether. Therefore, the measurement of cuff pressure is an important aspect of airway care.

A low-pressure cuff will produce an airtight seal with an intracuff pressure not exceeding 25 cm H_2O (measured during passive exhalation). A higher pressure is more likely to cause tracheal damage.[54]

Cuff pressures can be measured with the use of a three-way stopcock, a syringe, and a pressure manometer (Fig 4–31). The three-way stopcock is attached to the syringe, the manometer, and the cuff inflation line. While opened to all three ports, air is added or removed while the pressure changes are observed on the manometer. There are several manufactured systems available, such as the Pasey Cufflator by J.T. Pasey Co. (not shown) and Cuff-Mate II by DHD (also not shown), which eliminate the need for a separate syringe, manometer, and stopcock.

The two inflation techniques commonly used are minimal occluding volume and the minimal leak technique. With the minimal occluding volume technique, listen for an air leak as the cuff is slowly inflated during positive-pressure inspiration. Stop inflating at the minimum volume needed to eliminate an air leak via the mouth, nose, or tracheostomy stoma.

With the minimal leak technique, air is slowly injected into the cuff during positive-pressure inspiration until the

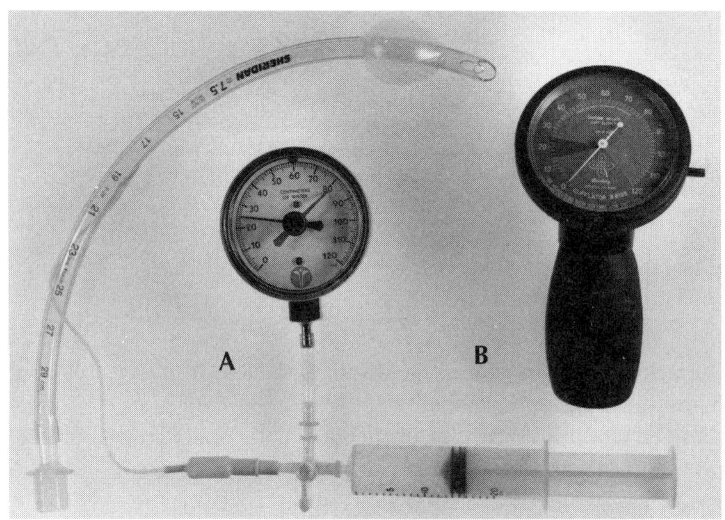

FIG 4–31
Cuff pressure manometer system **(A)** and Cufflator **(B)**.

leak stops. A small amount of air is then removed to allow a slight leak during peak inflation pressure.

Because the airways expand when positive pressure is applied, pressure on the trachea is less during inspiration. Therefore, the use of either the minimal occluding volume or the minimal leak technique does not eliminate the need for cuff pressure measurement to verify that pressure less than 25 cm H_2O is being used consistently.

Laryngoscopy Equipment

Laryngoscopes

A laryngoscope is a device to aid in visualizing the larynx. Generally, a laryngoscope has a battery-operated lighting system, a handle, and several types of detachable blades.

Today, the two commonly used laryngoscopes are direct-lighting or fiber-optic lighting systems. Direct-lighting laryngoscopes have several components (Fig 4–32). The handle comes in pediatric or standard sizes and is composed of a hollow metal chamber that houses the batteries. At one end of the handle is the blade attachment and battery contact point. When properly placed, the attachment blade locks into position and activates the light bulb attached to the threaded receptacle on the distal portion of the laryngoscope blade. This lighting system provides direct lighting to the laryngeal area when the blade is properly placed in the airway.

Fiber-optic laryngoscopes are similar in general appearance to direct-lighting laryngoscopes; however, mechanically they operate quite differently. The hollow handle may be metal or plastic in composition and houses batteries and a pressure-activated light bulb. When a blade containing a fiber-optic channel is seated on the handle, the pressure-activated light bulb turns on and transmits light through the fiber-optic bundle to illuminate the airway. A major advantage of the fiber-optic scope is that it is more flexible and therefore easier to use in small patients and/or those with massive facial or upper airway trauma.

Numerous laryngoscope blades exist for both the direct- and fiber-optic–lighted handles. Only the most commonly used blades will be discussed in this chapter. Each type of blade is usually available in five different

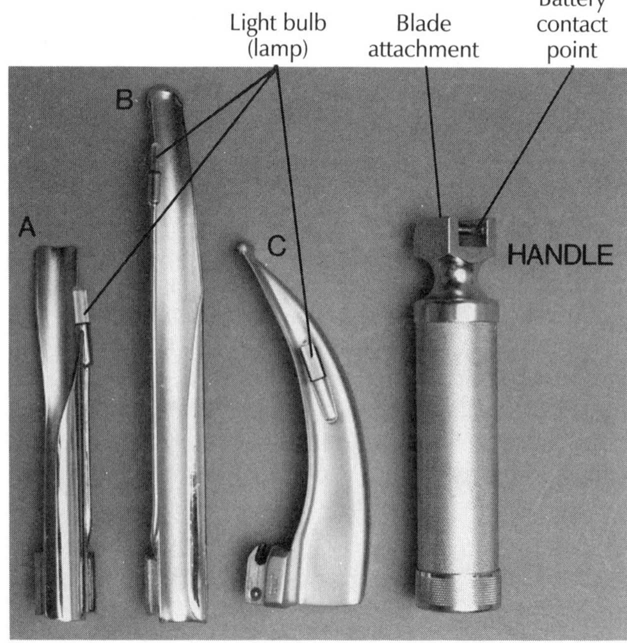

FIG 4–32
Rigid direct-lighting laryngoscope handle and blades. **A,** Wisconsin blade. **B,** Miller blade. **C,** MacIntosh blade.

sizes, 0 for neonatal, 1 for infant, 2 for child/small adult, 3 for adult, and 4 for large adult.

Curved (MacIntosh) blades (Fig 4–32, C) have a flat inferior surface that pushes the tongue to the left. At the tip, a smooth, rounded surface allows atraumatic insertion into the vallecula, the junction of the base of the tongue and the superior aspect of the epiglottis. The superior aspect of the blade is open to allow a larger space in the mouth for endotracheal tube insertion (Fig 4–33).

There are two commonly used straight blades, Wisconsin and Miller. Wisconsin blades (Fig 4–32, A) have a straight three-quarter cylindrical barrel with the light very near the distal tip of the blade. This design allows a straight channel of visualization to the larynx when the epiglottis is lifted from the inferior surface by the blade. Miller blades (Fig 4–32, B) have a smooth, rounded, downward-curved tip that also lifts the inferior surface of the epiglottis. Similar to the Wisconsin blade, it has a three-quarter cylindrical barrel; however, it is flatter in design.

Direct-lighting and fiber-optic laryngoscopy components are not compatible with each other since the direct-lighting system has the light bulb in the blade and the fiber-optic lighting system has the light bulb in the handle. The choice of blade is based on the user's experience and familiarity with a particular blade. Most laryngoscopists train with one blade predominantly and use an alternate blade occasionally when it would be more advantageous than the routinely used blade. In essence, personal preference of the user determines the blade used.

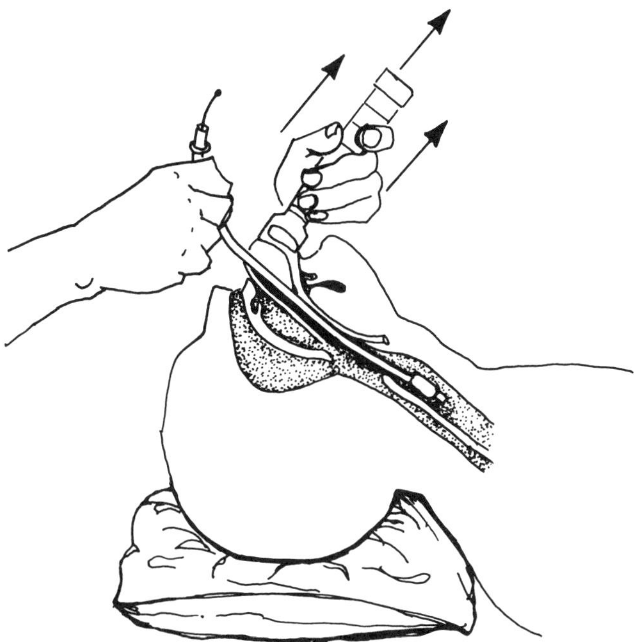

FIG 4–33
Using a direct-lighting laryngoscope to pass the endotracheal tube. To maintain a clear view while inserting the endotracheal tube, pass the tube gently just lateral to the path of the laryngoscope. Carefully maneuver the tube between the vocal cords until the distal end rests 2 cm above the carina. (From Eubanks DH, Bone RC: *Comprehensive Resp. Care* 2nd ed. Pg 567. Mosby–Year Book).

Laryngoscopes are used to visualize the pharynx and larynx, usually for endotracheal intubation to establish an airway in cardiopulmonary resuscitation, anesthesia, respiratory insufficiency/failure, and trauma (Fig 4–33). Intubation of the trachea does not mandate the use of a laryngoscope. Blind insertion, tactile insertion, and fiber-optic bronchoscopy are other alternative methods of endotracheal intubation. Laryngoscopy is popularly used for anesthetized/paralyzed patients because the tube can be visualized as it passes through the vocal cords into the trachea. When compared with fiber-optic bronchoscopy, the equipment is much less expensive, easier to use, and more readily available in an emergency, and it does not require a separate power source.

Patients who are awake or who have normal muscle tone may not tolerate the use of a laryngoscope without sedation and/or topical anesthesia. The key to proper use of the laryngoscope is patient selection and preparation. The minimum equipment necessary for intubation includes oxygen, an Ambu bag with a mask, suction with tonsil tip, laryngoscope, endotracheal tube, syringe, and tape.

In cardiopulmonary resuscitation, rapid establishment of the airway is vital, and very little time is allowed for preparation. Intubation for anesthesia is a much more controlled situation, with optimal conditions present through the use of topical anesthesia, sedatives, and/or muscle relaxants. Some of the most difficult situations for intubation include awake patients with respiratory insufficiency, semiconscious patients with respiratory insufficiency, semiconscious patients with impending respiratory failure, and patients with head, facial, or cervical spine trauma. In these situations laryngoscopy may be extremely difficult or impossible or may even worsen the condition of the patient.

Choosing a laryngoscope is comparable to a tennis player's choice of racquet or a carpenter's choice of hammer. Any of the choices can do the job, but to perform efficiently and successfully in most situations, the operator needs to be comfortable with the laryngoscope. Functionally, there are some advantages and disadvantages to the different types of systems. The direct-lighting laryngoscope is thought to provide better lighting because the light bulb is closer to the area to be illuminated. However, this system requires one light bulb for each blade in the set and also different-sized light bulbs for different-sized blades. Since the light bulbs are detachable, a bulb could potentially become detached while in the patient's airway. Cleaning of the equipment is also more difficult since cleaning solutions may penetrate into the contact areas and cause malfunction. The Propper fiber-optic laryngoscope system (not shown) provides adequate lighting and has the additional advantages of single-piece blades that are easily cleaned and only one light bulb that is located in the laryngoscope handle. Single-use disposable laryngoscopes are available and avoid the cleaning/sterilizing problems; however, many laryngoscopists do not feel as comfortable with the plastic construction as compared with the metal laryngoscope.

Bullard Intubating Laryngoscopes

The Bullard intubating laryngoscope (Fig 4–34) provides indirect visualization of the larynx by using two light bundles, one is the light carrier and the other is the image bundle. These bundles are incorporated into a fixed, curved, metal tongue-blade attached to a laryngoscope handle. A fiber-optic light source may also be used for greater illumination. A third port in the blade tip is the working port, which may be used for suction, local anesthetics, oxygen administration, or the use of intubating forceps. This laryngoscope was designed for use in patients when direct visualization of the larynx would be difficult or impossible. Trauma, limited neck extension, limited mouth opening, and other anatomic abnormalities of the upper airway are specific situations when a Bullard laryngoscope may be useful.

Since the Bullard laryngoscope uses indirect visualization of the larynx, it requires a considerable amount of practice to become proficient in its use. Occasionally the larynx can be visualized, but difficulty arises when trying to manipulate the tip of the endotracheal tube to a more anterior position in the larynx. The use of a stylet may facilitate proper positioning in this situation. The Bullard intubating laryngoscope is available in adult and pediatric sizes and is beneficial in the management of some difficult airway cases.

Flexible Fiber-Optic Laryngoscopes/ Bronchoscopes

Flexible fiber-optic laryngoscopes/bronchoscopes (Fig 4–35) are designed for endoscopic observation of the respiratory tract, management of endotracheal intubation in patients with difficult airways, and verification of endotracheal tube placement. The Olympus LF-2 is an example of a tracheal intubation fiberscope. It has high-resolution optics encased in a waterproof insertion tube with a 4-mm OD and a 600-mm working length. There are two fiber-optic light bundles, one to transmit light and the other to receive the image on the viewing scope. A 1.5-mm-ID working channel can be used for suction, gas administration, or administration of local anesthetics. This device requires an electrically powered light source.

Intubation with a flexible fiber-optic laryngoscope requires more training and skill than with the standard laryngoscope. In general, it is used in difficult airways as described previously for the Bullard Intubating Laryngoscope, but it can also be used for verification of endotracheal and endobronchial tube placement.[38] More detailed information on fiber-optic bronchoscopy will be presented in a subsequent chapter.

Initial capital costs, labor-intensive maintenance, and

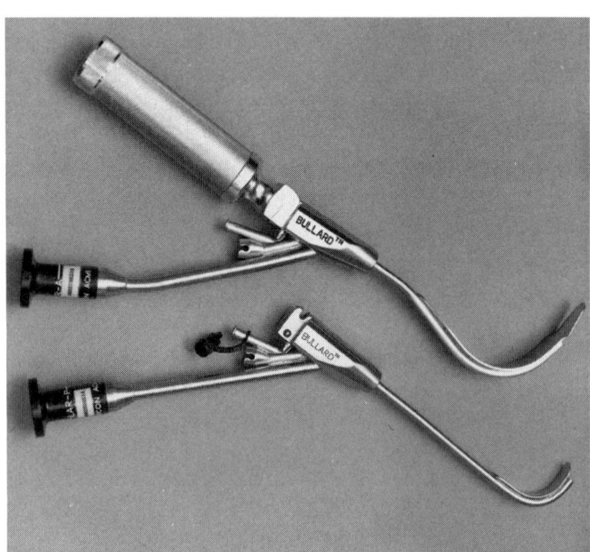

FIG 4–34
Bullard laryngoscope.

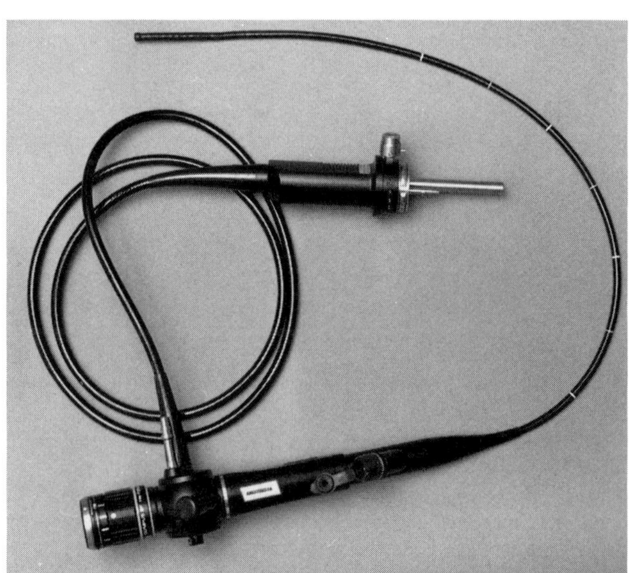

FIG 4–35
Flexible laryngoscope or bronchoscope.

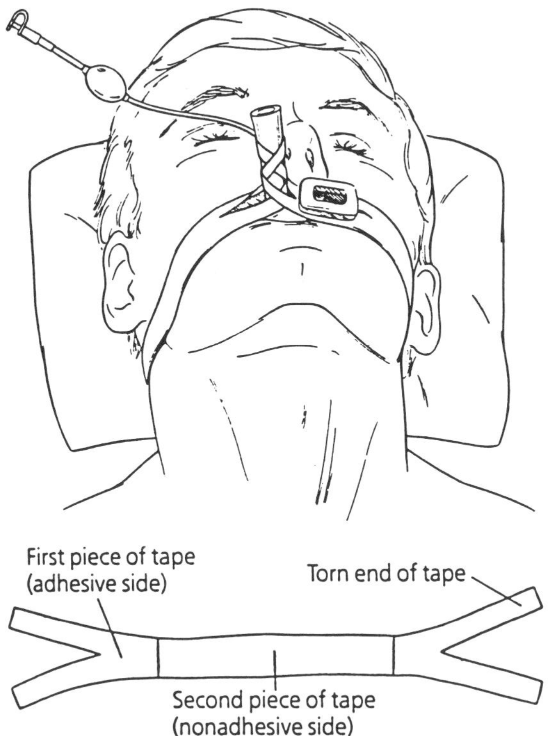

FIG 4–36
The best method for securing the tube's position involves nothing more complicated than two pieces of adhesive tape. The first is quite long (perhaps 2 ft) and split at both ends. The second piece of tape is roughly half the length of the first. Place the second piece of tape in the center of the first so that the adhesive sides of both pieces are pressed together. This will create a nonadhesive surface that can be wrapped around the patient's head without sticking to the hair. The ends of the first piece of tape are then wrapped around the endotracheal tube as shown. This creates a firm anchor for the tube. (From Gluck E, Eubanks DH, Bone RC: *J Crit Care Illness* 1992; 7:1323. Used by permission.)

rigorous training requirements limit wide-scale use of the flexible fiber-optic laryngoscope/bronchoscope for routine intubation. A disadvantage of using the fiber-optic laryngoscope only for emergency situations is that it requires frequent use in order for the practitioner to remain proficient—individuals who do not routinely participate in numerous emergency intubations may not insert enough tubes to maintain a desired level of competence.

Endotracheal Tube Holders

Methods of securing the endotracheal tube against movement in the trachea and/or accidental removal are problems that probably have been a topic of discussion and personal preference since the first tube was introduced. Traditional methods include the use of two pieces of water-resistant adhesive tape that are folded to prevent adherence to the patient's neck as they are passed around the neck and secured to the endotracheal tube (Fig 4–36).

A

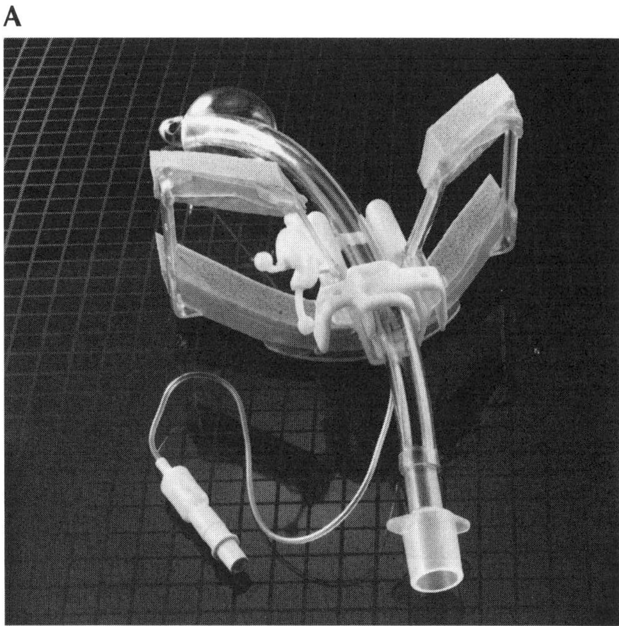

B

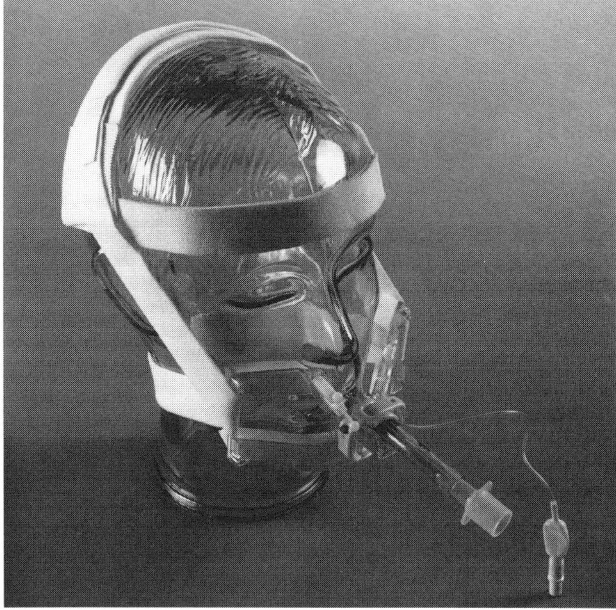

FIG 4–37
SecureEasy Endotracheal Tube Holder. **A,** SecureEasy before placement. **B,** SecureEasy in place with head harness. Endotracheal and nasogastric tubes are anchored without the use of tape. (Courtesy of IPI Medical Products, Chicago.)

A commercial system (SecureEasy) holds the endotracheal tube securely in place without adhesive taping and incorporates a soft bite block to prevent the patient from clamping down and occluding his own orotracheal tube (Fig 4–37, A and B). This tube holder is touted by the manufacturer to reduce the skin irritations caused by adhesive taping while securing the tube against accidental extubation.

SUMMARY

The selection and proper use of artificial airways is a competency that is essential to all respiratory care personnel. It is critical that physicians and others recognize which airway is best suited for a given clinical situation and, once it is placed, whether or not the airway is achieving the desired outcome. This knowledge and skill cannot be learned exclusively from a textbook and must be attained by many hours of working with patients who require artificial airways. Having achieved the objectives that were stated at the beginning of this chapter is a good start to becoming knowledgeable in airways.

REFERENCES

1. Berman RA, Lilienfeld SM: The Berman airway. *Anesthesiology* 1950; 11:136–137.
2. Kupp PJ, Crewe TC: An airway for the edentulous adult. *Anaesthesia* 1974; 29:601–602.
3. Carroll PF: Artificial airways = real risks. *Nursing* 1986; Aug, pp 56–59.
4. Collin VJ: *Principles of Anesthesiology*. Philadelphia, Lea & Febiger, 1966, pp 137–138.
5. Gallagher WI, Pierce AC, Powers SJ: Assessment of a new nasopharyngeal airway. *Br J Anaesth* 1988; 60:112–115.
6. Wanner A, Zighelboim A, Sackner MA: Nasopharyngeal airway: A facilitated access to the trachea for nasotracheal suction, bedside broncho-fiberoscopy and selective bronchoscopy. *Ann Intern Med* 1975; 75:593–595.
7. Haaf DP, Helms PJ, Diniwiddie R, et al: Nasopharyngeal airways in Pierre Robin syndrome. *J Pediatr* 1982; 100:698–703.
8. Schwatz AJ, Dougal RM, Lee WK: Modification of oral airway as a bite block. *Anesth Analg* 1980; 59:225.
9. O'Connor DCJ: A new airway-gag. *Lancet* 1958; 1:356–357.
10. Dorsch JA, Dorsch SE: *Understanding Anesthesia Equipment.* Baltimore, Williams & Wilkins 1984, pp 331–336.
11. Pollard BJ, O'Leary J: Guedel airway and tooth damage. *Anesth Intensive Care* 1981; 9:395.
12. American National Standard Institute: *Tracheal Tube.* ANSI Z79.14-1983. New York, 1983.
13. Cole F: A new endotracheal tube for infants. *Anesthesiology* 1969; 31:378–379.
14. Penlingon GN: Endotracheal tube sizes for children. *Anesthesiology* 1975; 24:494–495.
15. Canfield HMC: Orotracheal tubes and the metric system. *Br J Anaesth* 1963; 35:34.
16. Strong R, Passy: Endotracheal intubation: Complications in neonates. *Arch Otolaryngol* 1977; 103:329–335.
17. Brandstater B: Dilatation of the larynx with Cole tube. *Anesthesiology* 1969; 31:378–379.
18. Loeser EA, Stanley TH, Jordan W, et al: Postoperative sore throat: Influence of tracheal tube lubrication versus cuff design. *Can Anaesth Soc J* 1980; 27:156–158.
19. Dobrin P, Canfield T: Cuffed endotracheal tubes: Mucosal pressures and tracheal wall blood flow. *Am J Surg* 1977; 133:562–568.
20. Cooper JD, Grillo HC: Experimental production and prevention of injury due to cuffed tracheal tubes. *Surg Gynecol Obstet* 1969; 129:1235–1241.
21. Dunn CR, Dunn DL, Moser KM: Determinants of tracheal injury by cuffed tracheostomy tubes. *Chest* 1974; 65:128–135.
22. Lewis FR, Schlabohn RM, Thomas AN: Prevention of complications from prolonged tracheal intubation. *Am J Surg* 1978; 135:452–457.
23. Schwaf RJ, Schnader J: Ventilator autocycling due to an endotracheal tube cuff leak. *Chest* 1991; 100:1172–1173.
24. Heusner JE, Viscomi CM: Endotracheal tube cuff failure due to valve damage. *Anesth Analg* 1991; 72:262–270.
25. You G, Jong W, Oh TE: Failure of endotracheal tube cuff deflation. *Anesth Intensive Care* 1990; 118:425.
26. Patterson KW, Keane P: Missed diagnosis of cuff herniation in a modern nasal endotracheal tube. *Anesth Analg* 1990; 71:561–569.
27. Stark P: Inadvertent nasogastric tube insertion into the tracheobronchial tree. *Radiology* 1982; 142:239–240.
28. Ring WH, Adair JC, Elwyn RA: A new pediatric endotracheal tube. *Anesth Analg* 1975; 54:273–274.
29. Dorsch JA, Dorsch SE: *Understanding Anesthesia Equipment.* Baltimore, Williams & Wilkins 1984, pp 358–361.
30. McTaggert RA, Shustack AS, Noseworthy T, et al: Another cause of obstruction in an armored endotracheal tube. *Anesthesiology* 1983; 59:164.
31. Papulaire C, Robara S: An armored endotracheal tube obstruction in a child. *Can J Anaesth* 1989; 36:331–332.
32. ECRI: Airway fires: Reducing the risk during laser surgery. *Health Devices* 1990; 19:109–139.
33. Hawkins DB, Joseph MM: Avoiding a wrapped endotracheal tube in laser laryngeal surgery: Experience with apneic anesthesia and metal Laser-Flex endotracheal tube. *Laryngoscope* 1990; 100:1283–1287.
34. ECRI: Hazard. Xomed Laser-Shield endotracheal tubes: Flammable tubes still being used. *Health Devices* 1991; 20:444–445.
35. Barash PG, Deutsch S, Tinker J: Anesthesia for laser surgery. *ASA Refresher Course Anesthesiol* 1989; 17:215–226.
36. Miller RD: *Anesthesia,* ed 3. New York, Churchill Livingstone, 1990, p 1554.
37. Strange C: Double lumen endotracheal tubes. *Clin Chest Med* 1991; 12:497–506.
38. Benumof IL, Partriage BL, Salutierra C, et al: Margin of safety in positioning modern double-lumen endotracheal tubes. *Anesthesiology* 1987; 67:729–738.
39. Stauffer JL, Silvester RC: Complications of endotracheal intubation, tracheostomy, and artificial airways. *Respir Care* 1982; 27:417–434.
40. Jackson C: The technique of insertion of intratracheal insufflator tubes. *Surg Gynecol Obstet* 1913; 17:507.
41. An improved method for emergency cricothyrotomy. International Medical Devices, NU-TRAKE, 1980.

42. Downes JJ, Schreiner MS: Tracheostomy tubes and attachments in infants and children. *Int Anesthesiol Clin* 1985; 23:37–60.
43. Myer EN, Stool SE, Johnson JT: *Tracheotomy*. New York, Churchill Livingstone, 1988, pp 132–133.
44. Bach JR, Alba AS: Tracheostomy ventilation: A study of efficacy with deflated cuffs and cuffless tubes. *Chest* 1990; 97:679–683.
45. Scanlon CL, Spearman CB, Sheldon RL: *Egan's Fundamental's of Respiratory Care,* ed 5. St Louis, Mosby–Year Book, 1990.
46. Galoof HD, Toledo PS: Comparison of five types of tracheostomy tubes in the intubated trachea. *Ann Otol* 1978; 87:99–108.
47. Kamen JM, Wilkinson CJ: A new low-pressure cuff for endotracheal tubes. *Anesthesiology* 1971; 34:482.
48. Stauffer JL, Olson DE, Petty TL: Complications and consequences of endotracheal intubation and tracheostomy: A prospective study of 150 critical ill adult patients. *Am J Med* 1981; 70:65–76.
49. Sparker AW, Robin KT, Newland GN, et al: A prospective evaluation of speaking tracheostomy tubes for ventilator dependent patients. *Laryngoscope* 1987; 97:89–92.
50. Leder SB, Astrachan DE: Stomal complications and airflow line problems of the Communitrach I Cuffed Talking Tracheostomy Tube. *Laryngoscope* 1990; 100:1116–1121.
51. Leder SB: Verbal communication for the ventilator dependent patient: Voice intensity with the Portex "Talk" Tracheostomy Tubes. *Laryngoscope* 1990; 100:1116–1121.
52. American Heart Association: Standards for cardiopulmonary resuscitation and emergency cardiac care. *JAMA* 1986; 225:2843–2989.
53. Donen N, Tweed WA, Dashfsky S, et al: The esophageal obturator airway: An approval. *Can Anaesth Soc J* 1983; 30:194–200.
54. Selecky PA: Tracheostomy: A review of present day indications, complications, and care. *Heart Lung* 1974; 3:272–283.

5

Manual Resuscitators, Mechanical Ventilators, and Breathing Circuits

JOSEPH SORBELLO, M.S., RRT
RUSSELL A. ACEVEDO, M.D., F.C.C.P.

OBJECTIVES

- Appraise the performance characteristics of various self-inflating manual resuscitators.
- Differentiate between the clinical applications of self-inflating manual resuscitators, bag-and-valve resuscitators, gas-powered resuscitators, and demand valves.
- List the four basic functions of intermittent positive-pressure ventilation.
- Describe the four distinct phases of mechanical ventilation common to all mechanical ventilators.
- Define and explain the terms and definitions used in mechanical ventilation.
- Describe mechanical ventilator function based on the following categories: power input, power transmission or conversion, control, and output.
- Classify specific mechanical ventilators by power source, circuitry, control mechanisms, control variables, triggering mechanisms, inspiratory phase limits, cycling mechanisms, modes, and expiratory phase variables.
- Given a diagram or actual external ventilator breathing circuit, identify the component parts of the system.
- Given a diagram or actual external ventilator breathing circuit, trace the flow of gas through the system during inspiration and exhalation.
- Explain the potential effects of positive-pressure ventilation on various body systems.
- Describe the effects of various forms of positive pressure on the cardiopulmonary system.
- State the advantages and disadvantages of negative-pressure ventilation, control ventilation, assist/control ventilation, intermittent mandatory ventilation, pressure support ventilation, high-frequency positive-pressure ventilation, and inverse ratio ventilation.
- Discuss the work of breathing as it relates to the use of ventilator modes and patient circuitry.
- Describe factors that influence ventilation/perfusion relationships in the human lung.
- Explain the hemodynamic interaction that exists between the heart and lung.

The art of mechanical ventilation requires clinicians to combine their knowledge of normal cardiopulmonary physiology and pathophysiology, respiratory care techniques, and technical aspects of modern mechanical ventilators. This chapter is presented in two sections. The first section will cover the technical aspects and clinical application of some of the so-called second- and third-generation mechanical ventilators, ventilator circuitry, and manual resuscitators used in adult critical care. The second section focuses on the pathophysiology of the lung and how application of mechanical ventilation affects lung physiology.

POSITIVE-PRESSURE VENTILATION

Lung inflation is most easily accomplished by applying positive pressure to the airway, usually via oral/nasal endotracheal tubes and tracheostomy tubes. Positive-pressure ventilation may also be accomplished via face mask and nasal mask. In critical care units, lung expansion involving subatmospheric pressure (negative-pressure ventilation) is not as common as positive-pressure ventilation, and it will not be discussed here.

Positive-pressure ventilation can be accomplished mechanically by using a manual resuscitator, demand valves, and mechanical ventilators. When positive pressure is used to inflate the lungs, the process is termed intermittent positive-pressure ventilation[1] (IPPV) and usually refers to continuous mechanical ventilation. This differs from intermittent positive-pressure breathing (IPPB) in that IPPB describes the use of a ventilator to deliver aerosolized isotonic (normal) saline or other medication under positive pressure. IPPB is used as a short-term, periodic (16 to 20 minutes) breathing treatment for those otherwise spontaneously breathing patients who cannot generate adequate ventilation over extended periods of time.

MANUAL RESUSCITATORS AND DEMAND VALVES

As suggested by Pilbeam,[1] manual resuscitators are an integral part of the steps in beginning ventilatory support. These steps include patient preparation, establishment of an airway, manual ventilation, cardiovascular stabilization, ventilatory needs, and treatment of the cause of respiratory failure. Having established access to the airway, the manual resuscitator can be used to support the patient's ventilatory needs. The ideal manual resuscitator is easy to operate, troubleshoot, assemble/disassemble, and clean. The advantages of this device include its relative easy accessibility and portability and its ability to do the following: provide immediate ventilatory assistance, allow the clinician to monitor the patient's breathing efforts, and allow the clinician to respond to changes in airway resistance or lung-thorax compliance.

Manual resuscitators (also referred to as resuscitator bags or manually operated resuscitators) are devices using either a self-inflating or non–self-inflating bag, a one-way (nonrebreathing) valve system, an air/oxygen intake valve, an oxygen inlet nipple, and a high oxygen reservoir attachment. The basic purpose of a manual resuscitator is to provide positive pressure to the airway in conjunction with a face mask or artificial airway (endotracheal tube, tracheostomy tube, esophageal obturator airway, esophageal gastric tube airway, oral or nasal airways) while providing an oxygen concentration (fraction of inspired oxygen [F_{IO_2}]) range of 0.21 to 1.00. An excellent summary of the published reports on the performance of manual resuscitators along with standards/recommendations for design, testing, and clinical application was published recently by Barnes.[2]

The indications for the use of a manual resuscitator include

- Transport of a patient
- Emergency resuscitation (CPR)
- Stimulation of a cough
- Tracheobronchial aspiration (suctioning)
- Preparation for attachment to continuous mechanical ventilation
- Backup ventilation system for mechanical ventilators

Features of Manual Resuscitators

There are several types of manual resuscitators used throughout the United States and other countries. In general, the ideal manual resuscitator should

- Contain a true nonrebreathing valve system capable of 30-L/min (previous standard, 15 L/min) input flow without jamming
- Provide up to 100% oxygen at high delivered stroke volumes and ventilation rates without limiting delivered pressure
- Be constructed of materials that are easy to clean/disinfect/sterilize
- Have standard 15- and 22-mm connections that are available in adult and pediatric sizes

The standards for the design and construction of these devices were published by the American Society for Testing and Materials (ASTM)[3] from the results of national conferences on standards for cardiopulmonary resuscitation, which were published in the *Journal of the American Medical Association (JAMA)* in 1986 and 1992,[4, 5] and from the International Organization for Standardization (ISO).[6] These standards are important since they can be used as criteria for selecting the optimal manual resuscitator in terms of effectiveness, safety, and utility. Although there are many standards, below is a summary of those that are thought to be most relevant to a clinician's selection of a manual resuscitator for various uses.

An adequate bag-valve unit should have

- A self-refilling bag that is easily cleaned and sterilized
- A nonjam valve system allowing for a minimum oxygen inlet flow of 30 L/min
- A no–pop-off valve
- Standard 16-mm/22-mm fittings
- A system for delivering high concentrations of oxygen through an ancillary oxygen inlet at the back of the bag or by an oxygen reservoir
- A true nonrebreathing valve
- Satisfactory performance under all common environmental conditions and extremes of temperature (−180 to 600° C) and relative humidity (40% to 96%)
- Both adult and pediatric sizes
- A face mask provided with or intended for use

with a manual resuscitator; the mask shall have a body, face seal, and connector capable of receiving the patient connector of the resuscitator

Additionally, a manual resuscitator should have the following features:

- The body of the mask should be transparent.
- The face seal should provide an effective fit that minimizes leaks over the operating pressures and temperature.
- The apparatus dead space of the resuscitator, excluding the face mask, shall not exceed 30 mL for adults, 16 mL for children, and 7 mL for infants.
- The resuscitator shall be designed to facilitate effective operation by one person when used with a face mask to provide adequate ventilation of the patient's lungs.
- The resuscitator components in contact with the patient breathing mixture shall withstand sterilization or be labeled for single use only (disposable).
- The resuscitator shall be designed to minimize incorrect reassembly; for those designed to be disassembled, the manufacturer shall include disassembly and assembly instructions, which shall include a schematic showing correct assembly.
- If equipped with an overpressure limiting system, there should be an audible or visible warning to the operator when the pressure-limiting system is activated. *(Note that ASTM has not changed this general requirement as of this publication date to coincide with the American Heart Association (AHA) recommendations for a no–pop-off valve.)*
- The pressure-limiting system, if provided, shall be capable of being overridden by the user.
- The override mechanism shall be readily apparent and directions provided to the user.
- Adult resuscitators shall deliver a tidal volume of no less than 600 mL into a test lung set at a compliance of 0.02 L/cm H_2O and resistance of 20 cm H_2O/L/sec.
- The tidal volume shall be achieved at a respiratory rate of no less than 20 breaths per minute without inversing the inspiratory:expiratory (I:E) ratio.
- The resuscitator shall deliver an F_{IO_2} (F_{DO_2}) of at least 40% when an oxygen source is available and at least 86% with an oxygen reservoir.
- When disabled by vomitus, the valve should be capable of being restored to proper function within 20 seconds.
- ASTM recommendations state that resuscitators conform with pressure limit and minute ventilation requirements after a shock test (being dropped 1 m onto a concrete surface).
- The F_{IO_2} delivery should be at least 86%; resuscitators should also be capable of delivering other percentages of oxygen, as specified by the manufacturer. The manufacturers should also specify the conditions under which various percentages of oxygen may be delivered.
- The device's gas connection shall be noninterchangeable; with threaded connection, it shall conform to the appropriate Compressed Gas Association (CGA) V-6 1978 specification for diameter index safety system (DISS) connections and shall be capable of functioning at 66 psig, +20%, −26%.
- The manufacturer shall state the approximate duration of a "D" (approximately 369 L) and "E" (approximately 626 L) size cylinder when the resuscitator is delivering a minute volume of 10 L/min of at least 86% oxygen or the manufacturer's selected value less than 86% oxygen.
- The maximum delivery pressure shall not exceed 66 cm H_2O over the range of supply pressures.
- The devices shall have a flow capability of at least 100 L/min at 20 cm H_2O, and flows at 40 cm H_2O shall be stated in the labeling.

The manual resuscitators seen in Table 5–1 are a fair representation of the manual resuscitators used in the United States at the present time. All use self-inflating bags, bag inlet valves, and patient (or inflation) valves.

Application Principles of Self-Inflating Manual Resuscitators

According to Eubanks and Bone, there are 12 guiding principles related to the application of self-inflating manual resuscitators.[7]

Principle No. 1

In a pulmonary arrest situation, mouth-to-mouth or other methods of providing immediate ventilation should be initiated unless a manual resuscitator is readily available. The AHA discourages "mouth-to-mouth" ventilation in favor of "mouth-to-mask" ventilation (with a one-way valve for rescuer protection) in lieu of at least two trained persons familiar with manual resuscitator use. The procedure for assessing the operation of a self-inflating manual resuscitator is as follows:

1. Select a manual resuscitator.
2. Remove it from its container.
3. Squeeze the ventilator bag.
   a. Note the rise and fall of nonrebreathing valve and air intake valve.

TABLE 5–1

Summary of Characteristics of Adult Self-Inflating Manual Resuscitators*

Resuscitator	Maximum Suggested Oxygen Flow Rate	Type of Oxygen Reservoir	Maximum Oxygen Percentage Expected With Optimum Conditions
AMBU (early)	<10–15 L/min to avoid valve jamming	Tube or bag with inlet one-way valve such as Laerdal's reservoir assembly	Up to 100%
AMBU E-2	High oxygen flows will not affect proper function	Tube or oxygen reservoir assembly	Up to 100%
Hope	Is less than 15 L/min to avoid valve jamming	Sleeve with tube or bag	Up to 100%
Hope II	High oxygen flows will not affect proper function	"Elephant" bore tube	Up to 100%
Air Viva	5 L/min may cause chattering; 10–15 L/min may cause valve jamming	None	Up to 80%
Laerdal RFB-II, adult	High oxygen flows will not affect proper function	Tube or oxygen reservoir assembly	Up to 100%
PMR	Oxygen flows up to 20 L/min will not affect proper function; flows over 20 L/min may cause some resistance to patient's exhalation. High oxygen flows will not affect proper function	None commercially available	Up to 80%
High Oxygen PMR	Low oxygen flows (<12 L/min) decrease bag refill and available breathing rates (high or low oxygen flows will not affect operation on modified unit)	None (high F_{IO_2} with attached valve movement—see Fig. 5–7)	Up to 100%
PMR II	High oxygen flows will not affect proper function	"Elephant" bore tube	Up to 100%
AIRbird	High oxygen flows will not affect proper function	Tube or tube-with-bag assembly may be added as a modification; demand valve can also be attached	Up to 100%
Hudson Lifesaver II	High flows will not affect proper function	Hudson's reservoir assembly with safety inlet and outlet valves	Up to 100%
Hudson Lifesaver and Robertshaw bag resuscitators			

* From McPherson SP: *Respiratory Therapy Equipment*, ed 4. St. Louis, Mosby–Year Book, 1990, pp 122–123. Used by permission.

   b. Feel air leave the outlet port of the nonrebreathing valve.
4. Test the resuscitator for leaks.
   a. Occlude the outlet port of the nonrebreathing valve and squeeze the bag.
   b. If the bag empties (slow or fast), there is a leak that must be corrected.
5. Disassemble the manual resuscitator according to the manufacturer's instructions and/or hospital procedure. Remove major components:
   a. Nonrebreathing valve.
   b. Ventilator bag.
   c. Oxygen reservoir (if present).
6. Disassemble each component.
   a. Arrange the pieces so that they can be reassembled in reverse order and number.
   b. Name and number each part and give its function as it is disassembled.
7. Reassemble the manual resuscitator by using the manufacturer's directions.
8. Squeeze the bag and note movement of the valves. Feel air leave the outlet port of the nonrebreathing valve.
9. Retest for leaks and correct as necessary.
10. Practice with a test lung. Note the ventilation volume; count the breathing frequency. Add supplemental O_2 and use the manual resuscitator on a test lung. Note changes in bag response time or in operational characteristics.

Type of Pressure Relief	Spontaneous Breathing Opens Valve for Oxygen (Inhalator)	Type of Patient Valve	Type of Bag Inlet Valve	Approximate Volume of Full Bag (mL)
None	No	Spring disk	Spring disk	2,000
None	Yes	Diaphragm	One-way leaf valve	1,300
Optional magnetic ball set to open at 40 cm H_2O	No	Spring disk	One-way leaf valve	2,000
Optional magnetic ball set to open at 40 cm H_2O	No	Spring disk	One-way leaf valve	2,000
Spring ball	No	Spring disk	–	2,000
None	Yes	Diaphragm and duckbill	One-way leaf valve	RFB-II: 1,800 Adult: 1,600
None	Yes	Diaphragm and leaf valve	Diaphragm	2,000
None	Yes	Diaphragm and leaf valve	Diaphragm and one-way (air) or oxygen inlet	2,000
Optional spring-loaded ball set to open at 40 cm H_2O	Yes	Diaphragm (smile face)	One-way leaf valve	1,760
None	Yes	Diaphragm and leaf valve	One-way leaf valve	2,000
None	Yes	Duck bill	One-way leaf valve	1,600
		Diaphragm and leaf valve	Leaf valve	1,800

Principle No. 2

With a manual resuscitator, a leak-proof system must be maintained between the resuscitator and the patient. Emergency ventilation with a self-inflating manual resuscitator is performed as follows:

1. Gather the necessary equipment.
   a. Self-inflating bag.
   b. Mask or tracheal tube.
   c. Adapter.
   d. Oxygen flowmeter.
   e. Oxygen connecting tubing.
   f. Oral airway.
2. Wash hands and don gloves or other protective attire. (If splashing is likely, a gown and face shield [or acceptable eye protectors and mask] may be necessary for rescuer protection.)
3. Assemble the equipment.
4. Connect the flowmeter to an O_2 source, and turn to flush or 15 L/min.
5. Clear the airway if necessary.
   a. Hyperextend the head.
   b. Insert the oral airway.
6. Seal the mask over the patient's mouth and nose, and secure with one hand.
7. Ventilate the patient by intermittently squeezing the bag. Look for chest wall excursion and correct as necessary.
   a. Deliver adequate tidal volume.

b. Ventilate by using the proper frequency.
8. Continuously monitor the patient for effective ventilation.
9. Check for incidental emesis and prevent aspiration.
10. Continue ventilation until relieved or until the procedure is terminated.
11. Return all used equipment for decontamination.
12. Wash hands and remove gloves and other attire.

Principle No. 3

Effective ventilation must be visually assessed by observing the patient's chest expansion during a manual inflation. To secure a face mask with a one-handed grip, the following steps are used:

1. Gather the necessary equipment:
   a. Self-inflating bag.
   b. Assorted sizes of masks.
   c. Assorted sizes of oral airways.
2. Wash hands and don gloves or other protective attire. (If splashing is likely, a gown and face shield [or acceptable eye protectors and face mask] may be necessary for rescuer protection.)
3. Place the patient in the supine position with the shoulders slightly elevated. (NOTE: A modified position must be used in cases of spinal injury.)
4. Insert an oral airway with the correct technique (unnecessary for student practice).
5. With the mask *detached* from the resuscitator bag, place the bridge (nose portion) of the mask over the bridge of the patient's nose.
6. Place the thumb of the left hand over the bridge of the mask, above the mask connector.
7. Place the index finger opposite the thumb below the connector so that it rests just above the mask cushion.
8. Position the chin portion of the mask over the front of the lower jaw while keeping the mask in a straight line.
9. Place three fingers (middle, ring, pinky) along the ridge of the mandible.
   a. Secure the mask by lifting the jaw to cause the face to be raised under the mask while simultaneously hyperextending the head.
   b. Adjust the thumb and index finger to correct for any leaks.
   c. Reposition the head as necessary to improve the airway.
10. Attach the resuscitator bag to the mask with the free hand, and squeeze the bag to deliver breath. (NOTE: In an actual patient situation, the resuscitator bag is not detached from the mask during mask placement.)
11. Do not attempt to correct for air leaks by pressing down on the mask. Proper technique is to rearrange the fingers and hyperextend the head while *lifting the face into the mask.*
12. Note the rise and fall of the patient's chest.
13. Readjust the hand position as necessary to prevent leaks.
14. Continue ventilation until relieved or until the procedure is terminated.
15. Return used equipment for decontamination.
16. Wash hands and remove gloves and other protective attire.

Principle No. 4

In nonintubated patients, care must be taken to protect the patient against possible regurgitation and aspiration of stomach contents. To operate a demand valve to assist and control ventilation, the following procedure is used:

1. Wash hands and don gloves or other protective attire. (If splashing is likely, a gown and face shield [or acceptable eye protectors and face mask] may be necessary for rescuer protection.)
2. Select the equipment:
   a. Demand valve.
   b. Pressure hose.
   c. Assorted sizes of masks.
   d. Assorted oral airways.
3. Connect the delivery hose to a 40- to 90-psi supply pressure source.
4. Depress the control button, and listen for flow of gas from the outlet.
5. Release the control button and note that gas flow ceases.
6. Attach the appropriate size of mask to the valve outlet.
7. Position the patient in the supine position. Insert an oral airway.
8. Apply the mask by hyperextending the head and lifting the patient's face into the mask.
9. Hold the mask in position with two hands.
10. If the patient is not breathing, depress the control button with a thumb until the chest rises; then remove the thumb. Note the fall of the chest. *Do not overinflate.*
11. If the patient is breathing, note the valve's re-

sponse to the patient's inspiratory efforts.
12. Check and correct for air leaks and stomach inflation.
13. Continue ventilation until relieved or until the procedure is terminated.
14. Turn off the supply gas.
15. Remove the demand valve and mask for decontamination.
16. Wash hands and remove gloves and other protective attire.

Principle No. 5

A manual resuscitator must always be tested for correct operation before use on a patient (see Procedures 1 to 4).

Principle No. 6

Excessive flow rates or inflation pressures (greater than 26 cm H_2O) should not be used. They can cause distension of the stomach and/or excessive lung volumes and lead to possible barotrauma. However true this may be in some cases, particularly in infants, the use of high flow rates and/or inflation pressures is often necessary in adults. The AHA now recommends that no pressure relief valves be placed on adult resuscitators so that adequate tidal volumes may be delivered despite the hazards of excessive inflation pressures and/or flow rates.[5] Distension of the stomach with air (usually because of excessive inflation pressures) may be obviated with proper opening of the airway (head tilt and chin lift) or modified jaw thrust/chin lift (see Fig 5–5).

Principle No. 7

Self-inflating units refill from the atmosphere and cannot be used in smoke-filled or other air-polluted environments.

Principle No. 8

Supplemental oxygen must be added to the unit if the patient requires an F_{IO_2} greater than 0.21.

Principle No. 9

The F_{IO_2} delivered (F_{DO_2}) by a manual resuscitator depends on the following parameters:

Stroke volume. The amount of volume squeezed out of the bag between the thumb and all the fingers after full inflation of the bag is the stroke volume. The larger the stroke volume, the larger the volume of oxygen that has to be used to refill the bag. If the oxygen flow rate (liters per minute) is insufficient to fill the reservoir with 100% oxygen, any deficit volume will be satisfied by entrained air, which when mixed with the 100% oxygen concentration in the reservoir bag, will decrease the F_{DO_2}.

Refill time of the bag. The slower the bag refills with oxygen, the smaller the amount of room air entrained, thus leading to a higher F_{DO_2}. Refill time is controlled by a slow release of the hand(s).

Rate. A fast ventilation rate will decrease the time available for the bag to refill and cause a decrease in oxygen concentration (a combination of stroke volume and refill time).

Flow rate of oxygen. The higher the flow rate of oxygen to the bag, the higher the concentration, provided that items are not beyond normal design limits. CAUTION: The use of high oxygen flow rates (above 15 L/min) is not recommended without a special attachment because it may interfere with the function of the valve in some units (the new standard/recommendation is 30 L/min).

The presence or absence of an oxygen reservoir bag (tube or attachment). The placement of an oxygen reservoir allows for the accumulation of more oxygen to be entrained into the bag during refill to increase the F_{DO_2}.

Principle No. 10

Resuscitators with various sized bags should be available for adult and pediatric use.

Principle No. 11

Relief ("pop-off") valves should be adjustable so that high airway pressure can be delivered when needed without the valve venting ("popping off"). NOTE: Relief valves are not used except on pediatric and infant units.

Principle No. 12

Positive end-expiratory pressure (PEEP) attachments should be available for use with patients who are not able to maintain adequate arterial oxygen tension (Pa_{O_2}) on a resuscitator without an attachment.

Additionally, the clinician should remember the following points in the operation of self-inflating manual resuscitators, as previously stated by Eubanks and Bone[7]:

1. The clinician should constantly assess the adequacy of ventilation along with the compliance and airway resistance offered by the patient. Decreasing compliance and/or increasing airway resistance is determined by the increasing difficulty in delivering the tidal volume. The immediate adequacy of ventilation is assessed through simple observation of bilateral chest movement and auscultation of breath sounds.
2. It is important that the clinician realize the limitations of any clinical assessment for predicting the effectiveness of ventilation. An accurate assessment of ventilation can be made only by

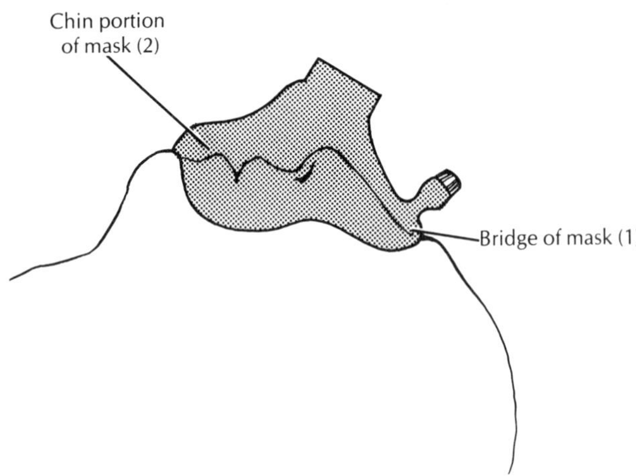
Chin portion
of mask (2)
Bridge of mask (1)

FIG 5–1
Proper placement of a resuscitation unit mask over a patient's face. (From Eubanks DH, Bone RC: Cardiopulmonary resuscitation, in Eubanks DH, Bone RC (eds): *Comprehensive Respiratory Care: A Learning System,* ed 2. St Louis, Mosby–Year Book, 1990, pp 638–639. Used by permission.)

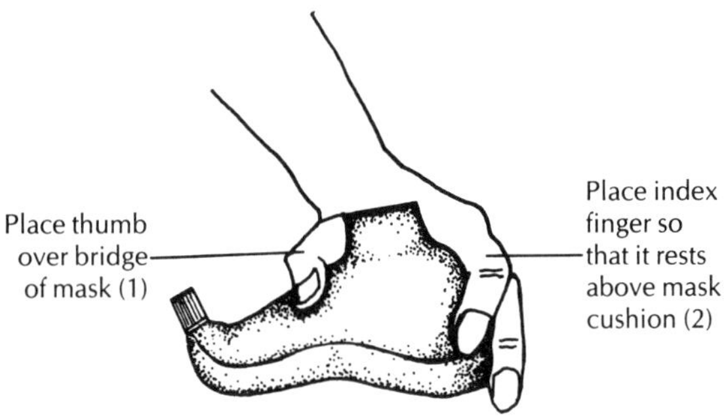
Place thumb
over bridge
of mask (1)
Place index
finger so
that it rests
above mask
cushion (2)

FIG 5–2
Proper hand positioning when holding a resuscitator mask to a patient's face. (From Eubanks DH, Bone RC: Cardiopulmonary resuscitation, in Eubanks DH, Bone RC (eds): *Comprehensive Respiratory Care: A Learning System,* ed 2. St Louis, Mosby–Year Book, 1990, pp 638–639. Used by permission.)

analyzing arterial blood gases or, in some cases, through noninvasive methods such as transcutaneous or end-tidal CO_2 monitoring devices.

3. Manual resuscitators are used when short-term ventilation is required. These include CPR efforts, transport of patients between points, hyperventilation techniques during suctioning, and while the patient is being prepared for attachment to a ventilator for continuous ventilation.
4. The hazards most frequently encountered when using manual resuscitators include the following:
   a. Leaks around the face or tracheal tube that prevent proper lung inflation.
   b. Improperly functioning equipment because of missing parts, improper assembly, or dirty and sticking valves.
   c. Poor ventilation techniques by the clinician such as failure to empty the bag enough to deliver a functional tidal volume, too-rapid or too-slow breathing frequency, failure to maintain a patent airway, and pausing too long between breaths while other procedures are being delivered.
   d. Failure to recognize and properly handle tension pneumothorax, aspiration, or acute episodes of hypoxia.
5. The clinician should master the difficult skill of proper positioning and securing an airtight seal of a face mask.

Constructed of black rubber or various combinations of transparent plastic and vinyl, these masks consist of three major parts: body, seal, and connector. The *body* forms the main structural portion of the mask and can frequently be molded to better fit the patient's face. The *seal* contacts the patient's face and prevents gas leaks between the face and mask. Mask seals may be inflatable air cushions or malleable material. Another type of seal is a rubber or plastic flange, which is a molded part of the mask body and is not inflatable. The *connector* is the small opening in the body that allows the mask to be attached to the resuscitator or other system. Masks have

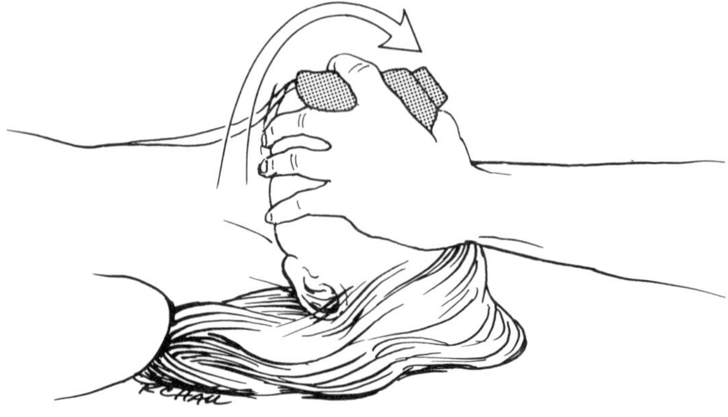

FIG 5–3
Proper placement of hands to hold a resuscitator mask to a patient's face and perform a head-tilt maneuver. (From Eubanks DH, Bone RC: Cardiopulmonary resuscitation, in Eubanks DH, Bone RC (eds): *Comprehensive Respiratory Care: A Learning System,* ed 2. St Louis, Mosby–Year Book, 1990, pp 638–639. Used by permission.)

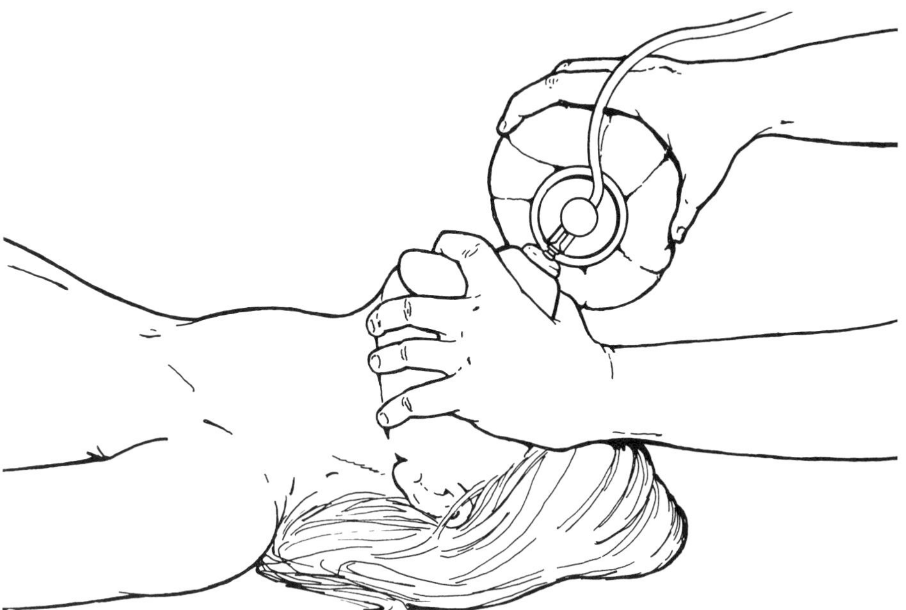

FIG 5–4
Ventilation using the bag-valve-mask and head-tilt/chin-lift method. (From Scanlon CL: Emergency life support, in Scanlon CL, Spearman CB, Sheldon RL (eds): *Egan's Fundamentals of Respiratory Care,* ed 5. St Louis, Mosby–Year Book, 1990, p 538. Used by permission.)

two types of connectors, a 22-mm outer diameter male and a 15-mm inner diameter female.

The "secret" to securing a proper seal with a face mask includes the following:

1. Selecting the proper mask size
2. Positioning the patient's head
3. Adjusting the seal
4. Fitting the mask to the face
5. Securing the mask in place

When selecting a face mask, a good rule is to select the smallest size that will provide a tight seal. This reduces dead space and is easier for the operator to secure in place. Masks are available in all sizes, from premature infant to large adult. Masks can be shaped to fit most patient's faces. Patients' faces that create the most difficulty are those that are edematous; those that are burned or have other types of trauma; those with beards, receding jaws, or flattened noses; or those that have nasogastric tubes in place. Figure 5–1 shows proper technique for mask placement. Figure 5–2 shows proper hand positioning when holding a resuscitator mask to a patient's face. Figure 5–3 shows proper placement of the rescuer's hands in holding a resuscitator mask to a patient's face while performing the head-tilt maneuver. Figure 5–4 shows proper technique for ventilation with a resuscitation bag and mask. The jaw-thrust (or chin-lift) maneuver is the "best first" approach to opening the airway of a victim with confirmed or suspected neck injury since it can usually be accomplished without extending the neck. Figure 5–5 illustrates this maneuver. The head should be carefully supported without tilting it backward or turning it side to side. The victim's lower jaw is lifted with both hands, one on each side, and the mandible is displaced forward without tilting the head backward. The rescuer's elbows should rest on the surface on which the victim is lying. Figure 5–6 shows proper positioning with an orotracheal tube in place.

The AHA states that in light of recent studies demonstrating the inability of clinicians to deliver adequate tidal volumes (10 to 15 mL/kg) to nonintubated manikins, bag-valve units (manual resuscitators) may actually provide less ventilatory volume than mouth-to-mouth or mouth-to-mask ventilation.[5, 8–12] Consequently, a lone clinician may be unable to provide a leak-proof seal to the face, deliver an adequate tidal volume, and maintain an open airway simultaneously. Therefore, manually operated, self-inflating bag-valve-mask units are used most effectively by at least two well-trained experienced clinicians working together.[13] To optimize bag-valve-mask performance, one clinician must be posi-

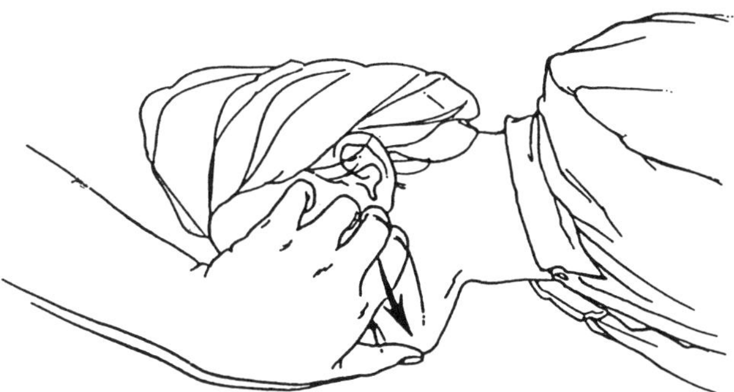

FIG 5–5
Jaw-thrust maneuver. (From American Heart Association: *Instructor's Manual for Basic Life Support.* Dallas Tx, American Heart Association, p 37, 1987. Used by permission.)

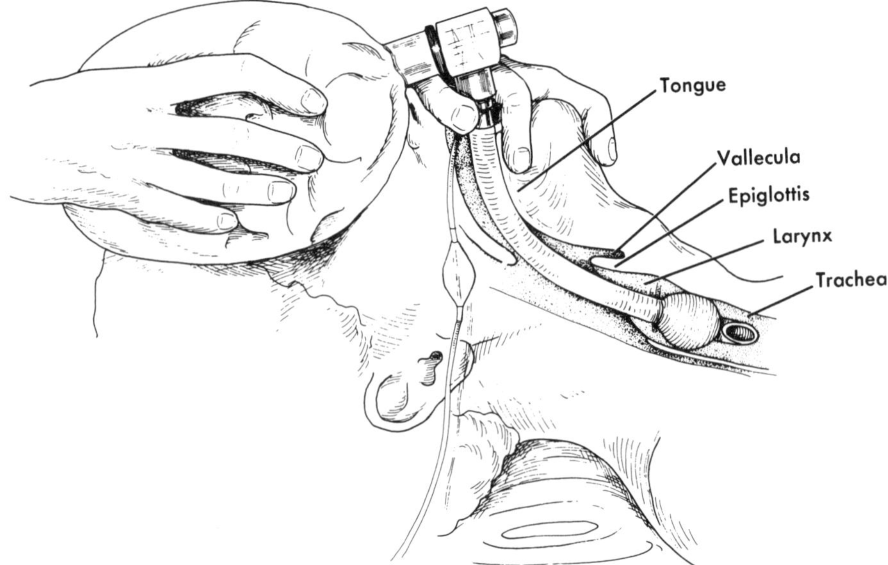

FIG 5–6
Orotracheal tube in place being used with a bag-valve resuscitator. (From Scanlon CL: Emergency life support, in Scanlon CL, Spearman CB, Sheldon RL (eds): *Egan's Fundamentals of Respiratory Care,* ed 5. St Louis, Mosby–Year Book, 1990, p. 533. Used by permission.)

tioned at the top of the victim's head. An oral airway should be inserted and the head elevated if no concern for neck injury exists (head tilt/chin lift). With the head in extension, the selected tidal volume (preferably 10 to 15 mL/kg in resuscitation efforts) should be delivered over 2 seconds. With two clinicians providing ventilation, one to hold the mask and one to squeeze the bag, more effective ventilation is likely. The addition of a third rescuer to provide cricoid pressure is suggested because providing bag-valve-mask ventilation *and* cricoid pressure with two clinicians is often awkward. The AHA is also quick to point out that proper use of a bag-valve device with other types of invasive airway adjuncts such as an esophageal obturator or esophageal gastric tube airway also depends on a proper mask fit and requires training, practice, and demonstrated proficiency. Figures 5–7 and 5–8 show a representative sample of adult manual resuscitators.

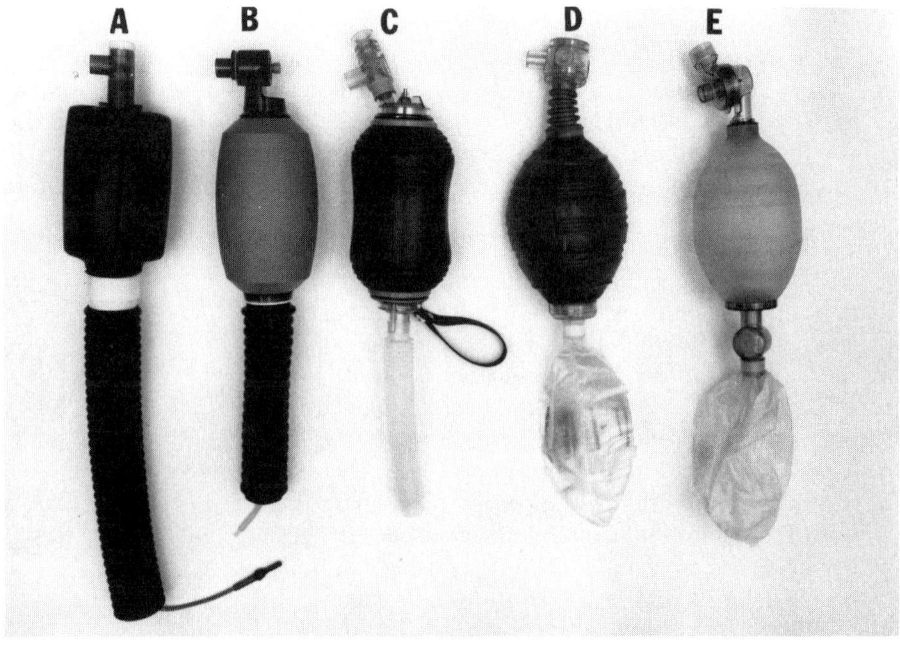

FIG 5–7
Adult manual resuscitators with reservoirs attached: Hope 2 **(A),** PMR **(B),** AMBU MS 30 **(C),** Air Viva **(D),** and Laerdal Silicone **(E).** (From TA Barnes: *Therapeutic and Emergency Modalities.* St Louis, Mosby–Year Book, 1988, p 264. Used by permission.)

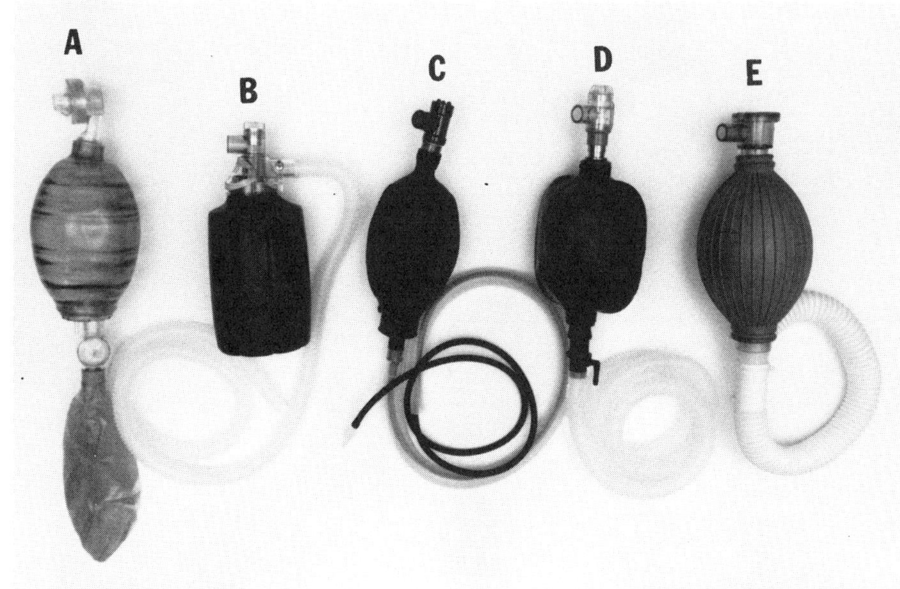

FIG 5–8
Adult manual resuscitators with oxygen reservoirs attached: **A,** Laerdal; **B,** Hope 1; **C,** Penior; **D,** Ambu; **E,** Vitalograph. (From TA Barnes: *Therapeutic and Emergency Modalities.* St Louis, Mosby–Year Book, 1988, p 264. Used by permission.)

OXYGEN-POWERED, MANUALLY TRIGGERED DEVICES (DEMAND VALVES)

Most of the manually triggered (time-cycled) devices and oxygen-powered breathing devices deliver high immediate flow rates with a manual control button. This contradicts the 1986 recommendation to limit their flow to 40 L/min.[4, 14–16] These devices can be used with a face mask, endotracheal tube, esophageal airway, or tracheostomy tube. With high inspiratory flow rates, gastric insufflation is probable when the devices are used with a mask. A particularly undesirable feature of current devices is that their flow rate is backpressure dependent, which causes gas flow to stop prematurely without alerting the rescuer. This is most likely to occur in those patients receiving chest compressions and those with high airway resistance and/or low lung-thorax compliance. Excessive inspiratory flow rates in intubated patients may also lead to maldistribution of ventilation and intrapulmonary shunting.

To obviate these problems, the 1992 AHA guidelines for oxygen-powered, manually triggered devices have been changed so that these devices should provide the following[5]:

1. One hundred percent oxygen at less than 40 L/min.

2. An inspiratory pressure relief valve that opens at approximately 60 cm H_2O and vents any remaining volume to the atmosphere or ceases gas flow; the valve may be set to 80 cm H_2O when used by advance rescuers, but only under medical direction.

3. An audible alarm that sounds whenever the relief valve pressure is exceeded to alert the rescuer that the victim requires high inflation pressures and may not be receiving adequate ventilatory volumes.

4. Satisfactory operation under common environmental conditions and extremes of temperature.

5. A demand-flow system that does not impose additional work; many oxygen-powered breathing devices currently used have restricted flow rates of 40 L/min, require unacceptably high triggering pressures in the demand mode, and should not be used for spontaneously breathing patients.

The AHA also suggests the following minimum design features for oxygen-powered devices:

1. Standard 15-mm/22-mm coupling for mask, endotracheal tube, esophageal obturator airway, tracheostomy tube, and other alternative invasive airways.
2. A rugged, breakage-resistant mechanical design that is compact and easy to hold.
3. A trigger positioned so that both hands of the rescuer can remain on the mask to hold it in position.

Additionally, the AHA states that these devices *must not be used* by untrained persons since the potential for complications is high and *must not be used* on pediatric patients.

Figure 5–9 shows a demand valve in the closed and open positions. Figure 5–10 shows a Robertshaw (demand) valve. Figure 5–11 shows a demand valve and its

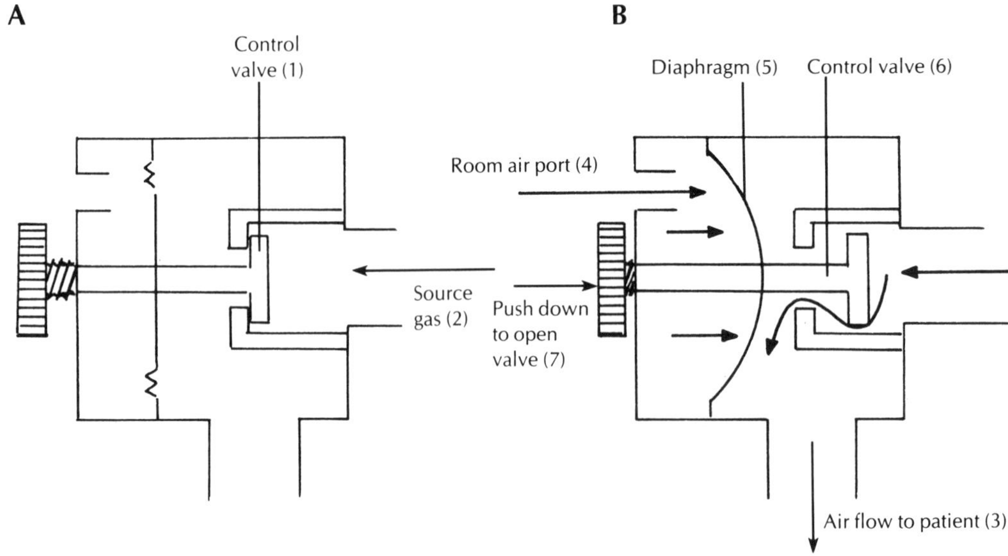

FIG 5–9
Demand valve. **A,** closed position; **B,** open position. (From Eubanks DH, Bone RC: Cardiopulmonary resuscitation, in Eubanks DH, Bone RC (eds): *Comprehensive Respiratory Care: A Learning System,* ed 2. St Louis, Mosby–Year Book, 1990, pp 638–639. Used by permission.)

general component parts. Hand positioning with the head-tilt/chin-lift procedure, as with manual resuscitators, is also recommended when using demand valves.

Procedures for self-inflating manual resuscitators, including assessing operation, emergency ventilation, securing a face mask by using a one-hand grip, and operation of a demand valve to assist and control ventilation, can be found at the end of the chapter. Procedures for the clinical application of these devices will vary depending on institutional/departmental policies. These procedures are meant as a *guideline only.* In addition to hand washing, the use of gloves, eye protection, splash-resistant gowns/aprons, and masks has

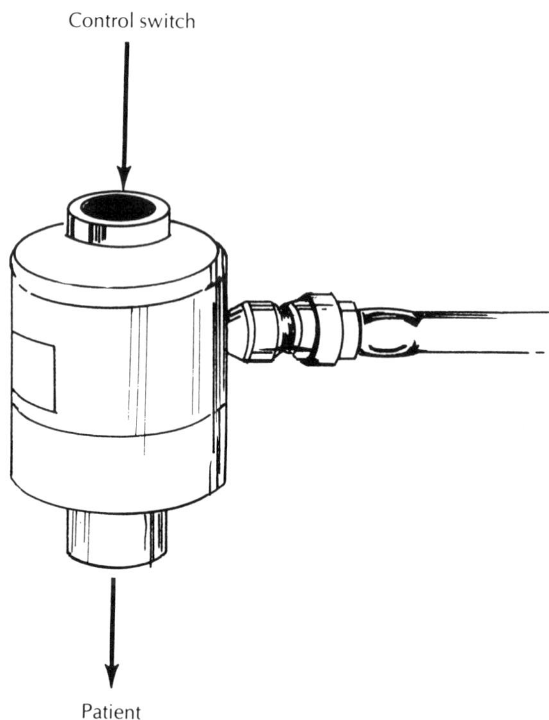

FIG 5–10
Robertshaw valve. (From Eubanks DH, Bone RC: Cardiopulmonary resuscitation, in Eubanks DH, Bone RC (eds): *Comprehensive Respiratory Care: A Learning System,* ed 2. St Louis, Mosby–Year Book, 1990, pp 638–639. Used by permission.)

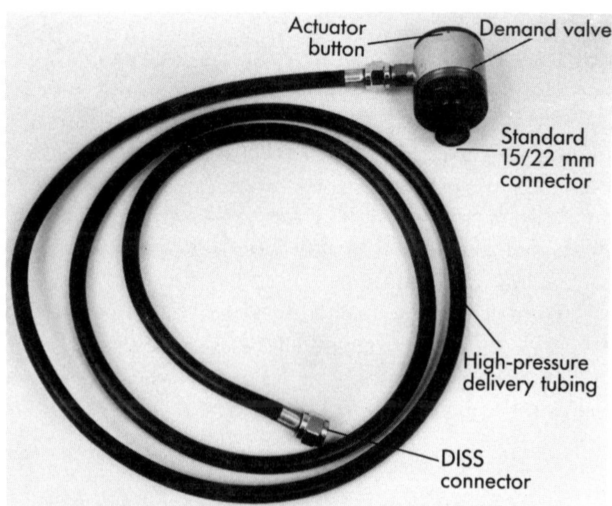

FIG 5–11
Parts of a gas-powered resuscitator demand valve. (*DISS* = diameter index safety system.) (From Scanlon CL: Emergency life support, in Scanlon CL, Spearman CB, Sheldon RL (eds): *Egan's Fundamentals of Respiratory Care,* ed 5. St Louis, Mosby–Year Book, 1990, p. 539. Used by permission.)

also become standard in many institutions since resuscitation devices are associated with situations that put the rescuer at some risk because of exposure to blood and body fluids. Manual resuscitator use is common in emergency and intensive care areas, where exposure to blood and body fluids is likely. The observance of universal precautions is mandatory, particularly in the emergency department where patients' preexisting diseases/organisms are unknown to rescuers. Furthermore, in some states it is considered unprofessional conduct subject to disciplinary action if appropriate protective precautions are not taken by licensed professionals in the practice of their profession. This certainly applies to licensed or unlicensed respiratory care practitioners performing patient care while operating resuscitation bags, gas-powered resuscitators, and mechanical ventilators.

MECHANICAL VENTILATORS

IPPV, also sometimes referred to as "controlled ventilation," must provide four basic functions:

1. Inflate the lungs
2. Terminate lung inflation
3. Provide for lung deflation
4. Initiate lung inflation

A mechanical ventilator works in much the same way, with these four functions, called phases, forming the heart of how mechanical ventilators are described or classified (see Fig 5–12). These four phases are as follows:

1. Inspiratory phase
2. Changeover from the inspiratory phase to the expiratory phase
3. Expiratory or exhalation phase
4. Changeover from the expiratory to the inspiratory phase

All mechanical ventilators must provide these four basic functions or phases. The functional characteristics among the many ventilators used today and the terminology used to describe those characteristics are varied.[17–26] How we choose to describe or "classify" mechanical ventilators is becoming increasingly important, particu-

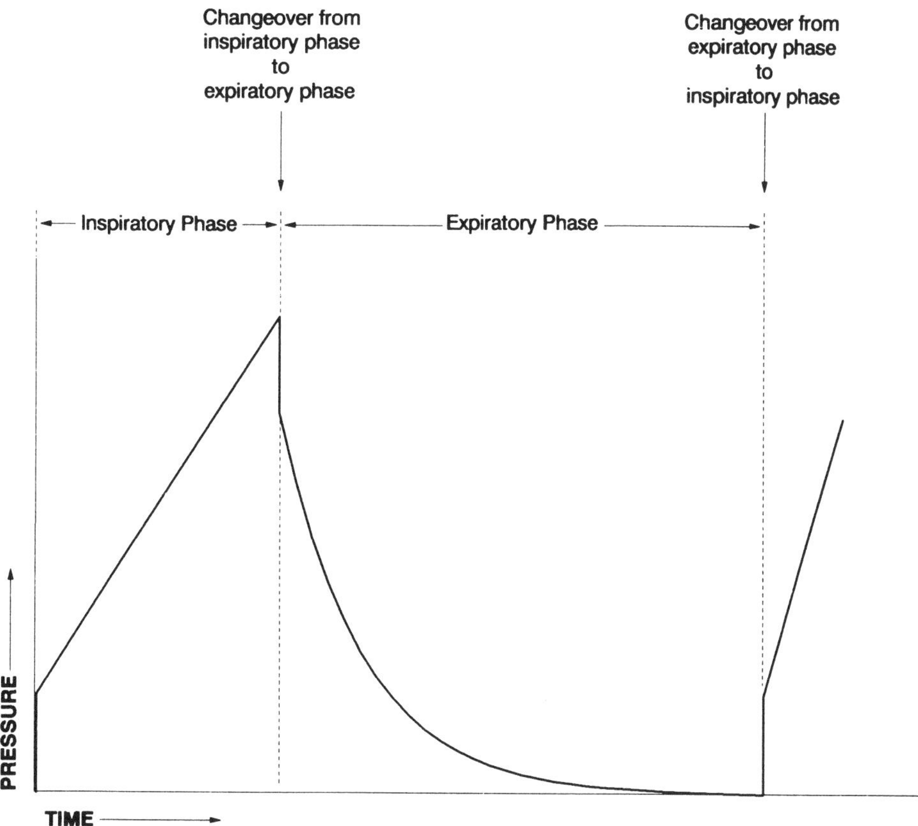

FIG 5–12
Four phases of the respiratory cycle. (From Dupuis YG: *Ventilators: Theory and Clinical Application,* ed 2. St Louis, Mosby–Year Book, 1992, p 7. Used by permission.)

larly with the tremendous performance options now available in microprocessor-controlled ventilators. Chatburn notes that ". . . classification schemes have been founded on descriptions of mechanical archetypes (such as constant vs non-constant pressure generator or constant vs non-constant flow generator). I believe the problem with this approach to be that it quickly becomes outdated and restrictive as technology evolves and archetypes become irrelevant or obsolete."[17] The article by Chatburn is intriguing and informative and may ultimately lead to a better system for describing mechanical ventilator function. The virtually limitless potential found in today's (and tomorrow's) microprocessor-controlled ventilators calls for a new and better classification system, thereby validating Chatburn's proposal. Unfortunately, this system has yet to be universally accepted by all clinicians in the medical and respiratory care communities. We feel, however, that it does provide clinicians with a better way to describe ventilator function.

Physical Features of Mechanical Ventilators

An essential feature of optimal care of the critically ill patient is a good, working knowledge of the particular mechanical ventilator being used with a given patient, how the ventilator interacts with the patient, and how changes in the patient's lung condition may alter ventilator function. This chapter presents Chatburn's classification system with a representative sample of modern mechanical ventilators and is not intended to be an exhaustive review of all mechanical ventilators available, as other texts have done.[23–26] Complete information on mechanical ventilators is best obtained in the following ways: manufacturer's literature, particularly operator's manuals; extensive, well-organized in-service programs, including demonstrations from trained manufacturers' representatives and return demonstrations by users; and probably most importantly, actual clinical/working experience with the ventilator while attached to a patient. Experience is, after all, often the best teacher.

A Classification System

A mechanical ventilator is a mechanism with a system of related elements designed to alter, transmit, and direct applied energy in a predetermined manner to perform useful work.[17] The energy input is in the form of electricity and/or compressed gas. The ventilator uses this energy to supplement or replace the patient's ventilatory muscles to accomplish the work of breathing. Therefore, the ventilator is a system that provides four universal functions:

1. Power input
2. Power transmission or conversion
3. Control
4. Output

Power Input

The input power or energy used to operate mechanical ventilators can be

- *Pneumatic:* usually a 50-psig source (range, 45 to 55 psig)
- *Electric:* alternating (ac or U.S. all current) or direct current (dc or battery)
- *Combination of pneumatic/electric*

Earlier-generation mechanical ventilators used only one of these power sources to function, with "first-generation" devices being pneumatically powered machines, such as the Puritan Bennett PR series and Bird Mark series, and electrically powered machines, such as the Emerson 3 PV and 3 MV. "Second-generation" machines were those using both electricity and pneumatics as the power source. "Third-generation" machines incorporate both electric and pneumatic power sources to function properly since they use advanced technology such as proportional solenoids and stepper motors in combination with microprocessor control.

Power Conversion and Transmission

Power conversion and transmission are the mechanisms used to drive the ventilator. These may consist of an internal or external compressor and output control valves (see Table 5–2).

Control

During mechanical ventilation, as with spontaneous ventilation, four separate but connected variables must be controlled and coordinated: volume, pressure, flow, and time. If any one or more of these variables are set to

TABLE 5–2
Power Conversion and Transmission*

External compressor
Internal compressor
Motor and linkage
Compressed gas, direct
Electric motor, rotating crank and piston rod
Electric motor, rack and pinion
Electric motor, direct
Output control valve
Pneumatic diaphragm
Pneumatic poppet valve
Electromagnetic poppet valve
Electromagnetic proportional valve

* Data from Chatburn RL: *Respir Care* 1991; 36:1123–1155.

TABLE 5–3
Mechanical Ventilator Control*

Control circuit
Mechanical
Pneumatic
Fluidic
Electric
Electronic
Control variables and waveforms
Pressure
Volume
Flow
Time
Phase variables
Trigger
Limit
Cycle
Baseline

* Data from Chatburn RL: *Respir Care* 1991; 36:1123–1155.

operate in a specific way, the others will and must respond in some manner. So, if a ventilator is set to deliver a tidal volume with a specified flow rate and waveform, airway pressure and inspiratory time would depend on the volume and flow chosen as well as on the patient's lung-thorax compliance and airway resistance. Table 5–3 shows the factors under ventilator control.

In order to establish control over the four variables, a "control circuit" must be built into the ventilator. The control circuit is the system that controls the driving mechanism and/or the output valve. Some ventilators may use one or more control circuits. Figure 5–13 shows the criteria for determining the control variable during a ventilator-supported inspiration.

Phase Variables. Once the control variables and the corresponding waveforms are identified, more information can be obtained by observing the events that occur during a ventilatory cycle (the period of time between the start of one breath and the start of the next breath). Mushin et al.[26] proposed that this time interval be divided into four phases:

1. The change from exhalation to inspiration
2. Inspiration
3. The change from inspiration to exhalation
4. Exhalation

These categorizations are useful in identifying how a ventilator begins, maintains, and ends an inspiration and what happens between inspirations. Within each phase, a given variable is measured and used to begin, maintain, and end the phase. Therefore, flow, time, pressure, and volume are referred to as phase variables. Figure 5–14 illustrates the criteria for determining the phase variables during a ventilator-supported breath.

Trigger. Trigger is the phase variable that initiates inspiration. Generally, mechanical ventilators are triggered to inspiration by time (set via a timing or rate control mechanism) or pressure (set via a pressure sensitivity mechanism). Some of the third-generation ventilators have incorporated flow triggering (Puritan-Bennett 7200 and Siemens 300).

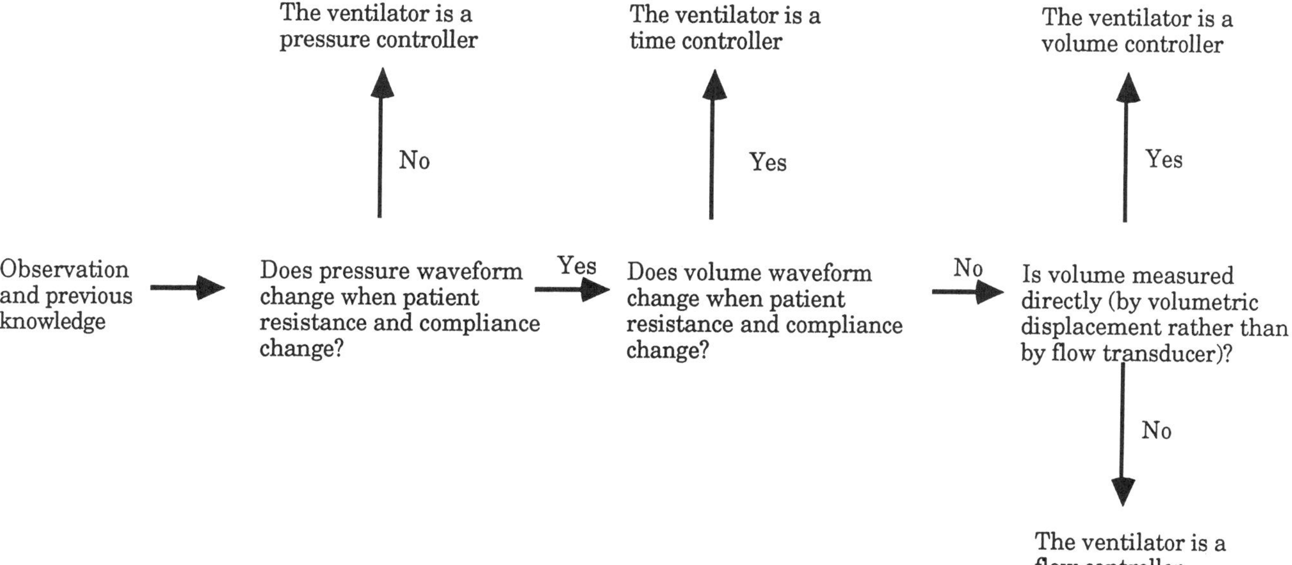

FIG 5–13
Criteria for determining the control variable during a ventilator-supported inspiration. Beginning with observations and previous knowledge of this ventilator, decisions are based on the effect of load on ventilator output. (From Chatburn RL: *Respir Care* 1991; 36:1123–1155. Used by permission.)

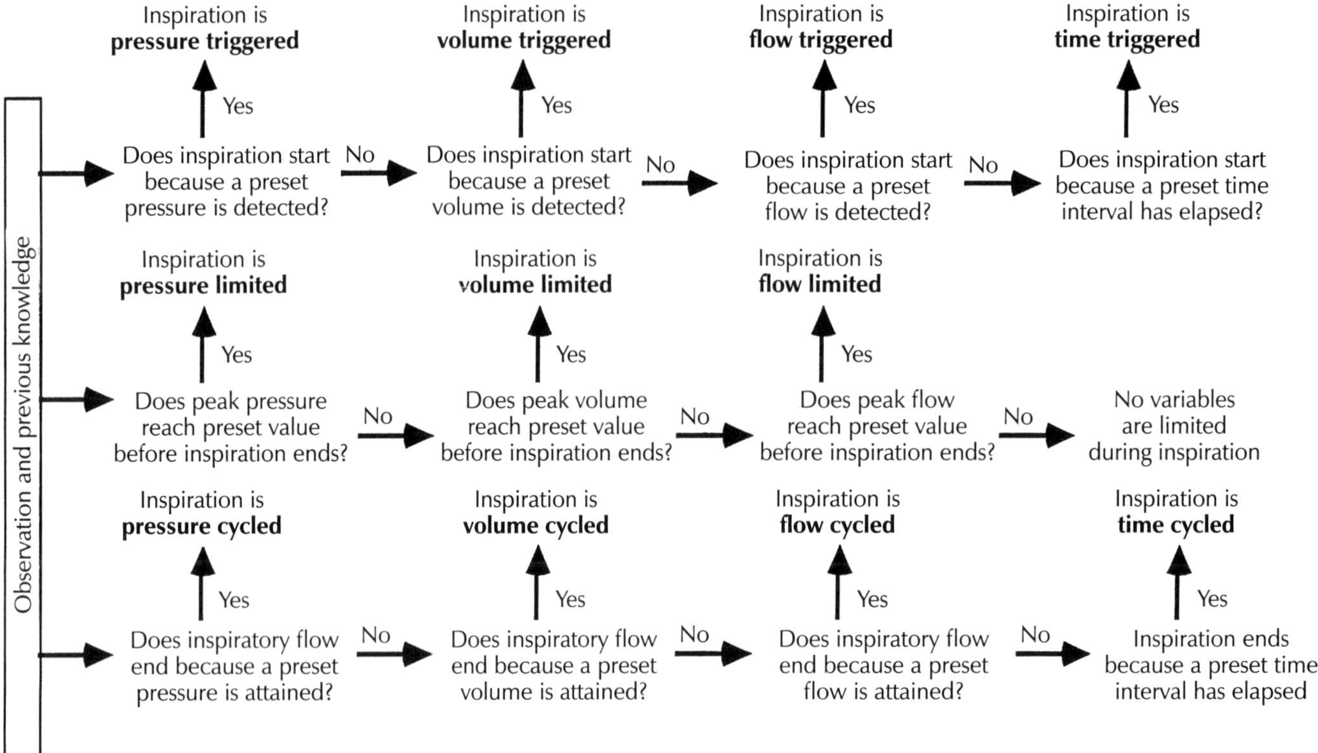

FIG 5–14
Criteria for determining the phase variables during a ventilator-supported breath. (From Chatburn RL: *Respir Care* 1991; 36:1123–1155. Used by permission.)

Limit. Inspiratory time is the time interval between the beginning of inspiratory flow to the beginning of expiratory flow. During inspiration, pressure, volume, and flow increase above their end-exhalation values. If one (or more) of these variables rises no higher than some preset value, the variable is termed a limit variable. This is different from a variable used to end inspiration (termed a cycle variable). So an additional criterion is added that inspiration not be terminated because a variable has met its preset limit value. A variable is limited if it increases to a preset value before inspiration ends.

Cycle. The end of inspiration occurs because some variable has reached a preset value. The variable measured and used to end inspiration is termed the cycle variable.

Baseline. Baseline is the variable that is controlled during the exhalation phase. This includes the ability to control expiratory pressures (constant positive airway pressure [CPAP] and PEEP).

Conditional Variables. These are the particular conditions under which variable patterns of ventilation are delivered. Each breath delivered by the ventilator contains a specified pattern of control and phase variables. This pattern may be constant and provide only one type of breath or pattern as with simple, earlier-generation ventilators, or it may be complex, as with the newer, microprocessor-controlled machines providing two or more types of breaths and limits.

Output

All clinicians are taught the importance of monitoring waveforms (outputs) such as electrocardiograms (ECGs) and hemodynamics. The same is true for mechanical ventilators where we observe pressure, volume, and flow waveforms. Table 5–4 lists the waveforms of interest when monitoring mechanical ventilator output. Although the actual waveforms produced may differ greatly, the ideal waveforms (Fig 5–15) help to define the capabilities of a particular ventilator.[27]

Clinicians have discussed the differences in control systems with emphasis on "open-loop" vs. "closed-loop" types. Figure 5–16 depicts the differences in these systems. Earlier-generation mechanical ventilators and even some ventilators manufactured currently incorporate both open- and closed-loop systems. A closed-loop, microprocessor-controlled (computer-controlled) feedback loop is now possible to enhance the performance of the driving/powering system. In order to achieve closed-loop control, the output must be measured and compared with a reference value. In a mechanical ventilator,

TABLE 5–4

Mechanical Ventilator Output (Waveforms)*

Pressure waveforms
Rectangular
Exponential
Sinusoidal
Oscillating
Volume waveforms
Ramp
Sinusoidal
Flow waveforms
Rectangular
Ascending ramp
Descending ramp
Sinusoidal
Effects of the patient circuit

* Data from Chatburn RL: *Respir Care* 1991; 36:1123–1155.

a transducer and electronic circuitry are needed to perform automatic closed-loop control. The advantage of this type of control is a more consistent output in the face of disturbances that might affect the delivery of pressure, volume, and flow such as changes in the patient's airway resistance or lung/thorax compliance, patient circuit leaks, pooled water from condensation in the patient circuit, and airway obstructions (kinking or mucous plugging of the endotracheal tube).

Effects of the Patient Circuit

It should be understood that what comes out of the ventilator outlet is not the same as what goes into the patient. The pressures, volumes, and flows measured inside the ventilator are always higher than those at the patient airway. Since the patient's circuit has a given compliance (the compliance of the tubing and the compressibility of the delivered gas), there is a pressure difference between the delivery point (the ventilator) and the receiving point (the patient's airway). Differences also occur between the set values for volume, pressure, and flow and the actual output from the ventilator because of errors in calibration.

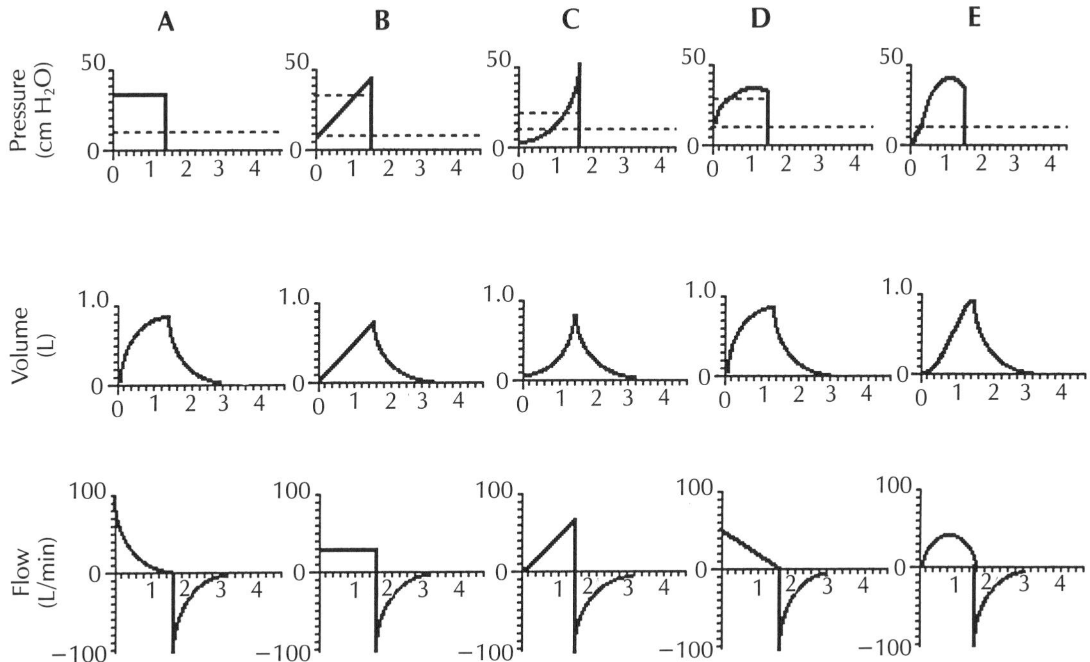

FIG 5–15

Theoretical waveforms. **A,** pressure-controlled inspiration with a rectangular pressure waveform, identical to flow-controlled inspiration with an exponential-decay flow waveform. **B,** flow-controlled inspiration with a rectangular flow waveform, identical to volume-controlled inspiration with an ascending-ramp volume waveform. **C,** Flow-controlled inspiration with an ascending-ramp flow waveform. **D,** flow-controlled inspiration with a descending-ramp flow waveform. **E,** flow-controlled inspiration with a sinusoidal flow waveform. The *short dashed lines* represent the mean inspiratory pressure, whereas the *longer dashed lines* denote the mean airway pressure (assuming zero end-expiratory pressure). For the rectangular pressure waveform in **A,** the mean inspiratory pressure is the same as the peak inspiratory pressure. These output waveforms were created by (1) defining the control waveform (e.g., an ascending-ramp flow waveform is specified as flow = constant × time) and specifying that tidal volume equals 644 mL (about 9 mL/kg for a normal adult); (2) specifying the desired values for resistance and compliance (for these waveforms, compliance = 20 mL/cm H_2O and resistance = 20 cm H_2O/L/sec, according to American National Standards Institute [ANSI] recommendations); (3) substituting the above information into the equation of motion; and (4) using a computer to solve the equation for pressure, volume, and flow and plotting the results against time. (From Chatburn RL: *Respir Care* 1991; 36:1123–1155. Used by permission.)

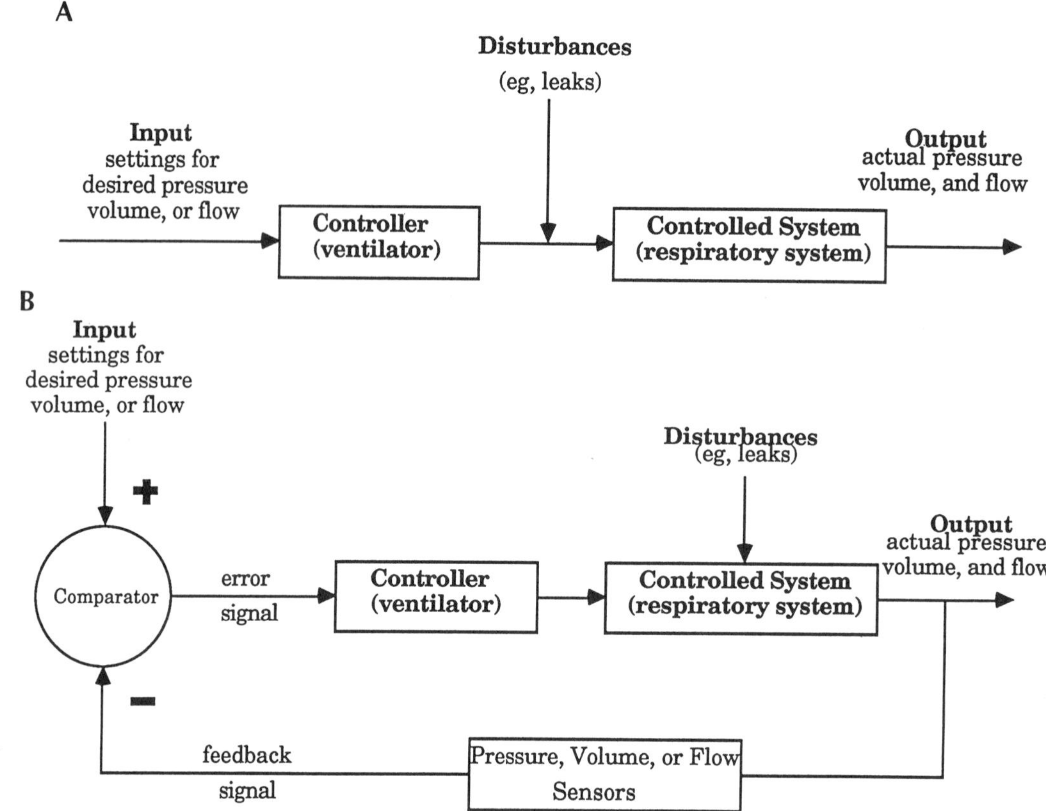

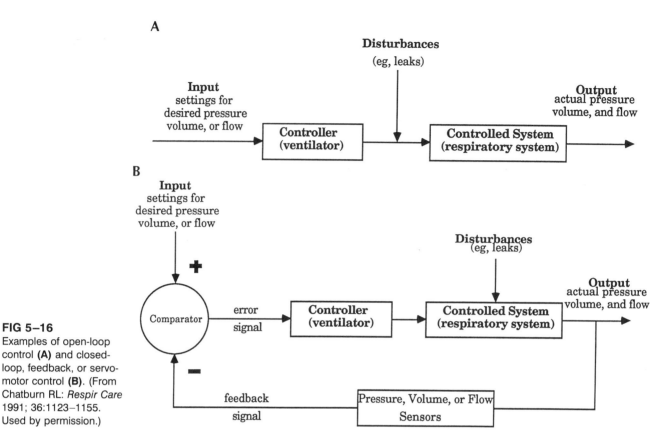

FIG 5–16
Examples of open-loop control **(A)** and closed-loop, feedback, or servo-motor control **(B)**. (From Chatburn RL: *Respir Care* 1991; 36:1123–1155. Used by permission.)

Alarm Systems

Mechanical ventilator alarms have increased in number and complexity. Day and MacIntyre[28] have previously stated that the goal of ventilator alarms is to warn of events. An event is defined as any condition or occurrence that requires clinician awareness or action. Technical events are those involving an inadvertent change in the ventilator's performance; patient events are those involving a change in the patient's clinical status.[29] A mechanical ventilator may contain any number of conceivable alarms. However, the most logical and appropriate would include the ventilator's mechanical-electronic operation and those variables associated with the mechanics of breathing (i.e., time, flow, pressure, and volume). Also included would be analysis of exhaled gas for oxygen and carbon dioxide concentration. Table 5–5 shows the type of alarm systems included in mechanical ventilators.

Alarms may be audible, visual, or both, depending on the critical nature of the alarm condition. Specifications for an alarm event should include the following:

- Conditions that trigger the alarm
- The alarm response in the form of audible and/or visual messages

TABLE 5–5
Mechanical Ventilator Alarm Systems*

Input power alarms
Loss of electrical power
Loss of pneumatic power
Control circuit alarms
General systems failure (ventilator inoperative)
Incompatible ventilator settings
Inverse I/E ratio
Output alarms
Pressure
High and low peak airway pressure
High and low mean airway pressure
High and low baseline pressure (PEEP or CPAP)
Failure of airway pressure to return to baseline within a specified period
Volume
Flow
Time
High or low ventilatory frequency
High or low inspiratory time
Long or short expiratory time (long expiratory time = apnea)
Inspired gas
High or low inspired gas temperature
High or low F_{IO_2}

* Data from Chatburn RL: *Respir Care* 1991; 36:1123–1155.

- Any associated ventilator response such as termination of inspiration or failure to operate
- Whether the alarm must be manually reset or resets itself when the alarm condition is rectified

Table 5–6 outlines the various levels of alarm priority along with characteristics and appropriate categories. This system is based on the ventilator classification scheme.

Input Power Alarms

Loss of electrical power. Mechanical ventilators typically contain a battery backup system in case of power failure, if only to power alarms. These alarm systems warn of electrical power cutoff while the machine is plugged in and switched on (e.g., power cord disconnect). If designed to operate on an external or internal battery, as with transport ventilators, an alarm (usually visual and audible) warns of a low-battery condition.

Loss of pneumatic power. Loss of pressurized gas input will activate alarms if either compressed air and/or oxygen is cut off or reduced below a specified inlet pressure. These alarms may be activated by an electronic pressure switch (e.g., Puritan-Bennett 7200 series) or pneumatically operated as a component of the blender (e.g., Siemens Servo 900C).

Control Circuit Alarms

These alarms are those that warn the clinician that set control variables are incompatible/unacceptable (e.g.,

TABLE 5–6

A Four-Level Classification of Ventilator Alarms*

	Level 1†	Level 2	Level 3	Level 4
Alarm characteristics				
Mandatory?	Yes	Yes	No	Yes
Redundant?	Yes	No	No	No
Noncancelling?	Yes	No	No	Yes
Audible?	Yes	Yes	Yes	No
Visual?	Yes	Yes	Yes	Yes
Automatic backup response?	Yes	No	No	No
Automatic reset				
Audible?	Yes	Yes	Yes	Yes
Visual?	No	Yes	Yes	Yes
Applicable alarm categories				
Input				
Electric power?	Yes	No	No	No
Pneumatic power?	Yes	No	No	No
Control circuit				
Inverse I:E?	No	Yes	No	Yes
Incompatible settings?	No	No	No	Yes
Mechanical/electronic fault?	Yes	No	No	No
Output				
Pressure?‡	Yes	Yes	Yes	Yes
Volume?§	Yes	Yes	Yes	Yes
Flow?¶	Yes	Yes	Yes	Yes
Minute ventilation?	Yes	Yes	Yes	Yes
Time?‖	Yes	Yes	Yes	Yes
Inspired gas (F_{IO_2}, temperature)?**	Yes	Yes	No	Yes
Expired gas (F_{EO_2}, F_{ECO_2})?	No	No	Yes	No

* From Chatburn RL: *Respir Care* 1991; 36:1123–1155. Used by permission.
† Level 1, critical ventilator malfunction; level 2, noncritical ventilator malfunction (not immediately life-threatening); level 3, patient status change; level 4, operator alert (inappropriate control setting or alarm threshold).
‡ Pressure alarms: high and low peak, mean, and baseline.
§ High and low inhaled and exhaled tidal volume. A leak alarm may be included.
‖ The alarm is triggered if expiratory flow does not fall below the set threshold (gas trapping).
¶ The alarm is triggered if the inspiratory or expiratory times are too long or too short.
** Tracer gases may be included for functional residual capacity calculation.

inverse I:E ratio) or that some aspect of a ventilator self-test has failed (e.g., microprocessor failure). The ventilator usually responds with a general message such as "ventilator inoperative."

Output Alarms

Output alarms are triggered by an unacceptable value of the ventilator's output in which the value of a control variable falls outside an expected range. These include values measured for pressure, volume, flow, time, or inspired/expired gas.

1. *Pressure*
   a. Peak airway pressure—indicating an endotracheal tube obstruction, pneumothorax or patient asynchrony (high), or leak in the patient circuit (e.g., external circuit disconnect or inadequate cuff inflation [low])
   b. Mean airway pressure—indicating air trapping, accumulating secretions, or a change in the ventilatory pattern leading to a change in the patient's oxygenation status (high) or a leak in the patient circuit (low)
   c. Mean airway pressure—indicating a patient-circuit, exhalation-manifold obstruction or inadvertent PEEP (high) or disconnection of the patient from the external circuit (low)
   d. Failure of airway pressure to return to baseline within a specified period—indicating patient-circuit obstruction or exhalation-manifold malfunction
2. *Volume:* exhaled tidal volume—indicating improvements in the patient's resistance and/or compliance
3. *Flow:* high and low exhaled minute ventilaion—indicating hyperventilation (or possible machine self-triggering) and possible apnea or disconnection of the patient from the patient circuit
4. *Time*
   a. High or low ventilatory frequency—indicating hyperventilation (or possible machine self-triggering) and possible apnea
   b. Inspiratory time too long or too short
      (1) Too long—indicating a possible patient-circuit obstruction or exhalation-manifold malfunction
      (2) Too short—indicating that adequate tidal volume may not have been delivered (in a pressure control mode) or that gas distribution in the lungs may not be optimal
   c. Expiratory time too long or too short
      (1) Too long—indicating apnea
      (2) Too short—warning of alveolar gas trapping (i.e., the expiratory time should be five or more time constants of the respiratory system)
5. *Inspired gas*
   a. High/low inspired gas temperature
   b. High/low F_{IO_2}
6. *Expired gas*
   a. Exhaled carbon dioxide tension. End-tidal carbon dioxide levels may reflect Pa_{CO_2} and reflect the efficiency of ventilation. Mean exhaled P_{CO_2} along with minute ventilation measurements could reveal additional information concerning CO_2 production, thus helping to determine the respiratory quotient and the tidal volume/dead space ratio (V_D/V_T)
   b. Exhaled oxygen tension. Analysis of end-tidal and mean exhaled P_{O_2} may provide information about gas exchange and could be used with CO_2 data to calculate the respiratory quotient[29]

CHARACTERISTICS OF RECENT "THIRD-GENERATION" MECHANICAL VENTILATORS

The distinguishing characteristic of the newer and more sophisticated critical care mechanical ventilators used today is the incorporation of microprocessor control. As stated by Kacmarek and Meklaus,[30, 31] these types of ventilators may have the following advantages:

- Flexibility and variability in gas delivery pattern
- Backup/apnea ventilation availability in all modes (i.e., assist/control, synchronized intermittent mandatory ventilation (SIMV), intermittent mandatory ventilation (IMV), pressure support ventilation (PSV), CPAP, volume support, pressure-regulated volume control)
- Ability to evaluate/monitor the overall function
- Need for fewer moving parts
- Extensive patient-ventilator system monitoring capabilities
- Ease of repair
- Ease of updating systems
- Improved spontaneous breathing capabilities
- RS-232 outputs capability of interfacing with computer systems

The disadvantages may include the following:

- Relatively expensive
- Increased complexity possibly causing difficulty in

clinician operation and resulting in considerable education and updating to ensure complete understanding of the machine's many functions/options.

- Because of the complexity in control panel configuration, misinterpretation by clinician-operators of how the patient is being ventilated (the exact mode and options are not readily apparent).
- In the most sophisticated models, possibly too many unneeded options and too costly and/or unnecessary for the majority of patients who require mechanical ventilation. Less complex versions of these ventilators are available (i.e., Puritan Bennett 7200e, Hamilton Amadeus, and the Bird 6400 ST)

External Mechanical Ventilator Circuitry

With the advent of better technology, the need for major adaptation, particularly that added to the external circuit of the ventilator, has been virtually eliminated. For example, Figure 5–17 depicts a typical modification made for continuous-flow IMV for a second-generation mechanical ventilator manufactured without the IMV (or SIMV) option (e.g., Puritan-Bennett MA-1 or the Emerson 3PV). This is similar in design to that proposed by Kirby in 1976.[34] This adaptation works well for many patients but illustrates the limitations of earlier-generation machines. Besides being cumbersome in some cases, these adaptations could be hazardous since each "adapter" or piece added to the circuit also increases the likelihood of operator errors leading to technical events (those involving an inadvertent change in the ventilator's performance). Figure 5–18 shows a generic external circuit that could be found on any of today's third-generation mechanical ventilators.

Modern Mechanical Ventilators

Below is a representative sample description of modern mechanical ventilators as adapted from Pilbeam[32] and other sources.[17, 18, 23–26, 30] A more detailed description of each ventilator, as defined by the classification system proposed by Chatburn, is found in Table 5–7.

BEAR 2

This ventilator (Fig 5–19), aside from an updated monitoring system and a few changes in the pneumatic components, is similar to the BEAR 1 in general performance. The display and control panels are illustrated in Figure 5–20, A and B. A listing of the display and control panel components is shown in Table 5–8 on p. 171.

- Power source: electric or compressed gas
- Control circuit: electronic
- Cycling control variable: volume, time, or pressure

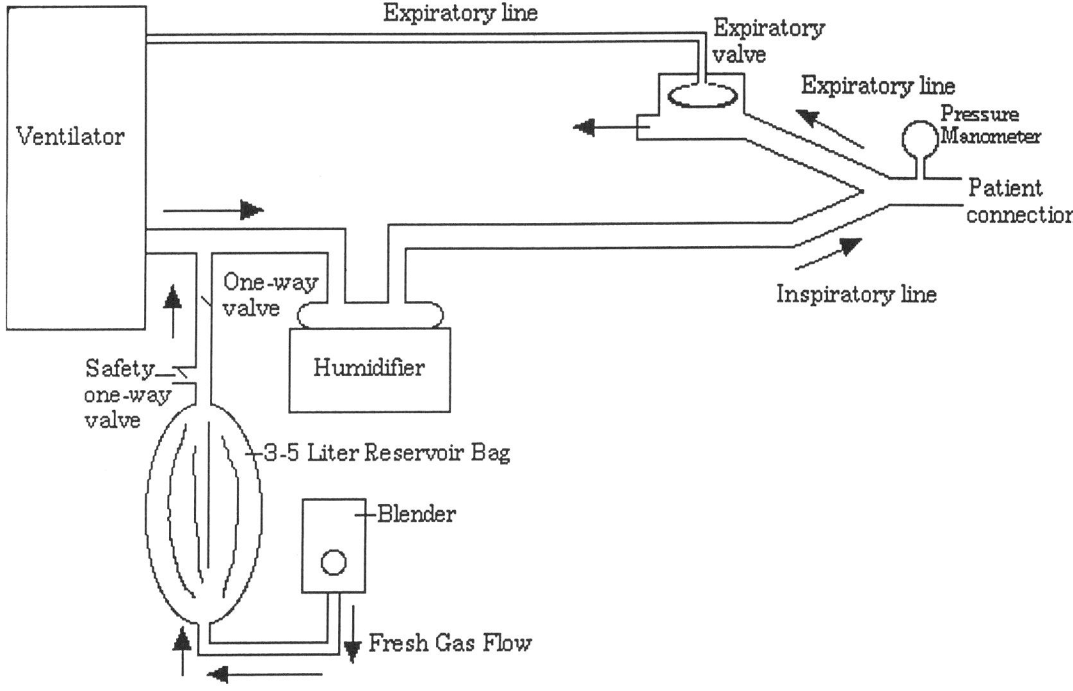

FIG 5–17
Continuous-flow IMV system with a reservoir bag and safety one-way valve. Fresh, continuous gas flow from the blender fills the bag and flows through the circuit for spontaneous breathing.

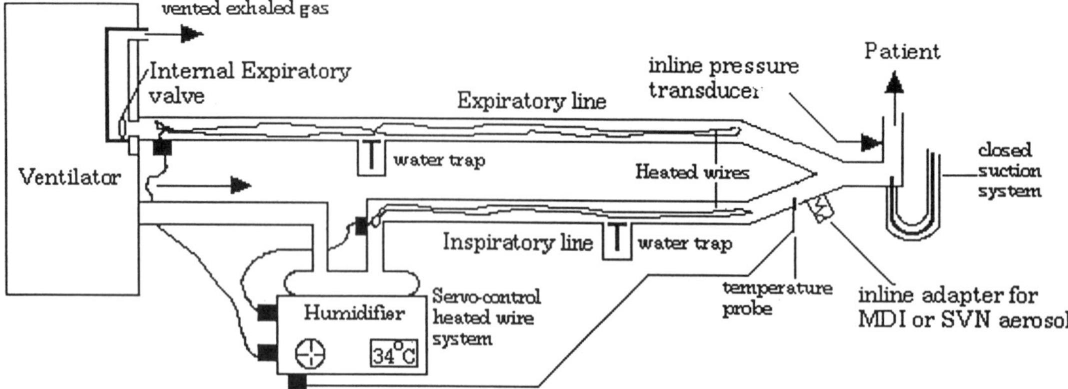

FIG 5–18
A generic external mechanical ventilator circuit. Modern circuits such as this are constructed to minimize frequent breaks or disconnections in the circuit to empty condensate or perform tracheobronchial aspiration, thus theoretically decreasing the opportunity for infection/cross-contamination and other patient events. Other modifications may be made to this circuit, including not using a heated wire system. For instance, some institutions may utilize an unheated humidifier along with a heat-moisture exchanging filter as reported by Suzukawa et al.[33] Modern circuits are often devoid of the external exhalation manifold and utilize an internal exhalation valve where gas flow and pressure are also measured. Some mechanical ventilators employ circuits with a pressure transducer at the patient wye (e.g., Hamilton Veolar), which may be a better and more accurate method of patient monitoring. (MDI = metered dose inhaler; SVN = small volume nebulizer).

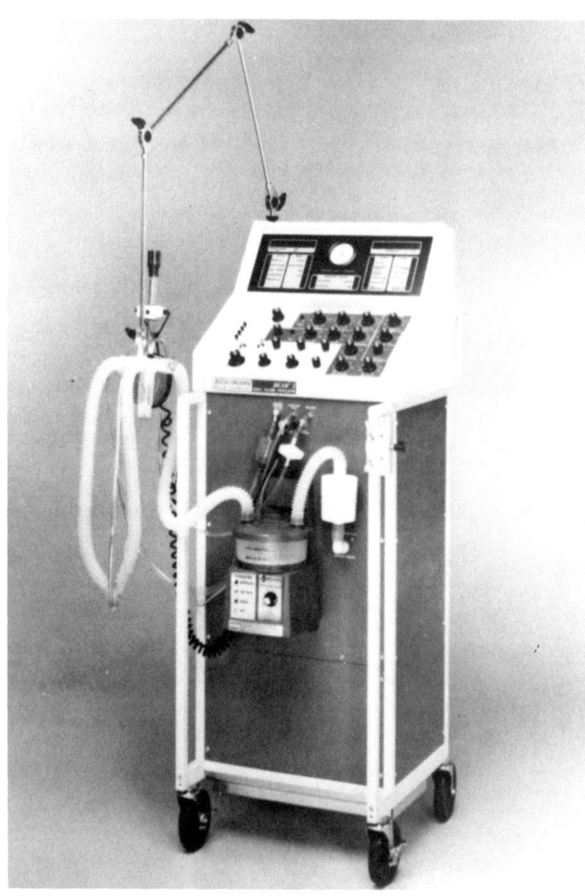

FIG 5–19
BEAR 2 adult volume ventilator. (Courtesy of BEAR Medical Systems, Inc, Riverside, Calif.)

- Inspiratory waveform: constant or nonconstant flow generator
- Pressure limit: 0 to 120 cm H_2O
- Tidal volume: 100 to 2,000 mL
- Flow range: 10 to 120 L/min
- Frequency: 0.5 to 60 breaths per minute
- Inspiratory time: 0.5 to 10 seconds
- Expiratory time: 0.95 to 120 seconds
- CPAP or PEEP: 0 to 50 cm H_2O
- F_{IO_2}: 0.21 to 1.00

Other features include sigh and SIMV modes; sensitivity setting from −1 to −5 cm H_2O; and alarms for high and low pressure, O_2 failure, low volume, I:E ratio, low PEEP or CPAP, loss of power, high temperature, high rate, and ventilator inoperative.

BEAR 3

This ventilator is essentially a BEAR 2 with pressure support (Fig 5–21). The display and control panels are illustrated in Figure 5–22. The display, indicator, and control panels are seen in Table 5–9.

- Power source: electric or compressed gas
- Control circuit: electronic
- Cycling control variable: volume, time, or pressure
- Inspiratory waveform: constant or nonconstant flow generator
- Pressure limit: 0 to 120 cm H_2O
- Tidal volume: 100 to 2,000 mL
- Flow range: 10 to 120 L/min
- Frequency: 0.5 to 60 breaths per minute

TABLE 5–7

Ventilator Classification*

Ventilator	Power Source	Circuitry	Control Mechanism	Control Variable†	*Tigger* Initiating Inspiration‡	*Limit* Inspiratory Phase Limit‡	*Cycle* Ending Inspiration‡	Modes§
BEAR 2	Pneumatic	Single	Electronic	F: constant, decelerating	P/T	V/F	P/V/T	C/AC/SIMV/PEEP/CPAP/IP/sigh
BEAR 3	Pneumatic	Single	Electronic	F: constant, decelerating	P/T	V/F	P/V/T/F	C/AC/SIMV/PEEP/CPAP/IP/sigh/PS
BEAR 5	Pneumatic	Single	Electronic	P: rectangular F: constant, decelerating, accelerating, sinusoidal	P/T	P/V/F	P/V/T/F, T	C/AC/SIMV/PEEP/CPAP/IP/sigh/ PS/MMV
BEAR 1000	Pneumatic	Single	Electronic	P: variable (exponential to rectangular) F: constant, decelerating, sinusoidal	P/T	P/V/F/T	P/V/T/F, T	C/AC/SIMV/PEEP/CPAP/IP/sigh/ PS/PC/MMV pressure slope, pressure augmentation
Servo 900C	Pneumatic	Single	Electronic	P: rectangular F: constant, decelerating	P/T	P/V/F	P/F/T	C/AC/SIMV/PEEP/CPAP/IP/sigh/ PS/PC
Servo 300	Pneumatic	Single	Electronic	P: rectangular F: constant, decelerating	P/T/F	P/V	P/F/V/T	C/AC/SIMV/PEEP/CPAP/IP/PS/PC/ volume support, pressure-regulated volume control
Hamilton Veolar	Pneumatic	Single	Electronic	P: rectangular F: constant, decelerating, accelerating, sinusoidal	P/T	P/V/F	P/F,V,T	C/AC/SIMV/PEEP/CPAP/IP/sigh/ PS/PC/MMV
Puritan Bennett 7200ae	Pneumatic	Single	Electronic	P: rectangular F: constant, decelerating, sinusoidal	P/T/F	P/V/T/F	V/P/T/F	C/AC/SIMV/PEEP/CPAP/IP/sigh/ PS/PC/flow-by

* Adapted from Pilbeam SP: Physical aspects of mechanical ventilation, in *Mechanical Ventilation: Physiological and Clinical Applications*, ed 2. St Louis, Mosby–Year Book, 1992, p. 158. Used by permission.

† P = pressure; F = flow.

‡ P = pressure; V = volume; T = time; F = flow.

§ P = pressure; V = volume; T = time; F = flow. C = control; AC = assist control; IP = inspiratory pause; PS = pressure support; PC = pressure control; SIMV = synchronized intermittent mandatory ventilation; MMV = mandatory minute ventilation; PEEP = positive end-expiratory pressure; CPAP = continuous positive airway pressure; sigh = periodic deep breaths.

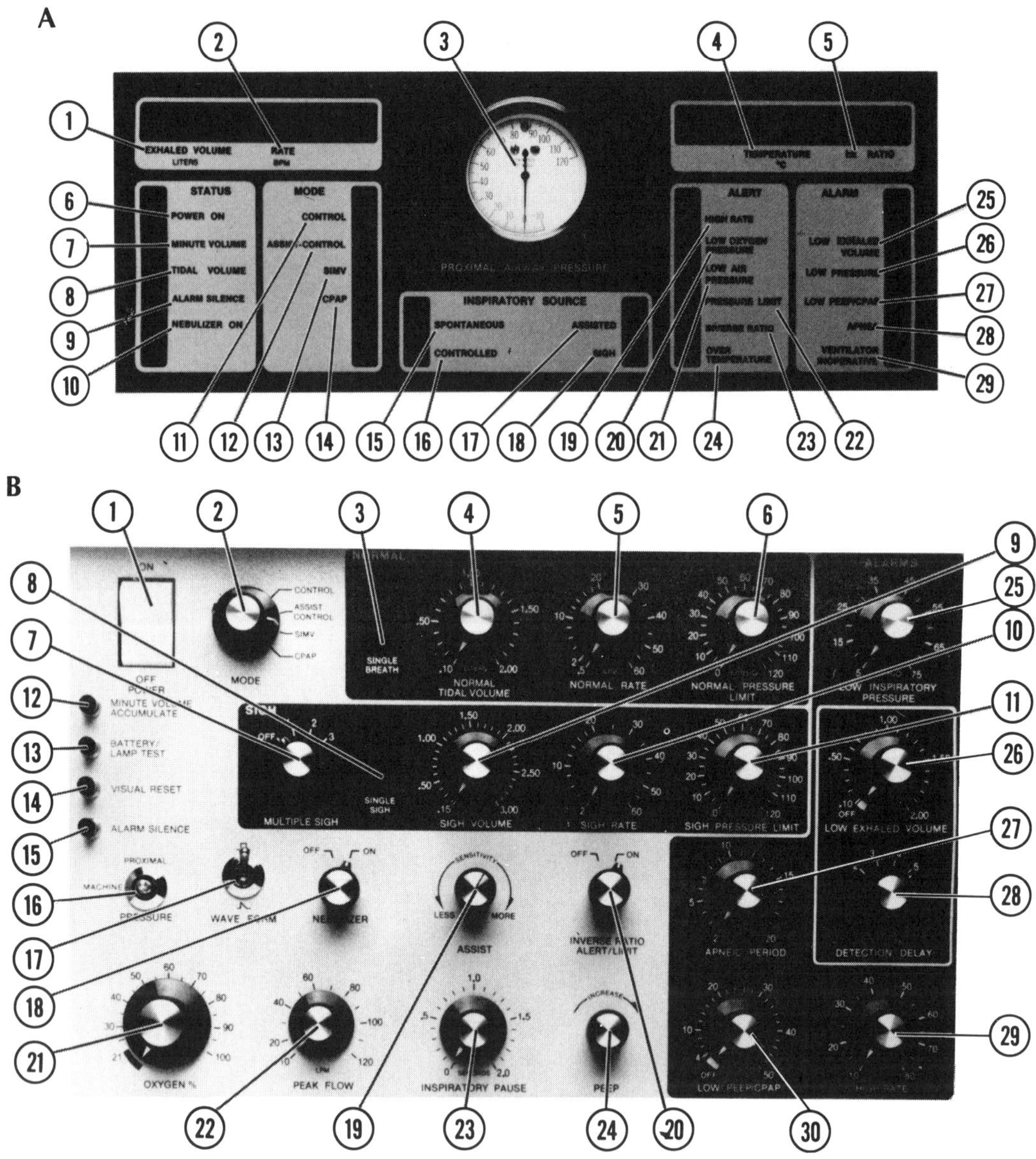

FIG 5–20
Display panel **(A)** and control panel **(B)** of the BEAR 2 ventilator. (Courtesy of BEAR Medical Systems, Inc, Riverside, Calif.)

- CPAP or PEEP: 0 to 60 cm H_2O
- F_{IO_2}: 0.21 to 1.00

Other features include sigh, SIMV with pressure support, and pressure support modes; sensitivity setting from −1 to −5 cm H_2O; inflation hold for 0 to 2 seconds; and alarms for high and low pressure, oxygen failure, low volume, I:E ratio, low PEEP or CPAP, loss of power, high temperature, high rate, and ventilator inoperative.

BEAR 5

This represents BEAR/Intermed's first move in microprocessor controlled ventilators (Fig 5–23). This was the first ventilator to incorporate a cathode ray tube (CRT)-based monitoring package while also allowing for infant, pediatric, and adult ventilation. The CRT interface allows for setting of alarms as well as access to other monitors including graphics and mechanics. The graphics page displays real-time flow, volume, and pressure. The mechanics page displays ventilation parameters including the patient's airway resistance, static compliance, and compliance compensation. Figure 5–24, A and B illustrate the BEAR 5 keyboard arrangement and CRT display with control keys. Table 5–10 shows the ventilator's control panel with controls, indicators, and CRT panel displays.

- Power source: pneumatic
- Control circuit: microprocessor-controlled stepper motor
- Cycling control variable: volume, time, or pressure
- Inspiratory waveform: rectangular, ascending, descending, sine wave

TABLE 5–8

BEAR 2 Ventilator Display and Control Panels*

Display panel	
1. EXHALED VOLUME, LITERS	Digital display of the breath-to-breath exhaled volume or minute volume
2. RATE, BPM	Digital display of the breathing rate per minute based on the average of the last 20 seconds. The display updates every second
3. PROXIMAL AIRWAY PRESSURE	Manometer calibrated between −10 and 120 cm H_2O. Displays proximal airway pressure or system (machine) pressure depending on the position of the PROXIMAL PRESSURE toggle switch
4. TEMPERATURE, °C	Digital display of gas temperature sampled at the patient wye
5. I:E RATIO	Digital display of breath-to-breath ventilator inspiratory time-to-expiratory time ratio in the CONTROL and ASSIST-CONTROL modes. A flashing display indicates that the expiratory portion of the ratio exceeds the inspiratory portion by at least 9.9. The display will also flash to indicate that inspiration time exceeds 6 seconds. The colon in the display will flash on and off to indicate an inverse I:E ratio.
6. POWER ON	Light indicates that the ventilator is plugged into an operating ac outlet and the power switch is on
7. MINUTE VOLUME	Flashing light indicates that the exhaled volume is being accumulated for 1 min. Continuous light indicates that the minute volume is being displayed.
8. TIDAL VOLUME	Light indicates that the digital EXHALED VOLUME display is displaying tidal volume
9. ALARM SILENCE	Light indicates that all audio alarms except VENTILATOR INOPERATIVE are canceled for 60 seconds
10. NEBULIZER ON	Light indicates that the nebulizer is on during a ventilator-delivered breath
11. CONTROL	Light indicates that the mode selector switch is set to the CONTROL mode
12. ASSIST-CONTROL	Light indicates that the mode selector switch is set to the ASSIST-CONTROL mode
13. SIMV	Light indicates that the mode selector switch is set to the SIMV mode
14. CPAP	Light indicates that the mode selector switch is set to the CPAP mode
15. SPONTANEOUS	Light blinks to indicate a patient-initiated spontaneous breath
16. CONTROLLED	Light blinks to indicate a ventilator-initiated positive-pressure breath
17. ASSISTED	Light blinks to indicate a patient-initiated positive-pressure breath
18. SIGH	Light indicates that a sigh breath is currently being delivered or that the previous breath was a sigh breath
19. HIGH RATE	Light and audio alarm indicate that the breath rate has exceeded the HIGH RATE alert control setting
20. LOW OXYGEN PRESSURE	Light and audio alarm indicate that the oxygen inlet pressure is below 27.5 ± 2.5 psi with the OXYGEN % selector above 21%
21. LOW AIR PRESSURE	Light and audio alarm indicate that the air supply pressure is below 9.5 psi
22. PRESSURE LIMIT	Light and audio alarm indicate that the system pressure has exceeded the setting of the NORMAL PRESSURE LIMIT control and the inspiratory phase is terminated
23. INVERSE RATIO	Light indicates that the inspiration time interval has exceeded the exhalation time interval. In the CONTROL mode the audio alarm activates, and the inspiratory phase is terminated when the INVERSE RATIO ALERT/LIMIT control is set to the ON position
24. OVER TEMPERATURE	Light and audio alarm indicate that the temperature of the gas at the patient wye exceeds 41°C or that the temperature probe is disconnected or malfunctioning
25. LOW EXHALED VOLUME	Light and audio alarm indicate that the exhaled volume has not exceeded the level set on the LOW EXHALED VOLUME alarm control for the number of consecutive breaths specified by the DETECTION DELAY switch
26. LOW PRESSURE	Light and audio alarm indicate that the inspiratory pressure has not exceeded the value set for the LOW INSPIRATORY PRESSURE alarm control or that the pressure has not dropped below that setting during the expiratory phase
27. LOW PEEP-CPAP	Light and audio alarm indicate that the PEEP-CPAP pressure is less than the setting of the LOW PEEP-CPAP alarm control
28. APNEA	Light and audio alarm indicate that the breath interval has exceeded the APNEA PERIOD alarm setting
29. VENTILATOR INOPERATIVE	Light and audio alarm indicate a total gas failure, ac power failure, an electronic malfunction in the internal volume measuring circuitry, or a sigh rate logic failure
Control panel	
1. POWER ON/OFF	Controls electrical power to the ventilator
2. MODE CONTROL	Selects the mode of operation: CONTROL, ASSIST-CONTROL, SIMV, and CPPA
3. NORMAL SINGLE BREATH	Push-button control; allows the delivery of 1 control breath as specified by the setting of the tidal volume control. 350-ms delay prevents stacking of breaths. Operational in all modes.
4. NORMAL TIDAL VOLUME (LITERS)	Calibrated between 0.10 and 2.00 L. Determines the tidal volume delivered during the inspiratory phase
5. NORMAL RATE (BPM)	Calibrated between 0.5 and 60 breaths per minute. Determines the number of ventilator-delivered breaths in 1 min
6. NORMAL PRESSURE LIMIT (CM H_2O)	Calibrated from 0 to 120 cm H_2O. Sets the inspiratory pressure limit for the normal breath. When the set pressure limit is reached, the audiovisual PRESSURE LIMIT ALERT activates, and the inspiratory phase ends
7. MULTIPLE SIGH	Calibrated between OFF, 1, 2, and 3. Determines the number of sighs delivered at specific intervals. Operational in the CONTROL and ASSIST-CONTROL modes only

(Continued.)

TABLE 5–8 (cont.)

8. SINGLE SIGH	Push-button control permits the delivery of a sigh volume as specified by the SIGH VOLUME control in all modes of operation provided that the MULTIPLE SIGH SWITCH is not in the *off* position. The control is disabled until 350 ms after exhalation begins
9. SIGH VOLUME (liters)	Calibrated between 0.15 and 3.0 L. Determines the volume delivered during the sigh period
10. SIGH RATE (sph)	Calibrated between 2 and 60 sighs per hour. Determines the interval between the sigh breath. Functional in the CONTROL and ASSIST-CONTROL modes only with the MULTIPLE SIGH switch set to the 1, 2, or 3 position. The fundamental time period is doubled during the sigh breath. For example, when the normal rate is set to 10 bpm, the respiratory cycle lasts 6 seconds. Following a sigh breath the ventilator will wait 12 sec before delivering a control breath
11. SIGH PRESSURE LIMIT (CM H_2O)	Calibrated between 0 and 120 cm H_2O. Sets the inspiratory pressure limit for the sigh period. When the set limit is reached, the audiovisual PRESSURE LMIT ALERT activates, and the inspiratory phase ends
12. MINUTE VOLUME ACCUMULATE	Push-button control initiates a 1-min time period in which the exhaled-tidal volume is accumulated. The minute volume is then displayed for the second minute. Push-button control allows immediate return to tidal volume display
13. BATTERY/LAMP TEST	Push-button control illuminates all digital display segments and LED indicators and tests the integrity of the rechargeable batteries and the power-loss audio alarm
14. VISUAL RESET	Push-button control resets all activated visual alarm and alert indicators
15. ALARM SILENCE	Push-button control disables the audio portion of the alarms and alerts for 60 sec (except VENTILATOR INOPERATIVE). Resets automatically after 60 sec or can be manually reset by depressing the button.
16. PROXIMAL PRESSURE	Toggle switch; spring loaded in the PROXIMAL position to sample the pressure at the patient wye. In the MACHINE position the pressure is sampled upstream from main-flow bacteria filter. The pressure is displayed on the PROXIMAL AIRWAY PRESSURE manometer
17. WAVE FORM	Influences the flow pattern during the positive-pressure breath
18. NEBULIZER	Turns the nebulizer compressor on/off
19. ASSIST SENSITIVITY	Adjustable between −1 and −5 cm H_2O. Allows the adjustment of the inspiratory effort required in triggering the ventilator for a positive-pressure breath
20. INVERSE RATIO ALERT/LIMIT	The OFF position allows inverse I:E ratios. The ON position terminates inspiration and activates the INVERSE RATIO ALERT when the ratio reaches 1:1
21. OXYGEN %	Calibrated between 21% and 100% oxygen. Selects the concentration of oxygen in the inspired gas
22. PEAK FLOW (LPM)	Calibrated between 10 and 120 L/min. Selects the peak unrestricted flow of the positive-pressure breath
23. INSPIRATORY PAUSE (seconds)	Calibrated between 0 and 2.0 sec. Determines the time in which the lungs are held inflated following a positive-pressure breath
24. PEEP	Adjustable between 0 and 50 cm H_2O. Selects the baseline pressure as displayed on the PROXIMAL AIRWAY PRESSURE manometer
Alarms	
25. LOW INSPIRATORY PRESSURE (cm H_2O)	Calibrated between 3 and 75 cm H_2O. Activates the audiovisual LOW PRESSURE alarm when the inspiratory pressure does not exceed the control setting or fails to drop below that setting during the expiratory phase
26. LOW EXHALED VOLUME (liters)	Calibrated between OFF/0.10 and 2.00 L. Activates the audiovisual LOW EXHALED VOLUME alarm when the exhaled volume does not exceed the control setting for the number of breaths selected on the DETECTION DISPLAY control
27. APNEIC PERIOD (seconds)	Calibrated between 2 and 20 sec. Activates the audiovisual APNEA ALARM if the interval between spontaneous or controlled breaths exceeds the alarm setting
28. DETECTION DELAY (breaths)	Selects the number of consecutive breaths of low tidal volumes required to activate the audiovisual LOW EXHALED VOLUME alarm
29. HIGH RATE (BPM)	Calibrated between 10 and 80 BPM. Activates the audiovisual HIGH RATE ALERT if the total rate exceeds the alarm setting
30. LOW PEEP/CPAP (cm H_2O)	Calibrated between OFF and 50 cm H_2O. Activates the audiovisual LOW PEEP/CPAP alarm when the baseline pressure drops below the control setting

* From Dupuis YG: Ventilators: *Theory and Clinical Application*, ed 2. St Louis, Mosby–Year Book, 1992, pp 316–317. Used by permission.

- Pressure limit: 0 to 160 cm H_2O
- Tidal volume: 50 to 2,000 mL
- Flow range: 5 to 150 L/min
- Frequency: 0.5 to 150 breaths per minute
- Inspiratory time: 0.10 to 3.0 seconds
- PEEP or CPAP: 0 to 50 cm H_2O
- Pressure support: 0 to 72 cm H_2O
- Minimum minute volume: 0.5 to 40 L/min (augmented minute ventilation [AMV])
- Continuous flow: 5 to 40 L/min
- F_{IO_2}: 0.21 to 1.00

Other features include IMV or SIMV, time-cycled or pressure-limited IMV, CPAP, and AMV modes available;

CRT able to display monitoring, alarms, mechanics, or graphs; and alarms for high and low pressure, low tidal volume, high and low minute volume, high and low rate, high and low mean airway pressure, high and low PEEP or CPAP, I:E ratio, low O_2 and air source, and ventilator inoperative.

Comprehensive BEAR 1000

This ventilator (Fig 5–25) incorporates microprocessor control with added features far beyond the BEAR 5. It contains a much more enhanced monitoring system and display with the additional functions of pressure control ventilation, pressure augmentation, and pressure slope. Table 5–11 shows the panel details and specifications, and Figures 5–26 and 5–27 illustrate the control and monitors alarms panels, respectively.

- Power source: pneumatic
- Control circuit: microprocessor-controlled stepper motor
- Cycling control variable: volume, time, flow, or pressure
- Inspiratory waveform: rectangular, descending, sine wave
- Pressure limit: 0 to 120 cm H_2O
- Tidal volume: 0.10 to 2.0 L
- Flow range: 0 to 150 L/min
- Frequency: 1 to 120 breaths per minute
- Inspiratory time: 0.1 to 5.0 seconds

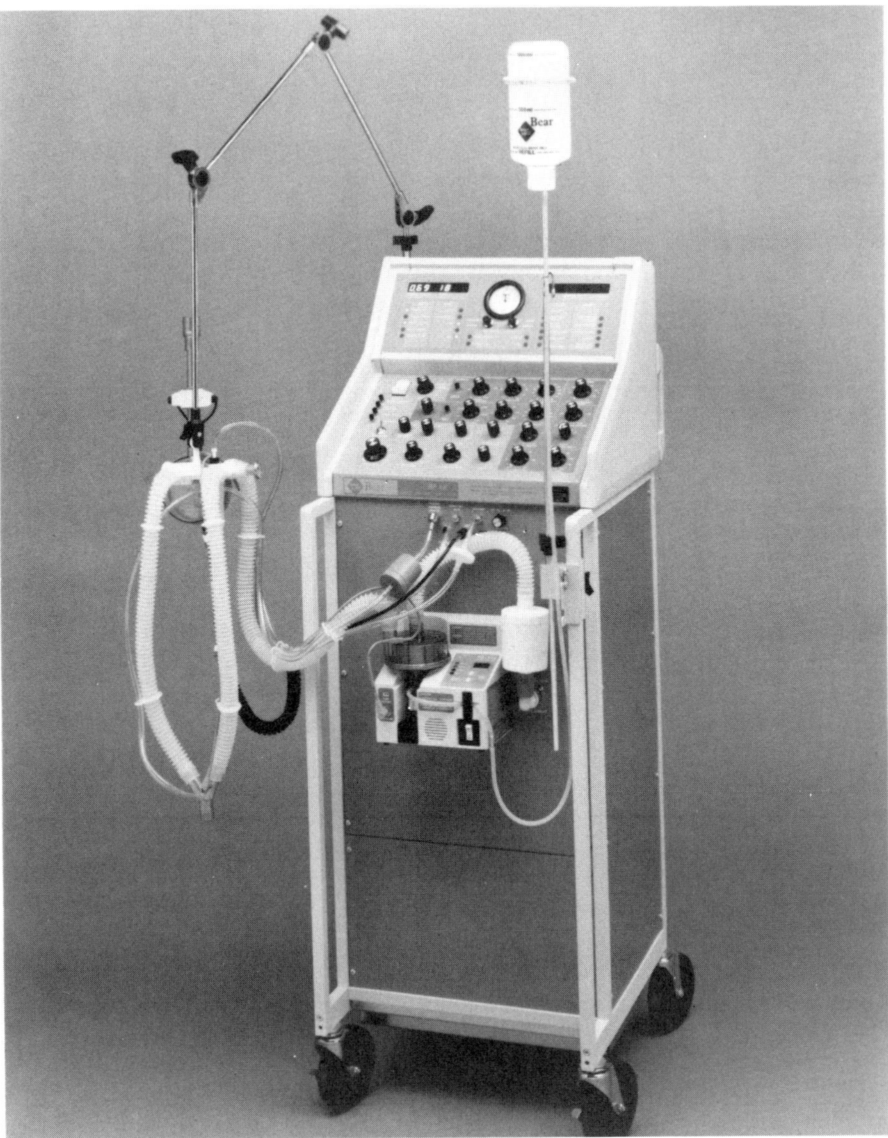

FIG 5–21
BEAR 3 ventilator. (Courtesy of BEAR Medical Systems, Inc, Riverside, Calif.)

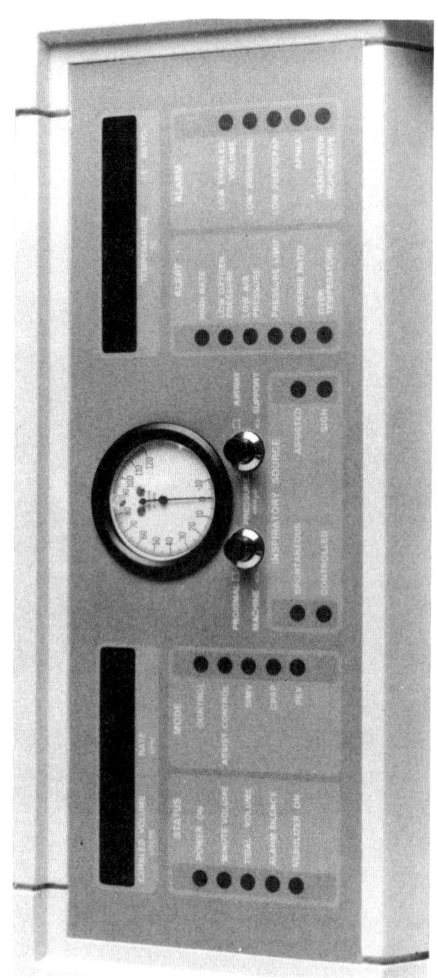

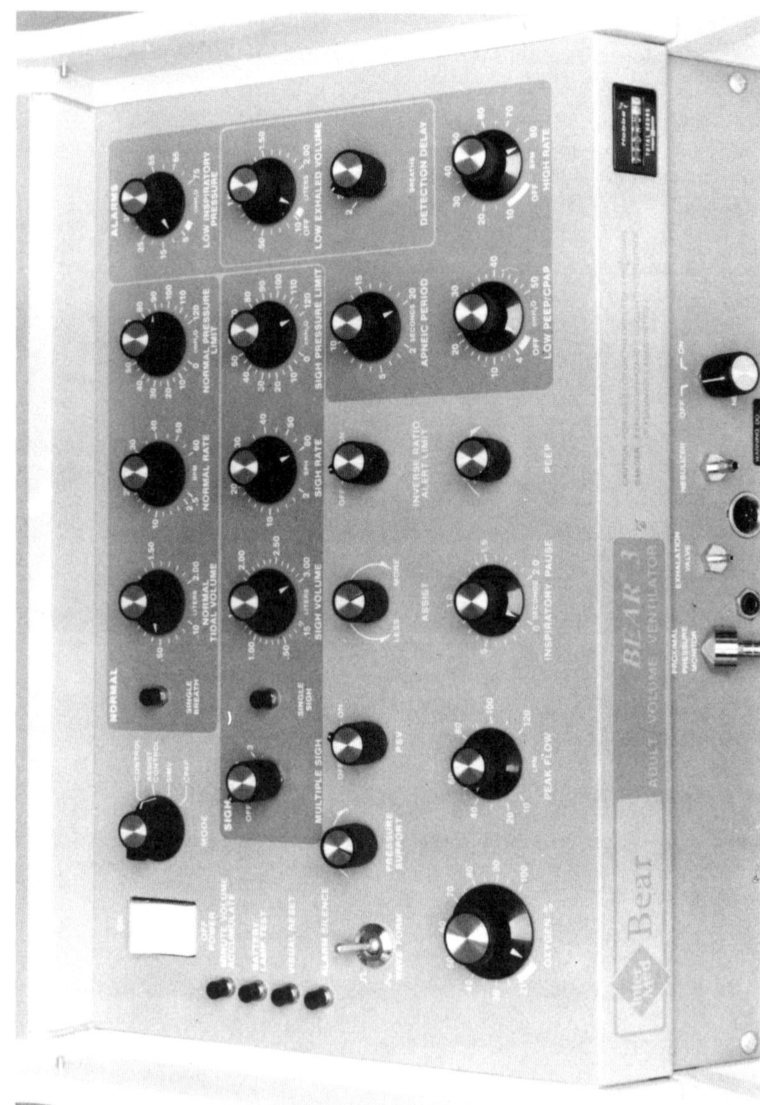

FIG 5–22
Display and control panel of the BEAR 3 ventilator. (Courtesy of BEAR Medical Systems, Inc, Riverside, Calif.)

- PEEP: 0 to 50 cm H_2O
- Pressure support: 0 to 80 cm H_2O
- Minimum minute volume: 0.0 to 50 L/min (augmented minute ventilation)
- F_{IO_2}: 0.21 to 1.00

Other features include inspiratory pause, expiratory pause, compliance compensation, pressure slope (pediatric and adult), pressure augmentation, and pressure control.

Siemens Servo 900C

This machine represents the updated version of the Siemens Servo 900B and was first introduced in the United States in 1981 (Fig 5–28). It has several modes of ventilation and was the first adult ventilator with pressure control and pressure support. Table 5–12 shows the ventilator's specifications, and Figure 5–29 illustrates the control panel.

- Power source: pneumatic
- Control circuit: electronic
- Cycling control variable: volume, time, or pressure
- Inspiratory waveform: rectangular and descending and ascending ramp
- Pressure limit: 0 to 120 cm H_2O
- Minute volume: 0.4 to 40 L/min
- Flow range: up to 120 L/min measured against 40 cm H_2O backpressure
- Frequency: 6 to 120 breaths per minute

TABLE 5–9

BEAR 3 Ventilator Display, Indicator, and Control Panels*

Display panel	
EXHALED VOLUME	Digital display of exhaled tidal volume in liters. When the MINUTE VOLUME ACCUMULATE button is depressed, the display accumulates tidal volumes for 1 minute and displays minute volume for an additional minute. After these 2 minutes the display is reset to tidal volumes.
RATE	Digital display of the total breaths per minute. The rate is calculated from last 20 sec and updates every second
PRESSURE	Monitors the selected pressure source from −10 to 120 cm H_2O. May be used to monitor proximal airway, machine pressure, or PSV set point
AIRWAY/SUPPORT	Depression of the button allows monitoring of PSV control
TEMPERATURE	Digital display of temperature sampled at the patient wye
I:E RATIO	Digital display of the ratio of inspiratory to expiratory times. The colon in the display flashes during inverse conditions. The display flashes on and off when 1. Ratio exceeds 1:9.9 2. Total inspiratory time exceeds 6 seconds
INLET PRESSURE GAUGES	Analog display of air and oxygen supply pressures between 0 and 100 psig
Indicator panel	
Status indicators	
POWER ON	Indicates power is switched ON
MINUTE VOLUME	Indicates EXHALED VOLUME digital display is showing minute volume. The indicator blinks while volume is accumulating and remains lit when minute volume is being displayed
TIDAL VOLUME	Indicates tidal volume is being displayed
ALARM SILENCE	Indicates all but VENTILATOR INOPERATIVE audio alarms are silenced for 60 sec
NEBULIZER ON	Indicates nebulizer compressor activated
Mode indicators	
CONTROL	Indicates ventilator set to CONTROL MODE
ASSIST CONTROL	Indicates ventilator set to ASSIST CONTROL mode
SIMV	Indicates ventilator set to SIMV mode
CPAP	Indicates ventilator set to CPAP mode
PSV	Indicates PSV control in ON position
Inspiratory source indicators	
SPONTANEOUS	Indicates a spontaneous or PSV breath. Functional in SIMV and CPAP modes
CONTROLLED	Indicates a ventilator-initiated breath
ASSISTED	Indicates a patient-initiated controlled breath
SIGH	Indicates sigh breath being delivered or previous breath was a sigh breath
Alert indicators	
HIGH RATE	Indicates HIGH RATE setting exceeded
LOW OXYGEN PRESSURE	Indicates O_2 source pressure less than 27.5 ± 2.5 psig and O_2 control set above 21%
LOW AIR PRESSURE	Indicates external air source less than 27.5 ± 2.5 psig and internal air compressor less than 9.5 psig
PRESSURE LIMIT	Indicates machine pressure limit reached and inspiration terminated
INVERSE RATIO	Indicates I:E ratio greater than 1:1 and inspiration terminated by INVERSE RATIO ALERT/LIMIT function
OVER TEMPERATURE	Indicates gas temperature at patient wye is 41°C or greater or probe disconnected
Alarm indicators	
LOW EXHALED VOLUME	Indicates exhaled volume is less than LOW EXHALED VOLUME alarm for the number of consecutive breaths set by the DETECTION DELAY switch
LOW PRESSURE	Indicates machine pressure less than the level set by LOW INSPIRATORY PRESSURE alarm control or below that during exhalation. Active for volume-controlled or PSV breaths
LOW PEEP/CPAP	Indicates PEEP/CPAP pressure less than level set on LOW PEEP/CPAP alarm control or leak exists during PEEP/CPAP mode
APNEA	Indicates interval between breaths exceeds APNEA PERIOD alarm setting
VENTILATOR INOPERATIVE	Indicates one of the following: 1. Electrical power failure or disconnect 2. Internal power supply failure 3. Insufficient gas pressure from all sources 4. Internal flow transducer failure 5. Sigh rate logic failure
LOW INSPIRATORY PRESSURE	Adjustable from 3 to 75 cm H_2O. Activates an audio/visual alarm when the inspiratory pressure does not exceed the control setting or fails to drop below that setting during the expiratory phase
LOW EXHALED VOLUME	Adjustable from OFF/0.10 to 2.0 L Activates an audio/visual alarm when the exhaled volume does not exceed the control setting for the number of consecutive breaths selected on the DETECTION DELAY control

(Continued.)

TABLE 5–9 (cont.)

DETECTION DELAY	Selects the number of consecutive breaths required to activate the LOW EXHALED VOLUME alarm
LOW PEEP/CPAP	Adjustable from OFF to 50 cm H_2O. Activates an audio/visual alarm when the baseline pressure drops below the control setting.
HIGH RATE	Adjustable from OFF to 80 BPM. Activates an audio/visual alert if the total rate exceeds the control setting
APNEIC PERIOD	Adjustable from 2 to 20 sec. Activates an audio/visual alarm if the interval between spontaneous or controlled breaths exceeds the alarm setting
CONTROL PANEL	
MODE	Selects the mode of operation: CONTROL, ASSIST CONTROL, SIMV, and CPAP
PRESSURE SUPPORT	Controls the level of PSV. Adjustable from 5.5 to 66 cm H_2O
PSV OFF/ON	Enables or disables PSV in SIMV or CPAP modes
SENSITIVITY	Adjust triggering sensitivity. Adjustable between −1.1 cm H_2O at 2 L/min and −8 cm H_2O at 70 L/min. PEEP/CPAP compensated
SINGLE BREATH	Delivers a tidal volume as determined by the setting of TIDAL VOLUME control unless the NORMAL PRESSURE LIMIT is reached
NORMAL TIDAL VOLUME	Adjustable from 0.1 to 2.0 L. Controls the volume delivered during positive-pressure breaths
NORMAL RATE	Adjustable from 0.5 to 60 BPM. Determines 1. Number of control breaths delivered during CONTROL and SIMV modes 2. Minimum number of breaths delivered in ASSIST-CONTROL mode
NORMAL PRESSURE LIMIT	Adjustable from 0 to 120 cm H_2O. Sets the inspiratory pressure limit for the NORMAL TIDAL VOLUME. Inspiration ends when the limit is reached
SIGH	Calibrated between OFF, 1, 2, and 3
MULTIPLE SIGH	Determines the number of sighs delivered at specified intervals. Operational in the CONTROL and ASSIST CONTROL modes. The normal breath interval is doubled during the sigh breath
SINGLE SIGH	Push-button control permits the delivery of a sigh volume as specified by the SIGH VOLUME and SIGH PRESSURE LIMIT settings Control disabled until 340 ms after exhalation
SIGH VOLUME	Adjustable from 150 to 3000 mL. Sets the volume of sigh breath
SIGH RATE	Adjustable from 2 to 60 sighs per hour. Operational in the CONTROL and ASSIST-CONTROL modes
SIGH PRESSURE LIMIT	Adjustable from 0 to 120 cm H_2O. Sets the pressure limit of the sigh breath. Inspiration ends when the set limit is reached and audio/visual alert activates
WAVE FORM	Influences the flow pattern of the volume-controlled breaths
INVERSE RATIO ALERT/LIMIT	The OFF position allows inverse I:E ratios. The ON position terminates inspiration and activates audio/visual alert when the ratio of controlled breath exceeds 1:1.
OXYGEN %	Adjustable from 21% to 100%. Selects the concentration of oxygen in the inspired gas.
PEAK FLOW	Adjustable from 10 to 120 L/min. Selects the peak unrestricted flow of the controlled breath
INSPIRATORY PAUSE	Adjustable from 0 to 2.0 sec. Determines the time in which the lungs are held inflated following a control breath
PEEP	Adjustable from 0 to 40 cm H_2O. Selects the baseline expiratory pressure. Circuit is compensated for up to a 25 L/min leak.
MINUTE VOLUME ACCUMULATE	Push-button control initiates a 1-min period in which all of the exhaled volumes are added and displayed on the EXHALED VOLUME display
BATTERY/LAMP TEST	Tests the internal, rechargeable battery
VISUAL TEST	Resets alarms and alert indicators after the cause is corrected
ALARM SILENCE	Silences all audio alarms except VENTILATOR INOPERATIVE alarm for 60 sec
NEBULIZER	Turns nebulizer compressor ON or OFF. Active for all positive-pressure breaths
Alarms	
LOW INSPIRATORY PRESSURE	Adjustable from 3 to 75 cm H_2O. Activates an audio/visual alarm when the inspiratory pressure does not exceed the control setting or fails to drop below that setting during the expiratory phase

* From Dupuis YG: *Ventilators: Theory and Clinical Application*, ed 2. St Louis, Mosby–Year Book, 1992, pp 320–322. Used by permission.

- Inspiratory time: 20% to 80% of the cycle time
- PEEP: 0 to 50 cm H_2O
- FIO_2: 0.21 to 1.00

Other features include SIMV; pressure support (0 to 100 cm H_2O); pressure control (0 to 100 cm H_2O); sensitivity of 0 to −20 cm H_2O; sigh mode; and alarms for high pressure, apnea, high and low minute volume, low source gas, high and low O_2 concentration, and loss of power. Additional options are inspiratory and expiratory pause buttons and a gas change button.

Servo 300 (SV 300)

This is the Siemens entry into microprocessor controlled ventilation (Fig 5–30). This machine is strikingly different in appearance and function as compared with other machines on the market today. Aside from its hefty price tag (approximately $30,000), this ventilator represents state-of-the-art technology with microprocessor control, portability, and ease of operation (the machine contains an automatic tutorial [autotutorial] that directs the clinician through setup for each mode in a step-by-step fashion). This ventilator is capable of ventilating neonatal, pediatric, and adult patients and also offers several new features including the new modes of ventilation, volume support and pressure-regulated volume control. Another new feature is the "touch pad" control offered to change and/or observe the ventilator's various functions. Figure 5–31 shows the front panel, and Figure 32, A through G shows each panel in more detail. Table 5–13 shows the specifications for the Servo 300.

- Power source: pneumatic
- Control circuit: electronic and microprocessor-controlled
- Cycling control variable: volume, time, flow, or pressure
- Inspiratory waveform: rectangular, descending ramp, exponential
- Pressure limit: 0 to 120 cm H_2O
- Frequency: 6 to 150 breaths per minute
- Inspiratory time: 10% to 80% of the cycle time
- Pause time: 0% to 30%
- PEEP or CPAP: 0 to 60 cm H_2O
- F_{IO_2}: 0.21 to 1.00

Other features include volume support, SIMV, volume control plus PSV, pressure control ventilation (PCV)

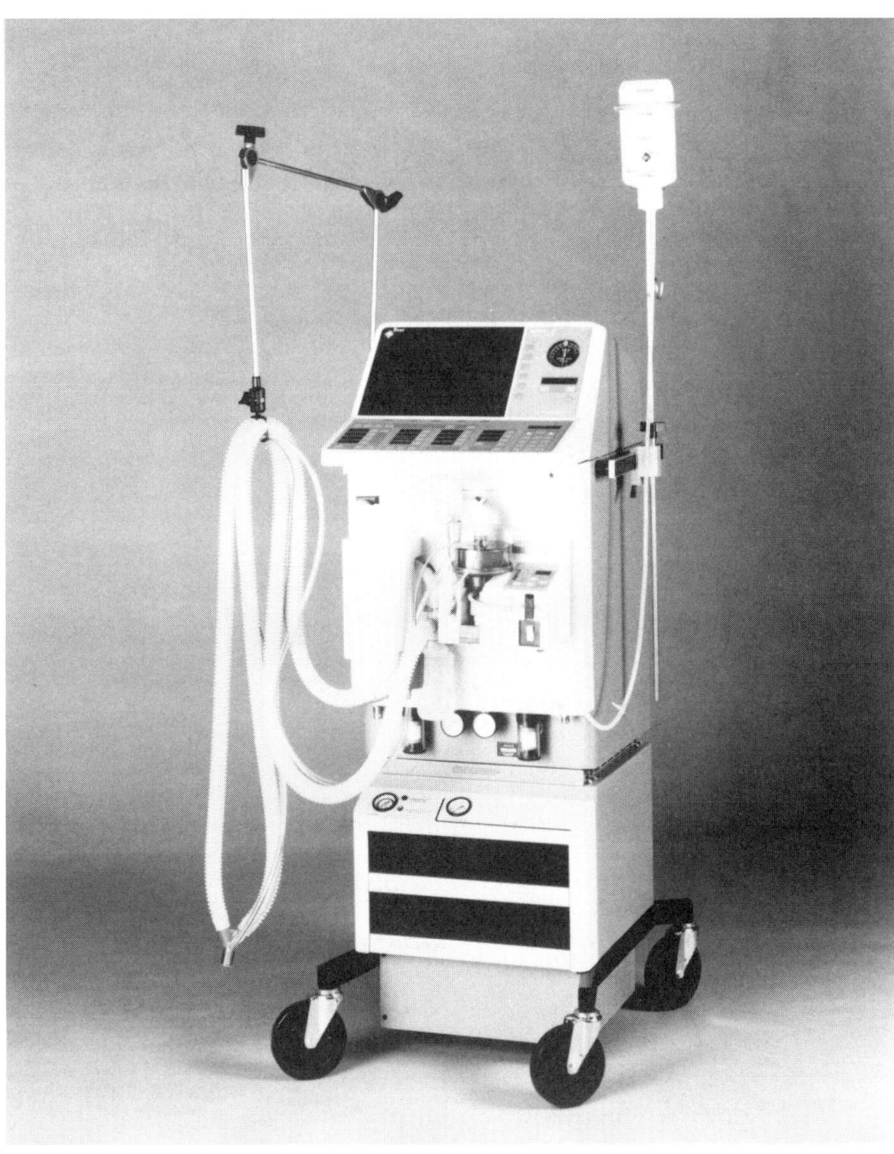

FIG 5–23
The BEAR 5 ventilator. (Courtesy of BEAR Medical Systems, Inc, Riverside, Calif.)

A

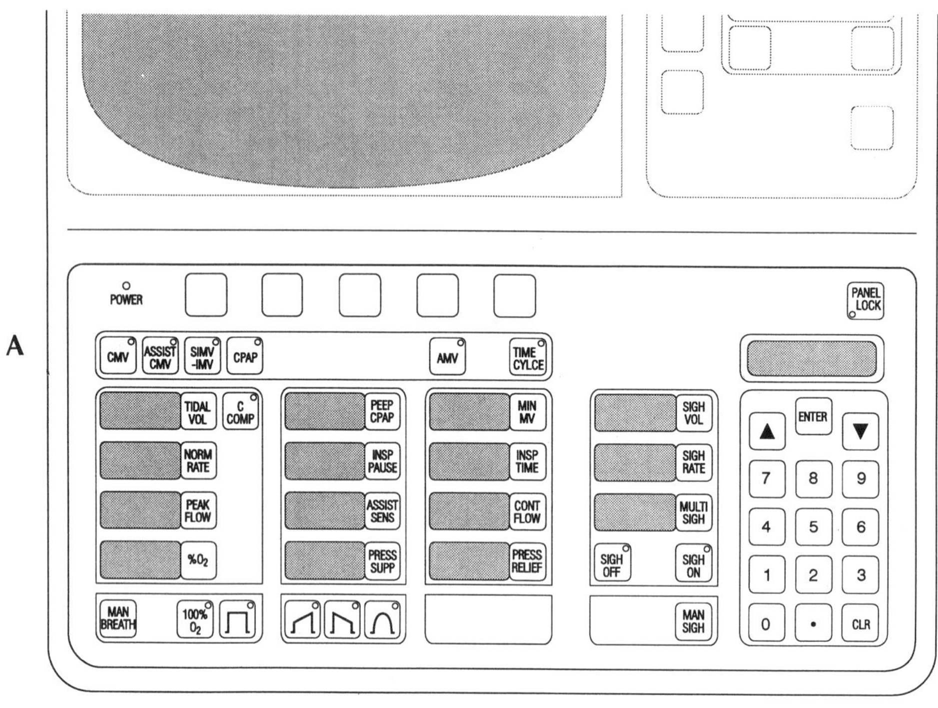

B

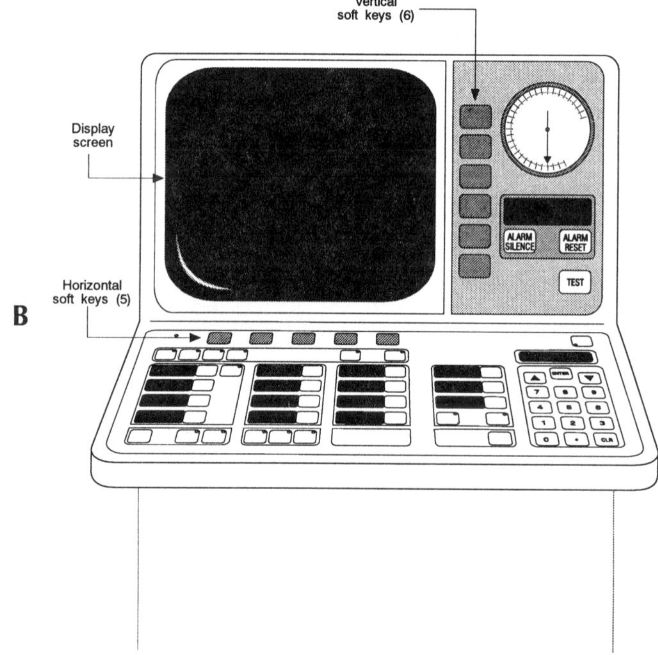

FIG 5–24
Keyboard arrangement of the BEAR 5 ventilator's control panel **(A)** and CRT display screen and associated control keys **(B)**. (Courtesy of BEAR Medical Systems, Inc, Riverside, Calif.)

TABLE 5–10
BEAR 5 Control and CRT Panels*

Control panel: controls and indicators	
POWER	Indicates ventilator turned ON
CMV	Indicates controlled mandatory ventilation mode
ASSIST CMV	Same as CMV except that breaths can be patient triggered
SIMV/IMV	Determines if the mandatory breath, as set by the NORMAL RATE control, will be synchronized with the patient's inspiratory effort. SIMV refers to demand flow. IMV occurs when continuous flow is selected
CPAP	Indicates continuous positive airway pressure mode
AMV	Augmented mandatory ventilation mode. Same as SIMV or CPAP mode except that the ventilator will ensure a clinician-selected minimum minute volume. When the average minute volume falls below the minimum level, the breath rate automatically increases to a level defined by Breath rate = Minimum minute volume ÷ Tidal volume Ventilator resumes normal operation when the average minute volume exceeds the preset by 1 L/min or 10%, whichever is less
TIME CYCLE	Indicates that the changeover from the inspiratory to the expiratory phase is time cycled. Used during continuous flow, pressure-limited mode, similar to pediatric ventilators
PANEL LOCK	When activated, no input can be made on the control panel
TIDAL VOL	Tidal volume, adjustable from 50 to 2000 mL, controls the volume of the mandatory breath. Available in the CMV, ASSIST CMV, SIMV/IMV, and AMV modes
NORM RATE	Normal rate, adjustable from OFF or 0.5 to 150 BPM. Available in the CMV, ASSIST CMV, SIMV/IMV, and TIME CYCLE modes
PEAK FLOW	Adjustable from 5 to 150 L/min (up to 170 L/min during pressure support). Available in the CMV, ASSIST CMV, SIMV/IMV, AMV, and CPAP (SIGH) modes
$\%O_2$	Selects the inspired oxygen concentration from 21% to 100% during all modes
MAN BREATH	Manual breath, activates one ventilatory cycle. Available in the CMV, ASSIST CMV, SIMV/IMV, AMV, and TIME CYCLE modes
100% O_2	Delivers 100% oxygen for 3 min and automatically resets. Available in all modes
Waveforms	*Square:* Selects the constant flow waveform *Accelerating:* Selects the increasing flow generator waveform *Decelerating:* Selects the decreasing flow generator waveform *Sine:* Selects the nonconstant flow generator waveform
C COMP	Compliance compensation, adjustable from 0 to 7.5 mL/cm H_2O. Clinician input of compliance factor on the keyboard. Adds the lost volume due to circuit compliance to the preset tidal volume. Available in the CMV, ASSIST CMV, SIMV/IMV, AMV, and CPAP (SIGH) modes
PEEP/CPAP	Adjustable from 0 to 50 cm H_2O. Available in all modes
INSP PAUSE	Inspiratory pause, adjustable from 0 to 2 sec. Available in the CMV, ASSIST CMV, SIMV/IMV, AMV and CPAP (SIGH) modes
ASSIST SENS	Assist sensitivity, adjustable from 0.5 to 5 cm H_2O and PEEP/CPAP compensated. Available in the ASSIST CMV, SIMV, AMV and CPAP modes. Must be set to initiate and monitor spontaneous breaths in SIMV/IMV, AMV, and CPAP
PRESS SUPP	Pressure support, adjustable from 0 to 72 cm H_2O. Available in the SIMV, AMV, and CPAP (DEMAND) modes
MIN MV	Minimum minute volume, adjustable from 0.5 to 40 L/min. Available in the AMV mode
INSP TIME	Inspiratory time, adjustable from 0.1 to 3 sec. Available in the TIME CYCLE mode
CONT FLOW	Continuous flow, adjustable from 5 to 40 L/min. Available in the IMV, CPAP, and TIME CYCLE mode
PRES RELIEF	Pressure relief, adjustable from 0 to 72 cm H_2O. Available in the TIME CYCLE mode
SIGH VOL	Sigh volume, adjustable from 65 to 3000 mL. Available in the CMV, ASSIST CMV, SIMV/IMV, AMV, and CPAP modes
SIGH RATE	Adjustable from 2 to 60 sighs per hour. Available in the CMV, ASSIST CMV, SIMV/IMV, AMV and CPAP modes
MULTI SIGH	Adjustable from OFF (MANUAL ONLY) to 1, 2, or 3. Available in the CMV, ASSIST CMV, SIMV/IMV, AMV, and CPAP modes
SIGH ON	Turns on the SIGH mode. Available in the CMV, ASSIST CMV, SIMV/IMV, AMV, and CPAP modes
SIGH OFF	Turns off the SIGH mode, including manual sigh
MAN SIGH	Manual sigh, activates one sigh cycle. Available in the CMV, ASSIST CMV, SIMV/IMV, AMV, and CPAP modes
Keypad	Used to enter all control parameters and alarm settings
CRT Panel	
ALARM SILENCE	Silences all but VENTILATOR INOPERATIVE audible alarm for 60 sec. Available in all modes
ALARM RESET	Cancels flashing video alarm and setting after the cause is corrected or self-corrected. Available in all modes
TEST	Activates all digital displays, which read 8s, all visual indicators, and nurse call. Available in all modes
VERTICAL SOFT KEYS (6)	On screen, identifies the line to be adjusted
HORIZONTAL SOFT KEYS (5)	On screen, identifies alarm to be adjusted, CRT operations, or action to be performed

(Continued.)

TABLE 5–10 (cont.)

ALARM INDICATOR	Activates with all alarm conditions. Available in all modes
VENT. INOP. INDICATOR	Activates with all inoperative conditions. Available in all modes
CRT monitors	
EXHALED TIDAL VOLUME	Displays from 0 to 999 mL EXHALED VOLUME monitors are based on trend information during CONTINUOUS FLOW
MANDATORY	Available in CMV, ASSIST CMV, SIMV, AMV, and CPAP (sigh demand flow)
SPONTANEOUS	Available in SIMV, AMV, AND CPAP (demand flow)
EXHALED MINUTE VOLUME	Displays 0 to 99.9 L/min. Available in CMV, ASSIST CMV, SIMV/IMV, AMV, and CPAP (demand flow)
TREND VOLUME INFORMATION ONLY	Displays 0 to 99.9 L/min. Available in IMV and CPAP (continuous flow), and TIME CYCLE
BREATH RATE (TOTAL)	Displays 0 to 999 BPM. Available in CMV, ASSIST CMV, SIMV/IMV, AMV, and CPAP
BREATH RATE (MECHANICAL)	Displays 0 to 999 BPM. Available in the TIME CYCLE mode
INSPIRATORY TIME	Displays 0 to 9.99 sec. Available in all modes for mandatory breaths
PEAK NORMAL/SIGH PRESSURE	Displays 0 to 150 cm H_2O. Available during positive-pressure breaths
MEAN AIRWAY PRESSURE	Displays 0 to 99 cm H_2O. Available in all modes
PEEP/CPAP	Displays 0 to 99 cm H_2O. Available in all modes
I:E RATIO	Displays 1.0.1 to 1.99.9. Available in all modes for mandatory breaths only
STATIC COMPLIANCE	Displays 5 to 200 mL/cm H_2O. Available in CMV, ASSIST CMV, SIMV/IMV, AMV, and CPAP for volume-delivered breaths only
RESISTANCE	Displays 2 to 100 cm H_2O/L/sec. Available in CMV, ASSIST CMV, SIMV/IMV, AMV, and CPAP
COMPLIANCE COMPENSATION ADDED VOLUME	Range is 0 to 750 mL. Available in CMV, ASSIST CMV, SIMV/IMV, AMV, and CPAP for volume-delivered breaths only
INSPIRATORY SOURCE	Identifies the source of the breath. A plus sign (+) after CONTROLLED +, ASSISTED +, or SIGH+ indicates that the patient's peak inspiratory flow has exceeded the preset setting or the patient has continued to inspire after the preset volume has been delivered
CONTROLLED	
ASSISTED	
SPONTANEOUS	
SIGH	
SUPPORTED	
Alarms	
LOW EXHALED VOLUME	Range is 0.3 to 2,000 mL. Alarms require 3 consecutive low volumes before activation
MANDATORY	
SPONTANEOUS	
LOW EXHALED MINUTE VOLUME	Range is 0.3 to 40.0 L/min. Available in CMV, ASSIST CMV, SIMV, AMV, and CPAP (demand flow)
HIGH EXHALED MINUTE VOLUME	Range is 1 to 80 L/min. Available in CMV, ASSIST CMV, SIMV, AMV, and CPAP (demand flow)
LOW BREATH RATE	Range is 3 to 155 BPM. Available in CMV, ASSIST CMV, SIMV, AMV, and CPAP (demand flow). The range is 0.3 to 155 in the TIME CYCLE, IMV, and CPAP modes
HIGH BREATH RATE	Range is 3 to 155 BPM. Available in all modes
LOW INSPIRATORY TIME	Range is 0.05 to 3 sec. Available in the TIME CYCLE mode
HIGH INSPIRATORY TIME (limit)	Range is 0.1 to 3.2 sec. Available in the TIME CYCLE mode
HIGH PEAK NORMAL PRESSURE (limit)	Range is 0 to 140 cm H_2O in the CMV, ASSIST CMV, SIMV/IMV, and AMV modes. Range is 0 to 80 cm H_2O in CPAP TIME CYCLE. Ventilator terminates the inspiratory phase when the threshold of the alarm is reached.
HIGH PEAK SIGH PRESSURE (limit)	Range is 0 to 140 cm H_2O. Inspiration is terminated when the threshold of the alarm is reached. Available in CMV, ASSIST CMV, SIMV/IMV, AMV, and CPAP
LOW INSPIRATORY PRESSURE	Range is 3 or preset PEEP/CPAP, whichever is greater, to 140 cm H_2O. Available in all modes
HIGH MEAN AIRWAY PRESSURE	Range is 0 to 75 cm H_2O. Available in all modes
LOW MEAN AIRWAY PRESSURE	Range is 0 to 75 cm H_2O. Available in all modes
HIGH PEEP/CPAP	Range is 0 to 55 cm H_2O. Available in all modes
LOW PEEP/CPAP	Range is 0 to 50 cm H_2O. Available in all modes
INVERSE I:E RATIO (mandatory breaths)	When set, limits the I:E ratio to 1:1. When overridden, limits the I:E ratio to 3:1. Inspiration is terminated when the I:E ratio limit is reached. Available in all mandatory breath modes
LOW OXYGEN PRESSURE	Activates alarm when O_2 pressure supply to the ventilator falls below 27 psig
LOW AIR PRESSURE	Activates alarm when air pressure supply to the ventilator falls below 27 psig
VENTILATOR INOPERATIVE	Activated when total gas supply is lost or in the event of an electrical power failure or system malfunction. Available in all modes
Preset values	
MINIMUM EXPIRATORY TIME	Set at 0.204 sec. Available in all modes
MAXIMUM INSPIRATORY TIME	Limited to 3.20 sec. Available in TIME CYCLE mode
MAXIMUM WORKING PRESSURE	Limited to 90 cm H_2O in the TIME CYCLE mode and 150 cm H_2O in all other modes

* From Dupuis YG: *Ventilators: Theory and Clinical Application*, ed 2. St Louis, Mosby–Year Book, 1992, pp 325, 326. Used by permission.

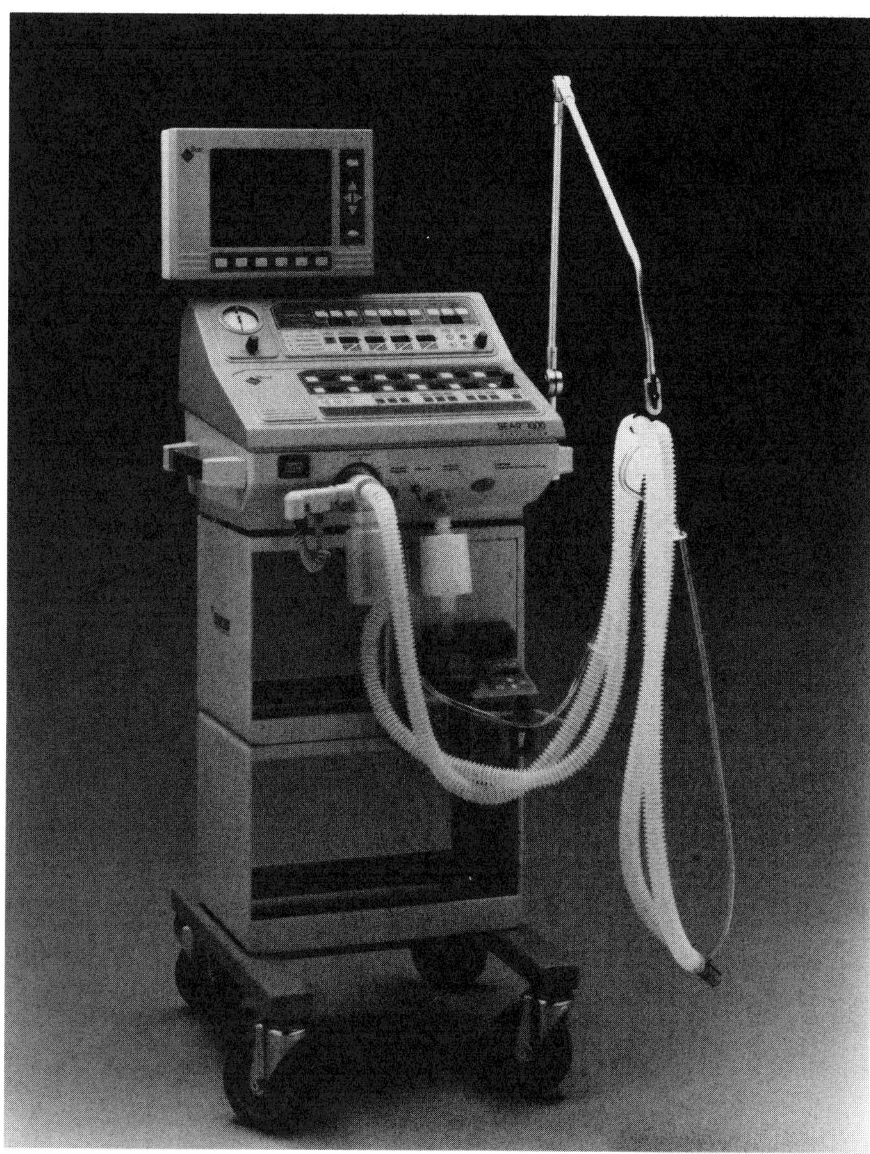

FIG 5–25
Comprehensive BEAR 1000 ventilator. (Courtesy of BEAR Medical Systems, Inc., Riverside, Calif.)

plus PSV, pressure support, pressure control, pressure-regulated volume control, PSV plus CPAP; inspiratory flow rise time percentage; sigh mode; and alarms for high pressure, apnea, high and low minute volume, low source gas, high and low O_2 concentration, technical alarm, and loss of power. Additional options are inspiratory and expiratory pause buttons and a gas change button.

Hamilton Veolar

The Veolar (Fig 5–33, A and B), like the Puritan Bennett 7200 series, the Siemens Servo 900 series, the BEAR 5, BEAR 1000, and other newer ventilators, uses electromechanical valves (solenoids) and microprocessor control to provide various ventilatory modes, flow patterns, and monitoring and alarm operations. Like the BEAR 6 and 1000, it offers mandatory minute ventilation (MMV), but in combination with pressure support only. The Veolar also utilizes a modern CRT monitoring system called Leonardo (optional package) along with a proximal airway pressure transducer. Specifications for the Veolar are shown in Table 5–14.

- Power source: pneumatic
- Control circuit: microprocessor
- Cycling control variable: flow, time, or pressure
- Inspiratory waveform: seven patterns, user selectable
- Pressure limit: 10 to 110 cm H_2O
- Tidal volume: 20 to 2,000 mL
- Flow range: 0 to 180 L/min
- Frequency: 0.6 to 60 breaths per minute

TABLE 5–11

BEAR 1000 Panel Details and Specifications*

Key	Range	Increment
Controls		
Upper controls		
TIDAL VOLUME	0.10–2.00 L	0.01
RATE	0.0, 0.5, 1–80, or 120 BPM†	1
PEAK FLOW	10–120 or 10–150 L/min†	1
O_2%	21–100	1
PRES SUP/INSP PRESS	0–65 cm or 0–80 cm H_2O†	1
ASSIST SENSITIVITY	0.2–5.0 cm H_2O	0.1
INSPIRATORY PAUSE†	0.0–2.0 sec	0.1
MMV LEVEL†	0–50 L/min	1
COMPLIANCE COMP	0.0–7.5 mL/cm H_2O	0.1
INSPIRATORY TIME†	0.1–5.0 sec	0.1
PRESSURE SLOPE	−9 to 0–9 and (pediatric) P-9 to P0–P9	P1
CONTROL LOCK	On, off	NA
SET KNOB	369 degrees	NA
Lower controls		
Mode keys		
ASSIST CMV	On, off, setup	NA
SIMV/CPAP (PSV)	On, off, setup	NA
PRESSURE CONTROL†	On, off, setup	NA
Waveforms		
SQUARE	On, off	NA
DECELERATING†	On, off	NA
SINE†	On, off	NA
Manual keys		
MANUAL BREATH	‡	NA
MANUAL INSP PAUSE	‡	NA
EXPIRATORY HOLD†	‡	NA
Other Control keys		
100% O_2	On, off	NA
SIGHS	On, off	NA
PRESSURE AUGMENT†	On, off	NA
NEBULIZER	On, off	NA
PEEP knob	0–50 cm H_2O	
Monitors		
Breath-type indicators§		
CONTROLLED BREATH	On, off	NA
SIGH BREATH†	On, off	NA
PATIENT EFFORT	On, off	NA
MMV ACTIVE†	On, off	NA
Exhaled volumes		
TIDAL VOLUME	0.00–9.99 L	0.01
TOTAL MV	0.0–9.99 L	0.1
SPONT MV†	0.0–9.99 L	0.1
Rates/ratio		
TOTAL	0–155 BPM	1
SPONT†	0–155 BPM	1
I-E RATIO†	1:0.2 to 1:99.0	0.1
MMV%†	0–100	1
Pressures		
PEAK†	0–140 cm H_2O	1
MEAN†	0–140 cm H_2O	1
PLATEAU†	0–140 cm H_2O	1

(Continued.)

TABLE 5–11 (cont.)

Key	Range	Increment
Alarms		
Built-in alarms§		
TIME/I:E LIMIT	On, off	NA
RUN DIAGNOSTICS	On, off	NA
GAS SUPPLY FAILURE	On, off	NA
FAILED TO CYCLE	On, off	NA
Adjustable alarms		
I:E OVERRIDE†	On, off	NA
TOTAL MINUTE VOLUME		
Low	0–50 L	0.1
High	0–80 L	0.1
TOTAL BREATH RATE		
LOW	3–99 BPM	1
High	0–155	1
PEAK INSP PRESSURE		
Low	3–99 cm H_2O	1
High	0–120 cm H_2O	1
BASELINE PRESSURE		
Low†	0–50 cm H_2O	1
High†	0–55 cm H_2O	1
Other alarm group keys		
ALARM SILENCE	On, off	NA
DIMMER	Low, high	NA
VISUAL RESET	‡	NA
ALARM LOCK	On, off	NA
TEST	‡	NA
SET KNOB	360 degrees	NA

* Courtesy of BEAR Medical Systems, Riverside, Calif.
† Depending on the ventilator model (BEAR 1000 vs. Comprehensive BEAR 1000).
‡ Active only while the key is pressed.
§ Machine established. Not set by the clinician.

- CPAP or PEEP: 0 to 50 cm H_2O
- Pressure support: 0 to 50 cm H_2O above PEEP up to an actual pressure of 50 cm H_2O
- Minimum minute volume: 1 to 25 L/min
- F_{IO_2}: 0.21 to 1.00

Other features include SIMV, CPAP, pressure support, pressure control, and MMV modes and alarms for high pressure, high rate, high and low minute volume, high and low O_2 percentage, low O_2 and air pressure, apnea, failure to cycle, and power failure.

Puritan Bennett 7200 Series

The 7200ae (Fig 5–34) fully loaded with options, like the Siemens Servo 300, carries a hefty price tag (approximately $28,000). Also like the Servo 300, the 7200ae represents state-of-the-art technology, with microprocessor control and such mechanisms as proportional solenoids providing gas flow. This ventilator offers many options, including a graphics package similar to that offered by Hamilton's Leonardo. With the addition of Flow-by 2.0, all breaths, both spontaneous and mandatory, can now be flow-triggered, thus offering the patient a lower work of breathing and the clinician a responsive and functional machine. An advantage in financial terms, as for some other ventilators, is the option to buy the basic machine with fewer options (i.e., the 7200e or the BEAR 1000 vs. the 7200ae and the Comprehensive BEAR 1000, respectively). Technical data and specifications are given in Table 5–15. The 7200 keyboard and international keyboard panels are illustrated in Figures 5–35 and 5–36, A and B.

- Power source: pneumatic
- Control circuit: microprocessor
- Cycling control variable: volume, time, pressure, or flow
- Inspiratory waveform: rectangular and descending and ascending ramp
- Pressure limit: 10 to 120 cm H_2O
- Tidal volume: 0.1 to 2.5 L
- Flow range: 10 to 180 L/min
- Frequency: 0.5 to 70 breaths per minute
- Inspiratory time: adjustable
- PEEP: 0 to 50 cm H_2O
- F_{IO_2}: 0.21 to 1.00

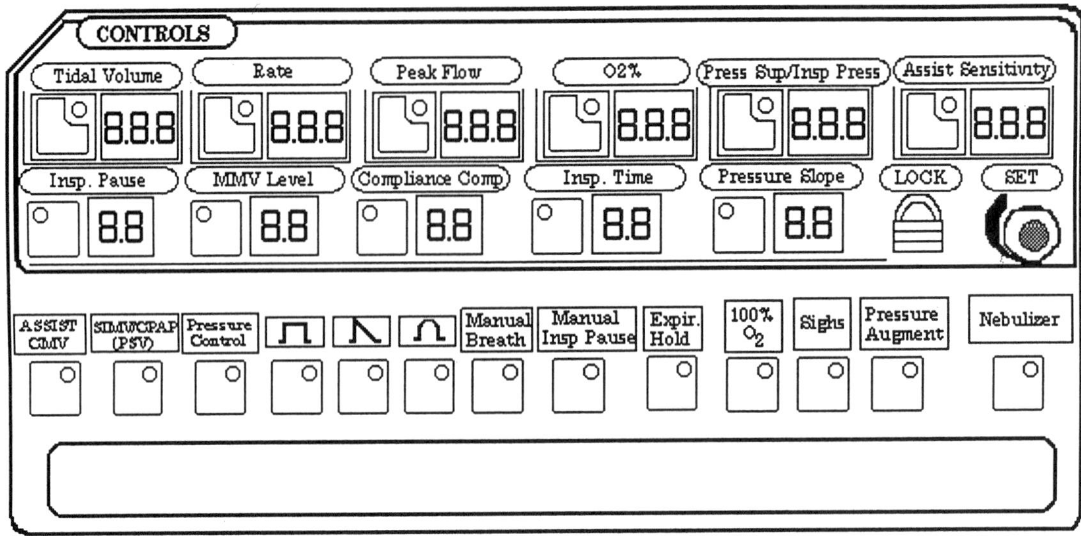

FIG 5–26
The BEAR 1000 control panel.

Other features include SIMV, CPAP, PSV (0 to 70 cm H_2O), pressure control (with SIMV, 0 to 100 cm H_2O), and sigh modes; 100% O_2 delivery for 2 minutes to suction; and alarms for high and low pressure, apnea, I:E ratio, power loss, exhalation valve leak, low volume, ventilator inoperative, O_2 failure, low rate, low CPAP or PEEP, and low battery. It also has a self-test mode, sensitivity of −0.6 to −20 cm H_2O, and inflation hold. Optional features are Flow-by (the new 2.0 version allows flow sensing of all breaths, mechanical and spontaneous), static and dynamic mechanics, spontaneous inspiratory flow rate, graphics, pulse oximeter, and plasma screen display.

Mechanical Ventilation Modes

Because of the expanded capabilities of modern mechanical ventilators due to microprocessor control, functional options are continuing to grow at an exponential rate. One of the growth areas has been in the number and types of modes offered.

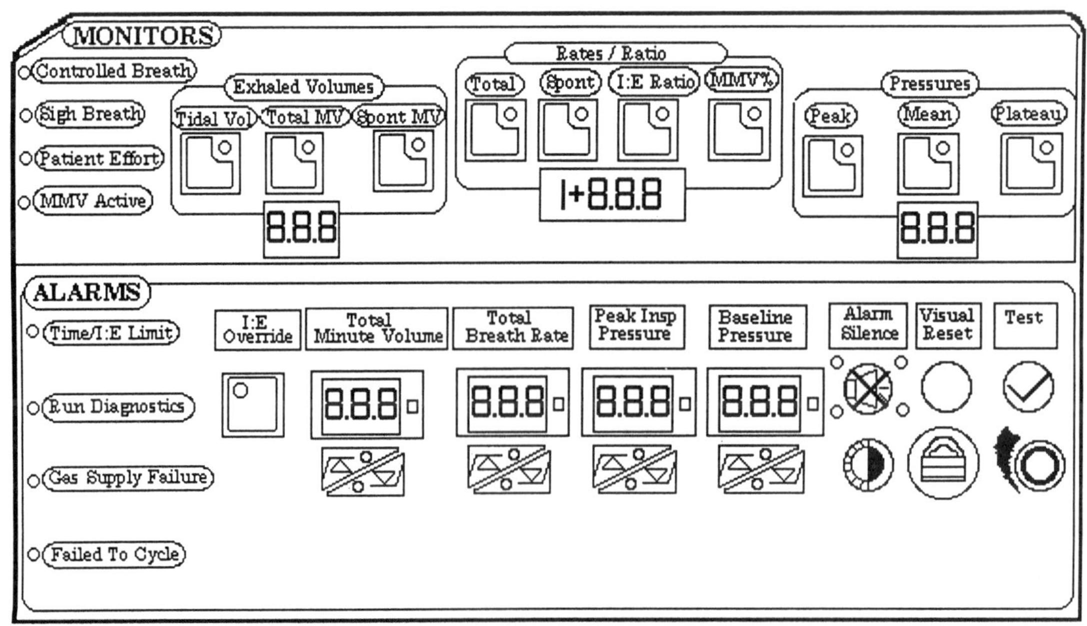

FIG 5–27
The BEAR 1000 monitors and alarms panel.

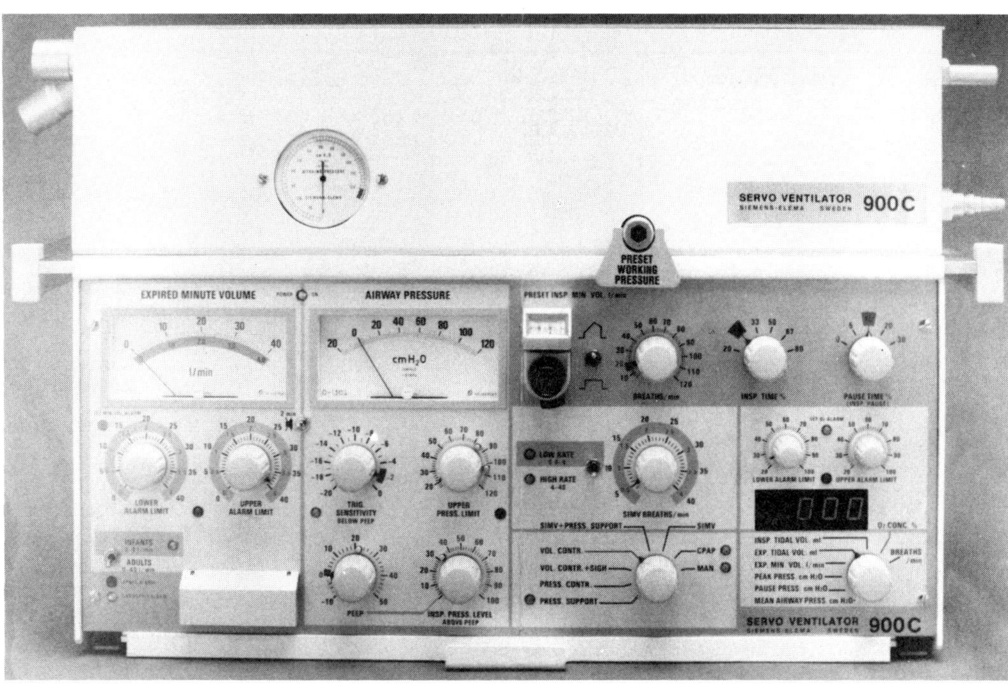

FIG 5–28
Servo 900C ventilator. (Courtesy of Siemens-Elema AB, Solna, Sweden.)

TABLE 5–12
Siemens Servo 900C Ventilator Specifications*

Minute volume	0.5–40 L/min
Rate	5–120 breaths per minute (SIMV, 0.5–40 breaths per minute)
Inspiratory time (%)	20, 24, 33, 50, 67, 80
Pause time (%)	0, 10, 20, 30
Sensitivity	−20 to 0 cm H_2O (PEEP compensated)
PEEP	0–50 cm H_2O
NEEP	0 to −10 cm H_2O (with extra equipment)
Pressure limit	16–120 cm H_2O
Working pressure	0–120 cm H_2O
Inspiratory pressure level	0–100 cm H_2O above PEEP (120 cm H_2O maximum)
Flow pattern	Square wave or sine wave in volume control modes; square wave in SIMV modes; decelerating taper in pressure control mode
Sigh	One sigh every 100 breaths at double the tidal volume and inspiratory time or *off*
Displays	
Pressure meter	−20 to 120 cm H_2O
Expired minute volume meter	0–4 (infants) or 0–40 L/min (adults)
Respiratory rate	In breaths/minute
Oxygen concentration	In percent
Inspired tidal volume	In liters
Expired tidal volume	In liters
Expired minute volume	in L/min
Peak pressure	In cm H_2O
Pause pressure	In cm H_2O
Mean airway pressure	In cm H_2O
Alarms	
Gas supply	Audible, visual
Power failure	Audible
Expired minute volume	High or low, audible, visual
Pressure limit	Audible, visual, 16–120 cm H_2O
Apnea	Audible, visual; occurs if no breath is detected for 15 sec
Oxygen (%)	Audible, visual; high: 30% to 100%; low: 18% to 90%

* From McPherson SP: *Respiratory Therapy Equipment*, ed 4. St Louis, Mosby–Year Book, 1990, p 333. Used by permission.

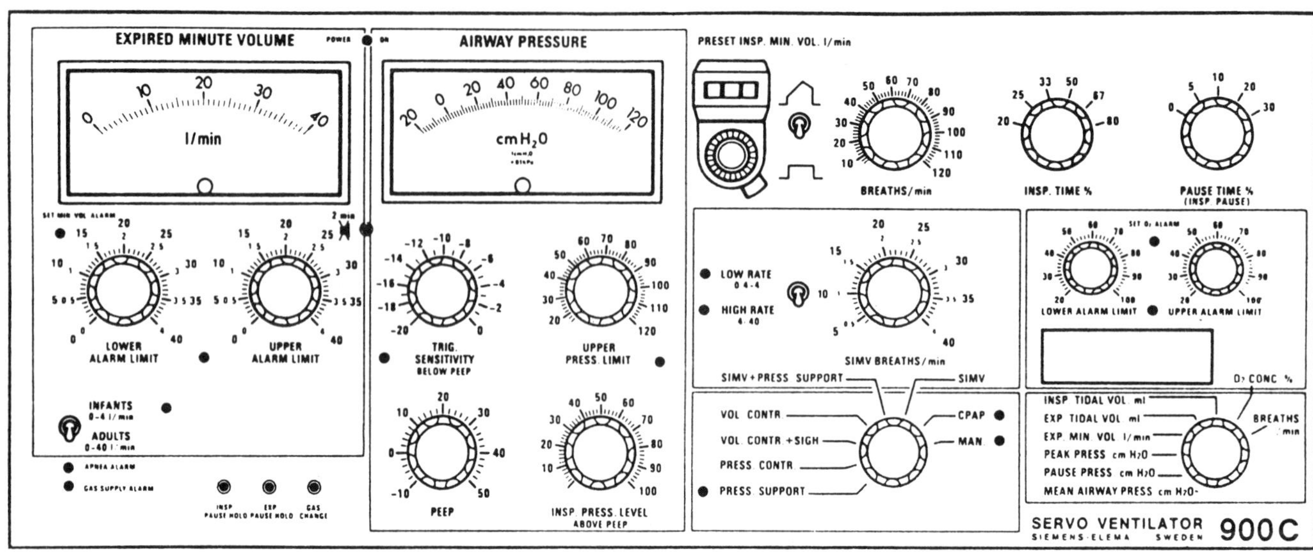

FIG 5–29
Control panel of the Servo 900C ventilator. (Courtesy of Siemens-Elema AB, Solna, Sweden.)

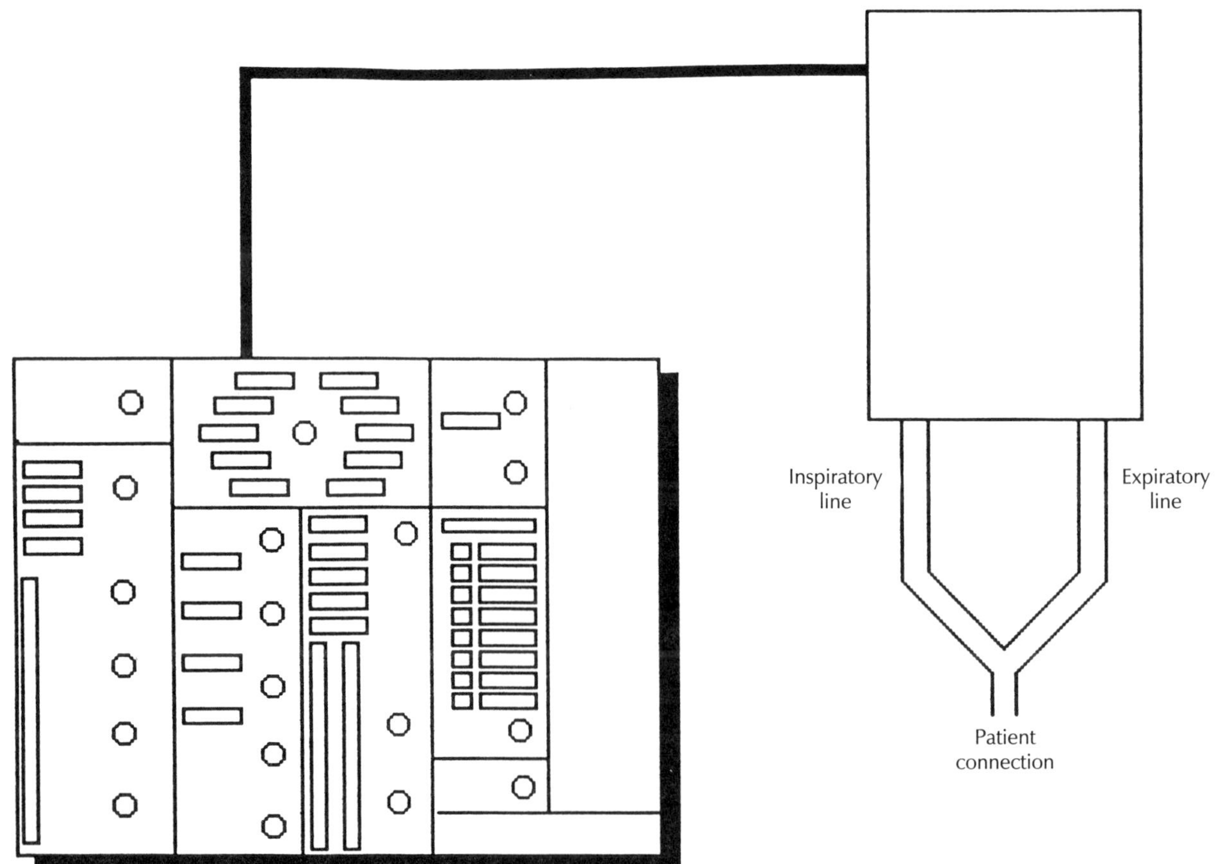

FIG 5–30
The Siemens Servo 300.

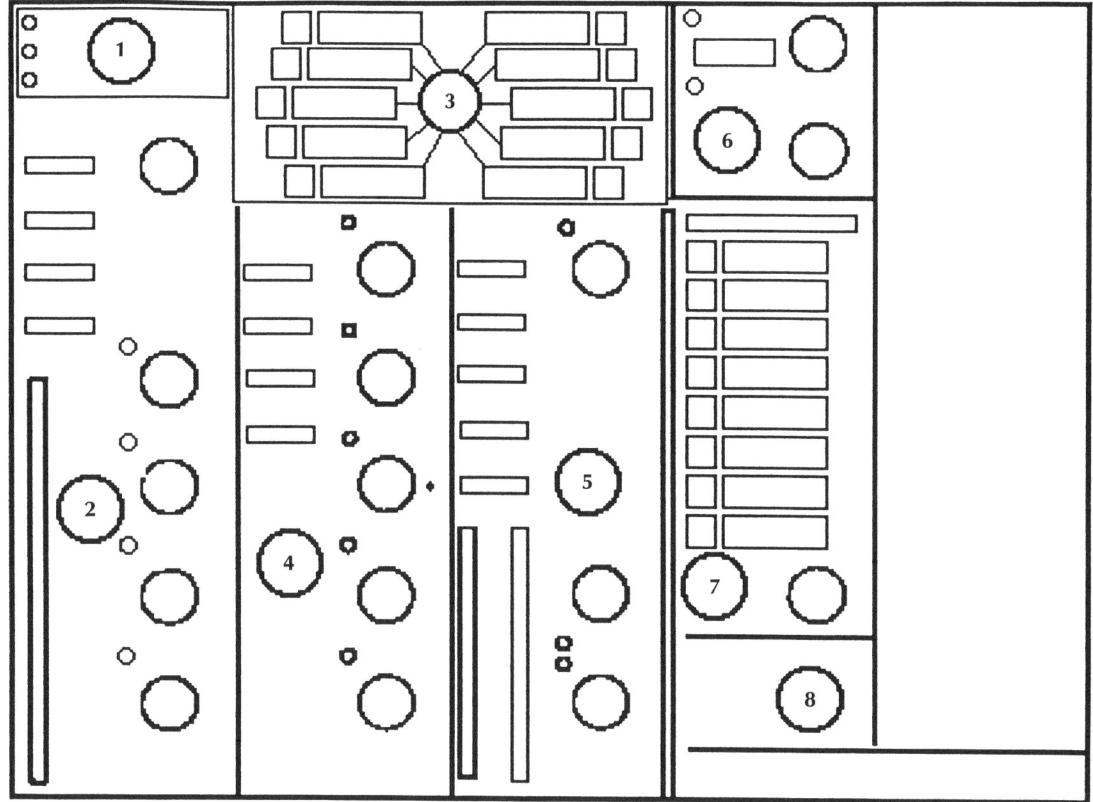

1 Patient range selection
2 Airway pressure
3 Mode selection
4 Respiration pattern
5 Volumes
6 Oxygen concentration and start breath
7 Alarms
8 Pause hold

FIG 5–31
Siemens Servo 300 front panel.

The term "mode" is used to represent the manner in which gas is delivered, regardless of whether the tidal volume is pressurized. Traditionally, all triggered breaths (mechanical or spontaneous) have been generated by the patient via a pressure differential sensing mechanism set by the clinician. Most recently, flow triggering for both spontaneous and mechanical breaths has been introduced (see the discussion on Flow-by later in this chapter). Pressure waves for each of the modes are illustrated in Figure 5–37.

Control

The machine is responsible for initiation and delivery of each tidal volume as preset by the clinician. The patient will not receive additional mandatory breaths despite efforts from the patient. Thus the patient is "locked out" and cannot increase minute ventilation. This is also referred to as "CMV" (continuous mandatory ventilation—Puritan-Bennett 7200 series, BEAR 5 and 1000) and "volume control" (Siemens Servo series: Siemens Servo 900C and Servo Ventilator 300).

Assist

The patient is totally responsible for initiation of the inspiratory phase, but the ventilator delivers the tidal volume. There is no backup mandatory rate set, so in the event of apnea, the patient will not receive ventilation unless there are factory default or clinician-preset backup settings to provide ventilation.

Assist/Control

The machine functions in the assist mode unless the patient's respiratory rate falls below a preset level, at which time the machine reverts to the control mode. It also reverts to the CMV mode, where the sensitivity is set to allow machine response with patient efforts if desired by the patient, thereby exceeding the preset base respiratory rate. This is also referred to as "CMV"

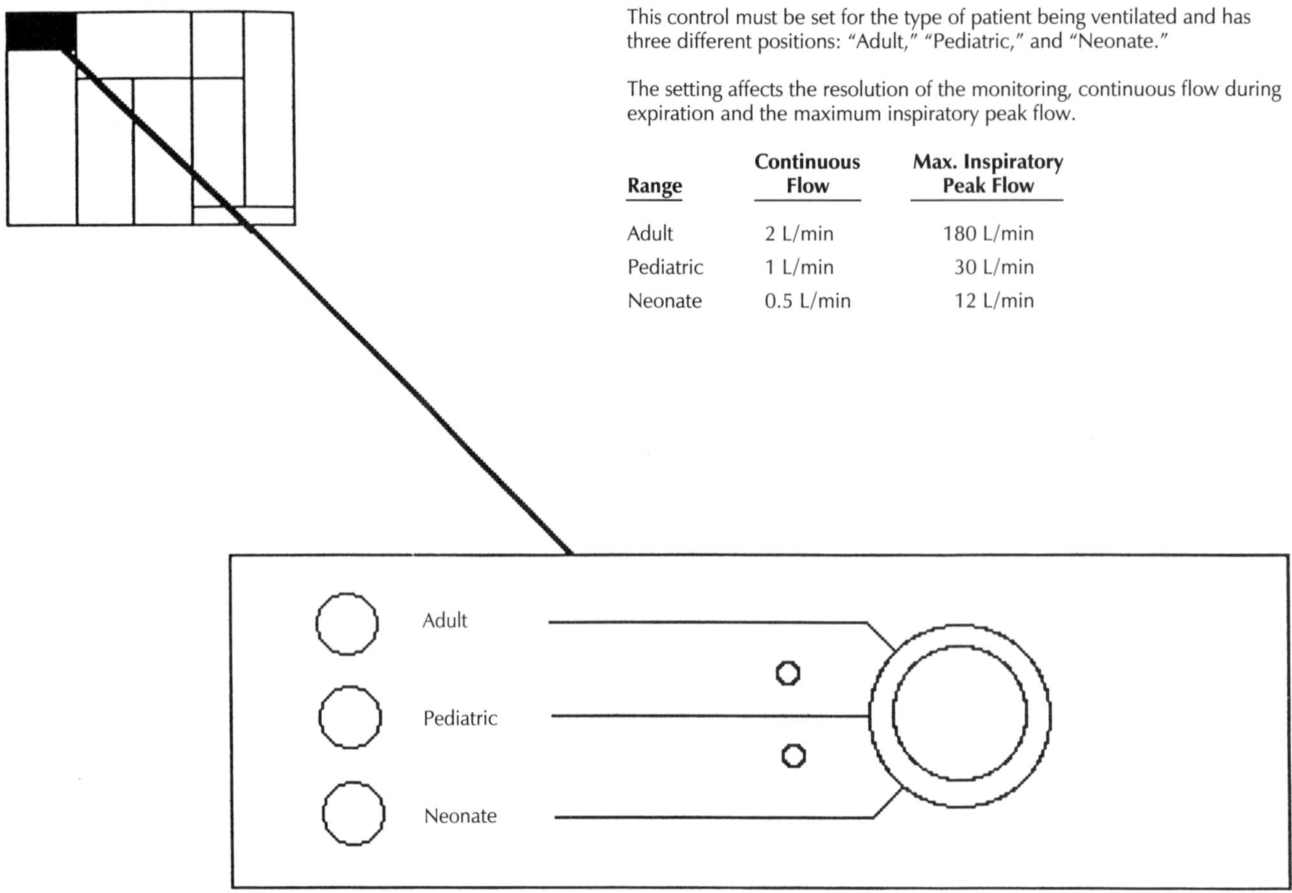

This control must be set for the type of patient being ventilated and has three different positions: "Adult," "Pediatric," and "Neonate."
The setting affects the resolution of the monitoring, continuous flow during expiration and the maximum inspiratory peak flow.
Range | Continuous Flow | Max. Inspiratory Peak Flow
Adult | 2 L/min | 180 L/min
Pediatric | 1 L/min | 30 L/min
Neonate | 0.5 L/min | 12 L/min
Adult
Pediatric
Neonate

FIG 5–32
Siemens Servo 300 ventilator. **A,** patient range selection panel.

(continuous mandatory ventilation—Puritan-Bennett 7200 series) and "volume control" (Siemens Servo series: Siemens Servo 900C and Servo Ventilator 300).

Intermittent Mandatory Ventilation

The patient is allowed to breathe spontaneously from an internal or external high-flow system or from the ventilator via a demand valve that provides fresh gas flow, and at preset intervals (at the preset mechanical respiratory rate) the machine functions in the control mode to deliver a preset tidal volume.

Synchronized Intermittent Mandatory Ventilation

The patient is allowed to breathe spontaneously from the ventilator, which provides fresh gas flow via a demand valve or constant flow rate, and at preset intervals, the machine functions in the assist/control mode to deliver a preset tidal volume.

Mandatory Minute Ventilation

A minimum minute volume delivery is set on the machine. The patient may receive this volume by the following:

1. Breathing totally spontaneously, thus achieving the set minute volume on his own.

2. While being mechanically ventilated exclusively by the ventilator because of respiratory depression or some other cause resulting in apnea.

3. A combination of 1 and 2. If the patient's spontaneous minute volume falls below the minimum level, mandatory positive-pressure breaths at predetermined tidal volumes make up the difference. It may be used in conjunction with or exclusively with inspiratory pressure support (IPS) such as with the Hamilton Veolar. This is also called AMV (augmented minute ventilation), as on the Intermed BEAR 5, or EMMV (extended mandatory minute volume), as on the Engstrom Erica.

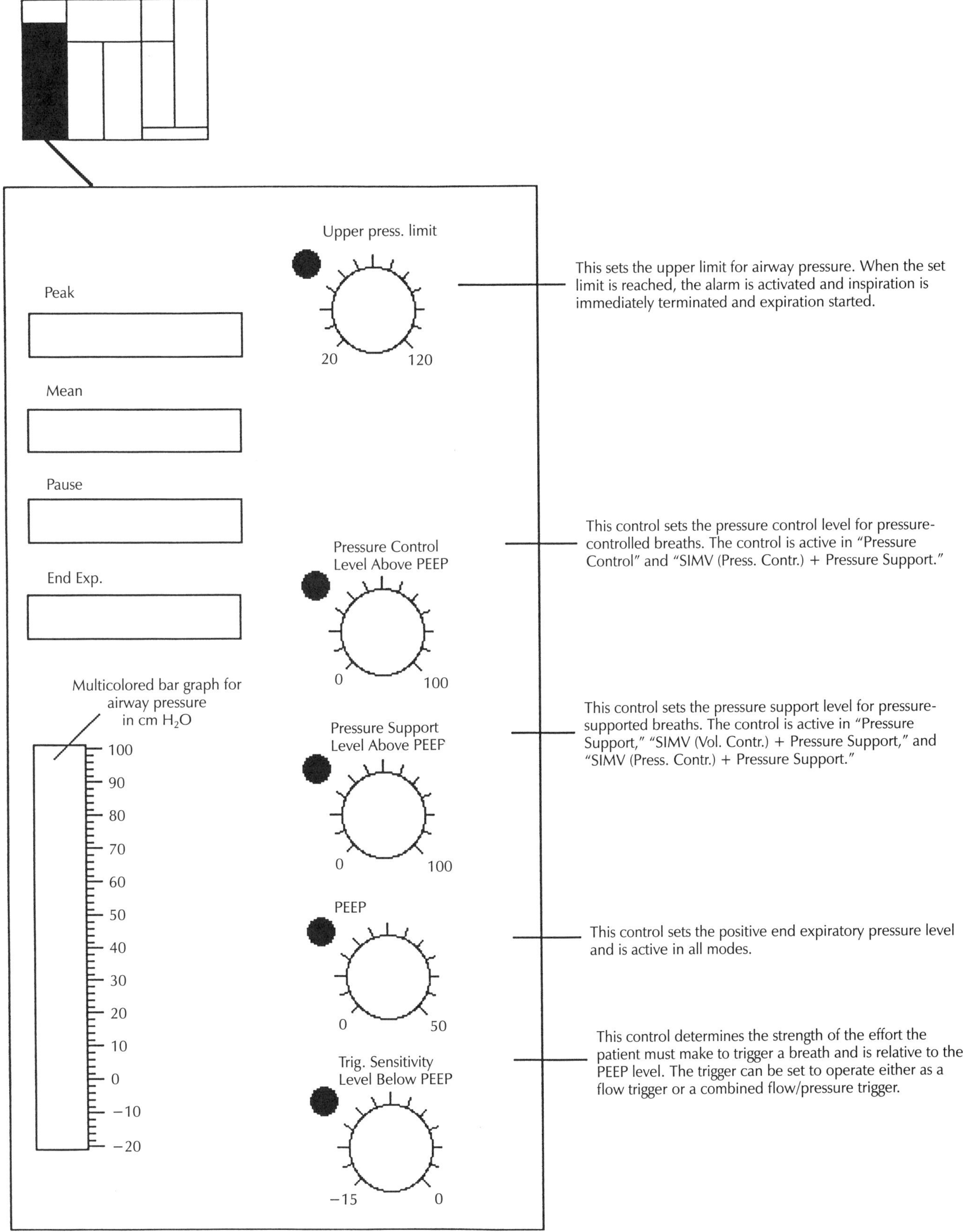
Upper press. limit
20
120
This sets the upper limit for airway pressure. When the set limit is reached, the alarm is activated and inspiration is immediately terminated and expiration started.
Peak
Mean
Pause
End Exp.
Pressure Control Level Above PEEP
0
100
This control sets the pressure control level for pressure-controlled breaths. The control is active in "Pressure Control" and "SIMV (Press. Contr.) + Pressure Support."
Multicolored bar graph for airway pressure in cm H_2O
100
90
80
70
60
50
40
30
20
10
0
−10
−20
Pressure Support Level Above PEEP
0
100
This control sets the pressure support level for pressure-supported breaths. The control is active in "Pressure Support," "SIMV (Vol. Contr.) + Pressure Support," and "SIMV (Press. Contr.) + Pressure Support."
PEEP
0
50
This control sets the positive end expiratory pressure level and is active in all modes.
Trig. Sensitivity Level Below PEEP
−15
0
This control determines the strength of the effort the patient must make to trigger a breath and is relative to the PEEP level. The trigger can be set to operate either as a flow trigger or a combined flow/pressure trigger.

FIG 5–32 (cont.)
Siemens Servo 300 ventilator. **B,** airway pressure panel.

(Continued.)

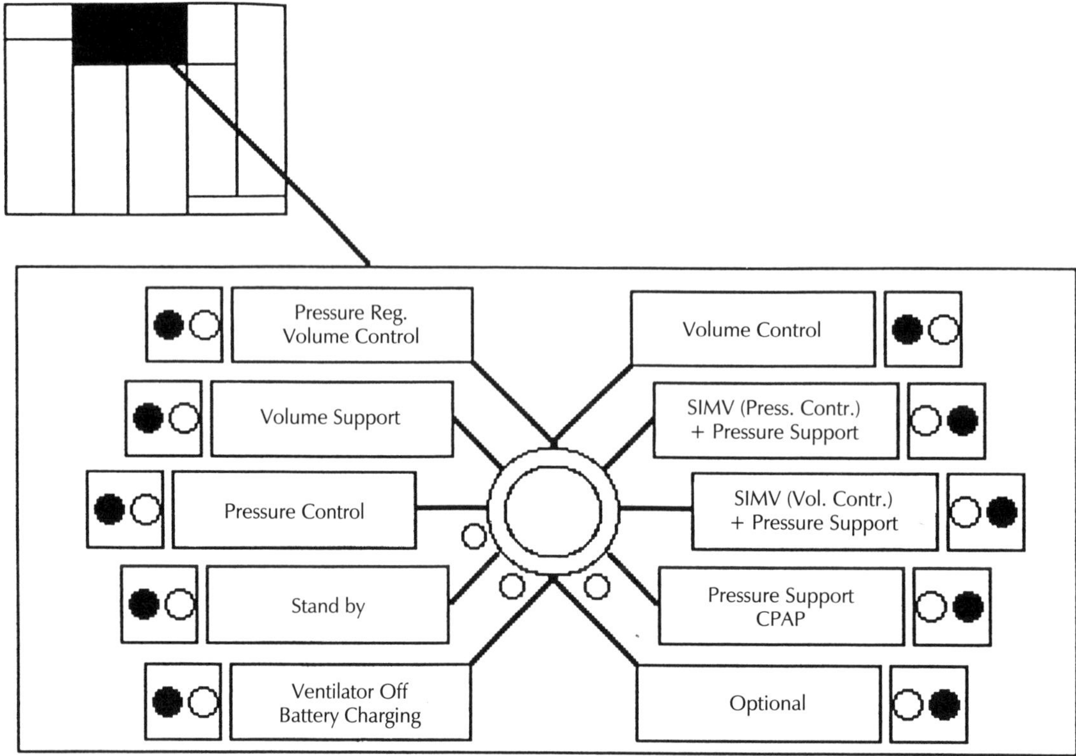

The mode selector can be set in 10 different positions, providing 8 different modes of ventilation.

Ventilatory Mode include:

Pressure Control: Pressure-controlled ventilation
Volume Control: Volume-controlled ventilation
Pressure Reg. Volume Control: Pressure regulated volume-controlled ventilation
Volume Support: Volume-supported ventilation
SIMV (Vol. Contr.) + Pressure Support: SIMV based on volume-controlled ventilation with pressure support
SIMV (Press. Contr.) + Pressure Support: SIMV based on pressure-controlled ventilation with pressure support
Pressure Support: Pressure-supported ventilation
CPAP: Continuous Positive Airway Pressure

FIG 5–32 (cont.)
Siemens Servo 300 ventilator. **C,** mode selection panel.

Constant (or Continuous) Positive Airwave Pressure

The patient breathes spontaneously via a high-flow system or demand valve that provides fresh gas flow. No mandatory or preset breaths are delivered with this mode. The set CPAP (baseline or resting level) pressure can be maintained at any level in the positive range down to and including zero. Ideally, the pressure in the patient's airway remains consistent at the set CPAP level and varies slightly, with each breath deflecting 1 or 2 cm H_2O below baseline (less positive) during inspiration and 1 or 2 cm H_2O above baseline during exhalation. Pressures achieved during inspiration and exhalation are sometimes referred to as inspiratory positive airway pressure (IPAP) and expiratory positive airway pressure (EPAP), respectively.

Inspiratory Pressure Support or Pressure Support Ventilation

During spontaneous ventilation only, the ventilator functions as a pressure generator (decelerating flow pattern). Pressure develops rapidly in the ventilator system and remains at that level until a certain flow rate is reached (a flow-cycled breath). On selected ventilators, the breath ends when the spontaneous inspiratory flow rate decreases to 25% of the peak inspiratory flow (or some other specific flow rate). This mode may be used independently or in conjunction with CPAP, SIMV, or

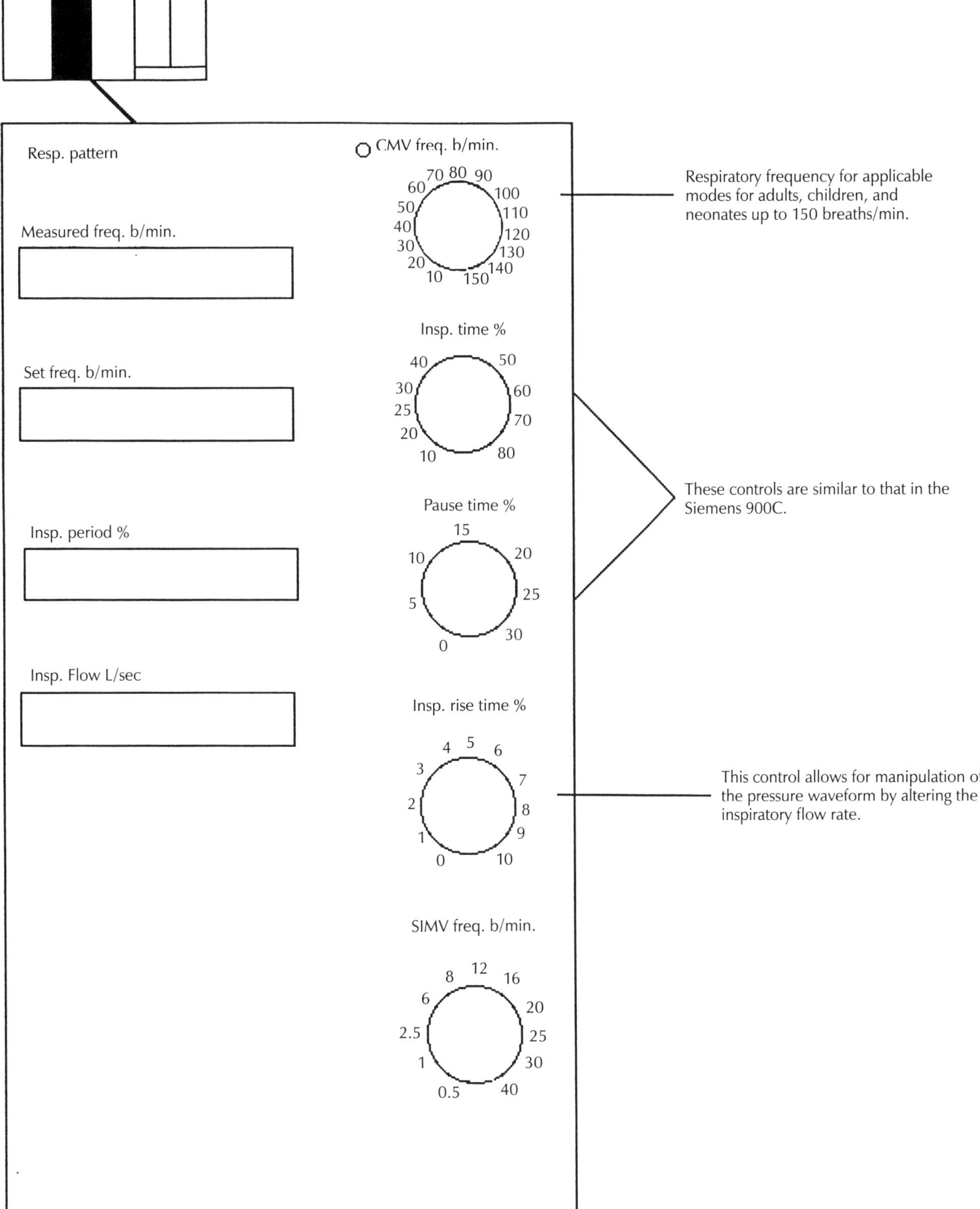

FIG 5–32 (cont.)
Siemens Servo 300 ventilator. **D,** respiration panel.

(Continued.)

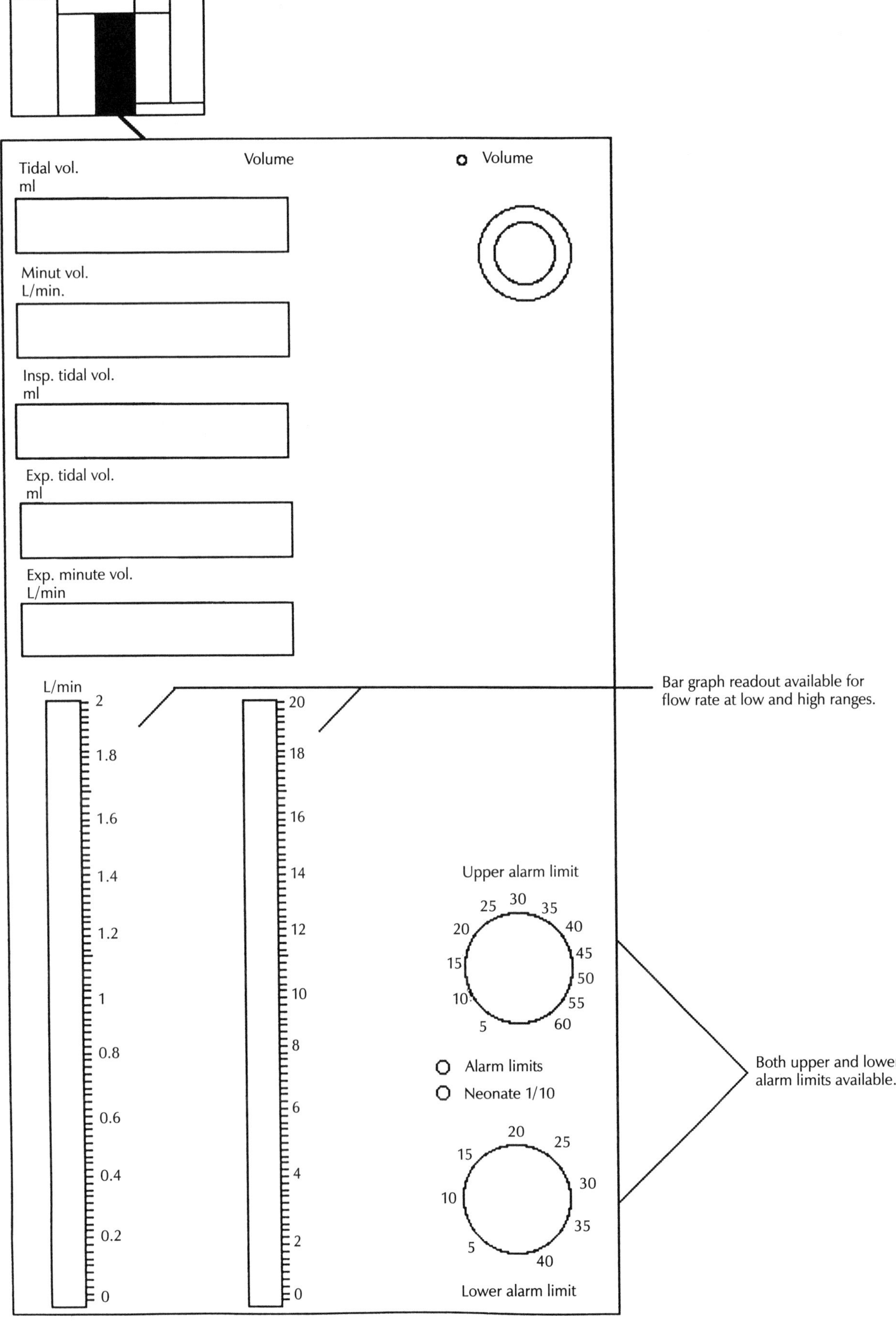

FIG 5–32 (cont.)
Siemens Servo 300 ventilator. **E,** volume panel.

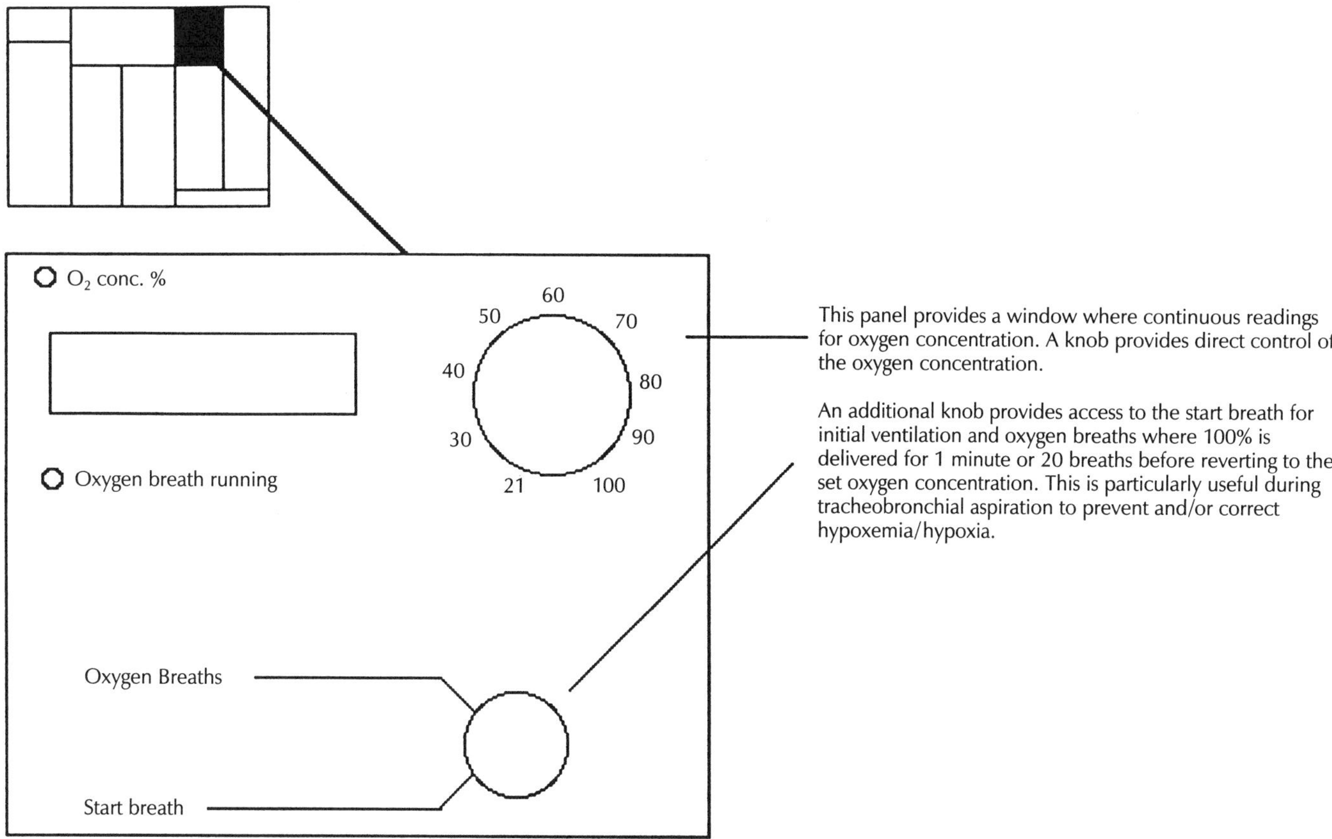
O₂ conc. %
50
60
70
40
80
30
90
21
100
Oxygen breath running
This panel provides a window where continuous readings for oxygen concentration. A knob provides direct control of the oxygen concentration.
An additional knob provides access to the start breath for initial ventilation and oxygen breaths where 100% is delivered for 1 minute or 20 breaths before reverting to the set oxygen concentration. This is particularly useful during tracheobronchial aspiration to prevent and/or correct hypoxemia/hypoxia.
Oxygen Breaths
Start breath

FIG 5–32 (cont.)
Siemens Servo 300 ventilator. **F,** oxygen concentration and start breath panel. *(Continued.)*

MMV. Tidal volume varies with lung-thorax compliance, airway resistance, pressure support level (peak pressure set), and the degree of patient effort.

Airway Pressure Release Ventilation

Alternating levels of CPAP are used in a spontaneously breathing patient. There are two levels of CPAP, and the patient is allowed to breathe spontaneously at each level. The clinician selects both the dual CPAP levels and the period of time that the patient spends at each level. Periodically, the pressure is "released" or dropped to a preset level (zero or ambient pressure is possible).

- A baseline CPAP level is set, normally at 2 to 10 cm H_2O.
- A secondary CPAP level is set to ensure a pressure-assisted tidal volume, normally at 10 to 30 cm H_2O(really a pressure support breath).
- The rate is dependent on the ventilation required.
- The expiratory time is kept short to prevent collapsing of alveoli.
- Frequently a reversal of the I:E ratio is used.
- At each level of CPAP the patient may breathe spontaneously.

This mode is presently only available on the PPG Irisa ventilator. By definition, airway pressure release ventilation (APRV) is similar to bilevel positive airway pressure (BiPAP). However, although "BiPAP" devices exist that allow for two levels of CPAP, both the inspiratory and expiratory pressures in these devices are preset for each respiratory cycle and do not change from breath to breath. In APRV, the patient may breathe for many cycles at one CPAP level, and then at a preset interval, the pressure is released to a lower CPAP level, where several more breaths are taken. There is "bilevel" breathing, but APRV is much more sophisticated. Respironics, Inc., has introduced a "mask ventilator" system ($BiPAP_{TM}$) that provides two levels of CPAP, one during inspiration (IPAP) and one during exhalation (EPAP), thereby fitting the basic definition of bilevel positive airway pressure. All breaths are flow-triggered (similar to Puritan Bennett's Flow-by 2.0 flow sensitivity) and require the patient's effort to be 40 mL/sec to initiate inspiration. Although not classified as a continuous mechanical ventilator, the more sophisticated unit ($BiPAP_{TM}$ S/T-D Ventilatory Support System) is marketed as providing four operating modes:

1. *CPAP.*—Inspiratory (IPAP) and expiratory (EPAP) pressures are the same during spontaneous breathing.

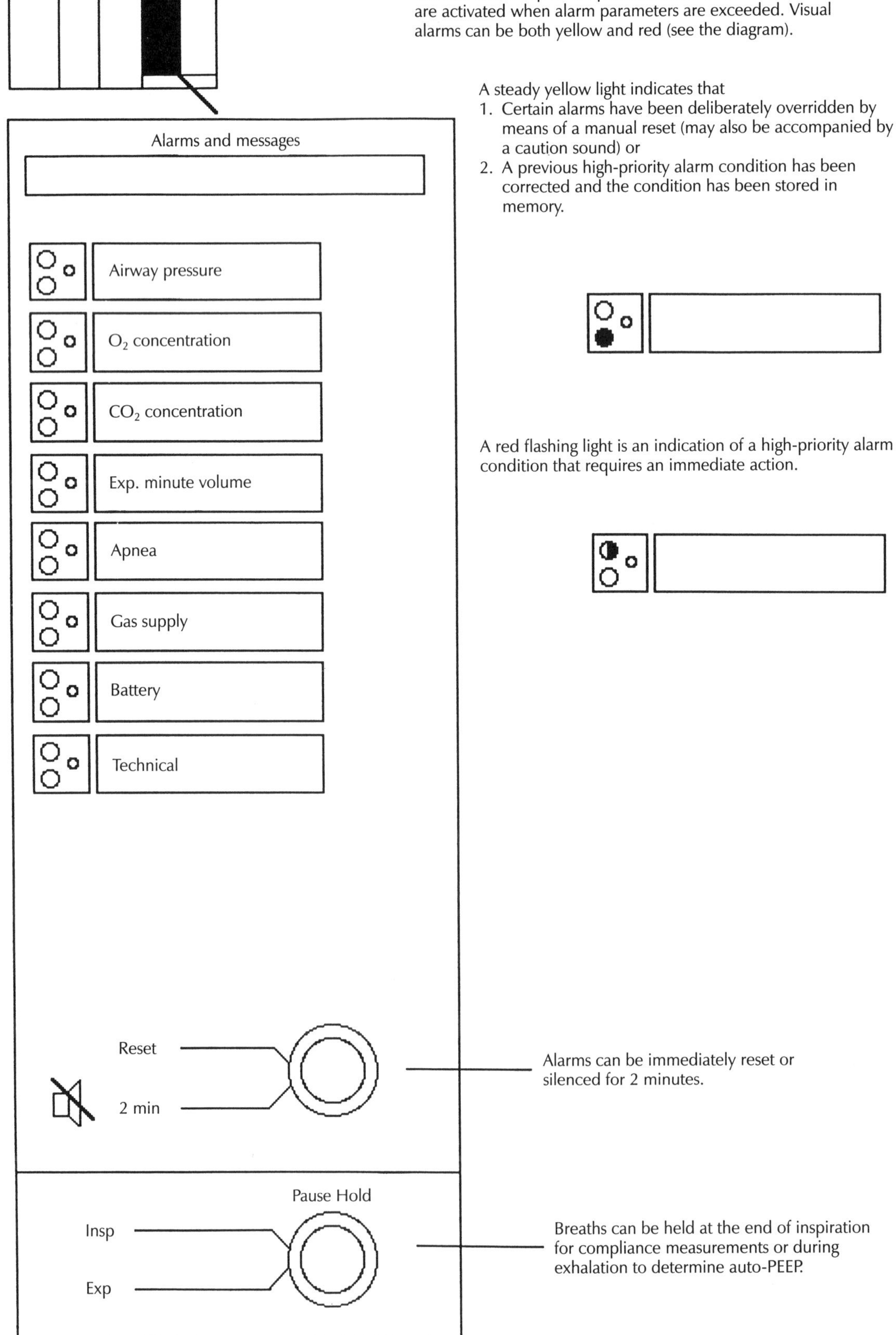

Alarm events are displayed in the "Alarms and messages" window at the top of the panel. Audible and visual alarms are activated when alarm parameters are exceeded. Visual alarms can be both yellow and red (see the diagram).
A steady yellow light indicates that
1. Certain alarms have been deliberately overridden by means of a manual reset (may also be accompanied by a caution sound) or
2. A previous high-priority alarm condition has been corrected and the condition has been stored in memory.
Alarms and messages
Airway pressure
O_2 concentration
CO_2 concentration
Exp. minute volume
Apnea
Gas supply
Battery
Technical
A red flashing light is an indication of a high-priority alarm condition that requires an immediate action.
Reset
2 min
Alarms can be immediately reset or silenced for 2 minutes.
Pause Hold
Insp
Exp
Breaths can be held at the end of inspiration for compliance measurements or during exhalation to determine auto-PEEP.

FIG 5–32 (cont.)
Siemens Servo 300 ventilator. **G,** alarms and messages window.

TABLE 5–13

Siemens Servo 300 General Technical Specifications*

Dimensions	Patient unit
	With rail: W242 × D370 × H240 mm
	Without rail: W230 × D320 × H240 mm
	Front panel: W427 × D110 × H321 mm
Weight	23.2 kg
Computer interface	RS-232C
Capabilities	Neonate/pediatric/adult
Pneumatic power	2–6.5 bar (29–100 psi) air and O_2
Mains power	100, 120, 220, and 240 V ac ± 10%, 50–60 Hz
Battery backup	Built-in rechargeable, 12 V, 1.9 A · h, × 2
Controls	
O_2 concentration	21%–100% ± 4%
Rate controlled ventilation	5–150 breaths/min
Rate SIMV	0.5–40 breaths/min
Inspiration time	10%–80% of breath cycle
Pause time	0%–30% of breath cycle
Inspiration pressure	0–100 cm H_2O
PEEP	0–50 cm H_2O
Upper pressure limit	15–120 cm H_2O
Trigger sensitivity	−17 to 0 cm H_2O with flow trigger
Method of triggering	Pressure and flow
Inspiratory rise time	0%–10% of breath cycle time
Preset minute volume	0.2–60.0 L/min for adult; pediatric: ± 5% ± 0.1 L/min; neonate: ± 5% ± 0.03 L/min
Tidal volume	2 ml to 4 L for adult; pediatric: ± 5% ± 1 mL; neonate: ± 5% ± 0.5 mL
Oxygen breaths	When activated: 20 or maximum of 1 min
Start breath	1 breath initiated in all modes
Alarm silence	2 min or reset
Pause hold	Inspiration and expiration
Apnea alarm	Adult, 20; pediatric, 15; and neonate, 10 sec
Continuous expiratory flow	0.5, 1.0, 2.0 L/min (neonate, pediatric, adult)
Modes	
Pressure control	
Volume control	
Pressure-regulated volume control	
Volume support	
SIMV (volume controlled) ± pressure support	
SIMV (pressure controlled) ± pressure support	
Pressure support	
CPAP	
Optional	
Stand by	
Ventilator off, battery charging	
Alarms	
Exhaled minute volume (high and low)	
Oxygen (high and low)	
Airway pressure	
Apnea	
Battery low	
Gas supply failure	
Power failure	
Technical alarms	
Monitors	
O_2 concentration	± 5% of read value
Pressure	Peak, pause, mean, end expiratory ± 5% or ± 2 cm H_2O
Volume	Tidal
	Adult: 5.0–3,999 mL
	Pediatric: 1.0–399 mL
	Neonate: 2.0–39 mL ± 5% ± 0.5 mL
	Minute
	Adult: 4.0–60.0 L/min ± 5% ± 0.1 L/min
	Pediatric: 1.0–5.0 L/min ± 5% ± 0.1 L/min
	Neonate: 0.2–1.5 L/min ± 10% ± 0.03 L/min
Frequency	± 10%, ± 0.5 bpm

* Courtesy of Siemens-Elema Life Support Systems, Solna, Sweden.

A

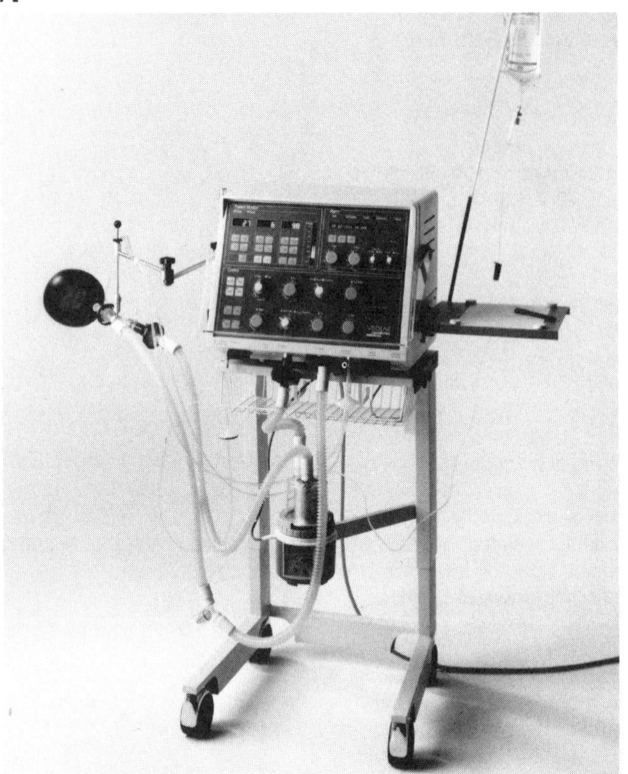

B

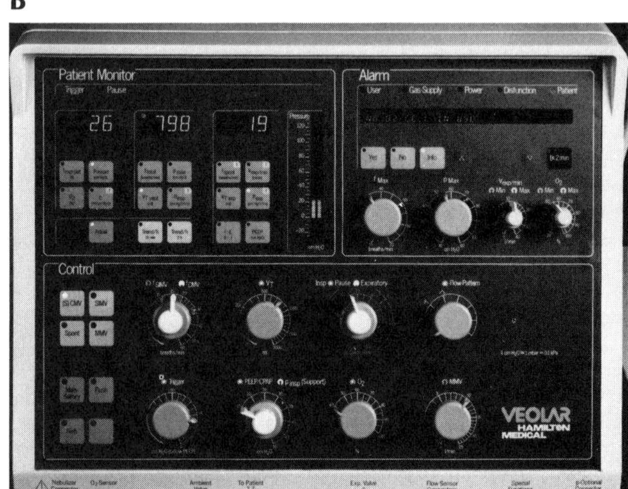

FIG 5–33
Hamilton Veolar volume ventilator **(A)** and control panel **(B)**. (Courtesy of Hamilton Medical, Reno, Nev.)

2. *S, or spontaneous.*—Two different pressure levels (IPAP and EPAP) are delivered during spontaneous breathing.

3. *S/T, or spontaneous/timed.*—A minimum respiratory rate is preset. If apnea occurs beyond the total cycle time or insufficient inspiratory effort is present, a breath is initiated, and the patient receives the preset IPAP and EPAP levels.

4. *T, or timed.*—The unit switches between the preset IPAP and EPAP levels at a fixed rate and I:E ratio.

Pressure Control Ventilation or Pressure Control and Pressure Control Inverse Ratio Ventilation (PCIRV)

The ventilator functions as a pressure generator (decelerating flow rate) with a preset, constant pressure delivered to the airway during a set time (a time-cycled breath). Both the mandatory respiratory rate and either the inspiratory time or the I:E ratio are set. The delivered tidal volume varies with lung-thorax compliance, airway resistance, the set pressure control limit (pressure control setting), inspiratory time, and probably auto-PEEP levels. The I:E ratio may be inversed for patients with severe adult respiratory distress syndrome (ARDS) with extremely low lung-thorax compliance.

Pressure-Regulated Volume Control

The respiratory rate, inspiratory time, and tidal/minute volume are preset. After the initial setup where the lung-thorax compliance is calculated after a test breath at 6 cm H_2O, the following three breaths are delivered at a pressure of 76% of the calculated pressure needed to deliver the preset tidal volume. For each of the following breaths, the inspiratory pressure is regulated to a value based on the volume/pressure calculation for the previous breath compared with the preset target tidal/minute volume. The pressure change is no more than 3 cm H_2O from breath to breath. If the measured tidal volume is too high, the pressure will decrease until the preset and measured volumes are equal. This mode is presently only available on the Siemens Servo Ventilator 300.

Volume Support

Volume support is a spontaneous breathing mode similar to pressure-regulated volume control (PRVC) in that the minimum tidal/minute volume and expected spontaneous respiratory rates are set. After the initial setup where lung-thorax compliance is calculated after a test breath at 6 cm H_2O, the following three breaths are delivered at a pressure of 76% of the calculated pressure

TABLE 5–14

Specifications for the Hamilton Veolar Ventilator*

Modes	Control, assist/control, SIMV, spontaneous (CPAP), pressure support, MMV
Tidal volume	20–2000 mL (infant flow sensor needed for TV <200 mL)
Rate	5–60 breaths/min on f CMV control; 0.5 to 30 breaths on f SIMV control
Pressure limit	10–110 cm H_2O
Peak flow	Up to 180 L/min (acquired by the interaction of various settings for mandatory breaths) for all types of breaths
Waveforms	Square, sine, decelerated taper, and accelerated taper
I:E ratio	1:4 to 4:1
Inspiratory hold (pause)	0–3 sec
PEEP	0–50 cm H_2O
Oxygen concentration	21%–100%
Sensitivity	Off to 15 cm H_2O below PEEP setting
Pressure support	0–50 cm H_2O above PEEP up to an actual pressure of 50 cm H_2O
Minimum minute volume	1–25 L/min
Alarms	
High rate	10–70 breaths/min
High pressure	10–110 cm H_2O
Low expiratory minute volume	1–40 L/min
High expiratory minute volume	1–40 L/min
Low oxygen percent	18–103%
High oxygen percent	18–103%
Apnea	15 sec
Fail to cycle	20 sec
Disconnection	2 breaths (sensed by flow sensor)
Tidal volume mismatch	3 breaths (flow sensor vs. setting error)
Flow out of range	Calculated flow needed during mandatory breaths, >180 L/min
Low O_2 and/or air pressure	<29 psig
Set trigger	SIMV, spontaneous, or MMV modes selected with sensitivity turned off
Alarm silence	2 min
Power failure	
Turn flow sensor	
Technical dysfunctions	

* Courtesy of Hamilton Medical: Reno, Nev.

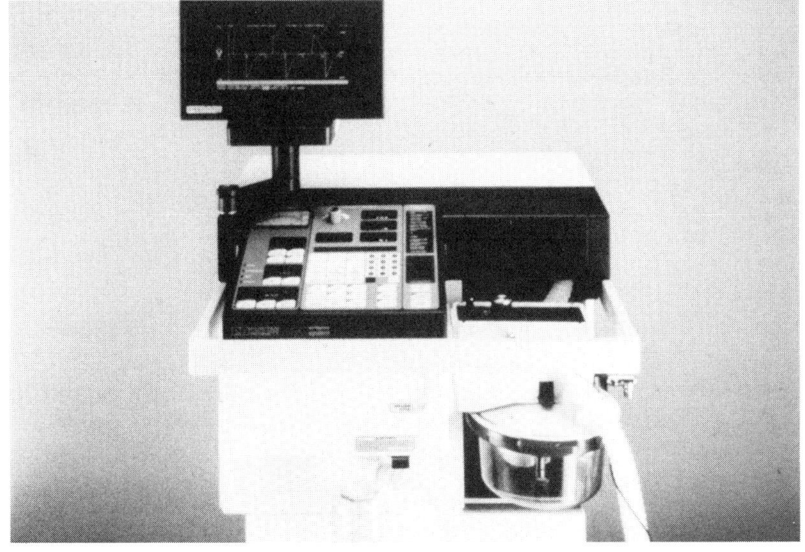

FIG 5–34

Puritan-Bennett 7200 series microprocessor ventilator with graphic screen and international keyboard. (Courtesy of Puritan-Bennett Corp, Santa Monica, Calif.)

TABLE 5–15

Technical Data and Specifications for the Model 7200 Ventilator*

Physical characteristics	
Dimensions	
Ventilator module	Height: 41.9 cm (16.5 in) Depth: 56.5 cm (22.5 in) Width: 55.9 cm (22.0 in)
Ventilator module with compressor pedestal	Height: 102 cm (40.0 in) Depth: 64.8 cm (25.5 in) Width: 55.9 cm (22.0 in)
Assembly weight	
Ventilator module	50.8 kg (112 lb)
Ventilator module with pedestal	95.3 kg (210 lb)
Ventilator module with compressor pedestal	114 kg (250 lb)
Pedestal	44.5 kg (98.0 lb)
Compressor pedestal	62.6 kg (138 lb)
Shipping weight (approximate)	
Ventilator module	79.4 kg (175 lb)
Ventilator module with pedestal†	
Ventilator module with compressor pedestal	172 kg (380 lb)
Pedestal	72.6 kg (160 lb)
Compressor pedestal	90.8 kg (200 lb)
Environmental requirements	
Altitude	
Operating	3,048 m (10,000 ft)
Storage/shipping	15,240 m (50,000 ft)
Environmental temperature	
Operating	16 to 41°C (60 to 105°F)
Storage	−34 to 71°C (−30 to 160°F)
Relative humidity	
Operating	0% to 90% noncondensing
Storage	0% to 100% noncondensing
Clearances for air circulation	Minimum of 15 cm (6.0 in) on all vertical sides
Storage requirements	
Less than 200 days	None
More than 200 days	Replace batteries (2) before returning to use

Electrical specifications

Model	Voltage (ac)	Amperes (rms)‡	Frequency (Hz)
Ventilator module	115 ± 10%	2.8	60 ± 5%
	100 ± 10%	§	60 ± 5%
	100 ± 10%	3.4	50 ± 3%
	220 ± 10%	§	50 ± 3%
	240 ± 10%	1.6	50 ± 3%
Compressor pedestal	115 ± 10%	4.7	60 ± 5%
	100 ± 10%	§	60 ± 5%
	100 ± 10%	6.4	50 ± 3%
	220 ± 10%	§	50 ± 3%
	240 ± 10%	2.6	50 ± 3%

Leakage current: ventilator module with compressor pedestal	Less than 100 μg amp at 115 V
Power cord	125 (240) V ac hospital grade, UL and CSA approved, 305 cm (10.0 ft)
Internal batteries (2)	Lead acid, 2.1 V dc typical, General Electric, sealed X-cell, 5 A · h rating
Pneumatic specifications	
Source pressure	
Oxygen (DISS 9/16-J8), medical grade, dry	241–689 kPa (35–100 psig)
Air (DISS 3/4–16), medical grade, dry	241–689 kPa (35–100 psig)
Source flow: air and oxygen	190 L/min, minimum at 35 psig

TABLE 5–15 (cont.)

Ventilator data	
Gas inlet protection	
Filtering capability, air and oxygen	Particle size, 0.3 μg with 99.8% efficiency
Water filter	Not intended to remove water vapor from gas. Use dry gas only
Operator-selected parameters	
Tidal volume	0.10–2.50 L
Respiratory rate	0.5–70 BPM
Peak inspiratory flow, maximum	10–120 L/min, operator selected 180 L/min during spontaneous breathing
Sensitivity, inspiratory	0.5–20 cm H_2O below PEEP
O_2%	21%–100%
Plateau	0.0–2.0 sec
PEEP/CPAP	0–45 cm H_2O
Operator-selected alarm thresholds	
High-pressure limit	10–120 cm H_2O
Low inspiratory pressure	3–99 cm H_2O
Low PEEP/CPAP pressure	0–45 cm H_2O
Low exhaled tidal volume	0.00–2.50 L
Low exhaled minute volume	0.00–60.0 L
High respiratory rate	0–70 BPM
Operator-selected modes	
CMV SIMV CPAP	Selects modes of ventilation
¶	(Reserved for future enhancements)
Inspiratory flow waveforms	
Square Descending ramp Sine	Selects waveform for mandatory breaths
Operator-selected submodes	
100% O_2 suction	Switches O_2 to 100 for 2 min
Manual inspiration	Commands the delivery of one mandatory breath
Manual sigh	Commands the delivery of one mandatory sigh breath (1.5 × tidal volume)
Automatic sigh	One sigh breath every 100 breaths
Nebulizer	Activates nebulizer for 30 min
Operator-selected alarm control keys	
Alarm silence	Silences audible alarm for 2 min
Alarm reset	Resets ventilator to prealarm state of alert
Alarm indicators	
High-pressure limit	Airway pressure exceeds alarm threshold
Low exhaled tidal volume	Tidal volume is below alarm threshold
Low pressure O_2 inlet	Supply O_2 pressure is below 35 psig
Low inspiratory pressure	Airway pressure during delivery of a mandatory breath is below alarm threshold
Low exhaled minute volume	Minute volume is below alarm threshold
Low pressure air inlet	Supply air pressure is below 35 psig
Low PEEP/CPAP pressure	Airway pressure is below alarm threshold
High respiratory rate	Actual respiratory rate exceeds alarm threshold
Low battery	Less than 1-hr reserve power for audible alarm
Apnea	No breath detected for 20 sec
I:E	Actual value greater than 1:1
Exhalation valve leak	Gas flow past the exhalation flow. Sensor during breath delivery is 50 mL or 10% of delivered volume, whichever is greater
Power disconnect alarm	ac power to the ventilator is interrupted
Alarm summary display	
Ventilator inoperative (red) Alarm (red) Caution (yellow) Backup ventilator (red) Safety valve open (red) Normal (blue)	Illuminates to indicate ventilator status
Operator-selected or monitored parameters	
Airway pressure	Continuous display, breath by breath
Exhaled volume	

(Continued.)

TABLE 5–15 (cont.)

Breath-type indicator lights (automatic)	
Assist Spontaneous Sigh Plateau	Illuminates during appropriate breath or breath cycle
Mean airway pressure Peak airway pressure PEEP/CPAP pressure Plateau pressure	In cm H_2O: three-digit display (maximum of two digits to the right of the decimal point)
Respiratory rate	In breaths per minute: three-digit display (maximum of one digit to the right of the decimal point)
I:E ratio	Two-digit display (maximum of one digit to the right of the decimal point)
Tidal volume Minute volume Spontaneous minute volume	In liters: three-digit display (maximum of two digits to the right of the decimal point)
Safety modes of operation	
Apnea ventilation Backup ventilator Disconnect ventilation	Temporary ventilatory support with factor preset parameters
Safety valve open	Patient breaths room air unassisted by ventilator
Self-diagnostics	
Power-on self-test (POST)	Automatic after power on (10-sec duration)
Extended self-test (EST)	Operator selected (2 to 3 min duration)
Ongoing checks	Automatic, continuous during ventilator operation
I:E ratio check	Automatic, with parameter changes
Lamp test	Operator selected
Output signals	
Remote nurse's call	For remote indication of alarm
Analog signals for pressure and flow	For display of parameters on separate recording device

* Courtesy of Puritan-Bennett Corp, Carlsbad, Calif.
† The ventilator module and pedestal will be shipped separately.
‡ Power consumption and amperage assume the connection of a Cascade II or equivalent humidifier.
§ Values not specified at this printing.
¶ Airway pressure is measured at the patient Y.

needed to deliver the minimum tidal volume. For each of the following breaths, inspiratory pressure is regulated to a value based on the volume/pressure calculation for the previous breath compared with the minimum tidal/minute volume. The pressure change is no more than 3 cm H_2O from breath to breath. If the measured tidal volume is too high, the pressure will decrease until the preset and measured volumes are equal. This mode is presently only available on the Siemens Servo Ventilator (SV) 300.

Flow-by or Continuous Flow

This option provides a predetermined flow of gas into the patient circuit before inspiration, with excess flow usually vented through the exhalation valve. The result is a fresh gas flow available to the patient as soon as an inspiratory effort is initiated. This feature minimizes the delay between the patient's inspiratory effort and the supply of gas to the patient wye. On some ventilators, such as the Puritan Bennett 7200 series, both a base flow and flow sensitivity are set. Base flow is the flow rate delivered during exhalation. This is effectively the available or fresh gas flow for the patient while breathing spontaneously during SIMV/IMV and CPAP. The Flow-by option is analogous to older "demand-flow" systems (as in the BEAR 1, 2, 3) or continuous-flow systems assembled externally for older-generation mechanical ventilators that had no internal provision for continuous gas flow.

Flow-by 2.0

This is the updated version of Puritan Bennett's "Flow-by" option and is now available on the Puritan Bennett 7200 series ventilators equipped with internal exhalation valves. This option allows for a lower inspiratory work of breathing for all breaths, regardless of mode. The Siemens Servo 300 has a similar system for flow triggering.

Additional Delivery Options

Sigh. Sigh mode entails periodic delivery of a mechanical tidal volume that is greater (commonly 50%) than the patient's set mechanical tidal volume.

Inflation hold (inspiratory hold, inspiratory pause). The incorporation of a static phase at the end

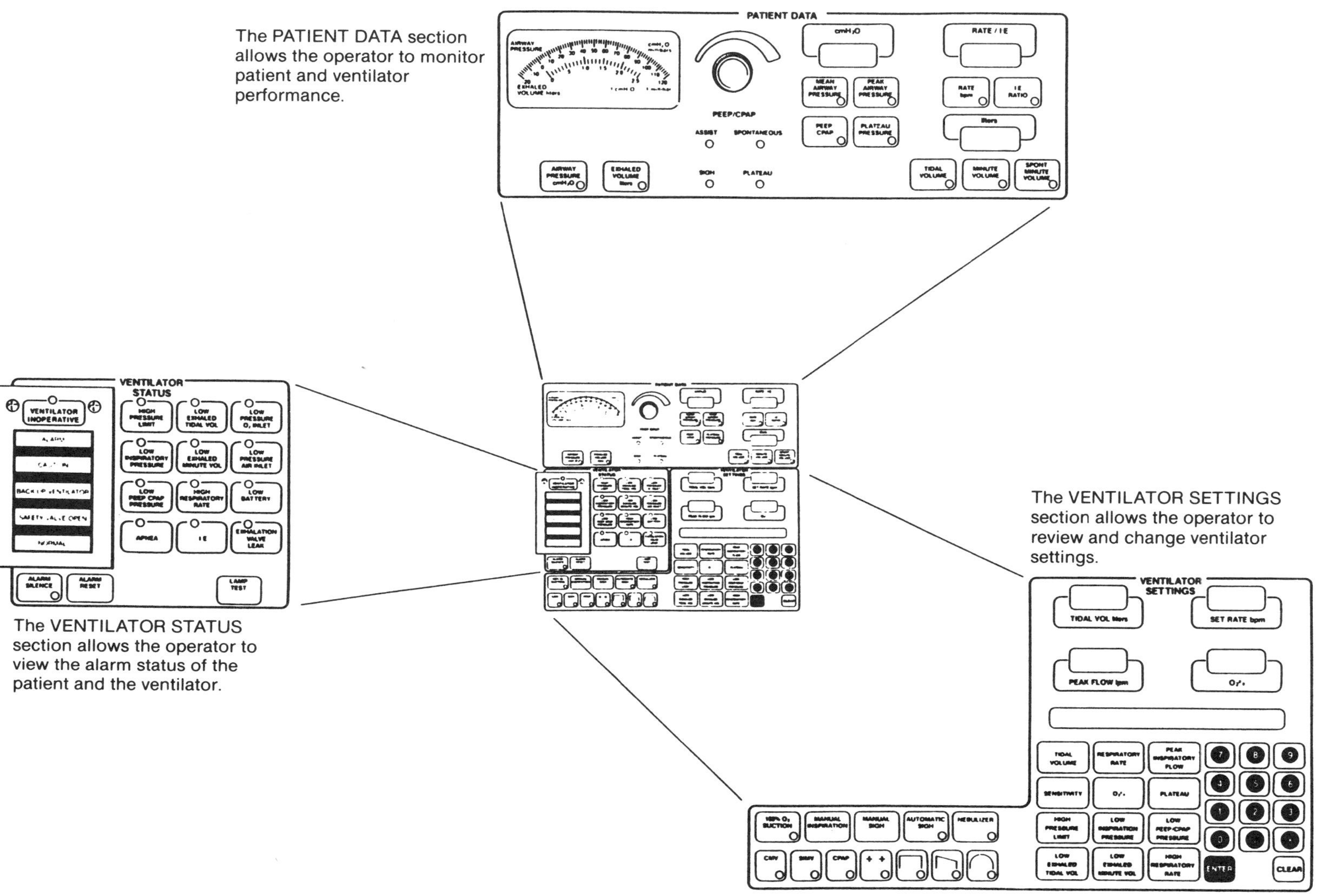

FIG 5–35
Sections of the keyboard display panel of the Puritan-Bennett 7200 microprocessor ventilator. (Courtesy of Puritan-Bennett Corp, Santa Monica, Calif.)

A

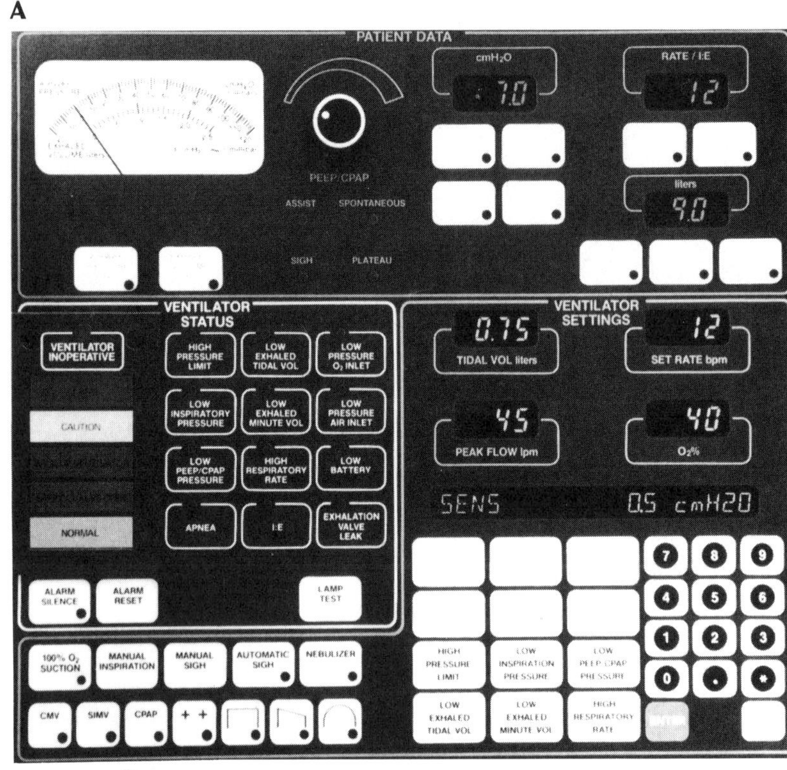

B

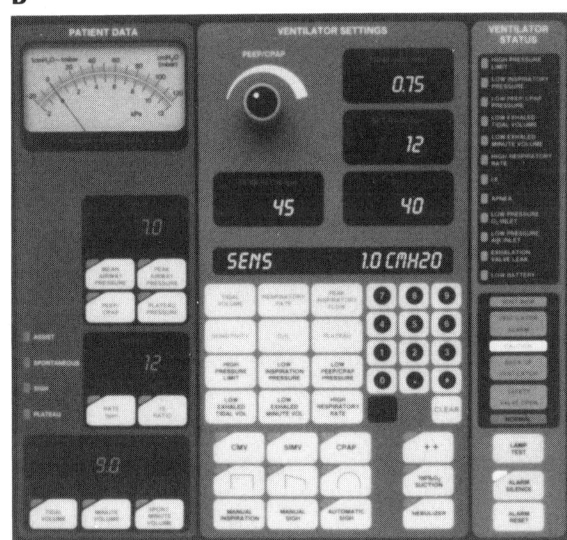

FIG 5–36
Control panel of the Puritan-Bennett 7200 microprocessor ventilator **(A)** and international keyboard **(B)**. (Courtesy of Puritan-Bennett Corp, Santa Monica, Calif.)

of inspiration, or inflation hold, can be achieved by holding the delivered tidal volume within the patient's airway or by maintaining a constant pressure at the patient's airway.

Pressure Augmentation. A "pressure boost" (only on the BEAR 1000 at this time), or pressure augmentation, can be used in conjunction with any mode where volume breaths are delivered, such as assist CMV or SIMV. A minimum tidal volume guarantee is set along with the desired pressure augmentation level (pressure support/inspiratory pressure setting), peak flow rate, and high peak inspiratory pressure alarm. The ventilator monitors the delivered tidal volume and will augment or add pressure to achieve that volume by "finishing off" the breath at the clinician-selected peak flow setting. The delivered inspiratory pressure may rise above the pressure support/inspiratory pressure setting that is required to achieve the desired delivered tidal volume given the patient's lung-thorax compliance, airway resistance, and demand. During this maneuver, an increase in patient

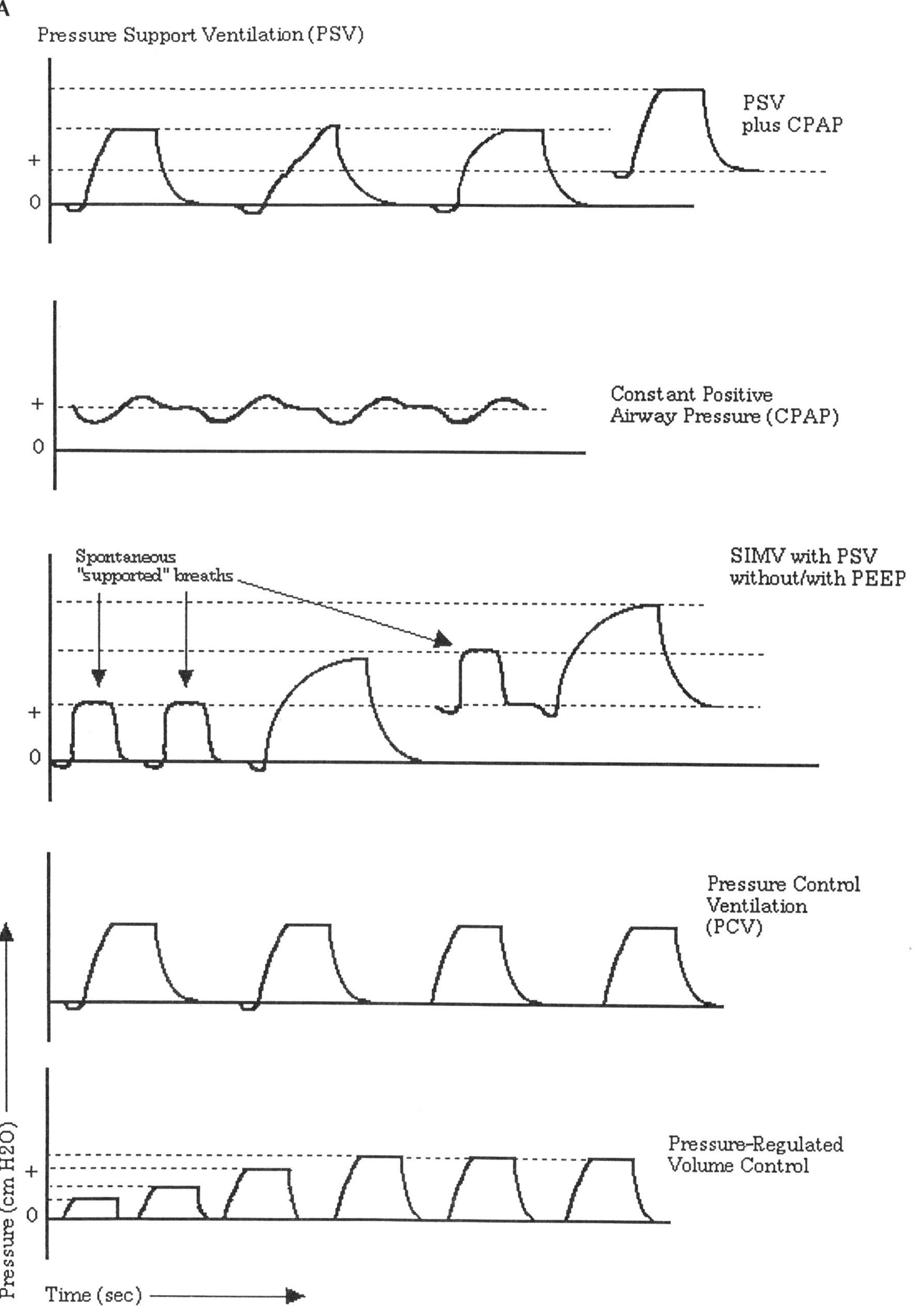

FIG 5–37
Pressure waveforms for various ventilatory modes. *(Continued.)*

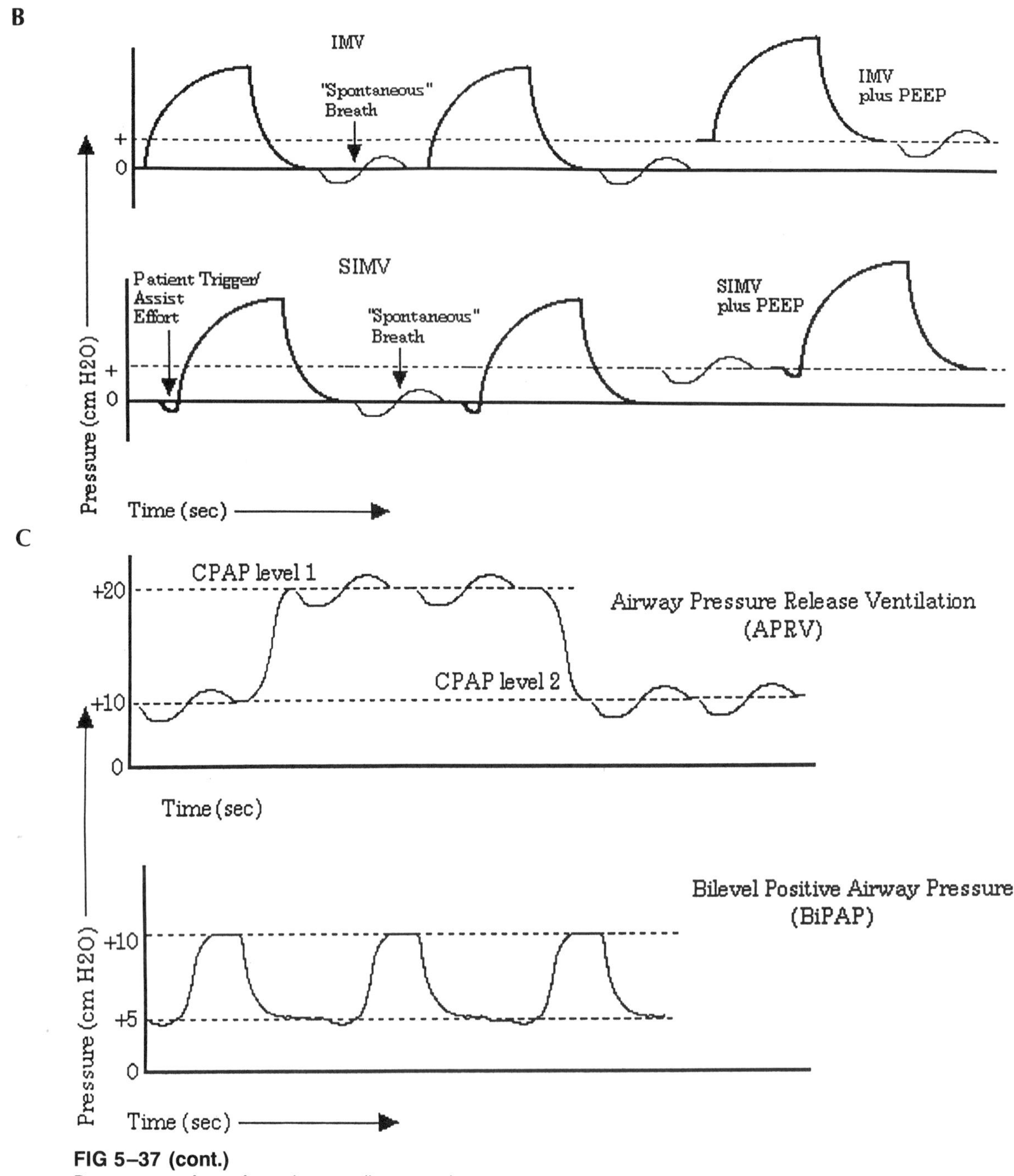

FIG 5–37 (cont.)
Pressure waveforms for various ventilatory modes.

demand for volume is rewarded by extra flow. Therefore, pressure augmentation will guarantee a minimum delivered tidal volume but does not limit the patient to this minimum setting.

Pressure Slope. By manipulating the inspiratory flow rate, this maneuver permits the clinician greater control in shaping the pressure waveform. This "fine tuning" changes the speed with which the inspiratory pressure level is achieved. The speed change is controlled by the initial flow rates and flow adjustment response rate, thereby affecting the degree of patient comfort (via improved ventilator-patient synchrony). This feature as "pressure slope" is available on the Comprehensive BEAR 1000. Functionally, the "inspiratory rise time" control on the Siemens Servo 300 accomplishes the same objectives. This pressure/flow function is available on all breaths regulated by pressure (which includes all modes if desired).

Expiratory retard (expiratory resistance). Expiratory retard entails establishing resistance to exhalation, decreasing expiratory gas flow, and hence lengthening the time that it takes the peak airway pressure to reach baseline.

Expiratory hold. This feature allows the clinician to lengthen the expiratory time primarily as a monitoring tool to detect auto-PEEP. This has been available on the Siemens 900C and is also available on the Servo 300 and the BEAR 1000.

Positive end-expiratory pressure. The maintenance of airway pressure above atmospheric at end exhalation, PEEP strictly refers to residual positive pressure during mechanical ventilation (as opposed to CPAP for a spontaneously breathing patient).

Negative end-expiratory pressure. The maintenance of airway pressure below atmospheric at end exhalation, or negative end-expiratory pressure (NEEP), is an option no longer offered as part of any modern mechanical ventilator system.

WORK OF BREATHING

Compliance

Compliance is defined as a change in volume associated with a change in pressure. In relationship to the lungs, compliance reflects the amount of pressure necessary to move a given tidal volume. Figure 5–38, A shows compliance curves of normal and diseased lungs. The functional reserve capacity (FRC) is the starting point for each inspiration. The chest wall has a natural tendency to expand, and the lungs have a natural tendency to collapse. Where those two forces are balanced determines the FRC. As compliance decreases, the amount of pressure necessary to distend the lungs increases no

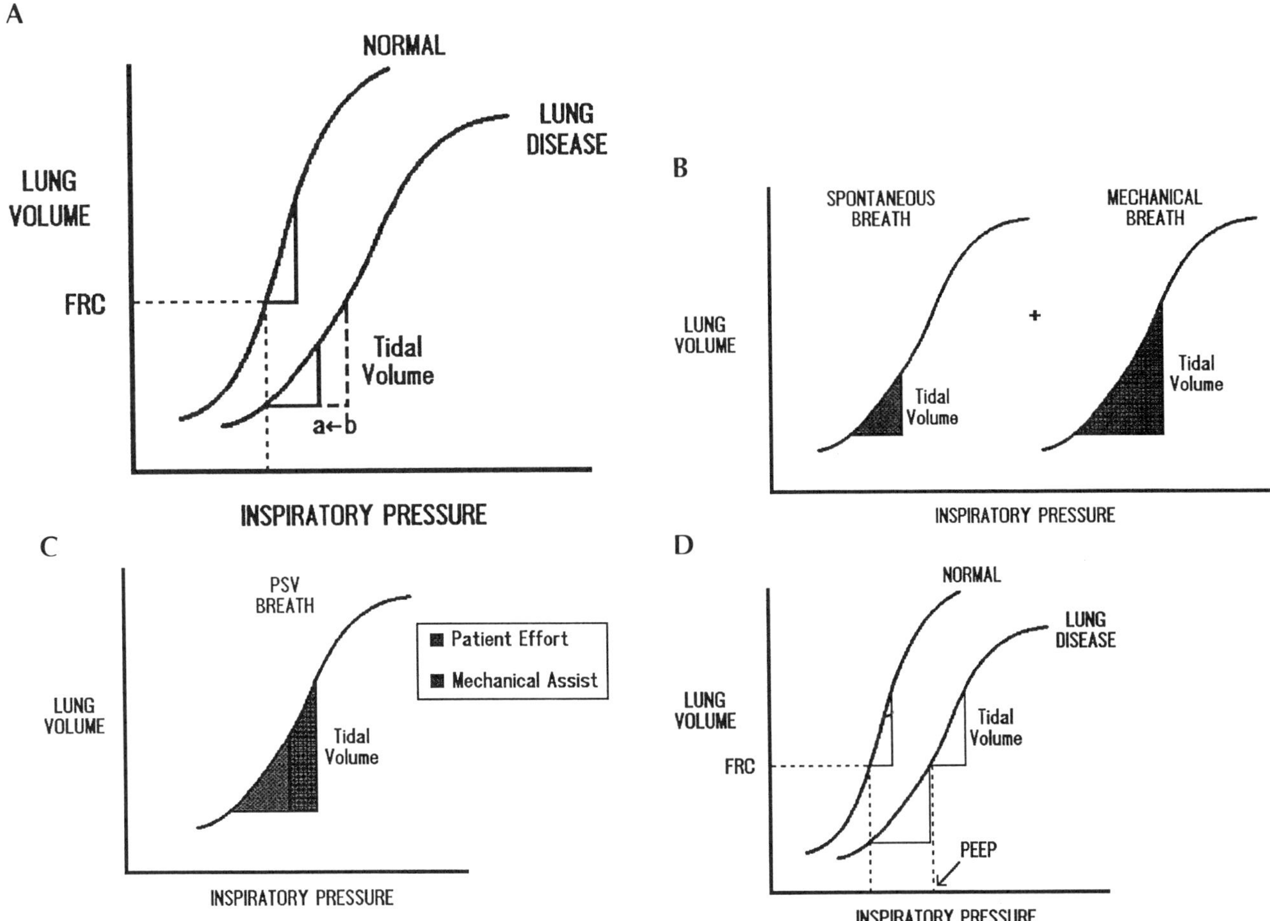

FIG 5–38
A, spontaneous breath—effects of decreasing compliance and inspiratory force or tidal volume.[38] **B,** SIMV/IMV—mechanical breaths and unsupported spontaneous breaths. **C,** PSV—patient and ventilator contribute to creating the breath. **D,** PEEP—decrease in work of breathing by improving compliance.

matter where you are on that compliance curve. In addition, the tendency of the lungs to collapse is increased while the chest tendency to expand remains the same, thus resulting in a drop in FRC. This drop in FRC places the patient in a less efficient part of the compliance curve, and this increases the distending pressure necessary to move that tidal volume. If the work associated with creating this distending pressure is too great for the patient, the patient will generate a smaller distending pressure and thus move a smaller tidal volume (b → a in Fig 5–38, A).

To maintain minute ventilation, the patient's respiratory rate increases to compensate for the decreased tidal volume. High-rate, low–tidal volume breathing is less efficient and consumes more oxygen than normal ventilation; this results in increased CO_2 production coupled with inefficient CO_2 elimination and puts a further load on the respiratory system, which if not relieved, will ultimately lead to respiratory failure. The role of mechanical ventilation is to unload the respiratory muscles and reestablish high–tidal volume, low-rate breathing. If the patient is on assist/control mode (A/C) or is on control ventilation (CMV), the machine is giving the patient full ventilatory support. Each time the breath is triggered (by the patient in A/C or by the ventilator in CMV), the patient receives the full tidal volume from the ventilator. This completely unloads the respiratory muscles.

Intermittent mandatory ventilation is the combination of spontaneous breaths and mechanical breaths (Fig 5–38, B). If the ventilator synchronizes the mandatory breaths with the patient's inspiratory effort, the mode is called SIMV. The set tidal volume and respiratory rate define a minute ventilation that the ventilator will do on a mandatory basis. The patient assumes the work necessary for the remainder of the minute ventilation. Since these breaths are not assisted, they will be small–tidal volume, high-rate breaths, as if the patient were not connected to the ventilator. The benefit gained with SIMV/IMV is from a reduction in the total minute ventilation that the patient is responsible for. If that reduction is inadequate (i.e., the SIMV/IMV rate is too low), the patient may be in ventilatory failure even while hooked up to the ventilator.

Figure 5–38, C illustrates a pressure support ventilation (PSV) breath. Where this differs from IMV is that the patient and the ventilator together produce the distending pressure that generates the tidal volume. All these breaths are high–tidal volume breaths, and the patient is not exposed to unassisted breaths. Each time the patient triggers the ventilator, the reservoir gas is pressurized to the set PSV level. This allows the patient to do less work to move a given tidal volume on a breath-by-breath basis. PSV can also be used in conjunction with SIMV to further decrease the patient's work of breathing. If on an SIMV/IMV mode or PSV, the patient may be receiving partial ventilatory support or full ventilatory support.

PEEP and CPAP can also be used to decrease the work of breathing (Fig 5–38, D). The presence of end-expiratory pressure will increase the patient's FRC and move it to a more favorable part of the compliance curve. By having the breaths start on the steep part of the compliance curve, the work for that breath would be decreased. This is illustrated by the decrease in area underneath the curve in Figure 5–38, D.

Endotracheal Tube Work

Pressure support can be used to compensate for additional inspiratory work resulting from the endotracheal tube and demand CPAP systems. Bolder et al.[35] reported that every 1-mm decrease in the diameter of the endotracheal tube results in a 34% to 154% increase in work, depending on the respiratory rate and tidal volume. Katz et al.[36] showed that Puritan Bennett 7200 ventilator circuits may result in a 10% to 40% increase in additional inspiratory work, depending on the inspiratory flow. Fiastro et al.[37] looked at using pressure support to compensate for inspiratory work resulting from the endotracheal tube and the demand CPAP circuit. They used a test lung model and looked at how much pressure support was necessary to bring the additional work down to zero while manipulating mean inspiratory flow and endotracheal tube size. They compared the pressure support level required for their test lung with that required for four subjects breathing through an endotracheal tube and found that the levels of PSV were the same. The amount of pressure support required to compensate for the endotracheal tube size and the mean inspiratory flow are shown in Table 5–16. By applying the level of pressure support in Table 5–16, the patient is not exposed to the additional work of the endotracheal tube

TABLE 5–16

Pressure Support to Compensate for Endotracheal Tube and CPAP System Work

	Inspiratory Flow Rate (L/min)				
ETT*	24	30	36	48	60
7.0	5	8	13	20	30
7.5	4	7	10	18	25
8.0	3	6	8	15	20
8.5	3	5	8	14	18
9.0	2	4	7	12	16

* ETT = endotracheal tube.

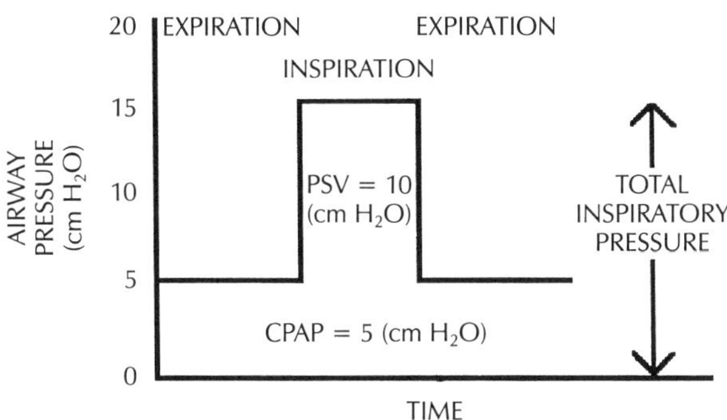

FIG 5–39
Airway pressure reflecting a PSV breath on a CPAP circuit.

or the CPAP circuit. This may be a more accurate assessment of the patient's ability to breathe spontaneously. This study was conducted with CPAP equal to zero, and it is unclear how much pressure support is necessary to compensate if there is continuous positive airway pressure in the circuit. If CPAP is used to improve lung compliance, then the overall work of breathing should decrease. Katz et al.[36] determined the work of breathing of several CPAP systems by using a test lung model and found that some systems increase the work of breathing and other ones decrease the work of breathing. These studies did not address the potential decrease in work of breathing resulting from the improved compliance from the CPAP itself.

The present generation of ventilators will add the pressure support on top of the existing CPAP level. In the example in Figure 5–39, the patient is receiving 5 cm H_2O of CPAP and 10 cm H_2O of PSV, resulting in a total inspiratory pressure of 15 cm H_2O. When performing a trial of spontaneous ventilation, it has been our practice to have the total inspiratory pressure equal the values in Table 5–16. To date there are no clinical studies addressing this question.

GAS EXCHANGE

Ventilation/Perfusion Relationships

The normal upright lung is an inhomogeneous collection of ventilation/perfusion (V/Q) ratios that are abnormally high at the top and much lower at the bottom (Fig 5–40).[39] The force of gravity augments perfusion to the bases, which in turn makes the bases less compliant and thereby harder to distend. Diaphragmatic activity compensates for this by creating a greater negative pressure at the bases and thus augmenting more ventilation to the well-perfused bases. When a patient is mechanically ventilated, the gas goes the path of least resistance, which tends to overventilate the more compliant apices and underventilate the less compliant bases. This creates a

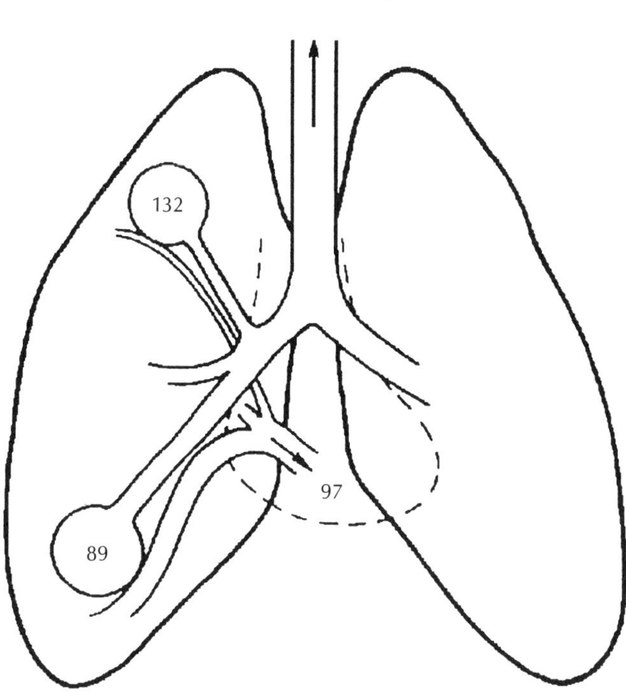

FIG 5–40
Regional differences in ventilation/perfusion relationships in a normal lung. (From West JB: *Lancet* 1963; 2:1055. Used by permission.)

ventilation/perfusion inequality that makes mechanical ventilation less efficient than spontaneous ventilation.

These ventilation/perfusion relationships can be used to advantage in the case of a patient with unilateral lung disease. Remolina et al.[40] demonstrated marked improvement in oxygenation by positioning the patient so that the good lung was in a dependent position and the sick lung was nondependent ("down with the lung"[41]).

Figure 5–41 depicts the relationship between airway pressure and vascular pressure in the lung. In zone 1, alveolar pressure exceeds both the arterial and venous pressures, and this results in complete collapse of the pulmonary vasculature and no blood flow. In zone 2, the alveolar pressure is less than the arterial pressure but greater than the venous pressure; the difference between the arterial and alveolar pressure determines the blood flow and results in a reduction in blood flow. In zone 3, the alveolar pressure is less than both the arterial and venous pressure; the blood flow is determined by the difference between the arterial and venous pressures, and blood flow is normal. As the amount of positive pressure in the chest is increased, zone 1 and zone 2 will also increase. All of zone 1 is dead space ventilation, and zone 2 represents areas with high V/Q ventilation, which will result in an increase in the dead space-to-tidal volume

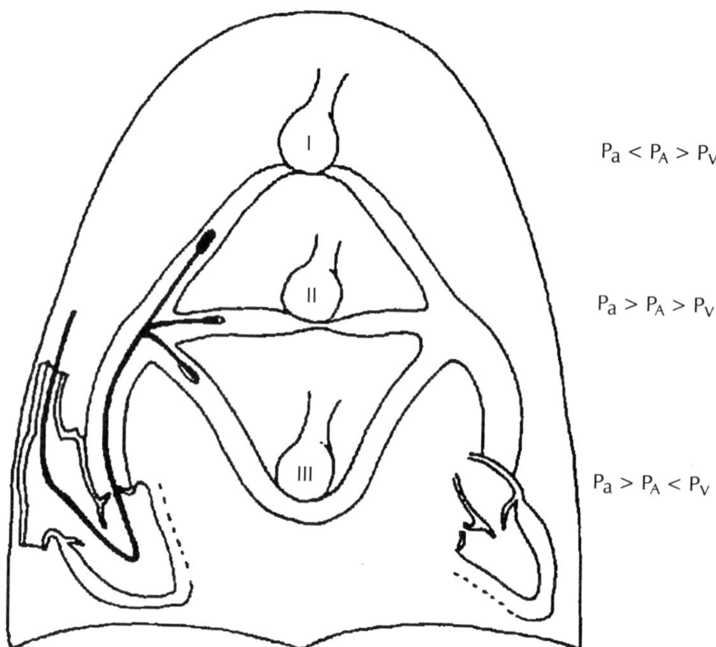

FIG 5–41
Effects of zoned ventilation on pulmonary vascular flow and hemodynamics. (From Marini JJ: *Respiratory Medicine,* ed 2. Baltimore, Williams & Wilkins, 1987, p 162. Used by permission.)

ratio (VD/VT). This is another reason why spontaneous ventilation is more efficient than mechanical ventilation.

Heart-Lung Interactions

The heart functions as a pump inside a pressure chamber, and the pleural pressure may have a significant effect on cardiac function. When going from negative-pressure spontaneous ventilation to positive-pressure ventilation, the preload to the right ventricle decreases. As the positive pressure increases in the chest, zone 1 and 2 ventilation is produced (Fig 5–41). These zones act as resistors in the pulmonary circuit and increase pulmonary vascular resistance, which increases right ventricular afterload. The right ventricle is not a very muscular structure, and it is very dependent on its afterload in order to preserve its stroke volume. Sibbald et al.[42] showed that patients with elevated pulmonary arterial pressures greater than 30 mm Hg had abnormally low right ventricular ejection fractions. In this study they also showed that the right ventricular ejection fraction correlated with pulmonary artery pressure (Fig 5–42).

To compensate for the decreasing ejection fraction, the right ventricle increases its end-diastolic volume.[43] This increase in end-diastolic volume will preserve right ventricular stroke volume until a critical right ventricular afterload is reached, after which the right ventricular pump starts to fail to provide adequate left ventricular filling. As the right ventricular end-diastolic volume increases, so does its end-diastolic pressure. The central venous pressure (CVP) is an estimation of the right ventricular end diastolic pressure. This is frequently used as an index of the patient's intravascular volume. In patients who are receiving a significant amount of positive-pressure ventilation, the assumption that the elevated CVP reflects an elevated intravascular volume is inaccurate. Shippy et al.[44] demonstrated in critically ill surgical patients that there was no correlation between CVP measurements and changes in blood volume measured by using an indicator dilution technique using ^{125}I-labeled human serum albumin (Fig 5–43).

Although the increase in right ventricular end-diastolic volume serves to preserve right ventricular stroke volume, it will reach a point that will impair left ventricular filling. As the right ventricle continues to dilate, the intraventricular septum shifts over in the direction of the left ventricle and impedes left ventricular filling (Fig 5–44). This ventricular interdependence results in an impairment in left ventricular compliance. This is one mechanism for the decrease in left ventricular preload that may be seen with positive-pressure ventilation.

If the right atrial pressure increases either because of positive-pressure ventilation or increases in right ventricular afterload, then the venous return to the right side of the circulation will decrease. This will eventually decrease pulmonary venous blood flow and left ventricular end-diastolic volume. In addition, as the lungs are inflated with positive-pressure ventilation, the heart is mechanically compressed by the lungs. This further decreases left ventricular compliance and impedes left ventricular filling. The pulmonary artery wedge pressure will reflect

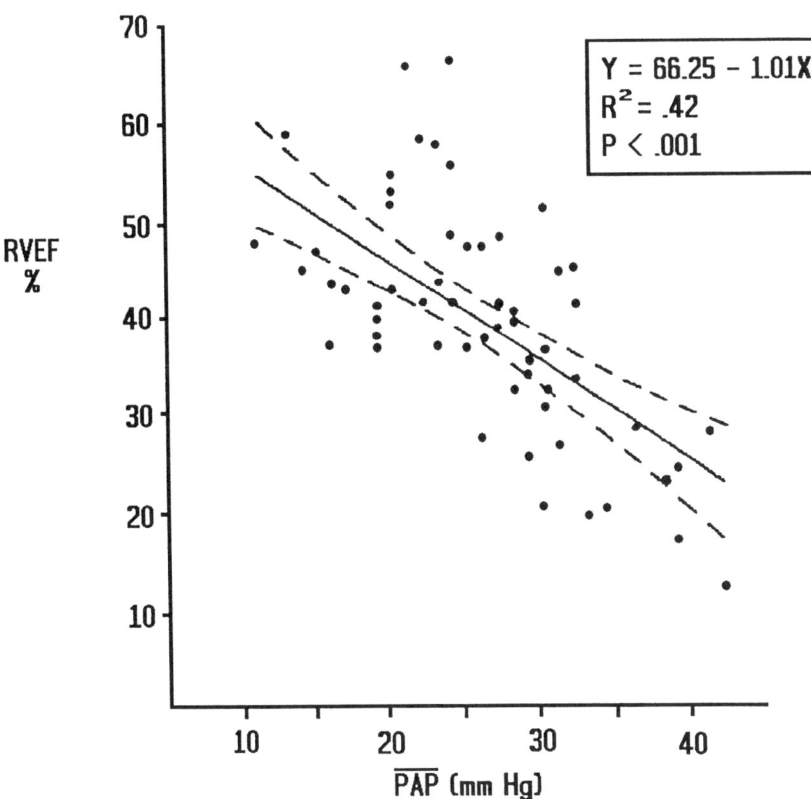

FIG 5–42
Relationship of right ventricular ejection fraction *(RVEF)* and mean pulmonary artery pressure *($\overline{PAP}$)* in patients with adult respiratory distress syndrome. (From Sibbald WT, Drieger AA, Myers MC, et al: *Chest* 1983; 84:126–134. Used by permission.)

these changes in left ventricular compliance in addition to changes in volume of the left ventricle. An elevated pulmonary artery wedge pressure may be related to the positive-pressure ventilation and may not reflect an increase in blood volume or left ventricular failure.[45]

Left ventricular afterload, defined as the peak transmural left ventricular pressure required to eject the stroke volume (left ventricular pressure − intrathoracic pressure), is improved with positive-pressure ventilation. Figure 5–45, A represents a patient with normal pleural pressures generating a systolic blood pressure of 120 mm Hg outside the thoracic cavity. This patient's left ventric-

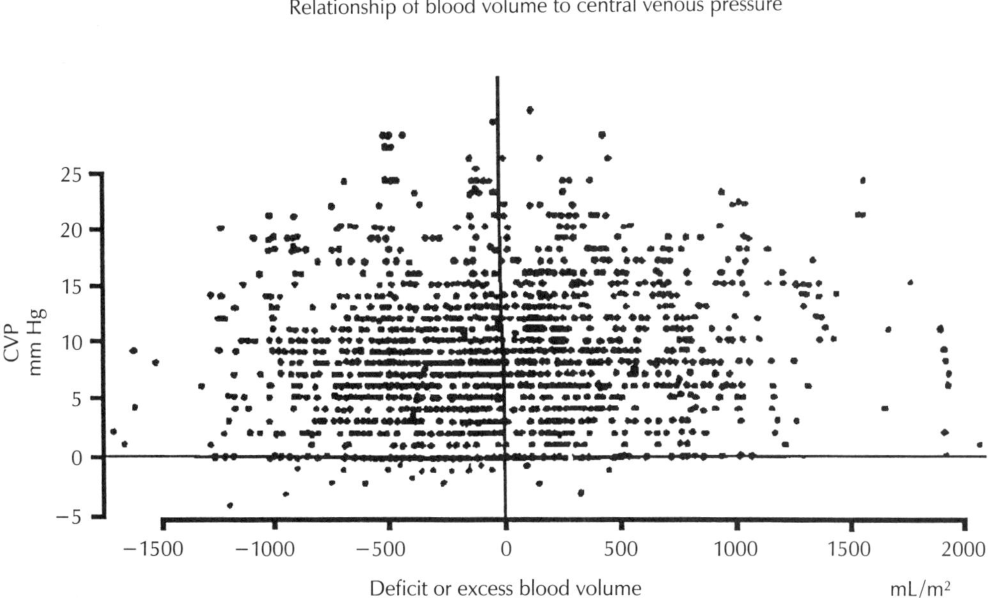

FIG 5–43
Blood volume measurements plotted against central venous pressure measurements. No correlation was found. (From Shippy CR, Appel PL, Shoemaker WCL: *Crit Care Med* 1984; 12:110. Used by permission.)

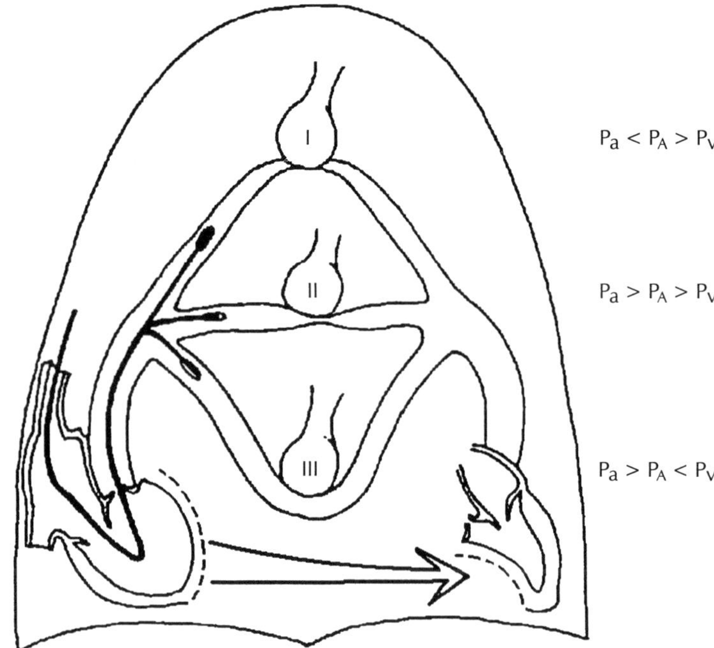

FIG 5–44
Effects of zoned ventilation on ventricular interdependence. (Adapted from Marini JJ: *Respiratory Medicine,* ed 2. Baltimore, Williams & Wilkins, 1987, p 162. Used by permission.)

ular end-diastolic pressure is 5 mm Hg, and the left ventricle needs to generate 115 mm Hg of pressure in order to eject its stroke volume.

The peak transmural left ventricular pressure is 125 mm Hg. Figure 5–45, B shows what happens if the pleural pressure is now raised to +20 cm H_2O. Some of that pressure will be transmitted to the left ventricle, and now the left ventricular end-diastolic pressure is 15. In order to get the same systolic blood pressure of 120 mm Hg, this ventricle now only needs to generate 105 mm Hg of pressure. The peak transmural pressure is now 100 mm Hg.

This decrease in left ventricular afterload may increase left ventricular stroke volume. Pinsky et al.[46] synchronized a high-frequency jet ventilator (HFJV) to the ECG and had the ventilator cycle only during systole. This allowed for augmentation of the stroke volume during systole with positive-pressure ventilation but avoided the preload reduction from a sustained increase in intrathoracic pressure. The study showed a significant improvement in cardiac output with the ECG-synchronized HFJV as compared with IPPB. Studies done on patients with end-stage cardiomyopathy, acute mitral regurgitation, and neonatal heart failure have shown significant improvement with this technique.[46–48] Clinical trials are ongoing to further evaluate this technique.

All forms of positive-pressure ventilation and not just PEEP illustrate these hemodynamic affects. Snyder and Powner looked at a series of dogs that had their cardiac output determined every 1 second while they were ventilated (Fig 5–46).[49] In this series of dogs, the cardiac output varied 47% from peak inspiratory pressure to end exhalation. This phenomenon would occur on a breath-to-breath basis; the more positive-pressure breaths that there are in the chest, the more hemodynamic embarrassment will be seen.

Another demonstration of this physiology may be seen on arterial tracings. Figure 5–47 is from a young patient who was a victim of a motor vehicle accident. ARDS developed, and the patient was ventilated on high levels of positive-pressure ventilation and PEEP. As the ventilator cycled, the patient's stroke volume and cardiac output dropped, as did the systolic blood pressure. The most common cause of pulsus paradoxus seen in a ventilated patient in an intensive care unit (ICU) is relative volume depletion. Zone 1 and 2 ventilation is a function of the relationship between airway pressure and vascular pressure. In a hypovolemic patient with the same degree of airway pressure, the patient will have more zone 1 and 2 ventilation than a euvolemic patient. This increases right ventricular afterload, decreases right ventricular stroke volume, and eventually decreases cardiac output. Treatment of ventilator-induced hemodynamic embarrassment consists of volume replacement and, if the patient is euvolumic, adding dobutamine to help right ventricular contractility. The efficacy of volume replacement can be monitored by following the pulsus paradoxus.

Auto-PEEP

Pepe and Marini[50] described the importance of auto-PEEP in mechanically ventilated patients with severe obstructive lung disease. This unintentional PEEP results from incomplete exhalation before the next breath occurs. The longer the expiratory time in patients with chronic lung disease, the greater the risk of auto-PEEP.

Figure 5–48 is from a patient in our unit who had severe chronic obstructive lung disease and unexplained hypotension. When the patient was removed from the ventilator for suctioning purposes, the systolic blood pressure rose from 60 to 140 mm Hg. The patient was ventilated on assist/control mode and zero PEEP. When the patient was returned to the ventilator, his blood pressure returned to the 60–mm Hg range. This patient's hypotension resolved by decreasing the mandatory minute ventilation.

Brown and Pierson[51] looked at 62 patients who were mechanically ventilated on control mode and another 10 patients with severe chronic obstructive lung disease. In the 62 patients who were on control ventilation and whose minute ventilation was above 10 L/min, 39% had measurable auto-PEEP. In patients with chronic obstructive lung disease, 50% demonstrated auto-PEEP.

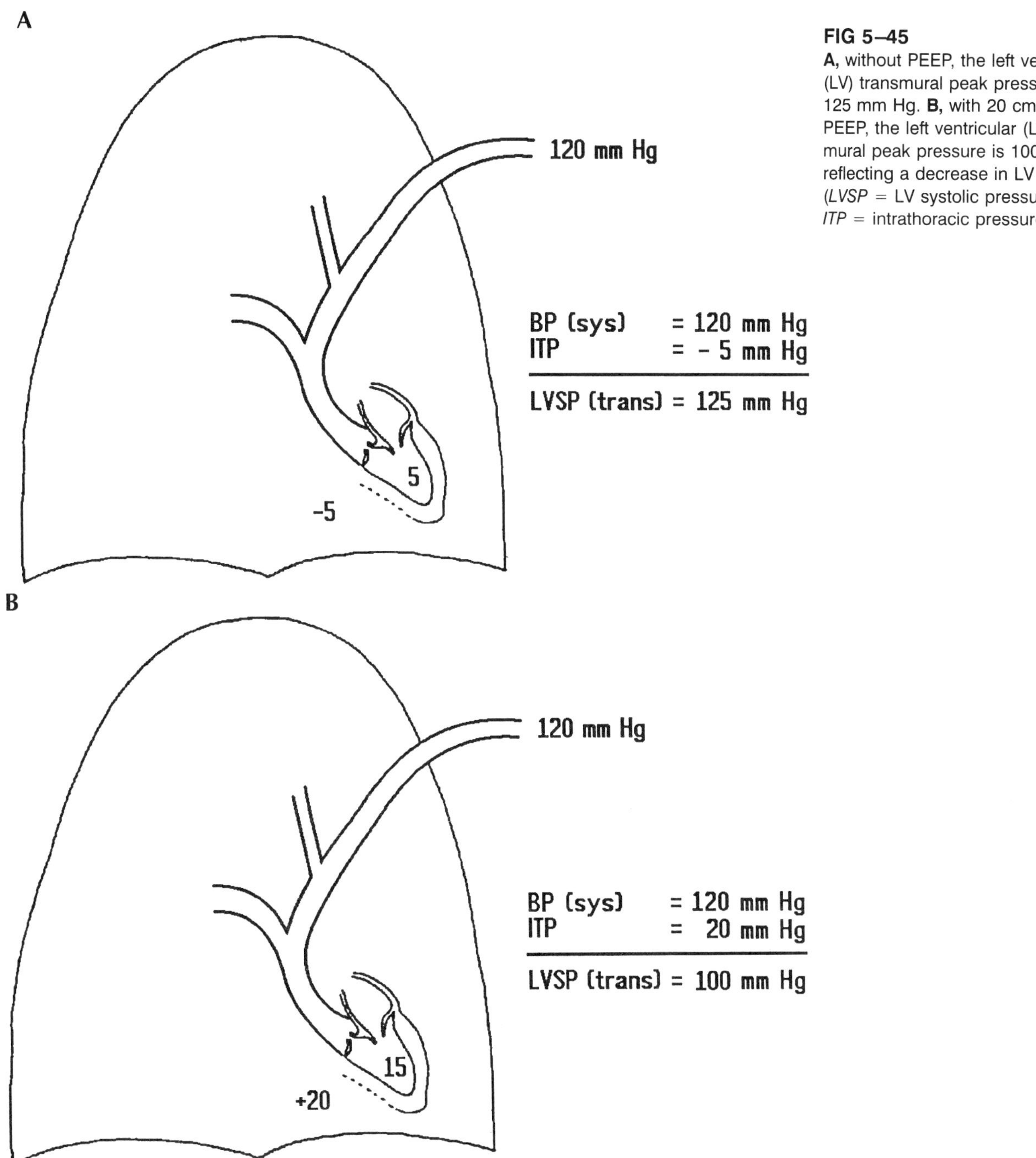

FIG 5–45
A, without PEEP, the left ventricular (LV) transmural peak pressure is 125 mm Hg. **B,** with 20 cm H_2O PEEP, the left ventricular (LV) transmural peak pressure is 100 mm Hg, reflecting a decrease in LV afterload. (*LVSP* = LV systolic pressure; *ITP* = intrathoracic pressure.)

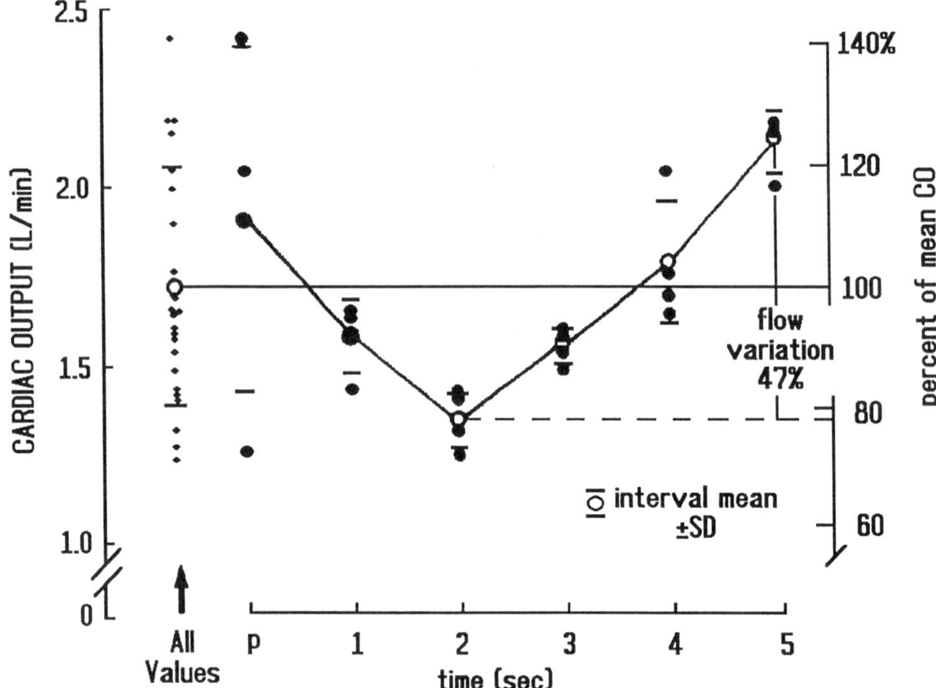

FIG 5–46
Thermodilution cardiac output measurements initiated at 1-second intervals after peak airway pressure *(p)*. (From Snyder JV, Powner DJ: *Crit Care Med* 1982; 10:677. Used by permission.)

If significant auto-PEEP is demonstrated, efforts should be made to decrease the inspiratory time to allow adequate time for exhalation. The most efficient way of doing this is to decrease the mandatory minute ventilation. This can be done by dropping the tidal volume and/or decreasing the respiratory rate. Dropping the tidal volume will decrease the inspiratory time, whereas decreasing the respiratory rate will increase time for exhalation. Other maneuvers include increasing the inspiratory flow rate to decrease the inspiratory time or using a larger endotracheal tube to decrease the resistance in exhalation.[52] Auto-PEEP should be considered any time that there is hemodynamic embarrassment in a mechanically ventilated patient, especially those with high minute ventilation needs and those with chronic obstructive lung disease.

The following are the potential effects of positive-pressure ventilation.

1. Ventilation/perfusion mismatch
2. Increased dead space/tidal volume ratio
3. Preload reduction
4. Increased pulmonary vascular resistance
5. Right heart pressure overload
6. Septal shift to the left impeding left ventricular filling
7. Auto-PEEP
8. Barotrauma

Positive pressure ventilation is less efficient because of the creation of ventilation/perfusion mismatches. Elimination of CO_2 is impaired by the increased dead space/tidal volume ratio resulting from creation of zone 1 and 2 ventilation. As the pressure in the chest increases, the venous return to the right ventricle decreases, and because of the creation of zone 1 and 2 ventilation, the pulmonary vascular resistance increases. This results in a

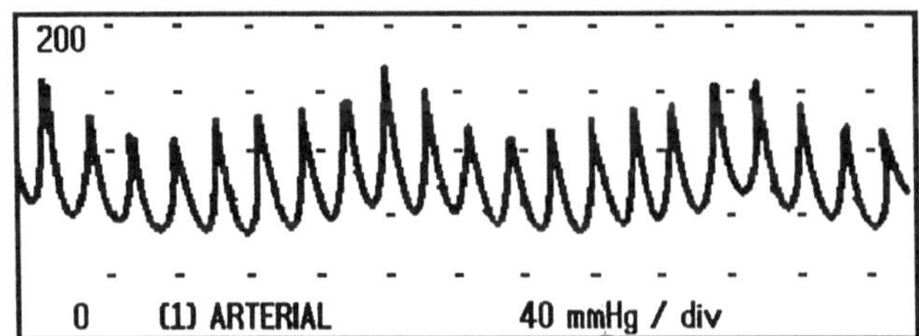

FIG 5–47
Pulsus paradox seen in a young trauma patient. Systolic blood pressure dropped 40 mm Hg with each ventilator cycle.

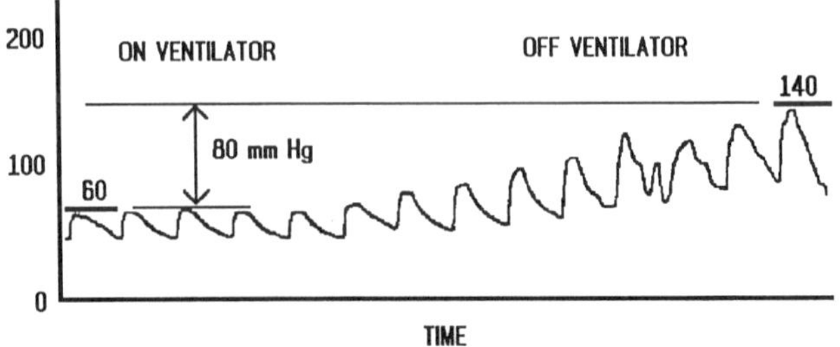

FIG 5–48
Auto-PEEP demonstrated by removal of mechanical support in a patient with obstructive lung disease.

drop in right ventricular ejection with right heart volume and pressure overload and may result in a shift of the intraventricular septum to the left and impede left ventricular filling. The left ventricle receives a smaller volume from the right ventricle along with a decrease in its compliance. This results in a smaller left ventricular end-diastolic volume, diminished stroke volume, and a diminished cardiac output. This pathophysiology is accentuated in patients who are hypovolemic and have normal lung compliance. Patients who have severe chronic obstructive lung disease and/or very high minute ventilation requirements may also have hemodynamic embarrassment because of auto-PEEP.

Positive-Pressure Ventilation and Oxygen Transport

One of the major responsibilities of the heart and lungs is to supply oxygen to the tissues to carry out their metabolic needs. The "job description" of the lungs is to extract oxygen from the inspired gas and combine it with the oxygen that has returned from the venous side of the circulation to saturate the blood on the arterial side. The heart's "job description" is to move that saturated blood from the lungs out to the tissues and to return the oxygen that was not consumed back to the lungs. Both organs are dependent upon each other to carry out their jobs. Patients who are severely hypoxic may have impairment of either the cardiac or pulmonary aspects of oxygen delivery. Ventilator management of these severely hypoxic patients must take into account this pathophysiology.

Table 5–17 is a summary of oxygen delivery variables. Oxygen content is the volume of oxygen measured in milliliters that is present in 100 mL of blood. Approximately 98% of the oxygen is bound to hemoglobin. The small fraction that is physically dissolved in the serum is not clinically significant in most circumstances. This allows an estimation of changes in content to be made with changes in saturation.

Oxygen transport (oxygen delivery) is the volume of oxygen in milliliters that is presented to the tissues per minute. The lungs are responsible for maximizing arterial content by saturating the arterial blood. The heart's responsibility is to maintain the cardiac output. If a significant amount of PEEP and mechanical ventilation is necessary to support lung function, then a drop in cardiac output may be seen, and the net effect may be a drop in O_2 transport.

For example, if an increase in PEEP results in a 5% increase in the Sa_{O_2} but the cardiac output drops by 10%, then the net change in O_2 transport is actually a decrease in O_2 transport to the tissues of 5%.

Oxygen consumption is the amount of oxygen in milliliters per minute that the tissues consume to meet their metabolic needs. Venous oxygen transport is the amount of oxygen in milliliters per minute that leaves the tissues and returns to the lungs. The venous O_2 transport is a function of the cardiac output and the venous content and will be directly related to the patient's oxygen consumption. Normal value for venous O_2 transport and arterial transport are 750 and 1,000 mL/min, respectively. Under normal conditions, 75% of the arterial oxygenation comes from the venous side of the circulation. If cardiac function is impaired, then arterial O_2 transport to the tissues will be diminished along with a decrease in venous O_2 transport to the lungs. This results in less oxygen being delivered to the lungs and impaired ability to saturate the arterial blood.

If the venous O_2 transport is subtracted from the arterial O_2 transport, an expression is derived that combines oxygen consumption, cardiac output, and $A\text{-}V_{O_2}$ content difference ("Fick equation"). If you assume that the oxygen consumption remains stable between two

TABLE 5–17

Oxygen Delivery Variables

Variable	Calculations	Normal
Sa_{O_2}		0.94–0.98
Sv_{O_2}		0.70–0.75
Ca_{O_2}	$(Hb \times Sa_{O_2} \times 1.34) + (0.0031 \times Pa_{O_2})$	20 vol%
Cv_{O_2}	$(Hb \times Sv_{O_2} \times 1.34) + (0.0031 \times Pv_{O_2})$	15 vol%
AV_{O_2}	$Ca_{O_2} - Cv_{O_2}$	3.5–5.0 vol%
O_2 transport		
Arterial	$Ca_{O_2} \times CO^* \times 10$	1,000 mL/min
Venous	$Cv_{O_2} \times CO \times 10$	750 mL/min
O_2 consumption		250 mL/min
Q_S/Q_T	$(Cc'O_2 - Ca_{O_2}) / (Cc'_{O_2} - Cv_{O_2})$ where $Cc'_{O_2} = (Hb \times 1.34) + (0.0031 \times P_{AO_2})$ $P_{AO_2} = (P_B - P_{H_2O}) \times F_{IO_2} - p_{CO_2}/R$	5% to 10%

* CO = cardiac output.

observations, then the change in cardiac output will be opposite the change in the A-VO_2 content difference. If the cardiac output drops, the A-VO_2 content difference should increase. Since there is not usually a big change in SaO_2, the arterial content generally stays the same, and most of the change is seen in the venous content. In this example, if the cardiac output drops, it is expected that the SvO_2 also will drop. The arterial-venous oxygen difference and venous saturation are good markers for the cardiac component in oxygen transport.

The clinical tool available to assess the pulmonary component of oxygenation is the venous admixture equation ("shunt fraction"). This model assumes that the pulmonary circulation is a two-compartment model where one compartment does not see gas-exchanging surfaces ("shunt") and a second compartment sees gas-exchanging surfaces (Fig 5–49). The alveolar oxygen tension is calculated from the alveolar air equation, and the assumption is made that the capillary pO_2 equals the alveolar pO_2. This allows for a calculation of capillary content. The arterial and venous contents are known from the arterial and mixed venous blood gas samples. This model assumes that the oxygen obtained from the inspired gas plus the oxygen that is obtained from the venous return equals the oxygen in the arterial system.

Patients with infiltrative lung disease or collapsed airways will have a large Q_S/Q_T. By opening alveoli and increasing gas-exchanging surfaces, PEEP should decrease Q_S/Q_T and improve arterial oxygenation. A normal Q_S/Q_T is approximately 5%. The average Q_S/Q_T for a first-day postoperative patient in the ICU is roughly 15%. Significant impairment in lung function is seen with a Q_S/Q_T in excess of 25%.

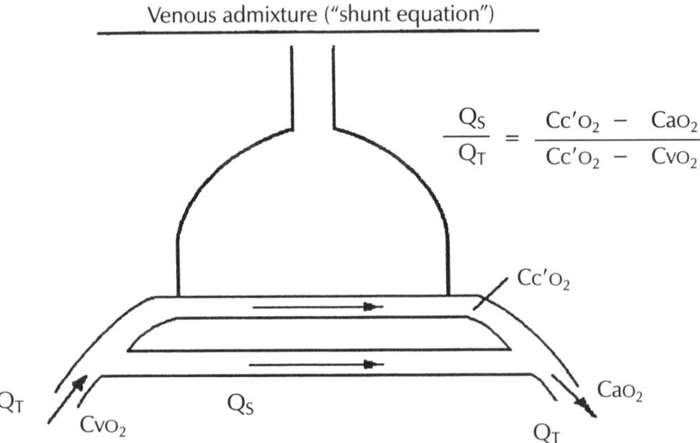

FIG 5–49
Measurement of shunt flow. The oxygen carried in the arterial blood equals the sum of the oxygen carried in the capillary blood and that in shunted blood. (From West JB: *Respiratory Physiology—The Essentials,* ed 2. Baltimore, Williams & Wilkins, 1982, p 56. Used by permission.)

Patients whose hypoxemia is refractory to increases in FIO_2 have large Q_S/Q_T values (Fig 5–50). With a 10% Q_S/Q_T, small changes in FIO_2 result in marked changes in arterial PO_2. When the shunt fraction approaches 40% to 50%, there is very small change in the PaO_2 with large changes in FIO_2.

As the Q_S/Q_T increases, a greater percentage of the arterial oxygen comes from the venous side of the circulation. These lungs are very dependent on venous oxygen transport, and marked decreases in venous oxygen tension and saturation will result in decreases in arterial oxygen saturation and content (Fig 5–51). Augmentation of cardiac output may be more efficacious in raising arterial PO_2 than trying to increase PEEP in these patients with markedly diminished SvO_2. Figure 5–52 shows the effect of changes in the A-VO_2 content

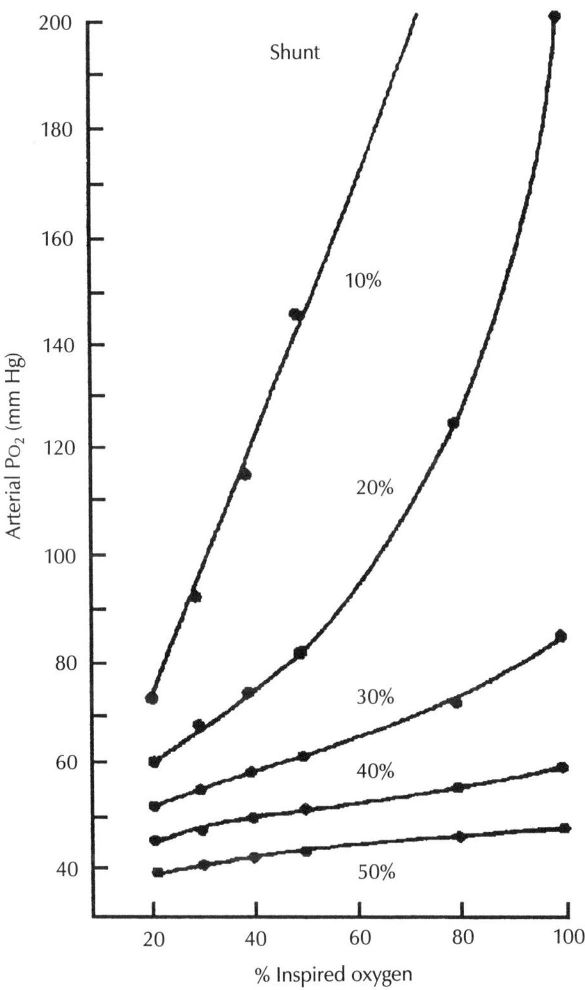

FIG 5–50
Relationship between arterial pO_2 and FIO_2 with different shunt fractions. As Q_S/Q_T increases, the change in pO_2 for a given change in FIO_2 decreases. (From Dantzker DR: *Clin Chest Med* 1982; 3:57–67. Used by permission.)

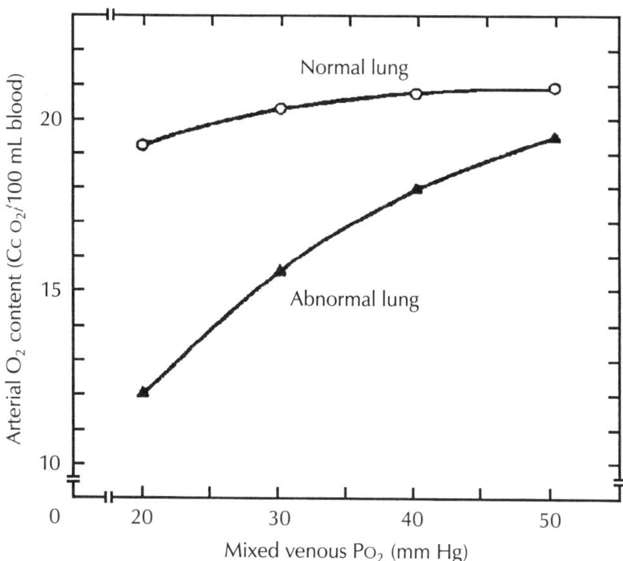

FIG 5–51
Relationship between arterial oxygen content and mixed venous oxygen tension. Q_S/Q_T = 40% in this abnormal lung. As the Q_S/Q_T value increases, a greater percentage of the arterial oxygen content is determined by the venous oxygen return. (From Dantzker DR: Gas exchange in acute lung injury, in *Critical Care Clinics: Acute Lung Injury.* Philadelphia, WB Saunders, 1986, pp 527–536. Used by permission.)

difference on Sa_{O_2} with different Q_S/Q_T values. As the shunt fraction increases, the arterial saturation becomes more and more dependent on the cardiac output and the A-V_{O_2} content difference. In patients who have a wide A-V_{O_2} content difference, intravenous dobutamine may be better than increasing PEEP to improve arterial oxygenation.

TABLE 5–18
Effects of Treatment Modalities on Cardiac and Pulmonary Function

Treatment	Heart	Lungs
PPV	– or ↓ CO, Sv_{O_2} – or ↑ A-V_{O_2}	↓ WOB* (V_{O_2}) ↓ Q_S/Q_T – or ↑ V_D/V_T ↑ barotrauma risk
PEEP/CPAP	– or ↓ CO, Sv_{O_2} – or ↑ A-V_{O_2}	↑ FRC (↓ WOB) ↓ Q_S/Q_T ↑ Sa_{O_2}, ↓ F_{IO_2}
Fluids	↑ CO, Sv_{O_2} ↓ A-V_{O_2}	– or ↑ pulmonary edema – or ↑ Q_S/Q_T
Dobutamine	↑ CO, Sv_{O_2}	No direct effects

* CO = cardiac output. WOB = work of breathing.

Putting It All Together

Table 5–18 outlines the effects of our therapeutic modalities on the heart and the lungs. Positive-pressure ventilation will decrease the work of breathing and decrease total oxygen consumption related to respiratory work. By better expanding the lung, arterial oxygenation is expected to improve. On higher levels of positive-pressure ventilation, dead space volume may increase, and the patient is at a higher risk for barotrauma. The heart, unless the patient is hypovolemic, may not see any adverse effects of positive-pressure ventilation until the level of positive pressure is quite high, and then the cardiac output may be impaired and result in a decrease in Sv_{O_2} and an increase in the A-V_{O_2} content difference.

PEEP and CPAP will improve pulmonary function by increasing the FRC, which will decrease the work of breathing and should also decrease Q_S/Q_T by opening up collapsed airways. This should result in an improvement

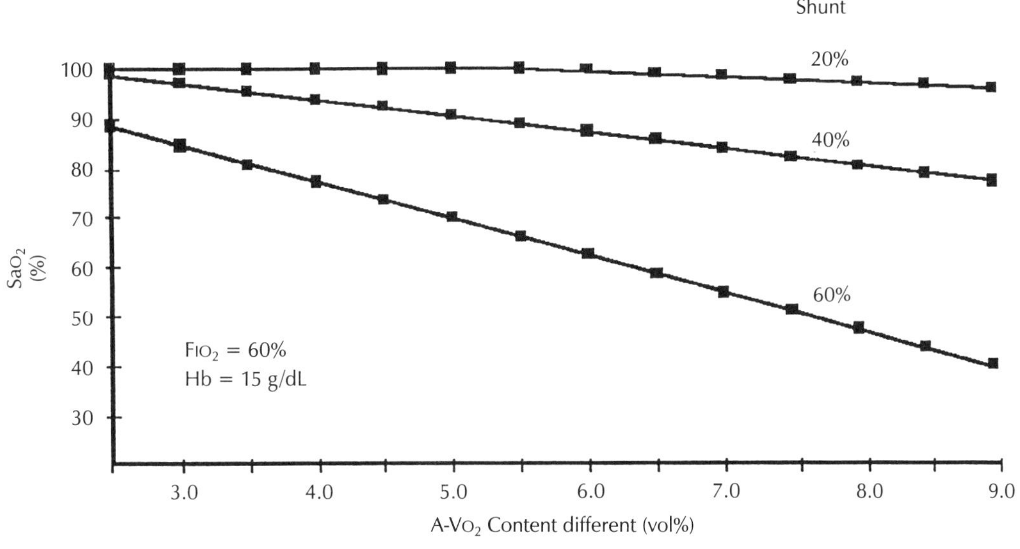

FIG 5–52
Relationship between Sa_{O_2} and A-V_{O_2} content difference, with F_{IO_2} and Hb kept constant. For large Q_S/Q_T values, increases in the A-V_{O_2} content difference will result in a decrease in Sa_{O_2}. Increasing cardiac output and decreasing A-V_{O_2} will increase Sa_{O_2} in patients with high Q_S/Q_T values.

in Sa_{O_2}. Lower levels of PEEP are not expected to have an effect on cardiac function, but as the end-expiratory pressure increases, the possibility for hemodynamic embarrassment also increases. With the exception of patients who are hypervolemic, fluid administration is likely to improve cardiac function and narrow the A-V_{O_2} content difference. This fluid may result in higher pressures in the pulmonary vasculature and potentiate a flux of fluid into the pulmonary interstitial space, which may be seen as or worsen pulmonary edema. In these patients an increase in shunt fraction may be seen. Although dobutamine is very effective in increasing inotropy and thus increasing cardiac output and decreasing the A-V_{O_2} content difference, it has no direct effect on pulmonary function.

The management of patients with acute respiratory failure, especially ARDS, must take into account all the effects of the different therapeutic modalities to ensure that oxygen delivery to the tissues is improved. A physiologic approach to these patients would be to use as much positive-pressure ventilation as necessary to decrease the work of breathing to an acceptable level and to use enough PEEP to decrease the F_{IO_2} to nontoxic levels, generally felt to be in the 50% to 60% F_{IO_2} range. Fluids are used to treat hypovolemia, although to maximize lung function, the circulation should be kept as dry as the heart will tolerate. If cardiac function is compromised by the positive-pressure ventilation and the patient is adequately volume-loaded, dobutamine should be used to augment cardiac function.

A pulmonary artery catheter, especially one with oximetric capabilities, is extremely helpful in managing these patients. As each maneuver is made, the effects on S_AO_2, SvO_2, Q_S/Q_T, cardiac output, and the A-V_{O_2} content difference can be measured. With the addition of a pulse oximeter, Sa_{O_2} and Sv_{O_2} can be measured continuously in these patients. Rasanen et al.[53] showed that estimation of Q_S/Q_T by the ventilation/perfusion index (VQI) allowed for titration of CPAP therapy in critically ill patients by using dual oximetry alone. A mathematical model can estimate partial pressures from the observed saturations, and the A-V_{O_2} content difference and Q_S/Q_T can be calculated very accurately from saturations alone (Acevedo R, unpublished data, 1991). The VQI, while being a very accurate trender of Q_S/Q_T, underestimates the Q_S/Q_T because of the assumption that all the partial pressures are zero.

The Baxter-Edwards explorer has a Nelcor oximeter along with its oximetric pulmonary artery catheter; this unit does on-line dual oximetry. It will measure Sa_{O_2}, Sv_{O_2}, and VQI and will estimate the oxygen extraction index on a continuous basis. Clinical studies are ongoing to assess the usefulness of this technology in treating patients with severe respiratory failure and ARDS.

Clinical Examples

Case 1

A 43-year-old woman was seen in the ICU, and a diagnosis of severe gram-negative pneumonia was made. The physical examination and x-ray findings were consistent with ARDS with a Q_S/Q_T of 50% and a requirement of 90% F_{IO_2} to maintain arterial saturation in the low 90% range. The patient was initially placed on 5 cm of PEEP. Throughout the first 24 hours, the PEEP was increased to try to improve her oxygenation and decrease the F_{IO_2} (Figure 5–53). We were asked to be involved because, by morning, the physicians "could not get her F_{IO_2} below 90%." Figure 5–54 shows that the PEEP was effective in dropping the Q_S/Q_T from 50% down to 30%, but it also increased the A-V_{O_2} content difference from just over 2 vol% up to 5 vol%. The improvement in lung function from the PEEP was completely offset by the decrease in cardiac output and O_2 delivery. Even though the lungs were using the inspired gas better, the amount of venous oxygen return to the lungs was markedly diminished with the net result of no change in arterial oxygenation.

At 10:00 hours, fluids and dobutamine were administered, with improvement in cardiac output and the A-V_{O_2} content difference. Even though the Q_S/Q_T did not change, the arterial saturation improved to the point that the patient was able to be weaned from 90% F_{IO_2} down to 60% F_{IO_2}. This is an example when inotropic support, instead of PEEP, was the best approach to treat hypoxemia.

Case 2

A 52-year-old woman had terminal cancer and hepatic failure. At the patient's prior request, mechanical ventilatory support was removed. At the arrow in Figure 5–54, she was changed from an SIMV of 10 and 40% F_{IO_2} to CPAP and room air. As expected, her arterial saturation dropped as well as her venous saturation. What was unexpected was that shortly afterward both of these parameters returned to baseline. Our initial impression at the bedside was that the Sv_{O_2} drop was due to her heart starting to fail as a result of the hypoxemia. By looking at both the Sv_{O_2} and Sa_{O_2} graphically it appeared that the A-V_{O_2} content difference was relatively well preserved (Figure 5–55). It looks like the drop in Sa_{O_2} occurred first, followed by a drop in Sv_{O_2}, which is why the A-V_{O_2} content difference dropped initially and then became wider. The low A-V_{O_2} content difference was felt to be the result of hepatic failure. Once the patient stabilized, there was

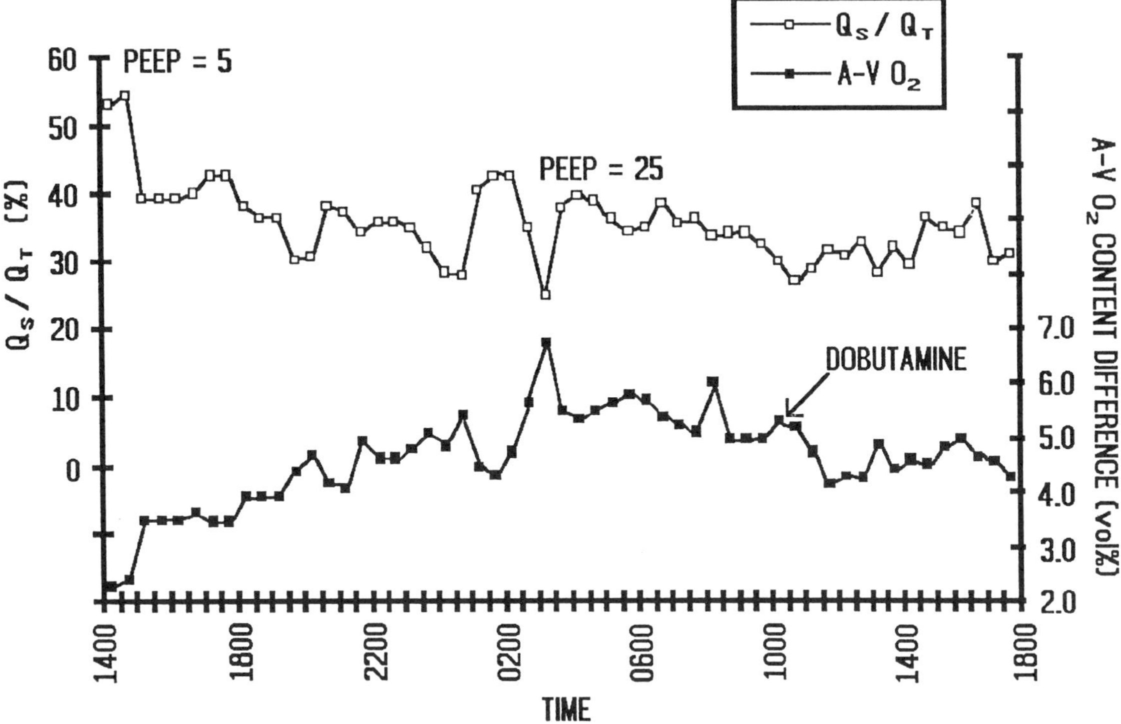

FIG 5–53
Case 1: Qs/QT and A-Vo_2 content difference trends in a patient with ARDS and cardiac compromise from positive-pressure ventilation (see the text).

no significant change in the A-Vo_2 content difference.

The marked changes in Qs/QT are what was of interest. She was controlled on the ventilator at a rate of 10, and when the rate was turned down to zero, this, in all likelihood, created a ventilation/perfusion mismatch where areas were being perfused but not well ventilated. This would worsen oxygenation and function as an increase in Qs/QT. As she picked up her own minute ventilation with her spontaneous breaths, she improved her ventilation/perfusion relationships closer to baseline so that by the end of the time frame in Figure 5–55, her Qs/QT and A-Vo_2 content difference were both fairly close to baseline. This demonstrated that the heart functioned better than what was initially suspected and that there was a transient change in pulmonary function that reverted close to baseline after a short period of time. It would be very difficult to sort out the physiology with just Svo_2 alone. Dual oximetry with continuous Qs/QT and A-Vo_2 content difference determinations may be helpful in defining hypoxemia from a cardiac or pulmonary standpoint. More investigation is needed to assess this monitoring tool.

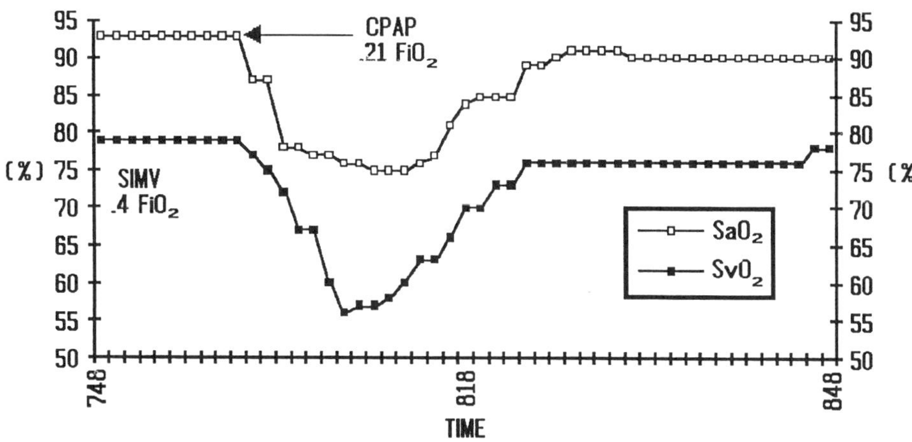

FIG 5–54
Case 2: dual oximetry in the patient in Figure 5–53 in whom mechanical support was withdrawn. Initial desaturation on the venous side was felt to be due to arterial desaturation and a failing, hypoxic heart (see the text).

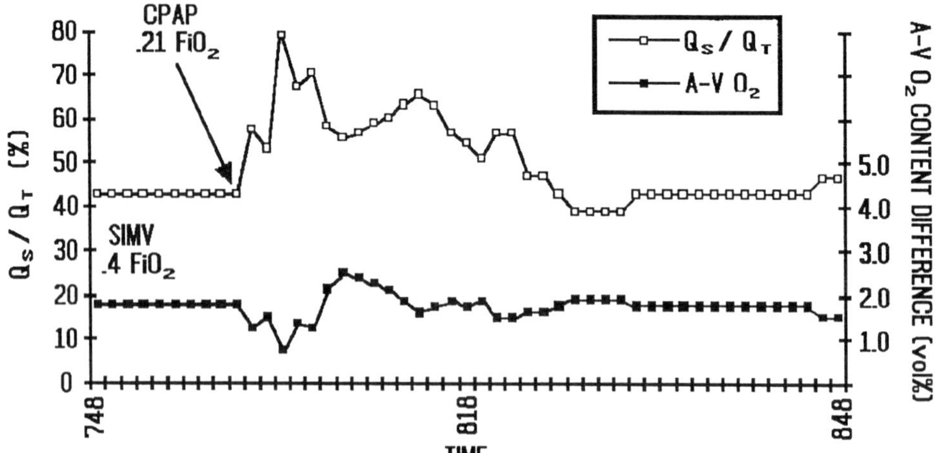

FIG 5–55
Case 2: Qs/QT and A-Vo_2 content difference trends show preserved cardiac function and marked transient impairment of pulmonary function. The low A-Vo_2 content difference was felt to be due to her hepatic failure (see the text).

Barotrauma

Gas escaping from the lungs during mechanical ventilation is a well-known complication of mechanical ventilation. If the gas tracks medially, the visible radiographic findings of pneumomediastinum and pneumoperitoneum may be seen. On examination subcutaneous emphysema may be appreciated. For a majority of patients these complications are of little clinical significance. If the gas tracks laterally, pneumothoraces may occur and, if formed under tension, can cause hemodynamic compromise and collapse. Tension air cysts may prevent the surrounding lung from adequately expanding and worsen lung function. Interstitial gas under pressure can rupture into pulmonary venules and cause systemic gas emboli, with possible myocardial and cerebrovascular damage.[54]

High peak airway pressures, requirements for high levels of PEEP, and the underlying pulmonary pathology are all risk factors for barotrauma. Presently data are emerging that look at alveolar volume and peak airway pressure as causes of ventilator-induced lung injury.[55] These animal models had a diffuse lung injury and edema that looked morphologically like ARDS.

Gattinoni et al.[56] demonstrated by computed tomographic (CT) scans that patients with ARDS may have regional overdistension if conventional tidal volumes are used. They showed that lung compliance was related to the amount of aerated lung that was contributing to ventilation and that the compliance of that aerated lung was relatively normal. This implies that patients with ARDS who have a low lung compliance may have only a small amount of functional lung tissue that is receiving a major percentage of the conventional tidal volumes. This would result in overdistension of these alveoli and thus ventilator-induced barotrauma. By increasing the PEEP in these patients, the amount of aerated lung tissue increases and distributes the tidal volume over a larger lung volume, thus decreasing overdistension.

Hickling et al.[55, 57] have addressed the question of our present high-volume, high-pressure management of ARDS being a cause of the persistent high mortality with that disease. They report a series of 50 patients with severe ARDS managed by reducing tidal volume, allowing spontaneous breathing with an SIMV circuit, and permitting hypercapnia. They attempted to keep the peak airway pressure less than 30 cm H_2O but always less than 40 cm H_2O. The hospital mortality rate in this group was significantly lower than what would have been predicted by Apache II (16% vs. 39.6%, $P < .001$).[57]

Marcy and Marini[58] reviewed the role of inverse ratio ventilation (IRV) in keeping peak airway pressure down. By prolonging the inspiratory time and adding PEEP, these authors were able to increase the mean airway pressure and improve oxygenation while not increasing peak airway pressure. IRV is used when therapeutic end points cannot be obtained with conventional ventilation.

Another maneuver to keep the peak airway pressure down is the use of high-frequency positive-pressure ventilation. This can be done on conventional microprocessor ventilators, where the goal is to drop the tidal volume down to approximately 4 to 5 cc/kg and increase the respiratory rate to the 40 to 60 range to maintain minute ventilation.

Permissive hypercapnia is well tolerated by patients without hemodynamic embarrassment. It may be necessary to support the pH with judicious use of bicarbonate or other buffering agents. These studies would suggest that maintaining a lower peak airway pressure is probably of greater benefit to patients than maintaining a "normal" Pco_2.

Figure 5–56 is a review of the maneuvers to decrease peak airway pressure. More clinical research is

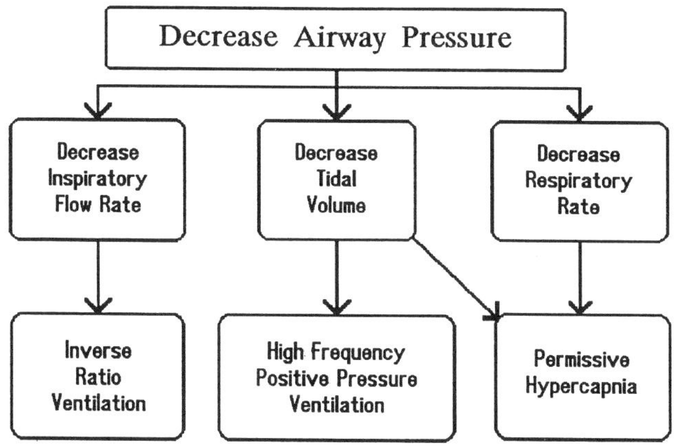

FIG 5–56
Maneuvers to decrease peak airway pressure and reduce the risk of barotrauma.

necessary to further define the usefulness of these procedures.

MODES OF VENTILATION

Negative-Pressure Ventilation

The present-day negative-pressure ventilators have eliminated many of the problems associated with the older models. They are simple devices and are very easy for home use. They improve chest compliance so that the patient has to draw a smaller negative pressure to move the same tidal volume. They are inexpensive, and as the health care dollar gets tighter, it is likely that more of this type of ventilation will be used in the home setting. If the patient does not require an airway for pulmonary toilet, the system can run without an endotracheal tube (Table 5–19)

The biggest drawback to this system is that it is unable to generate large tidal volumes with noncompliant lungs. It works very well in patients who have neuromuscular weakness or chronic obstructive lung disease, but it is not very effective for patients with acute pneumonia or an acute consolidative process. If copious secretions are present, an endotracheal tube may still be necessary for management.

TABLE 5–19
Negative-Pressure Ventilation

Advantages
- Simple devices
- Inexpensive
- Easy to use at home
- Does not require an airway

Disadvantages
- Secretions may necessitate an endotracheal tube
- Unable to generate large tidal volumes with noncompliant lungs

Control Mandatory Ventilation

In this mode the ventilator does all the work. It gives full ventilatory support and is quite effective in resting fatigued muscles. The demand valve is not initiated, so there is no work associated with it. Because this is all positive pressure, ventilation preload to the heart will be decreased. In hypervolemic patients this mode of ventilation can serve as a mechanical preload reducer. In volume-depleted patients a significant amount of hemodynamic embarrassment would be expected. A conscious patient does not like to be controlled. Heavy sedation or paralysis may be necessary in order to control the patient. Even with our "state-of-the-art" monitoring system, disconnection is still a problem and a risk to the patient. Since the patient has no input into the system, this mode of ventilation does not adjust to changes in the patient's clinical status. In a patient who is controlled at a rate of 10 and then becomes febrile, which increases CO_2 production, the hypercapnia will not be known unless routine blood gas studies are performed (Table 5–20).

Because the ventilator is doing all the work, prolonged periods on controlled ventilation may result in respiratory muscle atrophy. Barotrauma risk is increased with all positive-pressure breathing.

Assist/Control Ventilation

This is another mode of full ventilatory support, and it has advantages similar to those of control ventilation. In addition, by allowing the patient control over the respiratory rate, the need for sedation and paralysis is markedly decreased. In addition, this mode of ventilation will change as the patient's clinical status changes. If the patient is stable on an assist/control backup rate of 10 while breathing 20 times a minute and fever develops, the respiratory rate can be increased to 25 or 30 breaths per minute, with the machine delivering full tidal volume breaths with each initiation. This mode will serve as a

TABLE 5–20
Control Ventilation

Advantages
- Full ventilatory support
- Rests fatigued muscles
- Preload reduction in volume-overloaded patients
- Eliminates work of initiating demand volume

Disadvantages
- Patients do not like to be controlled!
- Sedation or paralysis necessary at times
- Disconnection risk (less now due to alarms)
- Preload reduction in volume-depleted patients
- Does not adjust to changes in clinical status
- Possible respiratory muscle atrophy
- Barotrauma risk

preload reducer in volume-overloaded patients and will rest fatigued muscles as long as the patient and the ventilator are in synchrony (Table 5–21).

As with control ventilation, preload reduction in volume-depleted patients may cause hemodynamic embarrassment. In a large number of these patients, respiratory alkalosis will develop, with a pH that can approach 7.48 to 7.50. This rarely becomes a problem clinically, and if the respiratory alkalosis is unacceptably high, switching to an SIMV/IMV circuit solves the problem.

Once a demand valve is added to the mode, it has its own set of possible complications. If the patient has a very fast inspiratory flow (i.e., severe acidosis, hypoxemia, high intracranial pressure), the patient may trigger the system appropriately at approximately 1 to 2 cm H_2O pressure. However, in the time that it physically takes for the valve to open, the patient may have drawn back an additional 5, 10, or 15 cm H_2O of negative pressure against the closed valve before it has had a chance to open. This markedly increases the work of breathing and negates one of the major advantages of being on full ventilatory support. Options to manage this problem include controlling the patient either by increasing the mandatory minute ventilation or by sedating the patient and treating the underlying cause of the high flow rate.

If the sensitivity is too high, the machine will sense nonrespiratory fluctuations, assume they are initiations, and hyperventilate the patient. These are patients who are breathing 30 to 40 times a minute with very severe respiratory alkaloses but who, on examination, appear quite comfortable and not in respiratory distress. I have seen pH values in the 7.6 to 7.7 range only with the ventilator hyperventilating the patient because of an oversensitive valve.

If the sensitivity is too low, the patient has to draw a greater negative pressure to initiate the machine, and this increases the work of breathing and further negates the major advantage of this mode of ventilation.

TABLE 5–21
Assist/Control Ventilation

Advantages
- Full ventilatory support
- Rests fatigued muscles
- Preload reduction in volume-overloaded patients
- Patient initiation decreases the need for sedation or paralysis
- Will respond to changes in clinical status

Disadvantages
- Preload reduction in volume-depleted patients
- Respiratory alkalosis
- Possible complications of demand volume
  - High inspiratory flow leading to increased work of breathing
  - Sensitivity too low leading to increased work of breathing
  - Sensitivity too high leading to hyperventilation

Intermittent Mandatory Ventilation Modes

By allowing spontaneous ventilation, IMV modes can give partial ventilatory support. The specific advantages of partial ventilatory support come with spontaneous breathing; therefore, to realize this, the patient must do a significant amount of spontaneous ventilation (Table 5–22).

With less positive pressure ventilation, less hemodynamic embarrassment and a lower risk for barotrauma are expected. With a more physiologic ventilation/perfusion relationship and less zone 1 and 2 ventilation, both oxygenation and CO_2 elimination should be more efficient. A continuous-flow IMV system is a system entailing lower work of breathing than SIMV; however, the SIMV system offers better monitoring and synchrony with the patient.

The cost of the advantages of partial ventilatory support is the increased work of breathing of the respiratory muscles. While there may be some conditioning of the respiratory muscles, if the amount of work that the muscles are required to do is excessive, the respiratory muscles may fatigue. The patient may go into ventilatory failure while on an SIMV/IMV circuit if the minute ventilation work required of the respiratory muscles is more than what they are able to handle. This is not a fault of the mode of ventilation but rather a problem resulting from having inadequately low levels set.

This mode of ventilation does not adjust to changes

TABLE 5–22
Intermittent Mandatory Ventilation

Advantages
- SIMV and IMV
  - Allows spontaneous ventilation
  - Less hemodynamic embarrassment
  - Respiratory muscle conditioning
  - More efficient ventilation
  - Lower airway pressure leading to decreased barotrauma
- IMV
  - Continuous-flow system leading to low work of breathing
- SIMV
  - Demand value leading to better monitoring and synchrony

Disadvantages
- SIMV and IMV
  - Increased work of breathing
  - Potential for respiratory muscle fatigue
  - Does not adjust to changes in clinical status
- IMV
  - Unable to monitor values on-line, asynchrony
- SIMV
  - Work associated with the demand value

TABLE 5–23
Pressure Support Ventilation

Advantages
Supports spontaneous work of breathing
Low airway pressures leading to decreased barotrauma risk
Less hemodynamic embarrassment
Compensates for work of the endotracheal tube
Better assessment of spontaneous ventilation
Allows facemask ventilation
Comfort!
Disadvantages
Requires a microprocessor machine (expensive)
System leaks result in "endless inspiration"

in the patient's clinical status. If a patient is stable on an SIMV of 10 per minute with a total respiratory rate of 20 per minute but then becomes febrile and the rate increases to 25 or 30 per minute, the additional 5 to 10 breaths per minute are spontaneous, and the total work is done by the patient. The ventilator solely gives the patient access to gas for this extra ventilation.

While the increase in work due to the demand valve is a specific disadvantage for the SIMV mode, this work can be compensated by the addition of PSV.

Pressure Support Ventilation

This mode of ventilation can deliver partial ventilatory support in addition to full ventilatory support. McIntyre[59] defines full ventilatory support on PSV (PSV_{max}) as enough PSV to maintain a spontaneous tidal volume of 10 to 12 mL/kg. As a mechanism of delivering partial ventilatory support, this mode of ventilation has the same advantages imparted with spontaneous ventilation. In addition, it can be used to compensate for the work of the endotracheal tube and, in this way, not expose the patient to some of the additional work of the ventilator system. A more accurate assessment of spontaneous ventilation may be CPAP plus PSV enough to compensate for the endotracheal tube (Table 5–23).

Brochard et al.[60] described a system whereby PSV can be administered by means of a tight-fitting face mask for short-term noninvasive ventilation. This is quite useful for short-term episodes of bronchospasm and for acute pulmonary edema.

Another major advantage of this mode is that patients tend to find this a comfortable method of ventilation. This may be because patients are never fully exposed to the work mandated by their pulmonary insufficiency. Pressure support ventilation is only available on the newer microprocessor machines, which cost more than those of prior generations.

For long-term ventilated patients with tracheostomies, PSV cannot be used with a leaking system. The ventilator has trouble sensing the drop in inspiratory flow through the leak, and inspiration continues until one of the alarms is triggered.

TABLE 5–24
High-Frequency Positive-Pressure Ventilation

Advantages
Lower airway pressures
Maintains ventilation in ARDS patients on high PEEP
Less hemodynamic embarrassment
Disadvantages
Easier on microprocessor machines
Frequently requires sedation or paralysis
Less efficient ventilation
Jet
Risk of obstruction to exhalation
Limited experience

High-Frequency Positive-Pressure Ventilation

Additional information is available in Chapter 6. On a conventional ventilator, high-frequency positive-pressure ventilation can be accomplished by setting the tidal volume to 4 to 5 mL/kg and the respiratory rate in the 40- to 60-per-minute range. This will allow ventilation at lower airway pressures and decrease the potential risk of barotrauma. The earlier-generation ventilators had trouble maintaining this performance, whereas the microprocessor machines do this effortlessly. Patients find this a very uncomfortable mode of ventilation, and sedation or paralysis is frequently necessary. The dead space/tidal volume ratio is quite high in these patients, which results in less efficient ventilation. In almost all of these instances, patients were controlled, which makes efficiency less of a problem (Table 5–24).

Ventilating a patient on a jet ventilator is further on in the same continuum. Jet breaths are of a small tidal volume, and rates are generally between 100 and 150 breaths per minute. Both peak airway pressure and mean airway pressure are quite low. Obstruction to exhalation is a serious problem and, if not recognized quickly, can have very serious effects. Everybody who works in a unit that has a jet ventilator needs to be aware that if there are problems with the jet, the patient needs to be removed from the ventilator and manually ventilated while the problems are sorted out. Many smaller nonuniversity ICUs may not have enough patients who are appropriate for jet ventilation in order to keep their staff proficient and to justify the cost of the jet ventilator.

Inverse Ratio Ventilation

This mode of ventilation still needs to be thought of as investigational. The major advantage of inverting the I:E

TABLE 5–25

Inverse Ratio Ventilation

Advantages
- Lower airway pressures
- Helpful in ARDS
- VC* IRV
  - Available on all ventilators
  - Minute ventilation controlled
  - Flow patterns controlled
- PC* IRV
  - Peak airway pressure controlled

Disadvantages
- VC IRV
  - Less strict peak airway pressure control
- PC IRV
  - Variable tidal volumes
  - Variable minute ventilation, less control over P_{CO_2}

* VC = volume cycled; PC = pressure cycled.

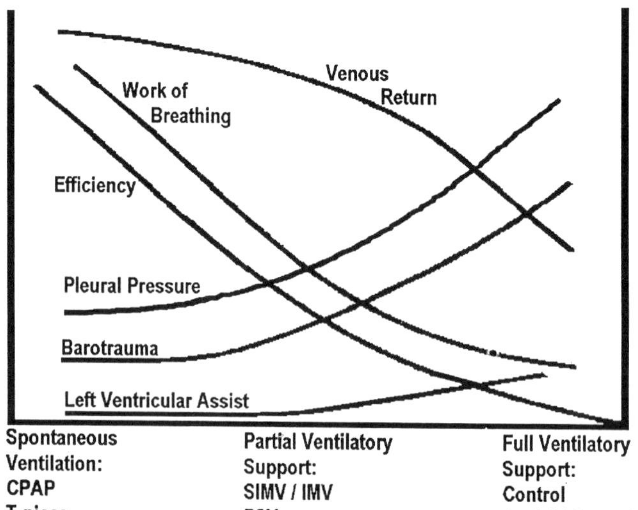

FIG 5–57
Spectrum of modes of ventilation as they affect cardiopulmonary physiology. (Adapted from Snyder JVL: *Curr Probl Surg* 1984; 21:43. Used by permission.)

ratio is to decrease the peak airway pressure while maintaining an adequate mean airway pressure. This may be of some benefit in patients with established ARDS. Both volume-cycled and pressure-cycled ventilators can administer IRV. Most adult ventilators are able to do volume-cycled IRV. This guarantees a minute ventilation and gives the clinician precise control over the flow pattern (Table 5–25).

Since the peak airway pressure is the dependent variable in this system, the pressures must be monitored carefully. Pressure-cycled IRV is available only on some ventilators. With this system, the peak airway pressure can be tightly controlled. Since the tidal volume is the dependent variable, the patient's minute ventilation must be monitored carefully. If the patient is permitted to become hypercapnic, close monitoring of minute ventilation is less of a problem.

CONCLUSION

In deciding what methods of ventilation are most appropriate for an individual patient, the beneficial and adverse effects of positive-pressure ventilation need to be evaluated. Figure 5–57 shows each of these effects as the degree of positive-pressure ventilation is increased. As the patient moves from spontaneous breathing to partial ventilatory support and then to full ventilatory support, there is an increase in pleural pressure, which results in a decrease in venous return. This, coupled with the effects on right ventricular function, may result in a decrease in cardiac output and blood pressure. As the amount of positive pressure increases, the work of breathing drops, as does the efficiency of ventilation. This is not a major problem since the ventilator is doing the bulk of the work and the inefficiency is not being transferred to the patient. When the machine is assuming most of the work of breathing by positive-pressure ventilation, it also exposes the patient to a greater risk of barotrauma. Increases in pleural pressure reduce left ventricular afterload and, under certain circumstances, may augment left ventricular ejection.

If the patient is unable to handle the work of breathing, full ventilatory support is needed. If the patient is able to handle some of the work of breathing, the benefits of spontaneous ventilation may outweigh the increased work of breathing. The actual mode of ventilation that the patient is placed on is less important than the physiology behind how much positive pressure the patient is exposed to. As far as barotrauma and circulatory embarrassment are concerned, it does not make a difference whether the patient is on control ventilation, assist/control ventilation, or a very high SIMV/IMV rate where the machine is doing almost all of the work. The clinician needs to individualize the mechanical support to the patient. The goal is to supply adequate mechanical ventilation for control of the patient's work of breathing while not exposing the patient to excessive amounts of hemodynamic embarrassment or barotrauma. A thorough understanding of the physiology behind mechanical ventilation will facilitate the clinician in making these decisions.

REFERENCES

1. Pilbeam SP: Selecting modes and initial settings, in Pilbeam SP (ed): *Mechanical Ventilation: Physiological*

and Clinical Applications, ed 2. St Louis, Mosby–Year Book, 1992, pp 165–213.

2. Barnes TA: Emergency ventilation techniques and related equipment. *Respir Care* 1992; 37:673–690.
3. American Society for Testing and Materials: *Standard Specification for Performance and Safety Requirements for Resuscitators Intended for Use With Humans. Designation: F-920-85.* Philadelphia, American Society for Testing and Materials, 1985.
4. Standards and guidelines for cardiopulmonary resuscitation (CPR) and emergency cardiac care (ECC). *JAMA* 1986; 255:2841–3044.
5. Guidelines for cardiopulmonary resuscitation and emergency cardiac care, Emergency Cardiac Care Committee and subcommittees, American Heart Association. *JAMA* 1992; 268:2171–2302.
6. International Organization for Standardization: *International Standard ISO 8382:1988 (E)—Resuscitators Intended for Use With Humans.* New York, American National Standards Institute, 1988.
7. Eubanks DH, Bone RC: Cardiopulmonary resuscitation, in Eubanks DH, Bone RC (eds): *Comprehensive Respiratory Care: A Learning System,* ed 2. St Louis, Mosby–Year Book, 1990, pp 638–639.
8. Elling R, Politis J: An evaluation of emergency medical technicians' ability to use manual ventilation devices. *Ann Emerg Med* 1983; 12:765–768.
9. Hess D, Varan C: Ventilatory volumes using mouth-to-mouth, mouth-to-mask, and bag-valve-mask techniques. *Am J Emerg Med* 1985; 3:292–296.
10. Cummins RO, Austin D, Graves JR, et al: Ventilation skills of emergency medical technicians: A teaching challenge for emergency medicine. *Ann Emerg Med* 1986; 15:1187–1192.
11. Johanningman JA, Branson RD, Davis K Jr, et al: Techniques of emergency ventilation: A model to evaluate tidal volume, airway pressure, and gastric insufflation. *J Trauma* 1991; 31:93–98.
12. Fuerst RS, Banner MJ, Melker RJ: Inspiratory time influences the distribution of ventilation to the lungs and stomach: Implications for cardiopulmonary resuscitation. *Ann Emerg Med,* in press.
13. Jesudian MC, Harrison RR, Keenan RL, et al: Bag-valve-mask ventilation: Two rescuers are better than one: Preliminary report. *Crit Care Med* 1985; 33:122–123.
14. Pearson W, Redding JS: Evaluation of the Elder demand valve resuscitator for use by first-aid personnel. *Anesthesiology* 1967; 28:623–624.
15. Osborn HH, Kayen D, Horne H, et al: Excess ventilation with oxygen-powered resuscitators. *Am J Emerg Med* 1984; 2:408–413.
16. Melker RJ, Banner MJ: Positive pressure and spontaneous ventilation characteristics of demand-flow valves: Implications for resuscitation. *Ann Emerg Med,* in press.
17. Chatburn RL: A new system for understanding mechanical ventilators. *Respir Care* 1991; 36:1123–1155.
18. Kacmarek RM, Mack CW, Dimas S: Technical aspects of mechanical ventilators, in Kacmarek RM, Mack CW, Dimas S (eds): *The Essentials of Respiratory Care,* ed 3. St Louis, Mosby–Year Book, 1990, pp 472–500.
19. Hayes B: Ventilation and ventilators. *J Med Eng Technol* 1982; 6:177–192.
20. Loh L, Venn PJH: Classifying mechanical ventilators. *Br J Hosp Med* 1987; 38(5):466–470.
21. Smallwood RW: Ventilators—classifications and their usefulness. *Anaesth Intensive Care* 1986; 14:251–257.
22. Young JD, Sykes MK: Artificial ventilation: History, equipment and techniques. *Thorax* 1990; 45:753–758.
23. Dupuis YG: *Ventilators: Theory and Clinical Application,* ed 2. St Louis, Mosby–Year Book, 1992.
24. McPherson SP: *Respiratory Therapy Equipment,* ed 4. St Louis, Mosby–Year Book, 1990.
25. Spearman CB, Sanders HG Jr: Physical principles and functional designs of ventilators, in Kirby RR, Banner MJ, Downs JB (eds): *Clinical Applications of Ventilatory Support.* New York, Churchill Livingstone, 1990, pp 63–104.
26. Mushin WW, Rendell-Baker L, Thompson PW, et al: *Automatic Ventilation of the Lungs,* ed 3. Oxford, Blackwell Scientific Publications, 1980, pp 101–103, 225.
27. Chatburn RL, Primiano FP Jr: Mathematical models of respiratory mechanics, in Chatburn RL, Craig KC (eds): *Fundamentals of Respiratory Care Research.* East Norwalk, Conn, Appleton & Lange, 1988, pp 59–100.
28. Day S, MacIntyre NR: Ventilator alarm systems. *Probl Respir Care* 1991; 4:118–126.
29. Weingarten M: Respiratory monitoring of carbon dioxide and oxygen: A ten year perspective. *J Clin Monit* 1990; 6:217–225.
30. Kacmarek RM, Meklaus GL: The new generation of mechanical ventilators. *Crit Care Clin* 1990; 6:551–578.
31. Kacmarek RM, Meklaus GL: Microprocessor controlled mechanical ventilators. *Probl Crit Care* 1990; 4:161–183.
32. Pilbeam SP: Physical aspects of mechanical ventilation, in Pilbeam SP (ed): *Mechanical Ventilation: Physiological and Clinical Applications,* ed 2. St Louis, Mosby–Year Book, 1992, pp 95–163.
33. Suzukawa M, Usada Y, Numata K: The effects on sputum characteristics of combining an unheated humidifier with a heat-moisture exchanging filter. *Respir Care* 1989; 34:976–984.
34. Kirby RR: IMV held satisfactory alternative to assisted, controlled ventilation. *Clin Trends Anesthesiol* 1976; Nov-Dec, p 4.
35. Bolder PM, Hedy TEJ, Bolder ER, et al: The extra work of breathing through adult endotracheal tubes. *Anesth Analg* 1986; 65:853–859.
36. Katz JA, Kraemer RW, Gjerde GE: Inspiratory work and airway pressure with continuous positive airway pressure delivery systems. *Chest* 1985; 88:519–526.
37. Fiastro JF, Habib MP, Quan SF: Pressure support compensation for inspiratory work due to endotracheal tubes and demand continuous positive airway pressure. *Chest* 1988; 93:499–505.

38. Snyder JV, Carroll GC, Schuster DP, et al: Mechanical ventilation: Physiology and application. *Curr Probl Surg* 1984; 21:57.
39. West JB: *Respiratory Physiology: The Essentials.* ed 2. Baltimore, Williams & Wilkins, 1982.
40. Remolina C, Khan AU, Santago TV, et al: Positional hypoxemia in unilateral lung disease. *N Engl J Med* 1981; 304:523–525.
41. Fishman AP: Down with the good lung. *N Engl J Med* 1981; 304:537–538.
42. Sibbald WT, Drieger AA, Myers ML, et al: Biventricular function in the adult respiratory distress syndrome. Hemodynamic & radionuclide assessment, with special emphasis on right ventricular function. *Chest* 1983; 84:126–134.
43. Sibbald WJ, Drieger AA: Right ventricular function in acute disease states: Pathophysiologic considerations. *Crit Care Med* 1983; 11:339–345.
44. Shippy CR, Appel PL, Shoemaker WC: Reliability of clinical monitoring to assess blood volume in critically ill patients. *Crit Care Med* 1984; 12:107–112.
45. Miro AM, Pinski MR: Hemodynamic effects of mechanical ventilation, in Tobin MJ, Grenvik A (eds): *Contemporary Management in Critical Care,* vol 1, *Mechanical Ventilation and Assisted Respiration.* New York, Churchill Livingstone, 1991, pp 73–90.
46. Pinsky MR, Marquez J, Martin D, et al: Ventricular assist by cardiac cycle–specific increases in intrathoracic pressure. *Chest* 1987; 91:709.
47. Stein K, Kramer D, Schlichtig R, et al: Effect of intrathoracic pressure (ITP) on ventricular performance during acute mitral regurgitation (abstract). *Am Rev Respir Dis* 1989; 139:22.
48. Killian A, Stein K, Guthrie RD, et al: Cardiac augmentation by cardiac cycle specific increases in intrathoracic pressure in a model of neonatal heart failure (abstract). *Am Rev Respir Dis* 1989; 139:21.
49. Snyder JV, Powner DJ: Effects of mechanical ventilation on the measurement of cardiac output by thermodilution. *Crit Care Med* 1982; 10:677–682.
50. Pepe PE, Marini JJ: Occult positive end expiration pressure in mechanical ventilator patients with airflow obstruction. *Am Rev Respir Dis* 1986; 126:166–170.
51. Brown DG, Pierson DJ: Auto-PEEP is common in mechanically ventilated patients: A study of incidence, severity and detection. *Respir Care* 1986; 31:1069–1074.
52. Scott LR, Benson MS, Bishop MJ: Relationship of endotracheal tube size to auto-PEEP at high minute ventilation. *Respir Care* 1986; 31:1080–1082.
53. Rasanen J, Downs JB, Dehaven B: Titration of continuous positive airway pressure by real time dual oximetry. *Crit Care Med* 1987; 15:395.
54. Marini JJ, Culver B: Systemic gas embolism complicating mechanical ventilation in the adult respiratory distress syndrome. *Ann Intern Med* 1989; 110:699–703.
55. Hickling KG: Ventilatory Management of ARDS: Can it affect the outcome? *Intensive Care Med* 1990; 16:219–226.
56. Gattinoni L, Pesenti A, Avalli L, et al: Pressure-volume curve of total respiratory system in acute respiratory failure. Computed tomography study. *Am Rev Respir Dis* 1987; 136:730–736.
57. Hickling KG, Henderson SJ, Jackson R: Low mortality associated with low volume pressure limited ventilation with permissive hypercapnia in severe adult respiratory distress syndrome. *Intensive Care Med* 1990; 16:372–377.
58. Marcy TW, Marini JJ: Inverse ratio ventilation in ARDS: Rationale and implementation. *Chest* 1991; 100:494–504.
59. MacIntyre NR: Weaning from mechanical ventilatory support: Volume-assisting intermittent breaths vs. pressure-assisting every breath. *Respir Care* 1988; 33:121–125.
60. Brochard L, Isabey D, et al: Reversal of acute exacerbation of COPD by inspiratory assist with face mask. *N Engl J Med* 1990; 232:1523–1529.

6

Nonconventional Mechanical Ventilation

ERIC GLUCK, M.D.
DAVID H. EUBANKS, Ed.D, R.R.T.

OBJECTIVES

- Discuss the operation and application of the various high-frequency ventilators on the basis of their operational characteristics.
- Differentiate between the bidirectional jet high-frequency ventilator and other high-frequency jet models.
- Compare the intravascular oxygenation (IVOX) and extracorporeal CO_2 removal ($ECCO_2R$) as to operational characteristics, sites for anatomic connection, and physiologic benefits.
- Explain the clinical inclusions and exclusions for use of a diaphragmatic pacer for assisted ventilation.
- Point out the advantages and disadvantages to using high-frequency ventilation, bidirectional jet ventilation, IVOX and $ECCO_2R$, and diaphragmatic pacing for supporting a patient's ventilation.

A review of the literature spanning the last 15 years indicates that there are four major concerns with traditional convective-type ventilator delivery systems[1]:

1. Undesirable influence of intermittent positive pressure on cardiac function
2. Inability to easily adopt new and special modifications
3. Inability to achieve desired oxygen and carbon dioxide levels with conventional ventilatory methods
4. Lung injuries that are precipitated by the use of conventional ventilators

Unconventional ventilators are defined as devices that do not provide ventilation or gas exchange according to usual or customary methods.

This chapter will present unconventional cardiopulmonary devices that are on the cutting edge of medicine and therefore in some cases may still be in various stages of clinical investigation.

High-frequency ventilation (HFV), bidirectional jet ventilation, intravascular oxygenation (IVOX), extracorporeal carbon dioxide removal ($ECCO_2R$), and diaphragmatic pacing will be discussed from the research and clinical perspective.

HIGH FREQUENCY VENTILATION

HFV is a generic term that describes various modes of mechanical ventilation using breathing rates greater than three times normal,[2] tidal volumes smaller than normal, and a ventilator circuit with negligible compressible volume.[3] The U.S. Food and Drug Administration (FDA) classifies any ventilator operating at a cycling rate of 150 beats per minute or any jet ventilator regardless of cycling frequency as a high-frequency device.[4]

An overview of the three general modes of HFV are presented below:

1. High frequency positive-pressure ventilation (HF-PPV) employs a time-cycled, positive-pressure, constant-volume ventilator with a low–compressible volume breathing circuit and a small tidal volume[4] (calculated dead space) at cycling rates of 60 to 100 breaths per minute.

2. High-frequency oscillatory ventilation (HFOV)[5] employs a piston, diaphragm, pump, or high-fidelity speaker to generate high-frequency pressure oscillations from 900 to 3,000 breaths per minute (50 Hz) with tidal volumes estimated to range from 5 to 80 mL. Both inspiration and exhalation are actively generated by the ventilator.

3. High-frequency jet ventilation (HFJV) is a subset of the high-frequency flow interrupter (HFFI) controlled by an electromechanical (solenoid) or fluidic cycling system to deliver small bursts of gas of 100 to 200 ms through an injector jet to the proximal or distal tip of an indwelling airway catheter tube at frequencies of 100 to 900 breaths per minute. Tidal volumes are small, usually 3 to 5 mL/kg of body weight.

Ideal High-Frequency Ventilator

Simon and Mitzner[5] describe the ideal HFV as having a wide range of frequency, easily controlled and reproducible tidal volume, minimum equipment dead space, independently controlled mean airway pressure of lung volume, variable inspiratory-to-expiratory time ratio (I:E ratio), and an effective high internal impedance.

History of High-Frequency Ventilation/ Oscillation

The first high-frequency oscillator (HFO) in the United States was designed and patented by John Emerson[6] in 1959 (Fig 6–1) as "an apparatus for vibrating portions of a patient's airway." Clinically, HFV was first reported by Butler et al. in 1980.[7]

Sjöstrand and other Scandinavian investigators[8] around 1969 began to report on a new form of mechanical ventilation for adults that incorporated breathing frequencies of 60 to 90 breaths per minute and small tidal volumes (V_T) of 200 to 300 mL. In order to deliver these unique ventilatory parameters, a special valve was attached to a time-cycled HFPPV with a small-volume and low-compression breathing circuit. In 1980 Carlon and his associates initially reported on the first clinically successful use of the HFJV.[9]

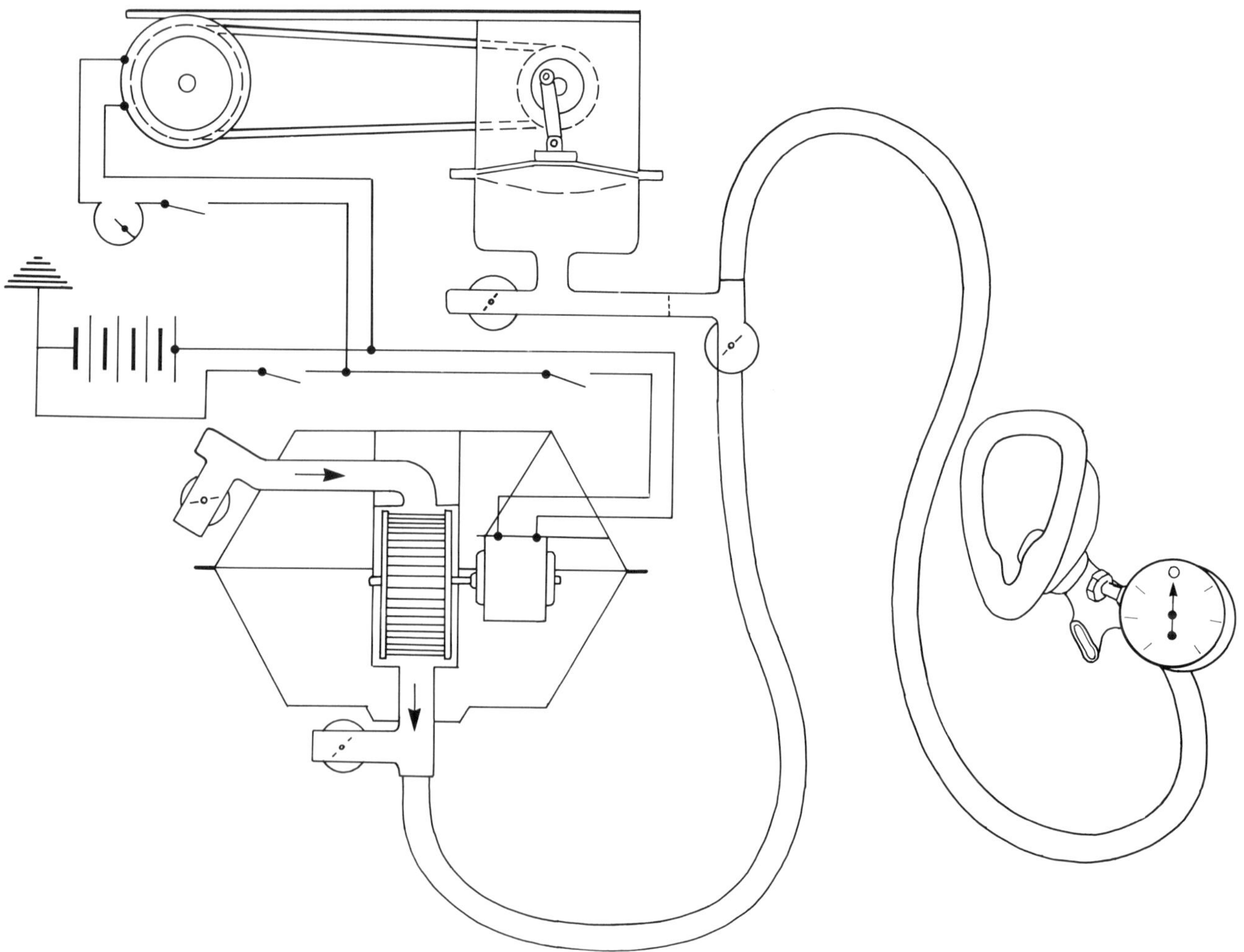

FIG 6–1
Emerson's high-frequency oscillator—"an apparatus for vibrating portions of a patient's airway." A rapidly cycling diaphragm *(26)* causes rapid oscillations to occur in the patient breathing circuit *(18)*.

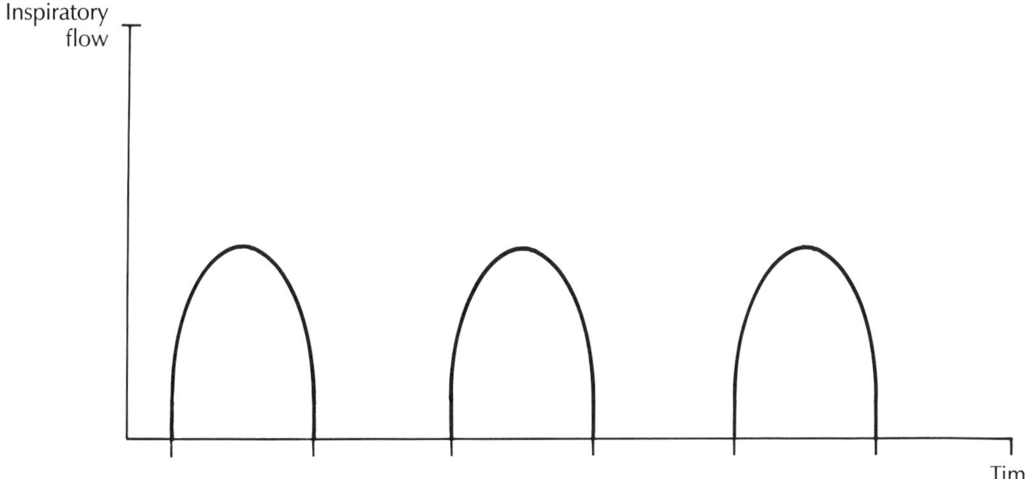

FIG 6–2
Sinusoidal inspiratory waveform as generated by a high-frequency oscillator.

Even though over 300 articles were published on HFV for the period of 1975 to 1985, only Carlon and his group approached their investigation as a randomized clinical trial.[10] Since Carlon and associates' report in 1980, more recent reports of HFV vs. conventional ventilation in randomized clinical trials include Hurst and his associates in 1990[11] and a multicenter trial by the OCTAVE Study Group[12] of the John Radcliffe Maternity Hospital and Oxford Region Hospitals.

High Frequency Oscillation

As was previously explained, HFO can be delivered by reciprocating pumps, cycling diaphragms, or oscillating high-fidelity speakers that rythmatically generate an approximate sinusoidal waveform (Fig 6–2). With HFOV the ventilator pushes gas into the lung on inspiration and withdraws it during exhalation. This type of active exhalation theoretically enhances the removal of CO_2 and prevents breath stacking leading to auto–positive end-expiratory pressure (auto-PEEP).[13] Cycling frequencies are from 1 to 15 Hz (900 cpm), and small tidal volumes are delivered at or at less than anatomic dead space. During inspiration a continuous flow of fresh gas is available at the proximal end of the endotracheal tube to flush out CO_2 and provide the desired fraction of inspired oxygen (F_{IO_2}).

HFO has been used in infants and adults with varying degree of success.[13–17] In infants, oxygenation is improved and carbon dioxide eliminated with relative ease when using HFO or HFJV.[18] However, in adults, carbon dioxide elimination remains a problem that clinicians are attempting to handle by building hybrid ventilators that can deliver a combination of HFV breaths that are superimposed on or interdispersed between conventional mechanical breaths (Fig 6–3). The VDR Oscillatron-1 amplifier device by Bird (Sand Point, Idaho) will be presented later in this section as an example of a unique device that enables the operator to convert a conventional ventilator to an HFO.

Gas Exchange Mechanisms With High-Frequency Oscillation

After nearly three decades of investigation the exact mechanisms by which HFV accomplishes gas exchange are still not clear. It is well documented that during spontaneous breathing or mechanical breaths by conventional ventilation, gas transport within the airways is primarily by convection (bulk flow) at the level of the upper airways and molecular diffusion at and below the level of the terminal bronchioles (at approximately the 17th bifurcation).[19]

The fact that CO_2 elimination can be achieved with HFO-delivered tidal volumes that are less than those of the calculated dead space defies the laws of respiratory physiology that state that, based on convective ventilation, in order for adequate alveolar ventilation to occur the individual must receive a tidal volume approximately three times that of the anatomic dead space, or 12 to 15 mL/kg of body weight. This is not the case with HFO, where tidal volumes are normally set at 5 to 80 mL.

Obviously gas exchange in the lung is dependent on more than just the size of the tidal volume. Froese and Bryan[1] have described six possible mechanisms that have an influence on CO_2 transport during HFO:

1. Bulk convection: Ventilation of alveoli that are directly exposed to the gas flow or receive contact via short bronchiolar pathways.

2. Pendelluft: Bulk movement of gas within the lung from fast-filling and fast-emptying units into slower units. Lehr et al. called this gross phase lag between the filling and emptying of lung regions "disco lung."[20]

3. Taylor dispersion: An application of the work by

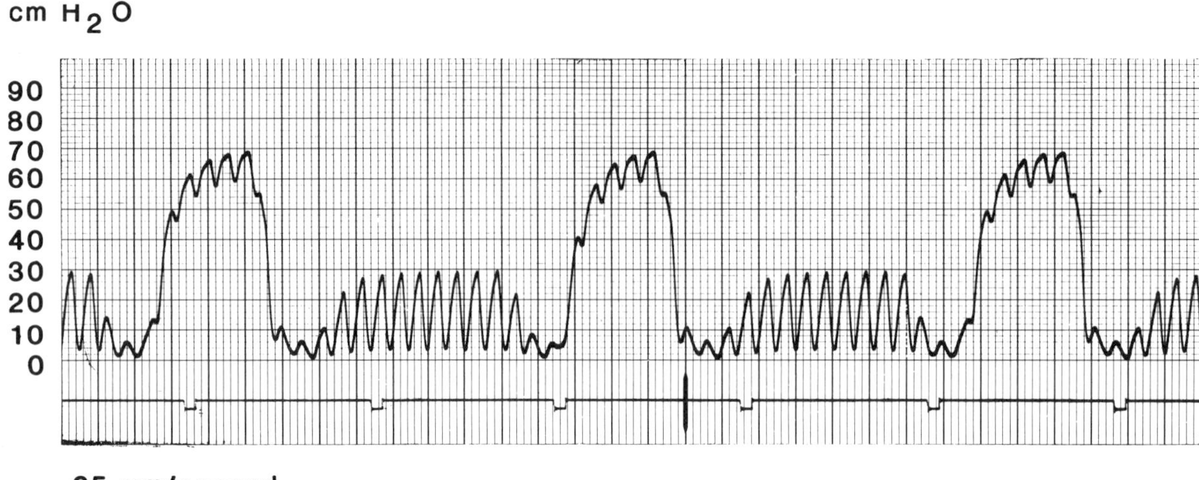

FIG 6–3
The use of oscillatory-demand continuous positive airway pressure during (high peak pressure) conventional tidal volume delivery will provide an oscillatory plateau decreasing the potential for barotrauma. (Courtesy of Percussionaire Corp., Sand Point, Idaho.)

Taylor[21] who showed that in laminar flow when a convective flow is superimposed on a diffusive process, there will be an increased dispersion of gas molecules by both radial and convective dispersion. As radial dispersion occurs, convective dispersion is reduced because the molecules in the central zones of higher axial velocity diffuse to the lateral zones of lower velocity, which impedes axial gas transport.

4. Asymmetrical velocity profiles: A theory by Hazelton and Scherer[22] that net convective transport of gas is accomplished as a result of the variance caused by the fact that in a straight tube the velocity profile during aspiration is parabolic and flat in the reverse direction. This mechanism may explain gas flow at bifurcations where the inspiratory gas profile is forced near the inner wall and the expiratory profile remains symmetrical. This asymmetrical profile may also explain how inspiration and exhalation may occur simultaneously during HFV.

5. Cardiogenic mixing: Enhancement of peripheral gas mixing caused by the vibrations of a beating heart—a sort of naturally occurring brownian motion.

6. Molecular diffusion: The prominent mechanism for gas movement in the terminal regions of the lung.

Research has shown that control of Pa_{CO_2} depends primarily on two factors: oscillatory flow into the lungs and the flow rate of fresh gas into the system. Mathematically, this may be explained by the following formula:

$$CO_2 \text{ elem } \alpha \text{ (f)} \times V_T \times 2 \text{ } (fV_T^2).^{23}$$

If the system is not provided with adequate fresh gas flow, rebreathing of carbon dioxide will occur. Banner[23] cites a report where the subject became hypercapnic when the fresh gas flow was reduced by 66% even though the frequency and V_T were held constant.

Oxygenation With High-Frequency Oscillators

Oxygenation during HFV indicated that pendelluft plays an even greater role in intrapulmonary gas mixing than it does in conventional ventilation.[19] Asymmetry profiles as explained above may contribute to gas mixing but could not be quantitated by Klocke et al.[19]

Taylor dispersion in turbulent flow is one of the primary factors for improved gas mixing.[19] In Klocke and associates' investigation of HFV, molecular diffusion exhibited little influence on gas transport and in fact played a much greater role in conventional ventilation than in HFV. Fredberg,[24] using a theoretical model, demonstrated in HFO that augmented diffusion was most influential in achieving gas transport in the central airways and that molecular diffusion was predominate at the alveolar level.

Slutsky et al.[25] noted from their work that in HFO the amplitude of the oscillatory flow, independent of frequency and stroke volume, is most significant in maintaining alveolar gas exchange.

As was stated at the beginning of this section, there are still conflicting theories as to the mechanisms that interact to provide adequate gas exchange with HFV.

One explanation that appears to summarize all the theories of gas exchange is the one given by McCarthy and Dillard III.[4] In their explanation, "airflow profiles whether oscillatory or not can be described as a continuum with turbulent flow at one extreme and laminar flow at the other extreme." In HFO, oscillatory flow causes gas exchange along this continuum that enables the alveoli to receive fresh oxygen and eliminate carbon dioxide.

Froese and Bryan[1] in their investigation were able to arrive at the conclusion that even though HFV is able to eliminate carbon dioxide by novel methods, oxygenation is still best achieved by using sufficiently high levels of PEEP or mean airway pressure to recruit for maximum oxygenation.

Evolution of the VDR Oscillatron-1 Amplifier

In 1979, Forrest M. Bird developed a new ventilatory technology called intrapulmonary percussive ventilation (IPV).* This technology incorporated the administration of aerosol and extrathoracic percussion into a small mechanical device.

As the name IPV implies, this device delivered percussion from within the airways as compared with the traditional chest physiotherapy technique (CPT) that applied clapping (percussion) and vibration to the outside of the thorax. Percussive impact frequencies could be programmed from approximately 100 to 200 cpm with the force of the percussion controlled by an adjustable pressure reduction valve. This unit, which was initially conceived as a viable substitute for intermittent positive-pressure breathing (IPPB) and CPT techniques, was expanded to evolve into a family of more sophisticated devices for use as short-term and continuous life support ventilators that delivered volumetric diffusive respiration (VDR).

These VDR devices were unique when compared with conventional mechanical ventilators because they could be programmed to initially deliver every form of

*The authors wish to thank Dr. Bird for his contribution to this section of the chapter. Dr. Bird is the founder, owner, and president of Percussionaire, Sand Point, Idaho.

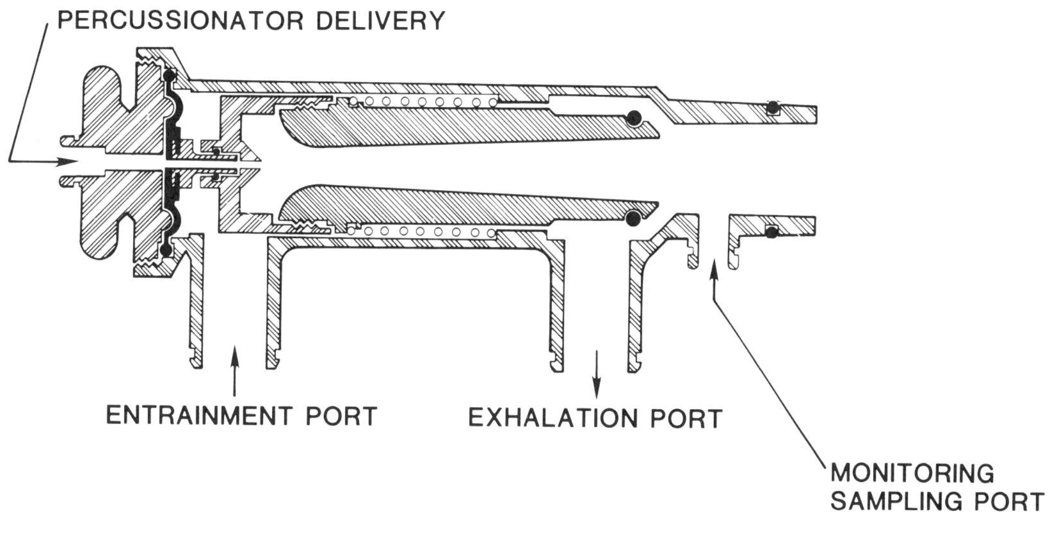

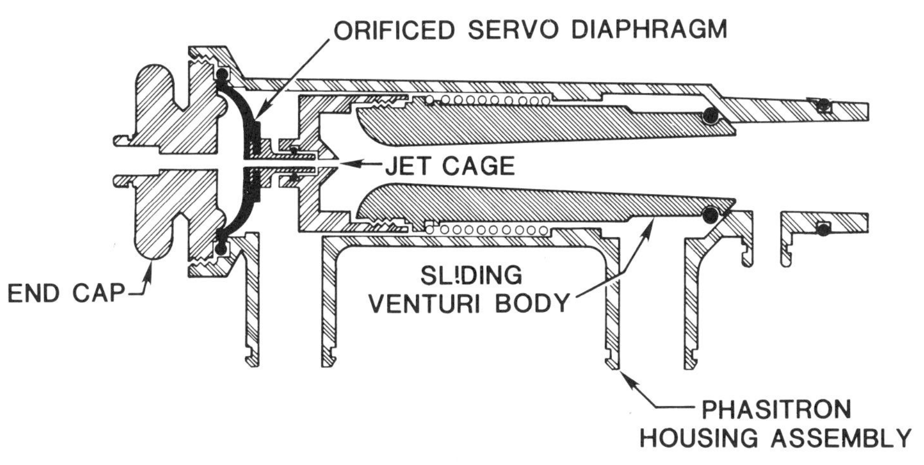

FIG 6–4
Open and closed Phasitron unit—a key operational unit that provides the physiologic mechanical interface between the percussive device and the patient. (Courtesy of Percussionaire Corp., Sand Point, Idaho.)

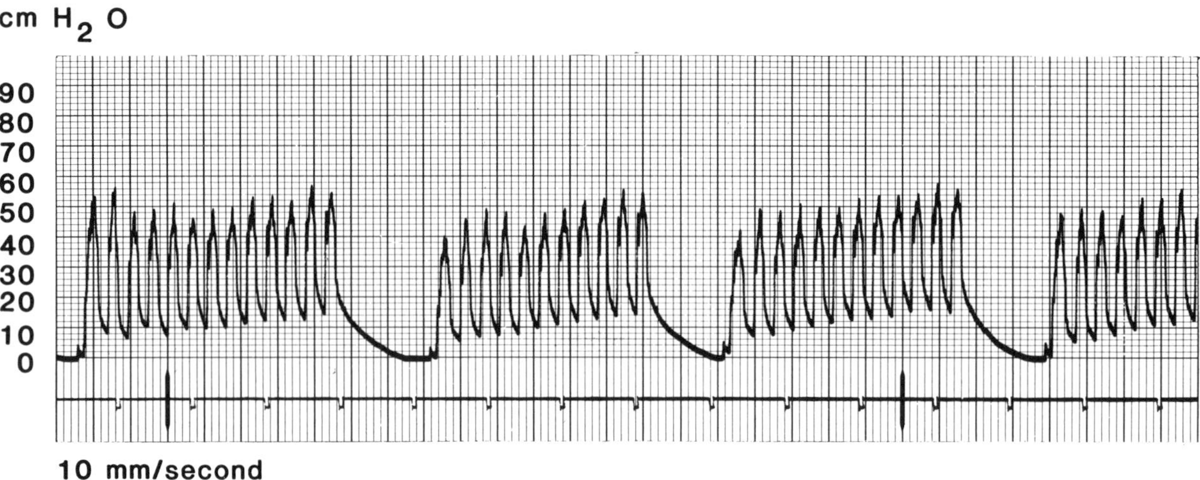

FIG 6–5
This classic intrapulmonary percussive ventilation static percussive waveform modified by dynamic flow against actual pulmonary structures resulted in a mean intrapulmonary wedge pressure of 10 cm H_2O. (Courtesy of Percussionaire Corp., Sand Point, Idaho.)

convective/diffusive ventilation with tidal volumes from 5 to 10,000 mL in a single device. The matrix VDR device allowed for conventional time-cycled intermittent mandatory ventilation (IMV) modes with total independence and/or combined diffusive/convection mechanical ventilation.

The key component in Bird's IPV/VDR devices is the Phasitron (Fig 6–4). This device is described as a physiologic mechanical interface to precisely profile the percussive cycled inflow of gases during the scheduled intrapulmonary mixing interval. By interposing the Phasitron between the percussive device and the patient's airway, a pneumatic clutch is provided to regulate and limit a buffered breath-stacking technique. The proximal airway pressure can be controlled to hold a mean intrapulmonary pressure wedge through which may be programmed repeated, percussive pressure rises followed by a baseline drop (Fig 6–5).

Essentially the lungs are maintained in a partial inspiratory position of function (inflated) while they are internally percussed by a pneumatic force. A peak percussive pressure can be selected that is automatically interrupted every 5 seconds with airway pressure returning to the ambient level.

This Phasitron technology is applied to all of Bird's fourth-generation ventilator devices including the Percussionaire Oscillatron-1 amplifier.

PERCUSSIVE OSCILLATRON-1 AMPLIFIER

The Percussionaire Oscillatron-1 amplifier (Fig 6–6) is a component of the VDR family of diffusive convective

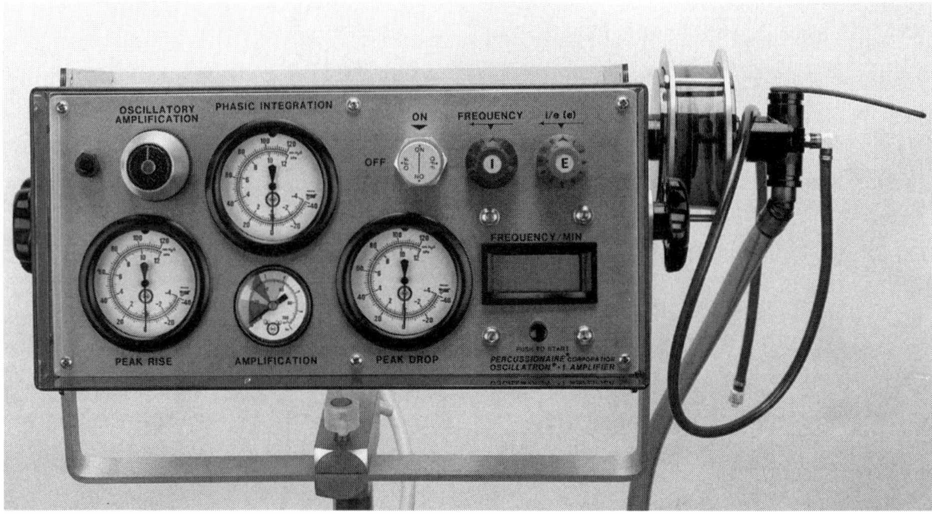

FIG 6–6
Bird VDR Oscillator-1 amplifier control panel. (Courtesy of Percussionaire Corp., Sand Point, Idaho.)

devices for IPV. The purpose of the device is to provide a means for the amplification of intrapulmonary diffusion when attached to a mechanical convective ventilator. Interfacing is accomplished by connecting transmission tubing to the patient's proximal airway Y-piece (Fig 6–7).

The Oscillatron-1 amplifier generates a dynamic percussive (push/pull) oscillation. Potential peak-to-peak pressure generation is factored by the programming of operational pressures (compressed air). With an operational pressure of 50 psig, peak-to-peak pressure potentials are above 100 mm H_2O. As operational pressures are reduced downward to 25 psig, peak-to-peak pressures are condensed toward 25 cm H_2O.

Frequency is determined by variable I:E ratios of from 1:1 to 1:3, which allows the scheduling of cyclic percussive frequencies of 200 to greater than 1,500 cpm.

The novel Oscillatron canister for sub–tidal volume delivery and recovery, with near instantaneous percussive positive/subambient pressure gradient reversal, is energized by the Pneumatic Phasitron, which serves as a fluidic percussive actuator (Fig 6–8). Therefore, the percussive pressure gradient transition is analog in nature, thus greatly decreasing the potential for barotrauma.

The Oscillatron-1 amplifier provides for operational ease with only three control knobs (Fig 6–9). One for percussive amplification (inspiratory flow rate) and another for I:E ratio programming used in conjunction with the third knob for frequency selection.

The direct monitoring of percussive potentials is presented on four conventional gauge/manometers. A color-coded gauge displays the programmed operational pressure (amplification) in pounds per square inch and/or bars. One manometer presents the peak cyclic pressure rise in centimeters of H_2O and kiloposcals; another, the peak pressure drop; and yet another, the integrated phasic pressure change over the mechanically programmed inspiratory and expiratory schedules.

When the Oscillatron-1 amplifier slaves a convective mechanical ventilator, it does not change the primary mass flow gradients in and out of the pulmonary structures. The Oscillatron-1 employs the programmed convective flow gradients of the enslaved ventilator as a carrier, which is modulated by attaching a percussive pressure rise and drop (through the transporting pressure waves) at the programmed frequency and amplitude (Fig 6–10). The percussive wave format can be symmetrical or asymmetrical (depending on I/E), with the carrier serving as a reference base line.

The greater the peak-to-peak pressure differential, the greater the percussive impact upon intrapulmonary gas flows. It follows that the greater the intra-airway mechanical gas mixing, the greater the intrapulmonary diffusion.

The propensity for the percussive wave formats to mobilize and then propel endobronchial secretions for cephalad intrapulmonary travel is based on several cardinal factors:

1. The percussive energy is imparted to a transporting positive-pressure carrier within the tracheobronchial tree.

2. The transporting inspiratory flow gradient has the ability to minimize the preferential airway.

3. Maximum endobronchial secretion mobilization is enhanced by the gradual pulsatile inflation of the pulmonary structures followed by a percussive oscillatory postinspiratory plateau (oscillatory equilibrium) to provide air distal to the retained endobronchial secretions. Then, for maximum cephalad secretion propulsion following the period of postinspiratory oscillatory equilibrium, the proximal airway pressurization (serving as a continuous positive airway pressure [CPAP] carrier) must be precipitously reduced to that of the stabilizing expiratory interval baseline. Essentially, a more rapid endobronchial expiratory flow than that produced during the pulsatile inspiratory uploading of the parenchymal structures serves to produce an expiratory mechanical ciliary escalator.

The ability of percussive shock waves to reduce the adhesive properties of endobronchial secretions is not currently known.

As previously cited, HFOs are not new, and their successes and failures have been detailed in countless publications. Many mechanical approaches have been employed to generate high-frequency intrapulmonary shock waves as well as sub–tidal volume delivery and recovery. Mechanically excited diaphragmatic membranes, pistons, solenoids, magnetic servoing of diaphragms (pistons), as well as other methodologies are among the principal means employed for oscillatory generation.

Previously described methods of generating intrapulmonary mechanical oscillation have been plagued with an ever-increasing inadvertent PEEP (mechanical-PEEP) as oscillatory frequency has been accelerated. Additionally, effective sub–tidal volume exchange, at cyclic frequency with an encroachment handicap, is secondary to the rate at which the reversal of inspiratory and expiratory flow gradients occurs. Finally, without a percussive reversal of inspiratory and expiratory flow gradients, the ability to effectively increase intrapulmonary diffusion and provide for endobronchial secretion mobilization, as well as propulsion, has been compromised.

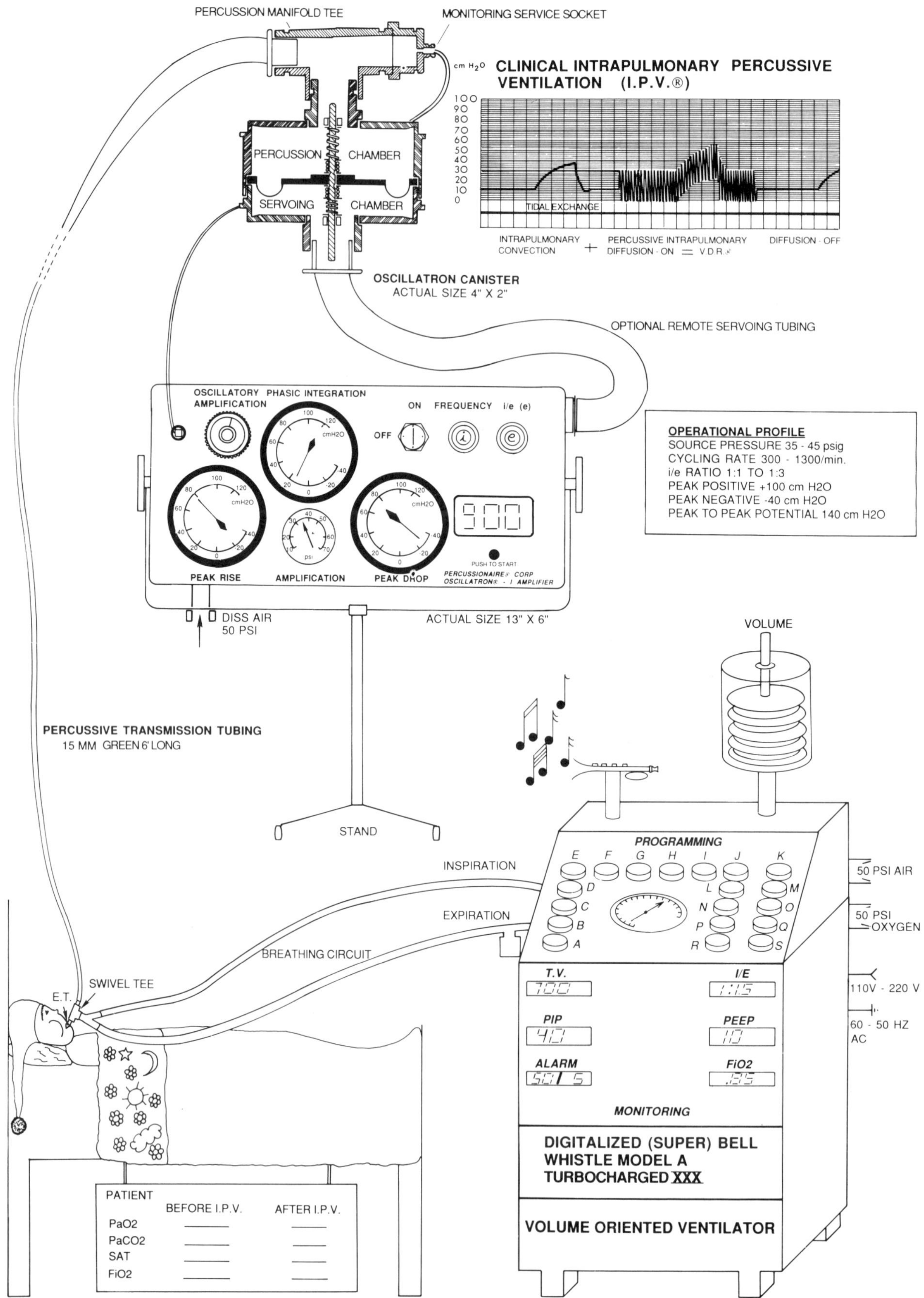

FIG 6–7
Oscillatron-1 amplifier connected to a conventional ventilator to deliver high-frequency oscillation. (Courtesy of Percussionaire Corp., Sand Point, Idaho.)

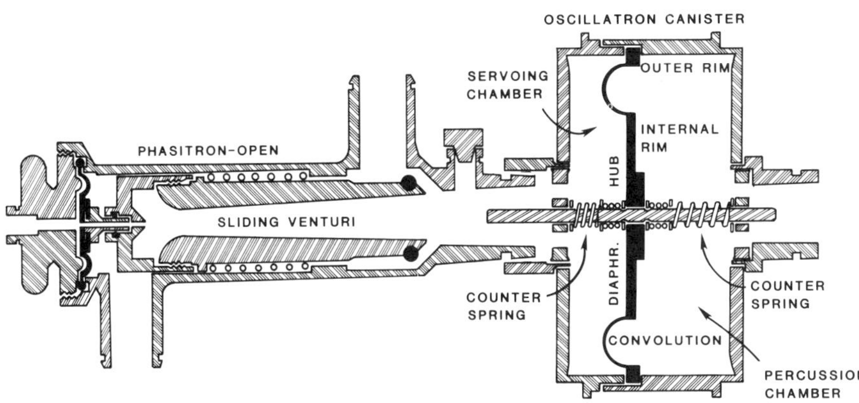

FIG 6–8
The Phasitron servoed canister generates dynamic percussive oscillation. (Courtesy of Percussionaire Corp., Sand Point, Idaho.)

Mechanically induced intrapulmonary diffusion without an adequate convective component to "wash out CO_2" can lead to the patient dying "nice and pink" secondary to metabolic acidosis.

The introduction of three pneumatic components and their integration into a mechanical ventilatory device allowed resolution of mechanical-PEEP penalties, as well as the inspiratory and expiratory flow gradient reversal retardations during high-rate diffusive ventilation.

The pneumatic flow timing logic cell with differential opening and closing pressures enabled a reliable means of flow interruption with (demonstraby) clean pulse generation at frequencies exceeding 3,000 cpm (Fig 6–11).

The Pneumatic Phasitron Monojet Injector/Exhalation Valve, with synchronous functions, reduced the mechanical-PEEP penalties to levels below clinical significance (Fig 6–12).

The advent of the Phasitron servoed pneumatic Oscillatron canister with a novel counterspring design for the servoing of commands eliminated the "state-of-the-art" clinical phase shift penalties associated with the available mechanical means for generating dynamic (push/pull) oscillation (Fig 6–13).

The Oscillatron-1 amplifier is capable of attaching a dynamic (push/pull) modulation to either a constant, ascending, and/or descending continuous or pulsatile carrier wave propagation. Peak-to-peak deflection potentials across the carrier wave can be amplified from 25 to greater than 100 cm H_2O over a wide percussive frequency range.

While the Oscillatron-1 amplifier is a member of the Percussionaire family of VDR devices directed at providing enhanced intrapulmonary percussion during volumetric diffusive respiration, there may be other applications for scheduling percussive diffusion during convective mechanical ventilation of the lung.

The Oscillatron-1 amplifier can be integrated into the VDR-1, 2, 3 or 4 Percussionator (Fig 6–14) and Monitron packages as well as ventilators by other manufacturers. All Percussionaire housings provide for interlocking facility.

General Description of the Oscillatron Features

The Oscillatron-1 is a universal, traditional time-cycled respirator used primarily as a cardiopulmonary intensive care and weaning device. It incorporates an

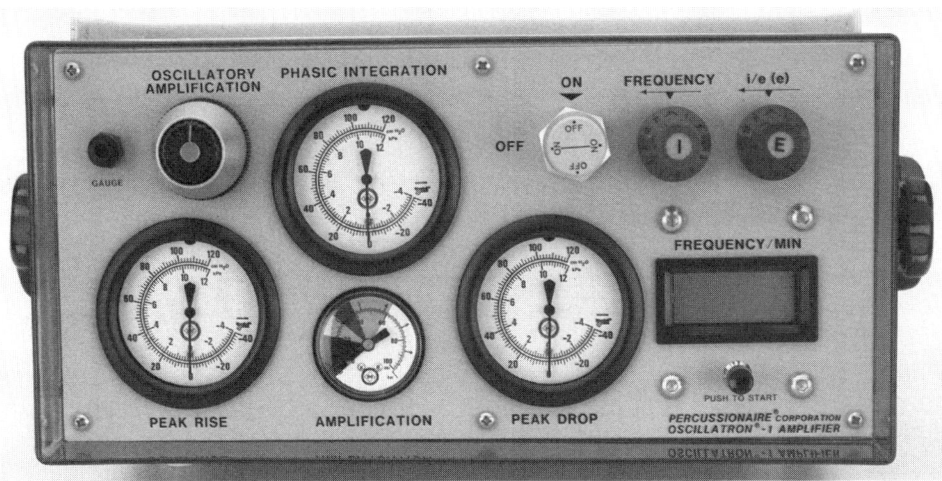

FIG 6–9
Oscillatron-1 amplifier showing three control knobs for ease of operation. (Courtesy of Percussionaire Corp., Sand Point, Idaho.)

A

cm H2O

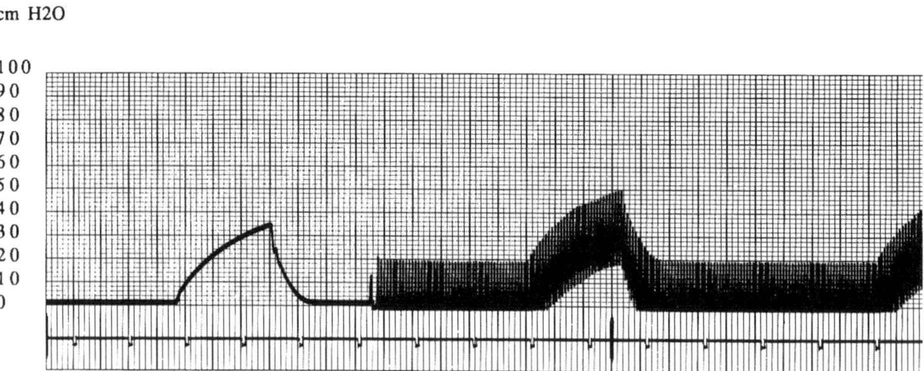

10 mm/sec

B

cm H2O

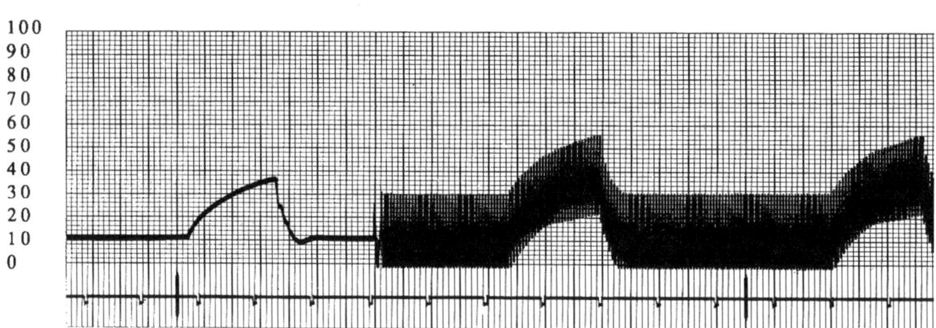

10 mm/sec

FIG 6–10
A, classic conventional mechanical ventilator (CMV) convective carrier for the VDR-3 modulated by percussive oscillation (at a frequency of 1,000 cpm) for the enhancement of intrapulmonary diffusion. **B,** classic CMV format as above, with demand continuous positive airway pressure (CPAP) (PEEP) modulated with the same percussive oscillation. (Courtesy of Percussionaire Corp., Sand Point, Idaho.)

independent closed-circuit, low-profile, self-monitored diaphragm oscillator with continuous dynamic (push/pull) cycling provision. The ability to deliver and retrieve sub–tidal volumes through an independent mean pressure suggests many ventilatory applications requiring enhanced diffusive ventilatory techniques. Essentially, a higher-rate positive/subambient percussive wave format is transmitted symmetrically or asymmetrically through the selected mean pressure. The Oscillatron-1 Percussionator can be employed as a "stand-alone" ventilator for universal cardiopulmonary management of neonates, children, and adults. Provisions designed into the Oscillatron-1 Percussionator allow isolated programming of traditional time-cycled ventilation. The time-cycled ventilator provides for independently selectable inspiratory and selectable (variable) expiratory times. Rate selection with standard calibration can be programmed from 5 to over 50 breaths per minute. I/E ratios from 10:1

FIG 6–11
The pneumatic flow timing logic cell interrupts gas flow with differential opening and closing pressures. (Courtesy of Percussionaire Corp., Sand Point, Idaho.)

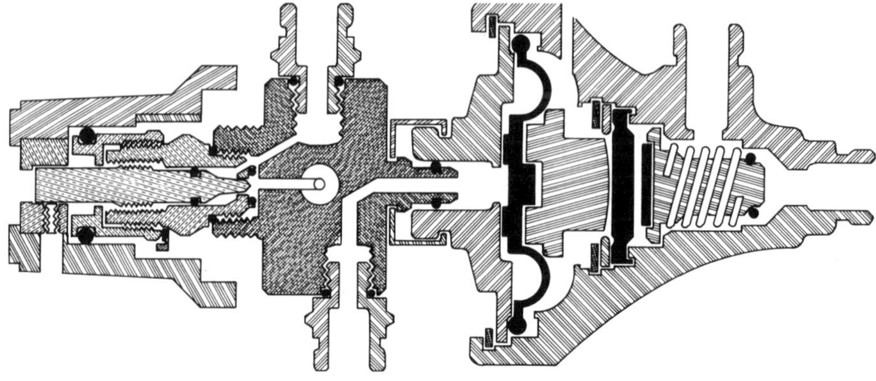

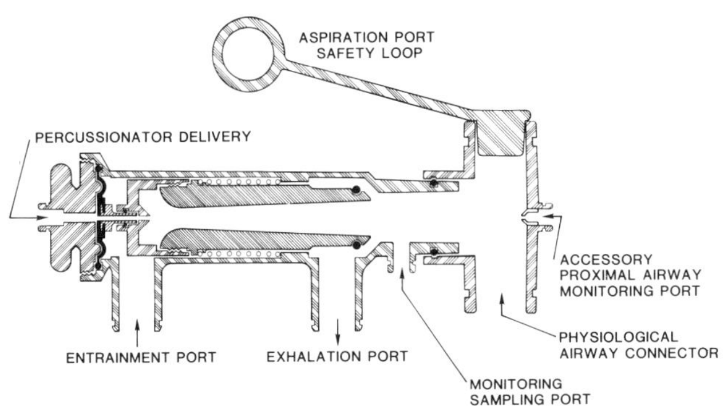

FIG 6–12
The pneumatic Phasitron Monojet Injector/Exhalation Valve maintains auto-PEEP levels below significant clinical levels. (Courtesy of Percussionaire Corp., Sand Point, Idaho.)

to 1:10 can be scheduled. The time-cycled respirator allows traditional tidal flow gradient control with secondary programmable diffusion during continuous diffusive percussive oscillation at cycling rates up to 1,300 per minute.

Universal neonatal, pediatric, and adult programming of the Oscillatron-1 Percussionator allowed by four distinct breathing circuits, one universal VDR fail-safe breathing circuit, two for neonates, and the other for pediatric and adult applications (Figs 6–15 to 6–18). The breathing circuits serve to dedicate the Oscillatron-1 to specific patient populations.

In the neonatal configuration (Figs 6–16 and 6–17) with the Oscillatron and/or Servotron breathing circuits, the Oscillatron-1 employs a traditional, minimal-volume, continuous-flow, hot or cold neonatal breathing circuit connected to a conventional endotracheal tube with a mechanical or pneumatic outflow valve to control demand CPAP, as well as a "backup" mean pressure rise governor. A traditional, positive cyclic amplitude-controlled, convective tidal exchange is delivered at programmable frequencies of 1 to 50 times per minute. A secondary separate identical timing circuit allows dynamic oscillatory rates up to 1,300 cycles per minute for diffusive/convective tidal exchange.

APT 1010

The APT 1010 (Fig 6–19) is classified as a microcomputer-controlled, pressure-preset, time-cycled HFV designed to provide ventilation of the lungs at frequencies from 60 to 600 beats per minute. The ventilator is connected to a multilumen endotracheal tube via a specialized patient circuit that provides for delivery of gas to the patient as well as monitoring of airway parameters. The effectiveness of the APT 1010 can be attributed to an open system and the high frequencies employed. Developed for the treatment of adults, the device has been evaluated in patients with adult respiratory distress syndrome (ARDS). Conventional positive-pressure ventilators have often been less than satisfactory in treating this disease because of the high peak inspiratory pressure and PEEP required for adequate gas exchange. These high pressures can lead to reduced cardiac output, barotrauma, and decreased oxygen delivery to the periphery. The ventilator's controls and alarm settings are input with a keypad via a menu-driven, user-controlled interface. Ventilator and patient parameters as well as alarm and diagnostic messages are displayed on a cathode ray tube (CRT) monitor and on a light-emitting diode (LED) display.

Background

As previously discussed, HFJV was developed in the 1970s as an alternative to conventional ventilation and provides ventilation at frequencies up to 150 breaths per minute. The motivation for developing HFJV was to decrease peak airway pressure and to better distribute gas throughout the lung. The APT 1010 differs in design and technology from other HFJVs in that it delivers gas pulses at higher frequencies—up to 600 breaths per

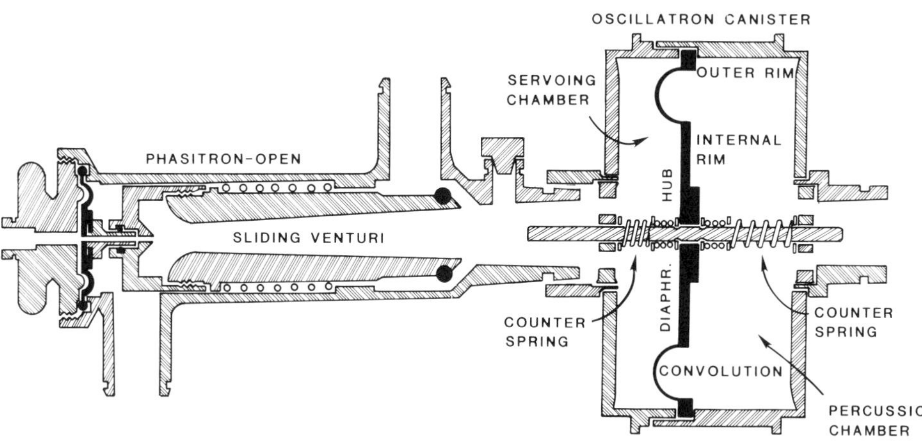

FIG 6–13
Phasitron Servoed Pneumatic Oscillatron Canister. (Courtesy of Percussionaire Corp., Sand Point, Idaho.)

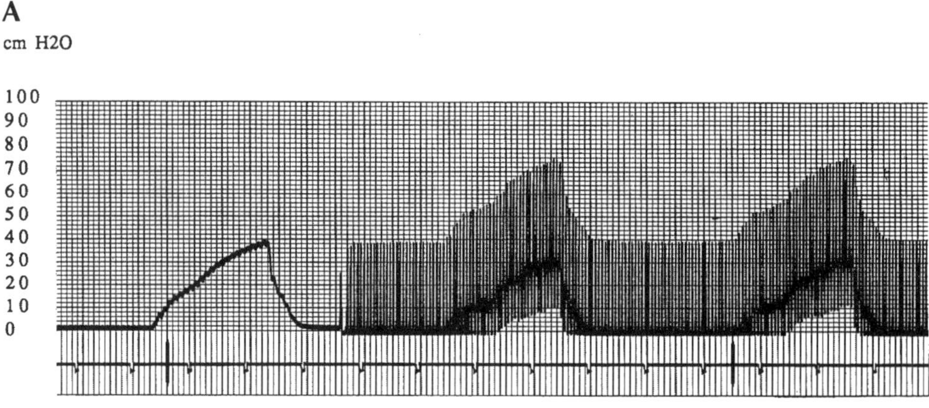

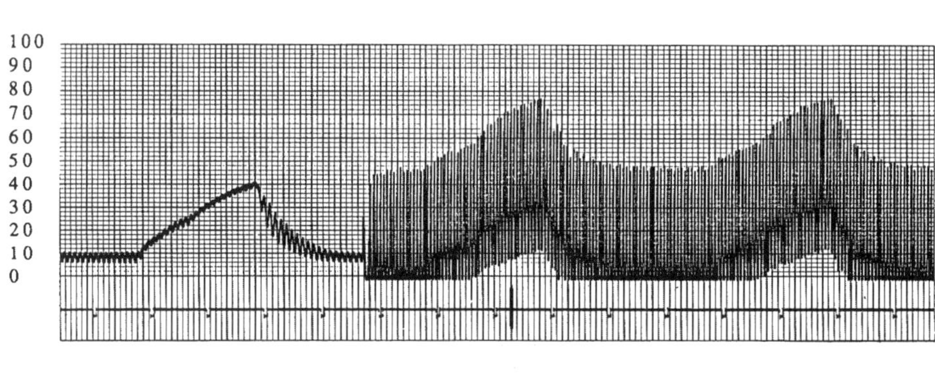

FIG 6–14
A, classic VDR-4 wave format enhanced by the Oscillatron-1 percussive amplifier with an oscillatory frequency of 1,000 cpm. **B,** VDR-4 format with 10 cm H_2O demand CPAP (PEEP) enhanced by the Oscillatron-1 percussive amplifier. CAUTION: The Percussionaire Oscillatron-1 amplifier is a VDR component for augmenting intrapulmonary diffusive ventilation only and does not provide for self-contained convective pulmonary exchange as does the VDR Oscillatron-1 Percussionator. (Courtesy of Percussionaire Corp., Sand Point, Idaho.)

minute (10 Hz). In addition, by utilizing a breathing circuit that is continuously open to the atmosphere (no exhalation valve) and a custom-designed gas delivery system, it is believed that the APT 1010 maximizes gas exchange with low intrathoracic pressure.

Theory of Operation

The method by which the exchange of O_2 and CO_2 occurs at high frequencies in lungs with damaged alveoli differs from that of conventional ventilation and HFJV. The APT 1010 is designed to improve oxygenation at lower peak airway pressures than conventional ventilators do. With damaged, fluid-filled alveoli presenting less surface area for effective O_2 transfer and CO_2 elimination, the problem has been to develop a means of delivering and removing gas from the alveoli while keeping them expanded during both inspiration and exhalation, thereby preventing their collapse. Conventional convective ventilators and other HFJVs transmit gas pulses to the alveoli at low to moderate frequencies (in a relative sense), which in turn causes the alveoli to expand and contract. This results in a nonconstant and time-varying pressure. Animal data[26] suggest that this volumetric change has been shown to be edemegenic. With leaking capillaries present already, additional extravascularization of water would worsen an already poor structure.

In contrast, the APT relies on a rapid succession of pulses, which by the time they reach the smallest airways and alveoli are damped to an almost *constant pressure* at or slightly less than the mean airway pressure measured at the distal end of the endotracheal tube. This *constant mean airway pressure* assists in recruitment and stabilization of the alveoli.

The ability of the APT 1010 to ventilate patients with ARDS is achieved in part by its high-velocity gas stream, which promotes convection through the large airways and allows the mean airway pressure to be established in the alveoli. Rather than moving gas in bulk quantities into the gas-exchanging areas of the lungs, as in the case of conventional ventilators, the APT 1010 delivers small quantities of gas and ventilates by enhancing gas transport in the lung through the increased frequency and kinetic energy of the mixed gas delivered. The extent of surface membrane available for diffusion can be con-

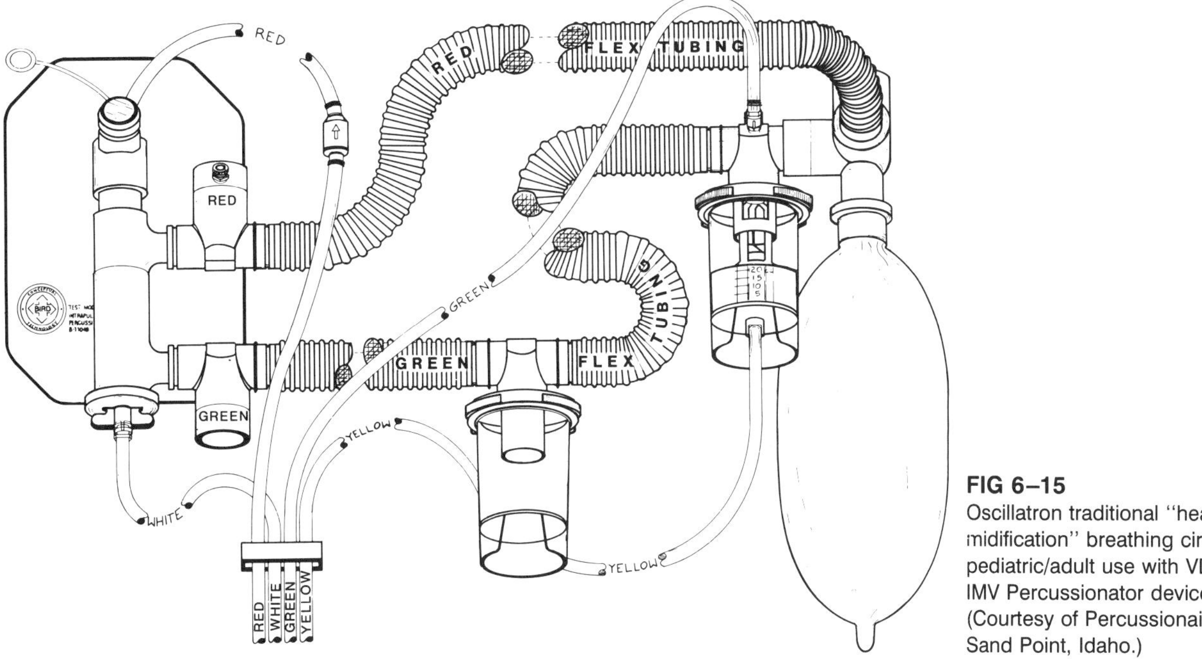

FIG 6–15
Oscillatron traditional "heated humidification" breathing circuit for pediatric/adult use with VDR/CMV/IMV Percussionator devices. (Courtesy of Percussionaire Corp., Sand Point, Idaho.)

trolled to a major extent by delivered gas, i.e., by the inspiratory time (I-time) and to a lesser extent by driving pressure and frequency. This process differs from positive-pressure conventional ventilation in that conventional ventilation relies on pressure gradients for gas transport. Thus a constant intra-alveolar pressure is not established, and the alveolar membrane changes in size and requires greater pressure for maintaining stability.

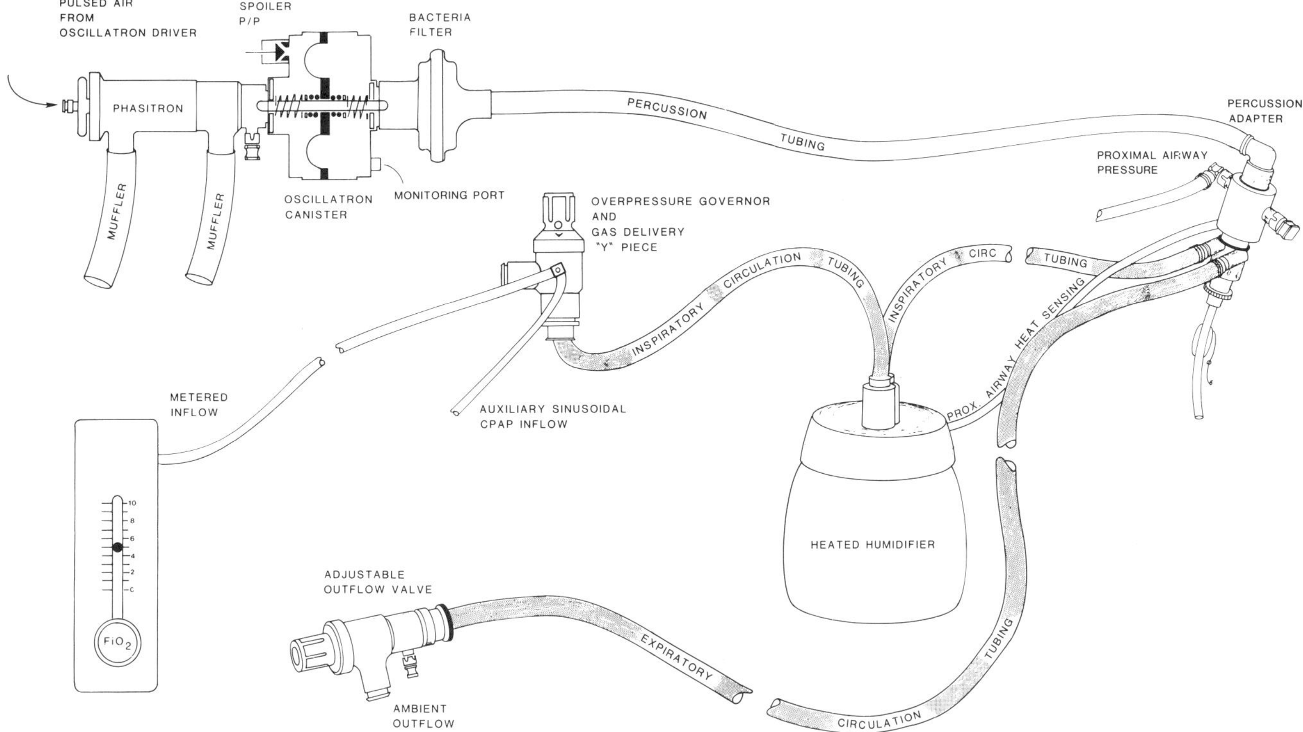

FIG 6–16
Oscillatron continuous-flow "heated humidification" breathing circuit for neonatal use with an Oscillatron-1 Percussionator. (Courtesy of Percussionaire Corp., Sand Point, Idaho.)

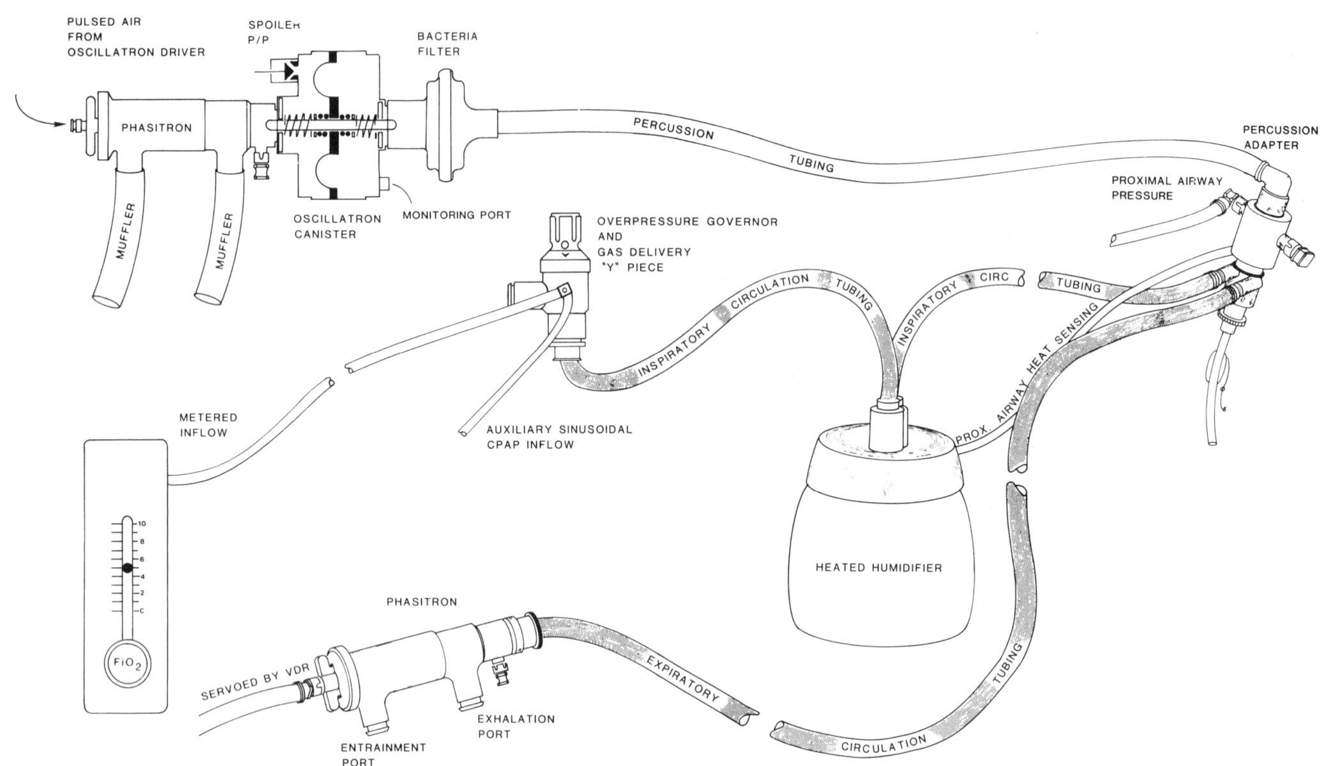

FIG 6–17
The Servotron neonatal continuous-flow breathing circuit for heated humidification with Phasitron-controlled outflow for the VDR Percussionator. (Courtesy of Percussionaire Corp., Sand Point, Idaho.)

The primary ventilation controls of the APT 1010 are frequency, I-time (percentage of the cycle that gas is delivered), and the driving pressure of the gas pulse. I-time is the most important determinant of mean airway pressure, although increasing the frequency and driving pressure will have a small effect on mean airway pressure as well. Increasing the I-time will improve O_2 loading by increasing the functional residual capacity (FRC) and establishing a larger surface area for gas exchange. Increased mean airway pressure will have a detrimental effect on cardiac output if allowed to become excessive.

In contrast, CO_2 elimination is most dependent on the driving pressure. Empirical data suggest that CO_2 elimination changes as an exponential function in relation to I-time. If tidal volume is kept constant, CO_2 elimination changes linearly with increasing frequency. Since there is an increase in volume per pulse with increased drive pressure and a subsequent concomitant increase in kinetic energy, the alveoli can be more easily "cleansed" of the CO_2. Increasing the mean airway pressure (by increasing the I-time) has a minimal effect on CO_2 elimination since the increased volume per pulse is counteracted by decreased available time for the CO_2 to escape. Increasing the frequency of the pulsations increases the arterial CO_2 because the volume per pulse decreases. Decreasing the frequency would have the opposite effect. The effects of various settings upon gas exchange parameters are shown below. Since PEEP has a similar effect on mean airway pressure, although achieving it in a slightly different manner from I-time, an estimate of the initial I-time setting directly follows the level of PEEP that the patient was receiving while on a conventional ventilator:

PEEP on a Conventional Ventilator	I-Time (&) On an APT 1010 Ventilator
0–5	34
5–10	36
10–15	38
15–20	40
>20	42

Control of Ventilator Parameters

I-time is adjustable from 15% to 60% of the inspiratory cycle.

Frequency is adjustable from 1.0 to 10 Hz (60 to 600 breaths per minute). This sets the number of pulses or cycles per second delivered to the patient.

Drive pressure is adjustable from 10 to 50 psi. This

sets the pressure delivered to the drive valve to within ±2 psi (supply pressure dependent). At a supply pressure of 50 psi, the maximum deliverable drive pressure is approximately 4 psi.

Secondary flow is adjustable from 10 to 65 L/min. This sets the flow of the bias flow gas to within 5 L/min or 10%, whichever is greater. The secondary flow passes through the humidifier and carries the heat and humidity to the nozzle gas.

O_2 concentration for the primary flow (nozzle flow) is adjustable to either high (100% O_2), mid (approximately 60% O_2), or low (21% O_2).

Endotracheal tube pressure is used to monitor airway pressure directly from the endotracheal tube

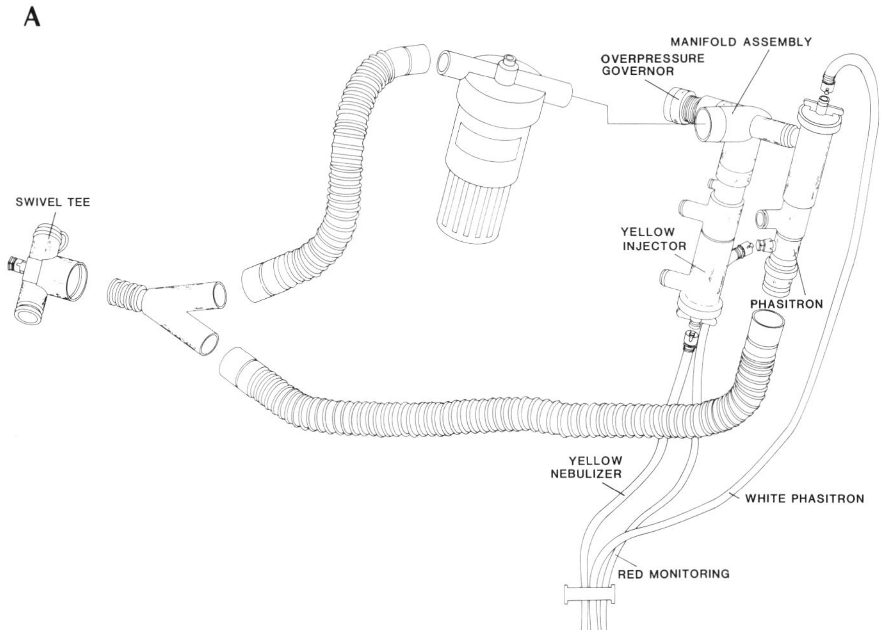

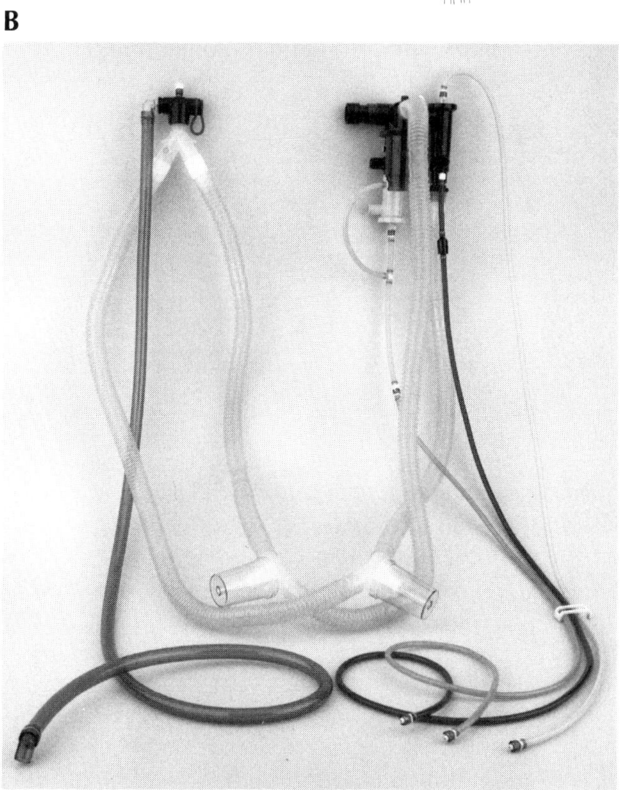

FIG 6–18
A and **B,** Oscillatron pediatric/adult constant-flow breathing circuit for the Oscillatron-1 Percussionator. (Courtesy of Percussionaire Corp., Sand Point, Idaho.)

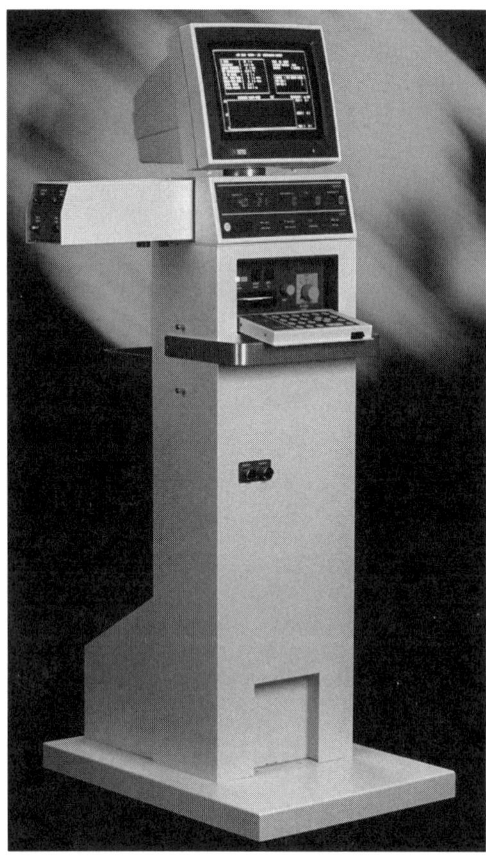

FIG 6–19
APT 1010 high-frequency jet ventilator showing a color monitor, display panel, front control panel, keyboard, and connections on the end of the arm.

through monitoring tubing to an amplified, solid-state differential pressure transducer. The sensitivity is ±0.1 cm H_2O with a response time of 1 ms.

Drive pressure monitoring is achieved by monitoring the primary gas drive pressure at the pressure regulator with an amplified, solid-state gauge pressure transducer. Its operating range is from 0 to 60 psi. The response time of the regulator is 1 ms. The pressure display is verified or updated every 17 seconds.

Alarms

1. *Valve open:* Indicates that the drive valve has remained opened longer than 1.8 seconds. This will *halt* the ventilator.

2. *Valve closed:* Indicates that the drive valve has remained closed longer than 1.8 seconds, the safety valve is closed longer than 1.8 seconds, or the pressure regulator is closed longer than 1.8 seconds.

3. *ET disconnect:* Indicates when the endotracheal tube pressure equals 0 for longer than 2.0 seconds.

4. *Drive pressure:* Indicates that the drive pressure is not within approximately 2 psi of the selected pressure.

5. *O_2:* Can be adjusted in 1% intervals.

6. *Temperature:* Maximum and minimum, adjusted in 1°C increments.

7. *MAP high:* Mean airway pressure adjustable in 1–cm H_2O increments.

8. *PIP high:* Peak inspiratory pressure adjustable in 1–cm H_2O increments.

9. *CPU:* Indicates that operation is no longer under software control (central processing unit failure).

Alarms are indicated via a beeping tone, an LED light, and a message on the screen.

RS 232 and parallel ports for inputting and outputting data are incorporated into the rear of the ventilator. The printer is a standard IBM PC (Centronics type) with graphics capabilities and calls for a 25-pin Sub-D female connection.

Backup Power Supply

A backup battery is incorporated into the electrical system so that the AC current charges the battery continuously while the device is not being powered by battery. The backup electrical supply will be initiated within 2 ms if the line voltage is less than 102 V AC. Once the line voltage is restored, the battery will immediately recharge in preparation for a subsequent power-out emergency. The battery provides full power for a maximum of 30 minutes and requires 12 hours for a full recharge.

Functional Description

For illustrative purposes the APT 1010 can be considered to consist of four functional modules (Fig 6–20): a pneumatic module, a control module, a patient module, and a humidification module. The pneumatic module consists of a gas blender, pressure and flow regulators, gas selector valves, and a drive valve. The control module consists of the microcomputer, data input and output systems, sensors, drive valve controller, and a safety/alarm system. The patient module consists of an entrainment chamber, nozzle, endotracheal tube, and connecting tubing to the APT 1010. The humidification system consists of a heated humidifier with associated water supply and tubing.

Pneumatic module. The pneumatic module (Fig 6–20) receives pressurized bulk gas from the hospital supply. The gas is filtered and then divided into primary and secondary flow paths. The primary flow provides high-pressure pulsed gas, whereas the secondary flow provides low-pressure continuous flow to the entrainment module.

TABLE 6-1
Effect of Ventilator Settings on Gas Exchange

Symptoms			Actions*
Major (Blood Gas Abnormal)	Referenced Other Gas	PAW†	(Freq $\Delta = 0.3$ Hz; I-Time $\Delta = 2\%$; DP $\Delta = 2$psi)
HIGH‡ P_{CO_2}	$P_{O_2}A$	> 50	↓ Frequency
		< 50	↑ Drive Pressure
	$P_{O_2}UA$†	> 50	↑ I-time†, may need to ↓ frequency
		< 50	↑ Drive pressure
LOW P_{CO_2}	$P_{CO_2}A$	> 50	↑ Frequency
		< 50	↑ Frequency
	$P_{O_2}UA$	> 50	↑ I-time, may need to ↓ frequency
		≤ 50	↑ I-time, may need to ↓ frequency
LOW P_{O_2}	$P_{CO_2}A$ low	> 50	↑ I-time
		< 50	↑ I-time
	P_{CO_2} high	> 50	↑ I-time, may need to ↓ frequency
		< 50	↑ Drive pressure

*If the patient is hemodynamically unstable, the addition of an inotropic agent may be necessary. If this is impossible increase the F_{IO_2}.
†PAW = pulmonary artery wedge; UA = unacceptable P_{O_2} or $F_{IO_2} > 50$. I-time = inspiratory time.
‡$P_{CO_2} > 55$ will require a reduction in frequency of 0.5 Hz to start.

After the supply gas is divided, the primary flow passes through a safety shutoff selector valve assembly that selects either 21%, 60%, or 100% O_2 concentration. The flow is then pressure-regulated to an operator-determined value, accumulated, and reaches an electronically controlled solenoid-driven drive valve. The valve, in response to a prescribed frequency, I-time, and waveform, interrupts the flow of high-pressure gas and delivers a pulsed high-velocity stream to tubing connected to a nozzle in the entrainment chamber. The

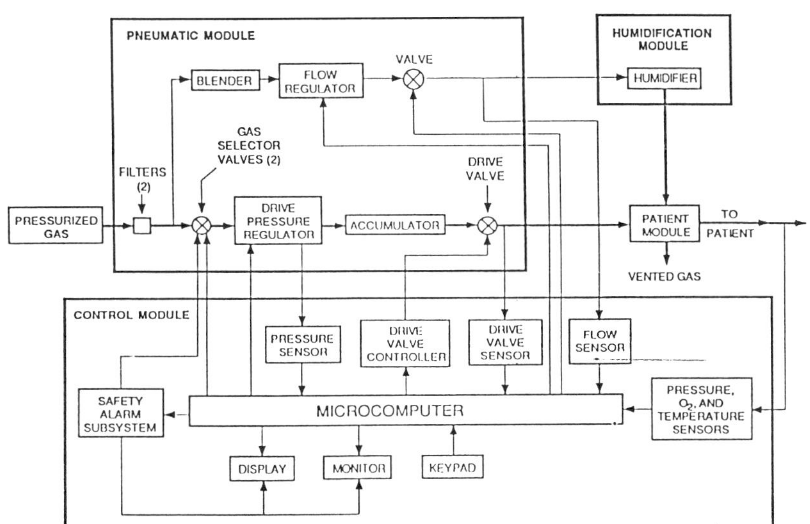

FIG 6–20
Block diagram of an ultrahigh-frequency system showing the four modules of the APT 1010 jet ventilator.

operation of the drive valve is monitored by an internal sensor that in the event of an open failure of the drive valve will close the safety shutoff selector valve to stop the primary flow.

The secondary flow passes through a mechanical blender that allows continuous settings from 21% to 100% O_2. This flow is then regulated and monitored with a flow sensor before entering the humidification module. Delivered F_{IO_2} is controlled by adjusting both the primary flow and the secondary flow. When the flows are mixed in the patient module, any F_{IO_2} can be obtained.

Drive valve. As described above, the function of the drive valve is to interrupt the flow of the high-pressure supply gas at a preset frequency and I-time and deliver the pulsed flow to the patient. Since the frequency of pulsation is to exceed 2.0 Hz (120 beats per minute), both the drive valve and the supporting circuitry must respond quickly to faithfully reproduce the waveforms desired. It should be noted that a crisp response of the drive valve has a significant effect not only on the character of the pulsations produced but ultimately on the gas exchange in the patient. This requirement translates into choosing a valve that will open and close rapidly and allow large peak flows and into designing circuitry that would aid and augment this process.

In view of the large number of cycles that would accumulate on these valves during their normal operation, it is also necessary to ensure that the valves will perform properly and reliably during their life. Methods for determining the performance characteristics of the valves before and during their use have been developed.

The pressure signal downstream from the valve is used to characterize the performance of the valve. In this technique, the output pressure signal between the valve and the nozzle is monitored. Based on the output characteristics described below, the valves are classified as being suitable or not. A valve's performance can be defined by four key elements:

1. Rise time—the amount of time from a fully closed to a fully open state.
2. Fall time—the amount of time from a fully open to a fully closed state.
3. Effective I-time—how faithfully the electronic drive signal is reproduced by the valve to achieve the appropriate duty cycle.
4. Peak pressure—indication of the valve's flow performance.

These four parameters demonstrate that the mechanics to open and close the valve are intact and without defect.

Safety/Selector Valves. The two safety/selector valves serve two purposes. First, they act as a safety system that allows the primary flow to be shut off in the event of a failure of the drive valve in an open or partially open position. Second, the valves control the O_2 concentration (either 21%, 60%, or 100%) of the primary flow by opening the valve connected to the desired gas source and closing the other.

These valves are identical to the drive valve and therefore have adequate flow capabilities.

Drive pressure regulator. The drive pressure regulator is a 2- to 60-psig (output) electronically (current) controlled pressure regulator that is used to automatically control the pressure delivered to the drive valve or change its value as requested by the user via keypad input. The actual output pressure of the regulator is measured with a pressure sensor whose output is used to control the pressure to the desired value via closed-loop software control.

Mechanical blender. A mechanical blender is used to control the O_2 concentration of the secondary flow from 21% to 100%. The blender as integrated into the APT 1010, is designed for medical application, and is commercially available. The input and output connections to the blender are made internally in the ventilator, with the only operator interaction being the control knob to adjust the percentage of O_2 needed.

Flow regulator. The secondary flow regulator is an electronically (current) controlled pressure regulator that is used to automatically control the secondary flow to a rate determined by operator input via the keypad. The actual flow is measured with a flow sensor whose output is used to regulate the flow to the desired value. Since the output of the secondary flow is open to the atmosphere and the flow is continuous, the flow is easily regulated via this technique.

Control module

Functional description. The control module (Fig 6–21) contains control systems (microcomputer, drive valve controller), monitoring systems (sensors), user interface systems (keypad, CRT monitor, and panel), and the power supply system.

By employing a software-controlled microcomputer to manage the operation of the ventilator, various features have been included as part of the APT 1010. Among these are a data acquisition and recording system, readily accessible diagnostics, and maintenance functions.

With the exception of the mechanical blender, drive valve controller, and microcomputer watchdog circuitry, all systems are controlled and/or monitored via the microcomputer under software control.

As described earlier, the mechanical blender is manually adjusted by the operator. The drive valve is controlled by a dedicated microprocessor that is pro-

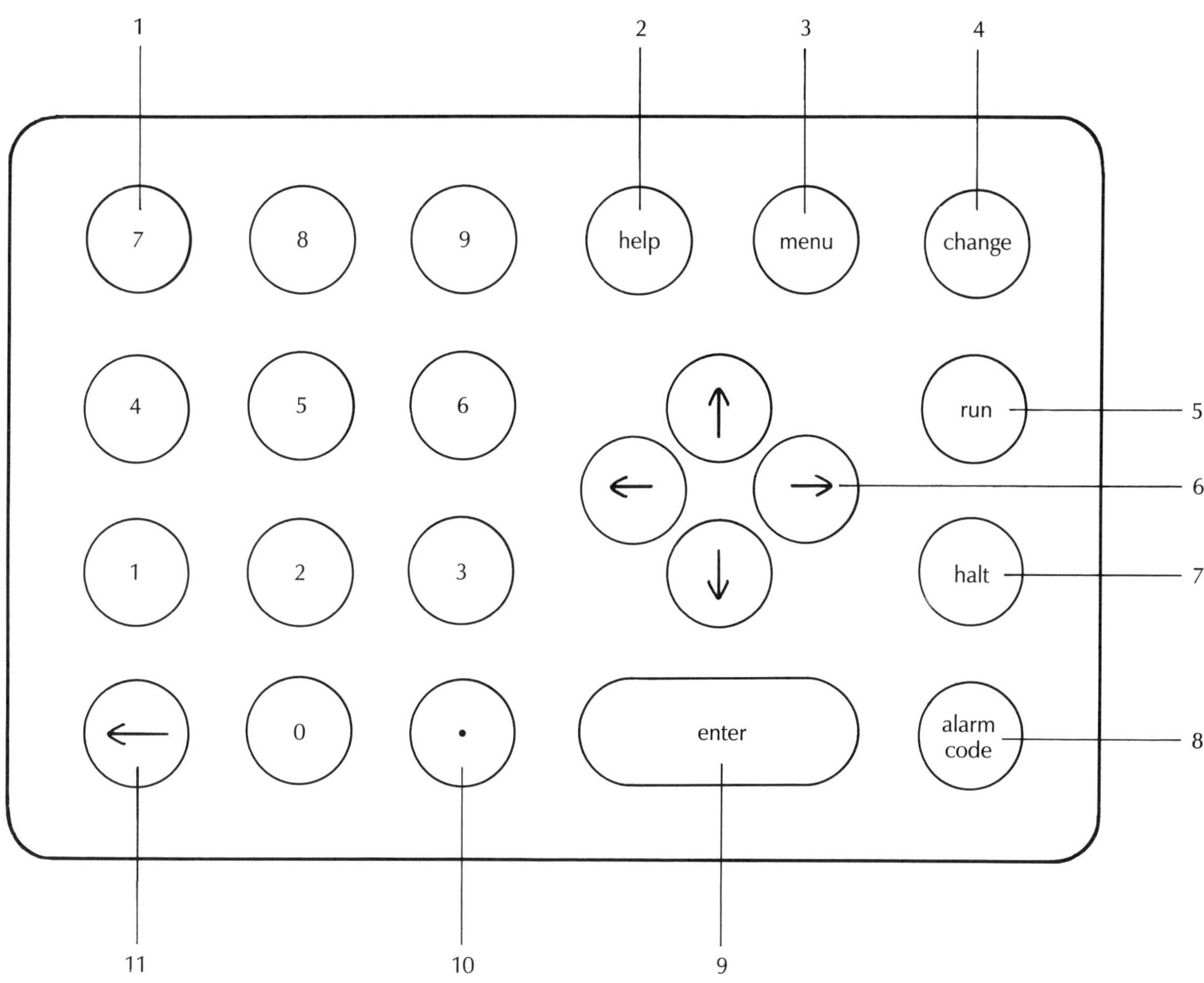

FIG 6–21
Keypad for the APT 1010 ventilator showing input options.

grammed by the microcomputer. Once programmed, the microprocessor allows for independent control of the device valve, although the microcomputer continuously and independently monitors the operation of the drive valve as previously described.

The characteristics of the gas supplied to the patient are monitored in the endotracheal tube. These include airway pressure, O_2 concentration, and temperature. These are interfaced to the ventilator through monitoring lines connected directly to the endotracheal tube.

The user can select menu options or input numerical data via keypad. The output to the user is presented on a CRT monitor and an LED panel that displays ventilator settings and status and key alarms in large LEDs. In addition, a graphic display of airway pressure is displayed on the CRT.

Monitoring the function and operation of the control module as well as issuing warnings of changes in patient conditions to the operator is provided by the safety/alarm system. This system monitors and provides fail-safe conditions to ensure patient safety and support while being ventilated.

The power supply system requires connection to a standard 120-V supply. The humidification system is powered through a connection on the ventilator.

A backup power system is integrated into the ventilator via an internal battery and inverter system. This allows for uninterrupted ventilation in the event of a power failure or brownout. The backup power system supports all ventilator functions, with the exception of the humidification system, which is deactivated since backup power is short-term and used only under emergency conditions.

Control module components

MICROCOMPUTER. The microcomputer utilized is an IBM PC–compatible system. It is configured with 512K random access memory (RAM) and dual disk drives where drive A is the nonvolatile RAM for main program storage and drive B (3½-in. floppy drive) is used for logging patient and ventilator data. A printer port is utilized for obtaining hard copies of selected screens.

DRIVE VALVE CONTROLLER. The drive valve is not driven directly by the microcomputer but by an independent intelligent waveform synthesizer that is programmed by the microcomputer. Once programmed by user input of the frequency and I-time, the synthesizer independently outputs the waveform necessary to control the drive valve as previously discussed.

DRIVE VALVE SENSOR. The drive valve sensor monitors the status of the drive valve to determine whether it is operating normally or has failed in a closed, open, or a partially open manner. If a nonstandard operating condition is detected, an alarm is activated. In the event of an open or partially open drive valve, the primary gas supply is shut off by closing the safety/selector valves.

The drive valve sensor is a high–frequency response (approximately 1 ms), 0- to 60-psig transducer that is temperature compensated. The sensor is mounted in line between the drive valve and the exit port on the ventilator.

FLOW SENSOR. The flow sensor measures the secondary gas flow and provides an electronic signal proportional to flow. This in turn is used in a closed-loop control system to control the flow rate.

The sensor uses an orifice plate within a tube to create a pressure differential that is related to flow. The pressure differential is measured with a solid-state differential pressure transducer that operates in the 0- to 15-psi range, which corresponds to a 0- to 5-V DC full-scale linear output.

AIRWAY PRESSURE SENSOR. The airway pressure sensor is required to measure airway pressures at the rate of 500 times per second. From these data the minimum, mean, and maximum pressures are determined and the airway pressure waveform constructed. These pressure values are also used to initiate alarms, including the endotracheal disconnect alarm. Mean pressure is determined by averaging the 500 readings taken in 1 second.

The airway pressure sensor utilized is a solid-state, 20– to 120–cm H_2O differential transducer that is internally temperature compensated. The amplified output (1 to 60 V dc) is linearly related to pressure. The input to the sensor comes from a port located distally in the endotracheal tube via pressure pulses transmitted through polyvinylchloride (PVC) tubing.

OXYGEN SENSOR. Since the gas supplied to the patient comes from two sources (primary and secondary flow) that can be of different O_2 concentrations, the actual concentration delivered to the patient is measured by sampling gas from a port in the endotracheal tube. The sampled gas flows to an oxygen sensor in the ventilator where its concentration is measured. The sensor is a galvanic fuel sensor typically used in respiratory applications with an operating life of approximately 1 year. The sensor is user replaceable and can be calibrated by following simple instructions displayed on the CRT along with a calibration adjustment knob on the rear of the ventilator.

TEMPERATURE SENSOR. Since the gas supplied to the patient comes from two sources (primary and secondary flow) that are of different temperatures, the actual temperature delivered to the patient is also measured in the endotracheal tube with a thermistor embedded in the inside wall of the main lumen. The thermistor is 2,252 Ω at 25°C, which is a standard (400 series) used in medical applications. The thermistor is connected to the ventilator via an adapter cable. The resistance, measured on an internal Wheatstone bridge circuit, is digitally converted and displayed on the CRT and display panel. Since the thermistors are interchangeable, it is not necessary to calibrate the ventilator for each individual thermistor.

KEYPAD. The keypad (Fig 6–21) provides the primary user input to control the ventilator through menu selections and numerical input. The keypad is a custom-designed membrane switch array that provides tactile feedback and durability. A Motorola 68000–based microprocessor is programmed to translate the custom array into a format recognized by the microcomputer.

MONITOR AND DISPLAY PANEL. A 12-in. CRT monitor is used to present all information including menus, alarms, and ventilator and patient data. The monitor is mounted on top of the ventilator and can be rotated for optimal viewing. On the display panel (Fig 6–22) key alarms (red LEDs) and ventilator parameters (amber seven-segment LEDs) are displayed. This display allows for continuous viewing of key parameters regardless of the screen displayed on the CRT. It also allows for viewing key parameters from a distance.

SAFETY/ALARM SYSTEM. The safety/alarm system is used to alert the operator of changes in patient conditions and connection, loss of ventilator inputs (i.e., gas supply or power), equipment malfunctions, and the unlikely event of a microcomputer failure. Alarms are indicated by being displayed on the display panel and/or the monitor and by an audible alarm. Contained within the safety/alarm system is a "watchdog" timer. This is a built-in function that independently monitors the function of the microcomputer. In the remote chance of a microcomputer malfunction, the operator is alerted. In

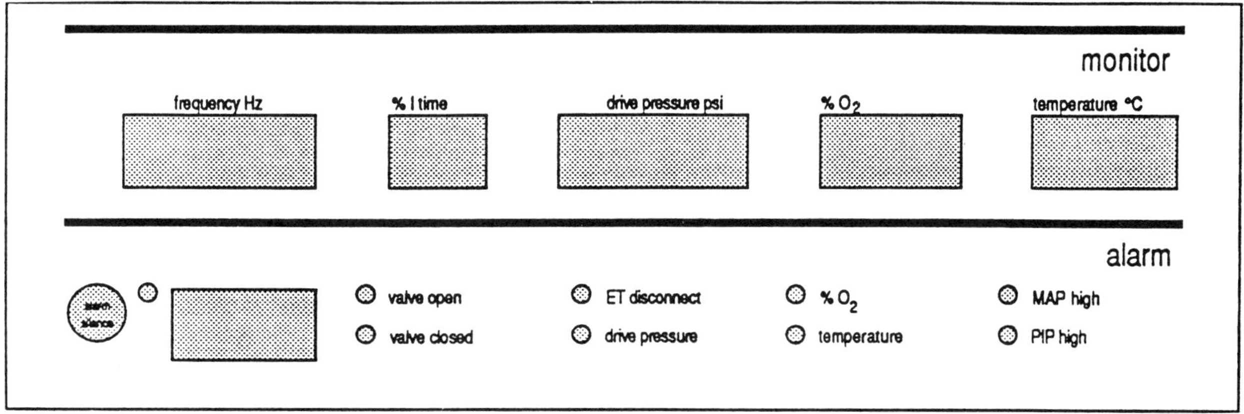

FIG 6–22
APT 1010 display panel showing key ventilator operating parameters in addition to display on the monitor.

this case, ventilation will continue at preset conditions since the drive valve is independently controlled.

POWER SUPPLY. With the exception of the CRT monitor and the humidification system, all electronic components in the APT 1010 run off low voltage (+5, +12, +24 V) supplied by a variable-input, 80-W switching power supply.

Patient module

Functional description. During the inspiratory phase of the ventilation cycle, the patient module takes the pulsed primary flow from a port on the ventilator through a custom-designed nozzle, entrains the secondary (heated/humidified) constant flow, and delivers it to the patient through the endotracheal tube. The high-velocity jet of dry pulsed gas mixes with secondary flow to provide the patient with gas at an adequate humidity and temperature.

During the expiratory phase of the ventilation cycle the gas exhaled by the patient returns through the endotracheal tube into the entrainment chamber where it, in turn, is entrained by the secondary flow and exhausted from the entrainment chamber, which is open to the atmosphere (Fig 6–23).

The continuous supply of low-pressure, humidified secondary flow functions to alternatively supply humidified gas for entrainment and remove expired CO_2 from the chamber without the use of mechanical valves, which would otherwise tend to deteriorate the entrainment process and would result in lower tidal volumes. Conversely, for the same reasons, the use of mechanical valves could lead to a buildup of CO_2 in the patient. Since the entrainment chamber is always open to the atmosphere, patient safety is enhanced by preventing excess pressure buildup in the lungs, which can take place with closed systems. Also, in the event of ventilator or gas supply failure, room air is available to the patient.

Patient module components

TUBING FROM THE VENTILATOR TO THE NOZZLE. From the exit port on the ventilator to the nozzle of the entrainment chamber, surgical-grade Tygon tubing is used. The tube is 36 in. long with an outer diameter (OD) of 0.25 and an inner diameter (ID) of 0.125 in. The ratio of the diameter of the tubing to the exit diameter of the nozzle is 2.12.

ENTRAINMENT CHAMBER. The entrainment chamber (Fig 6–23) consists of a T-shaped cylindrical connector that has been fitted with a stainless steel nozzle and an access port to allow for patient suctioning. A 15-mm male conical fitting at the output end connects to the fitting provided on the endotracheal tube. The other two connectors, one for the input of secondary flow and the other for exhaust, are stan-

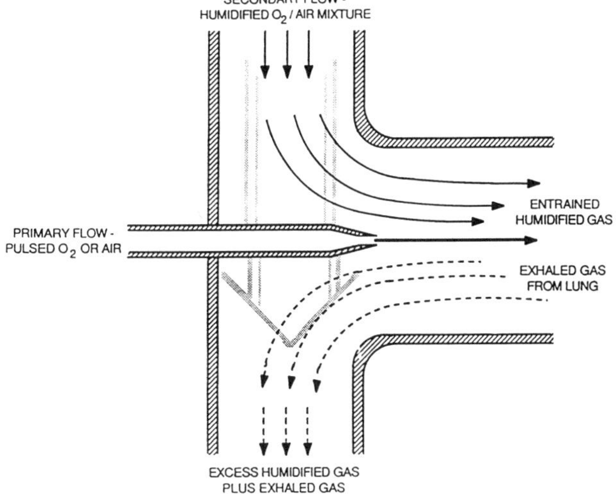

FIG 6–23
Entrainment chamber showing gas flow during cycling of the ventilator.

dard 22-mm connections that fit standard breathing tubing.

The nozzle, which is manufactured to APT's specifications, is designed and located within the entrainment chamber to optimize entrainment, flow, and gas exchange. It was found that placing the nozzle immediately downstream from the transverse inlet and outlet ports accomplished this optimization. The nozzle is positioned along the axis of the entrainment chamber and is oriented toward the axis of the endotracheal tube. In contrast to typical jet ventilators, the nozzle is located outside the endotracheal tube and therefore offers no resistance to the flow in the tube. Furthermore, the nozzle will not occlude the tube or be a surface on which mucus buildup can occur.

MONITORING LINES. The O_2- and pressure-monitoring lines are PVC tubing 36 in. long, 0.162 in. in OD, and 0.110 in. in ID. One end of the line is fitted with a male slip Luer fitting for connecting to the endotracheal tube, and the other end is fitted with a 0.2-μm filter that attaches to inlet ports on the ventilator. The monitoring lines may occasionally fill with water or mucus and must be purged. This is accomplished by injecting air or saline into the tubing with a syringe.

ENDOTRACHEAL TUBE. The endotracheal tube (Fig 6–24) used is an APT Ultracheal tube that is cuffed and has a main lumen, a cuff inflation/deflation lumen, a pressure-monitoring lumen, an O_2-monitoring lumen, and an embedded thermistor for temperature monitoring. Tubes with an ID of 7.0, 8.0, and 9.0 mm may be used. All connectors are marked and color-coded for ease of use. The tube also has a radiopaque line for radiologic visualization. The pressure port is located 0.875 in. from the distal tip of the tube. The O_2 port is located 1.75 in. from the tip of the tube, and the thermistor is located 0.377 in. from the tip of the tube. It should be noted that this tube can also be used with conventional ventilation.

Humidification module.

Functional description. The humidification module heats and humidifies the dry, continuous flow of blended gas provided by the pneumatic module and directs this flow into the entrainment chamber via insulated, corrugated, 22-mm breathing tubing.

Humidification is essential to protect the airways and to prevent desiccation, which could result in tracheitis. Since the APT 1010 nozzle delivers dry gas at somewhat lower than room temperature (as a result of the primary jet expansion), the primary gas that reaches the patient must obtain heat and humidity from the secondary gas flow. The design of the nozzle and the entrainment chamber ensures that sufficient humidified and heated gas is entrained at any permissible ventilator setting so that the resulting mixture of gases that reaches the patient is adequately humidified. Clinical trials have demonstrated this to be the case. In order to achieve adequate humidification of the gas reaching the patient, the humidified secondary flow should be nearly fully saturated and sufficiently heated so that when mixed with

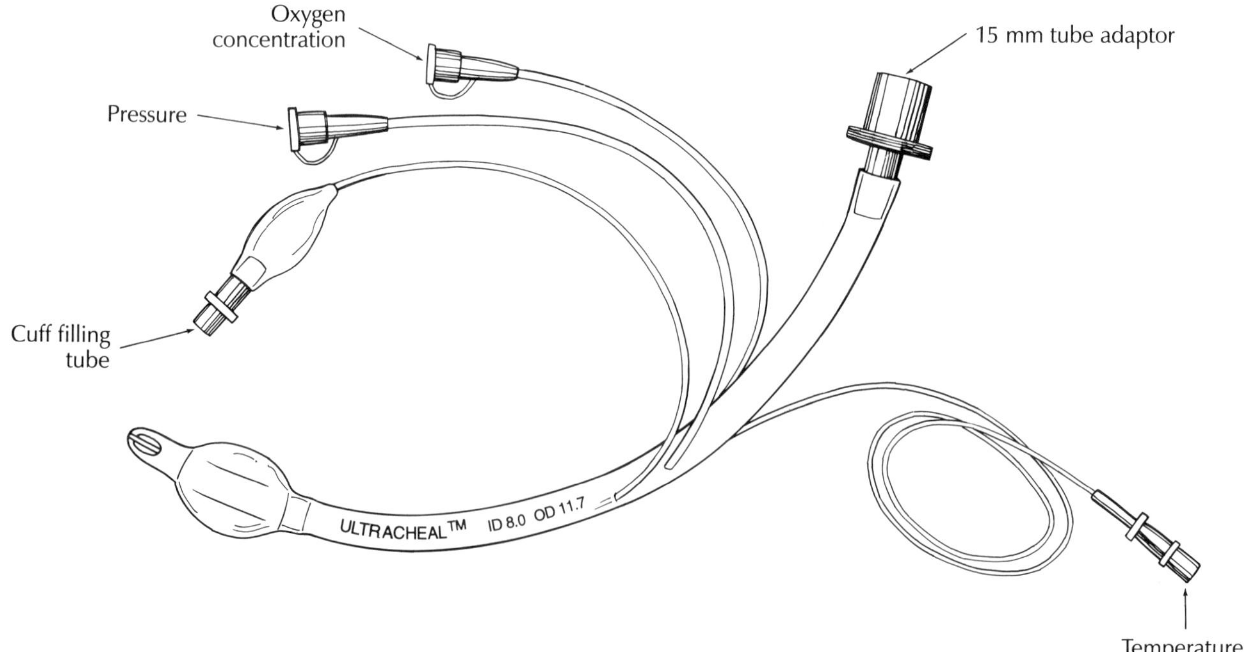

FIG 6–24
APT Ultracheal tube with an oxygen tube, pressure monitoring line, and cuff filling tube.

the cooler primary flow, the resulting mixture remains close to body temperature. As the temperature of a gas is increased, it can hold more water. Therefore it is desirable to have the humidifier produce humidified gas at as high a temperature as possible (the only limitation being that the gas delivered to the patient not be so hot as to cause thermal injury). The resulting secondary gas flow will remain fully humidified (at 100% relative humidity) as long as the temperature is not lowered and raised again. As the temperature is lowered, fully humidified gas (100% relative humidity) will "rain out" and retain only that amount of water allowable at that temperature. The gas will be fully saturated again (at 100% relative humidity) but with less water vapor than in its initial state. However, raising the temperature of the gas after it has been lowered will result in a relative humidity that is less than 100% since at that temperature it is holding less water than is possible.

Measuring the inhalation gas and confirming that the temperature in the endotracheal tube is close to body temperature ensure that totally humidified gas will be entrained since it would be holding the maximum water vapor allowable at that temperature. As noted above, clinical trials have confirmed these results.

Humidification components.

HUMIDIFIER. The humidifier system utilized is a standard, commercially available system that is widely used in conventional ventilator systems. This system is manufactured by Hudson RCI as model no. 380-55. The system, which is self-contained, provides continuously heated molecular high humidity at flows up to 100 L/min. Sterile water is gravity-fed from a replaceable reservoir.

At secondary flow rates specified for the APT 1010, humidifier output is approximately 50°C at 100% RH. The output of the humidifier is controlled by the operator with an adjustment knob on the humidifier. Output is adjusted to achieve the desired airway temperature as measured in the endotracheal tube and displayed on the CRT monitor and display panel. If the airway temperature should rise or fall beyond preset limits, an alarm will be activated.

As an additional safety measure, should the airway temperature rise above 41°C, power to the humidifier will be shut off to protect the patient.

The humidifier is equipped with a disposable chamber that is periodically replaced and disposed of after each patient.

PATIENT CIRCUIT. The patient circuit (Fig 6–25) consists of disposable tubing that is used to supply gas to and exhaust gas from the patient and to monitor airway parameters. The corrugated tubing is standard polyethylene 22-mm breathing tubing. As indicated in Figure 6–25, two sections are fitted with Raincoat sleeves that

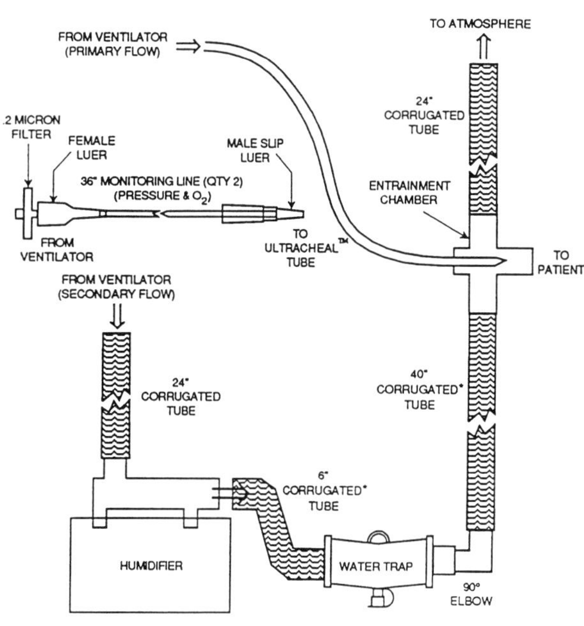

FIG 6–25
APT 1010 patient breathing circuit with various components identified.

coaxially enclose the breathing tubing inside a thin clear flexible casing in such a manner that an insulating dead air space is created between the outside of the circuit and the inside of the casing. This reduces temperature loss and associated rainout between the humidifier and the entrainment chamber.

Clinical Trials

The study was designed to prove the following hypothesis: the APT 1010 can improve oxygen loading, maintain adequate ventilation, and reduce airway pressures while maintaining an acceptable adverse reaction profile.

Each patient served as his own control, thus removing any bias that might occur if a matched group were required. Safety was evaluated by looking at the incidence of pneumothorax, mucus desiccation, hemodynamic compromise, and necrotizing tracheal bronchitis (Table 6–2). Routine bronchoscopies were obtained on the first 24 patients, at which time there was sufficient data to preclude further routine examination of the airways.

Summary of results. One hundred thirty-one patients were admitted into the study. Of these, 106 met the restrictive criteria for failing conventional ventilation. Those that were excluded from the study were found not to have ARDS or were on the ventilator for less than 24 hours; these are summarized in Table 6–3. Table 6–4 contains the descriptive data for the patient population, and Table 6–5 contains the sex and age distribution. Ages

TABLE 6–2
Adverse Reactions

	Indication					
	Barotrauma (Pneumothorax)		Mucus Dessication		Tracheitis	
Center	Number of Patients	Incidence on APT 1010 (%)	Number of Patients	Incidence on APT 1010 (%)	Number of Patients	Incidence on APT 1010 (%)
Hartford Hospital (53 patients)	4	8	10	19	2	4
U Mass (20 patients)	4	20	3	15	2	10
Maricopa (17 patients)	3	18	0	0	0	0
Others (16 patients)	1	6	3	19	0	0

ranged from 14 to 82 years. ARDS developed in the majority of the patients as a result of sepsis. The second largest group consisted of trauma. A statistical analysis for the population showed that they were similar from center to center and when compared with the literature.[27]

One hour after the change to the APT 1010, the above measurements were repeated. The protocol also required the above measurements to be repeated 24 hours after changing ventilators to ensure that the changes were not transient. Measurement 1 hour after the switch allowed us to see the ventilator effect without other competing causes for changes in clinical status.

Ventilation variables. Changes in the principal parameters were evaluated statistically by using a one-sided t-test. The results for the change in a/A ratio, F_{IO_2}, peak inspiratory pressure, mean airway pressure, P_{CO_2}, pH, and hemodynamic parameters are shown in Tables 6–6 to 6–10. Significant improvements were found for the a/A ratio and reductions in F_{IO_2}, peak inspiratory pressure, and mean airway pressure. Adequate alveolar ventilation

TABLE 6–3
Patients Excluded from Analysis

Center	Total Number of Patients	Did Not Meet Criteria of Failing CV*	Was Not on Machine For 24 hr	Did Not Have ARDS*
Hartford Hosp.	9	6	3	0
U Mass	7	3	4	0
Maricopa	0	–	–	–
Loyola	3	3	0	0
Brompton	2	1	1	0
Vanderbilt	0	–	–	–
Mt. Sinai	1	0	0	1
Duke	3	1	2	0
Sum	25	14	10	1

*CV = conventional ventilation; ARDS = adult respiratory distress syndrome.

TABLE 6–4
Patients Enrolled in the Study

			Etiology		
Center	Total Patients	Qualified Patients	Sepsis	Trauma	Other
Hartford Hosp.	62	53	24	11	18
U Mass	27	20	16	4	0
Maricopa	17	17	9	6	2
Loyola	9	6	2	3	1
Brompton	9	7	3	3	1
Vanderbilt	1	1	0	1	0
Mt. Sinai	3	2	2	0	0
Duke	3	0	–	–	–
Sum	131	106	56	28	22
Percentage	100	81	53	26	21

TABLE 6–5
Distribution of the Sex and Age of Patients in the Study*

		Sex		Age Distribution						
Center	Total No.	M	F	10–19	20–29	30–39	40–49	50–59	60–69	70–79
Hartford Hosp.	53	28	22	8	5	5	5	4	8	3
U Mass	20	9	10	2	6	2	2	2	3	2
Maricopa	17	10	7	1	4	2	5	2	1	2
Other centers	16	11	4	3	3	1	4	3	0	1
All multicenters	52	16	10	4	6	2	7	4	0	3
Total	106	37	27	12	11	7	12	8	8	6

* Totals may be different from subset; some patients were excluded because they did not have ARDS.

TABLE 6–6
Comparison of Oxygen Loading by Multicenter

	a/A Ratio				F_{IO_2}				
Center	CV*	1 hr	24 hr	Δ 24 hr	CV	1 hr	24 hr	Δ 24 hr	Success Meeting Safe F_{IO_2} (%)
Hartford Hospital									
N	53	52	52	52	53	52	52	52	
Mean	0.13	0.22	0.27	0.14	0.86	0.82	0.56	−0.30	
Std. Dev (±)	0.05	0.17	0.12	0.13	0.14	0.16	0.14	0.19	75 (39/52)
U Mass									
N	20	20	20	20	20	19	20	20	
Mean	0.17	0.20	0.26	0.09	0.79	0.84	0.64	−0.15	
Std. Dev. (±)	0.09	0.13	0.18	0.14	0.20	0.19	0.22	0.23	55 (11/20)
Maricopa									
N	17	16	17	17	17	16	17	17	
Mean	0.17	0.22	0.21	0.05	0.89	0.85	0.66	−0.23	
Std. Dev. (±)	0.08	0.13	0.12	0.14	0.16	0.19	0.21	0.24	47 (8/17)
Others									
N	16	16	16	16	16	16	16	16	
Mean	0.12	0.13	0.22	0.10	0.83	0.83	0.65	−0.19	
Std. Dev. (±)	0.06	0.08	0.17	0.16	0.21	0.18	0.21	0.18	56 (9/16)

*CV = conventional ventilation.

TABLE 6–7
Comparison of P_{CO_2} by Multicenter

	P_{CO_2}				
Center	CV*	1 hr	24 hr	Δ 24 hr	Success (%) ($20 < P_{CO_2} \leq 45$)
Hartford Hospital					
N	53	52	52	52	
Mean	38.30	32.90	31.58	−6.50	
Std. Dev. (±)	11.23	10.64	9.65	12.92	77 (40/52)
U Mass					
N	20	19	20	20	
Mean	40.90	38.42	35.95	−4.95	
Std. Dev. (±)	8.78	13.38	7.07	5.87	90 (18/20)
Maricopa					
N	17	17	17	17	
Mean	42.18	38.00	41.71	−0.47	
Std. Dev. (±)	12.23	16.76	10.03	10.71	82 (14/17)
Others					
N	16	16	16	16	
Mean	44.83	41.50	40.35	−4.48	
Std. Dev. (±)	11.03	17.23	13.82	12.63	56 (9/16)

*CV = conventional ventilation.

TABLE 6–8
Comparison of pH by Multicenter

Center	pH				Success (%) (7.30 < pH < 7.55)
	CV*	1 hr	24 hr	Δ 24 hr	
Hartford Hospital					
N	53	52	52	52	
Mean	7.36	7.42	7.45	0.09	
Std. Dev. (±)	0.10	0.11	0.08	0.13	90 (47/52)
U Mass					
N	20	20	19	19	
Mean	7.40	7.41	7.43	0.03	
Std. Dev. (±)	0.08	0.12	0.08	0.06	95 (18/19)
Maricopa					
N	17	17	17	17	
Mean	7.38	7.42	7.40	0.02	
Std. Dev. (±)	0.08	0.11	0.08	0.09	82 (14/17)
Others					
N	16	16	16	16	
Mean	7.38	7.42	7.40	0.03	
Std. Dev. (±)	0.10	0.14	0.10	0.10	81 (13/16)

*CV = conventional ventilation.

was established in the majority of patients, and there was no significant hemodynamic compromise seen. The goal of a ventilator is to oxygenate and ventilate a patient without causing an unacceptable amount of adverse reactions at the lowest possible airway pressure.[28, 29] Table 6–11 shows the number of patients who achieved clinically significant improvements in these parameters. The results demonstrate an improvement of ventilation parameters in critically ill adult patients with ARDS.

Survival. For this study a patient was considered a survivor if he was weaned from all positive-pressure ventilation for 24 consecutive hours (Table 6–12). In fact, all but two of the patients left the hospital. One must keep in mind that the survival rate that is reported in the literature is for nonstratified studies.[30] Those patients were not necessarily required to be failing conventional ventilation, as was the case for patients entered into this study. Therefore, the expected survival rate of patients in the current clinical trial should be lower than what is reported in the literature.

Follow-up data were obtained in 17 of the survivors at Hartford Hospital. The data showed typical post-ARDS

TABLE 6–9
Comparison of Airway Pressure by Multicenter

Center	PIP*				MAP*				Success at Reducing PIP by 10 cm (%)
	CV*	1 hr	24 hr	Δ 24 hr	CV	1 hr	24 hr	Δ 24 hr	
Hartford Hospital									
N	50	50	50	47	34	50	49	33	
Mean	52.8	44.9	42.1	−11.00	26.4	24.3	22.0	−5.70	
Std. Dev. (±)	12.0	8.0	10.7	11.46	5.5	5.0	5.6	6.11	53 (25/47)
U Mass									
N	18	18	19	18	11	19	18	9	
Mean	63.2	47.4	49.0	−13.61	33.4	29.7	29.6	−6.00	
Std. Dev. (±)	15.3	15.4	17.8	18.91	7.3	10.8	7.3	9.73	67 (12/18)
Maricopa									
N	17	16	14	14	9	15	14	8	
Mean	63.7	48.6	55.1	−9.86	29.2	27.9	30.0	2.00	
Std. Dev. (±)	8.9	11.6	14.9	10.36	5.5	7.6	6.5	3.30	57 (8/14)
Others									
N	15	15	15	15	7	15	15	7	
Mean	54.7	47.9	49.4	−5.33	28.6	24.7	26.5	−3.43	
Std. Dev. (±)	11.8	9.7	14.5	12.98	8.9	6.0	5.7	10.83	33 (5/15)

*PIP = peak inspiratory pressure; MAP = mean arterial pressure; CV = conventional ventilation.

TABLE 6–10
Comparison of Hemodynamic Data by Multicenter

	Blood Pressure				Heart Rate				Cardiac Output			
Center	CV*	1 hr	24 hr	Δ 24 hr	CV	1 hr	24 hr	Δ 24 hr	CV	1 hr	24 hr	Δ 24 hr
Hartford Hospital												
N	43	46	47	40	49	50	50	48	36	43	44	33
Mean	85.12	84.78	84.84	−1.41	117.49	114.24	109.54	−7.92	5.84	5.55	6.01	0.32
Std. Dev. (±)	15.98	14.22	15.06	15.24	22.52	20.71	20.25	21.27	2.16	1.96	2.00	1.71
U Mass												
N	20	19	19	19	19	19	20	19	15	18	19	14
Mean	80.08	83.09	92.26	12.25	116.37	115.37	110.00	−4.84	7.63	7.06	7.50	0.12
Std. Dev. (±)	8.38	12.87	15.78	13.12	17.67	15.95	20.63	17.17	1.92	2.71	2.60	2.91
Maricopa												
N	16	17	17	16	16	17	17	16	13	14	16	13
Mean	80.75	84.92	91.02	11.33	119.06	120.24	115.00	−2.06	7.51	7.75	8.69	1.55
Std. Dev. (±)	15.30	16.20	14.09	15.14	13.38	12.91	14.31	17.06	1.17	2.19	3.20	3.33
Others												
N	8	13	14	7	8	12	13	6	10	10	11	8
Mean	85.00	67.97	90.38	10.52	116.88	120.08	111.92	−8.00	7.26	7.97	7.74	0.05
Std. Dev. (±)	17.02	26.73	26.78	16.77	19.05	20.54	15.84	26.02	2.93	2.65	2.10	2.85

*CV = conventional ventilation.

diffusion defects that gradually cleared over a period of 6 months. Flow volume loops obtained on these patients did not demonstrate any upper airway obstruction. Only 1 patient had moderate obstruction to airflow. Thus the study did not reveal any increased risk with this form of ventilation when compared with conventional ventilation. At the same time, it clearly showed clinically significant improvement.

In summary, our experience has shown that the APT 1010 is safe and effective in the ventilatory management of adult patients with ARDS who have failed to respond to conventional ventilation:

1. Significant improvements in oxygen loading occurred.
2. Significant reductions in F_{IO_2} could be made.

TABLE 6–11
Percentage of Patients with a Satisfactory Response at 24 hr for Four Criteria of Response

	Response Criteria			
Center	$F_{IO_2} \leq 0.60$, $Pa_{O_2} \geq 60$	$25 \leq P_{CO_2} \leq 50$	$7.30 \leq pH \leq 7.55$	Δ PIP* ≥ 10 cm H_2O
Hartford Hospital	75% (39/52)†, 63–87†	76.9% (40/52), 65.9–87.9	90.3% (47/52), 82.3–98.3	53.2% (25/47), 39.2–67.2
U Mass	55% (11/20), 33–77	90% (18–20), 77–100	94.7% (18/19), 84.7–100	66.7% (12/18), 44.7–88.7
Maricopa	47.1% (8/17), 23.1–73.1	82.4% (14/17), 64.4–100	82.4% (14/17), 64.4–100	57.1% (8/14), 31.1–83.1
Others	56.3% (9/16), 32.3–80.3	56.3% (9/16), 32.3–80.3	81.3% (13/16), 62.3–100	33.3% (5/15), 9.3–57.3

*PIP = peak inspiratory pressure.
†Ranges represent the 95% confidence interval.

TABLE 6–12
Survival Rate

Patients	HH*	U Mass	Maricopa	Other Centers	Total
No. of patients in study	53	20	17	16	106
No of patients qualified†	44	16‡	16	15	91
No of patients surviving	29	8	7	6	50
Patients surviving (%)	65.9	50.0	43.8	40.0	55.0

* HH = Hartford Hospital.
† Number of patients in the study minus the number of patients with no decisions
‡Outcome pending.

3. Adequate ventilation could be obtained.
4. Clinically significant reductions in airway pressures occurred.
5. No adverse hemodynamic effects were noted.
6. No unusual reactions to this form of ventilation were found on autopsy.
7. The incidence of pneumothorax was comparable to the reported incidence in the literature.
8. The incidence of mucus desiccation was acceptable and did not result in significant patient compromise.
9. When compared with literature controls there was a significant improvement in survival.

Conclusions to be drawn from this study. The laboratory, animal, and human studies provide reasonable assurance that the APT 1010 ventilator is safe and effective for its intended use in adult patients with ARDS who are not responding to conventional ventilation. Bench testing of this device suggests that it should be able to run trouble free for a period of 1,500 hours. Although there are adverse reactions to this form of ventilation, they are not excessive when compared with conventional ventilation. The benefits of this form of ventilation clearly outweigh the risks.

Rationale for the Use of High-Frequency Ventilation

HFV in the United States has been used for laboratory investigation since 1959 when Emerson first described his unique HFO.[6] However, it was during the 1980s that an exponential growth of reports on the use of HFV appeared in the literature. Unfortunately, these reports were dominated by experiences with primarily HFPPV and HFJV, with little information about HFO. Clinical roles for HFV include[31, 32] its use during anesthesia for bronchoscopy, endoscopy, airway management of laryngeal microsurgery, and neurosurgical procedures. It is also used to ventilate neonates who are refractory to conventional ventilatory techniques. Other applications include ventilation of adults with ARDS, bronchopleural fistulas, and upper airway obstructions and ventilation of patients undergoing microneurosurgery and cardiac surgery.

HFO is primarily used to improve pulmonary gas exchange and/or to rest a lung to allow spontaneous ventilation to occur. It also may improve mucus clearance when the cilia are injured or destroyed by inducing an artificial cough.[33] The rationale for selecting HFV over conventional ventilation includes the following:

1. To ventilate patients refractory to conventional controlled ventilation[34]
2. To reduce the incidence of pulmonary infection and iatrogenic barotrauma[35]
3. To maintain normocapnia and a Po_2 saturation of greater than 90% on an Fio_2 of 0.6 or less[36]
4. To reduce the negative effect in cardiac output[36]
5. To reach the same therapeutic end point as conventional mechanical ventilation with a lower level of mean airway pressure and PEEP[34, 35]
6. To improve the deposition of aerosol to the peripheral regions of the lung in patients with chronic airway obstruction[37]
7. To improve the survival rate and decrease the incidence of pneumonia in patients with inhalation injury[38]

Even though the above reports are promising, clinicians are still reluctant to use HFV except in cases where conventional ventilation is not successful.

Clinical Experience

Clinical experience with HFJV is quite varied. Much of the difficulty in interpreting the studies stems from two major problems: first, the study design was poor in that most studies were done in an attempt to salvage patients who were already failing conventional ventilation, and second, the hypotheses of these studies had not yet been proved. Most investigators[37] conducted their evaluations under the hypothesis that lowering peak and mean airway pressures would be beneficial to patients with ARDS. Unfortunately, animal data generated years after the onset of these clinical trials did not support this premise. These animal experiments suggested that mean airway preservation was important in decreasing lung injury and that it was the change in volume that was more harmful, as far as parenchymal lung injury was concerned, than the actual change in pressures associated with conventional ventilation. Barotrauma, however, still appears to be related to the level of peak airway pressure achieved during ventilation. It seems that certain animals will achieve more benefits from HFJV than other animals. This created more confusion in assessing the efficacy of HFJV. Those animals with better collateral ventilation demonstrated a better response with respect to gas exchange that did the animals who had poor collateral ventilation.

Looking at all the studies combined, one would arrive at a conclusion that overall there is no significant benefit to HFJV when compared with conventional ventilation; however, anecdotal reports and our own personal experience have demonstrated that in a given patient who is failing conventional ventilation, HFJV may be a lifesaving therapeutic option. In the largest prospective randomized study to date, Carlon et al.[39] demonstrated that there was an improvement in airway pressure and oxygenation in a large group of patients with ARDS. He was unable to demonstrate an improvement in mortality predominantly because his underlying population had a very high mortality rate to begin with. One other prospective randomized study[40] also showed similar results in that oxygenation seemed to be improved, airway pressures were lower, but there was never any demonstrated improvement in the mortality rate. Several studies were performed with HFJV to determine whether in fact there was some benefits for patients with established barotrauma.[41] Two animal studies demonstrated significant improvement when animals were ventilated by HFJV vs. conventional ventilation.[42] However, in a very small study[43] consisting of five human subjects, jet ventilation produced no consistent benefit to patients with established bronchopleural fistulas when compared with conventional ventilation. The implication of lower airway pressures was that there would be less significant impairment of cardiovascular function during HFJV vs. conventional ventilation; however, when mean airway pressures were held constant, there was no significant difference between cardiac outputs or any other hemodynamic parameters in any of the studies where these parameters were measured. Recently, workers at the University of Pittsburgh have demonstrated that when HFJV pulsations are synchronized to cardiac cycles such that no impairment in left ventricular filling occurs, there is an augmentation in cardiac output. Unfortunately, devices such as this are not currently available except under research situations.

In summary, one would conclude that on a case-by-case basis some benefit may be achieved by HFJV when compared with conventional ventilation. Oxygenation and airway pressures seem to improve with this form of therapy as opposed to conventional ventilation; however, to date there has not been any prospective randomized study that has shown a decrease in morbidity and mortality associated with this type of therapeutic intervention. The adverse effects of HFJV appear to be similar to those of conventional ventilation. In the largest prospective study that looked at HFJV (previously cited), there was no significant difference between the new onset of barotrauma in the group receiving HFJV when compared with conventional jet ventilation. The incidence of upper airway colonization and respiratory infection, however, has not been measured on a large-scale basis but appears to be similar between the two groups. Additionally, the nature of the high flow employed by HFJV requires that a very sophisticated method of humidification be employed. If this methodology fails, desiccation of the airway becomes a very significant problem. Before desiccation of the airways per se occurs, there is usually inspissation of mucus resulting in tenacious sticky sputum that may cause obstruction of the endotracheal tube or the upper airways and can result in trauma to the upper airways as well. Therefore, careful attention to both temperature and humidity of the inspired gases during HFJV is required to ensure that no adverse effects can occur. As has been previously mentioned, malignant tracheobronchitis is an infrequent but very severe complication of HFJV and has a significant mortality rate associated with it. The initial problems associated with poorly designed devices with inadequate monitoring capabilities have largely been taken care of by the manufacturers and the FDA. The available devices on the market today employ sophisticated monitoring systems that ensure patient safety. The respiratory clinician is therefore left with some uncertainty as to the role of HFJV in the care of patients with acute lung injury. At least anecdotal data suggest that this has significant benefit in certain patient populations.[34,39,40–43] Unfortunately, at the present time the studies that have looked at HFJV have been tainted by poor design or unproven hypotheses. It also appears at the present time that with the advent of other respiratory therapy techniques improving oxygenation and CO_2 elimination, there has been a paucity of investigators who are interested in pursuing research in this field, which makes it unlikely that in the future we will see further studies that employ high-frequency generator devices to answer the question of their role in the treatment of patients with severe hypoxemia.

Potential Hazards With High-Frequency Ventilation

The greatest clinical hazard with any lifesaving device such as a ventilator is if it fails to provide the expected physiologic support. For this reason care must be taken by all clinicians to closely monitor patients receiving HFV. Dependence on ventilator alarms warning the operator that an undesired event has already occurred leave patients exposed to a potential problem even if *immediate* corrective action is taken.

Potential hazards with the use of HFV are similar to those experienced with conventional ventilation, compounded by the fact that this new technology is not understood as well as conventional ventilation. For this reason, patients receiving HFV must be cared for by a round-the-clock team of specifically trained clinicians in the operation and basic troubleshooting of HFV.

Specific problems most frequently encountered with the use of HFV include the following:

1. Unfamiliarity with operation of the device leading to a failure of the ventilation to provide adequate ventilatory support.
2. Carbon dioxide accumulation resulting from airway obstruction, inadequate entrainment of fresh air in the HFJV, and/or inadequate cycling frequencies in the HFJV and HFOV.
3. Barotrauma associated with obstructed airways and/or gas trapping leading to excessive auto-PEEP.
4. Improper humidification causing dehydration of the airways, mucus plugging, and subsequent air trapping.
5. In HFJV, damage to tracheal mucosa caused by sheer forces of the jet pulses against the tracheal wall.

BIDIRECTIONAL JET VENTILATION

One of the significant clinical difficulties associated with HFV in adult patients has been adequate alveolar ventilation. There are many possible explanations for the elevation in arterial P_{CO_2} often encountered in these patients. Since the physiology of gas exchange at frequencies less than 200 breaths per minute involves the same concepts of alveolar ventilation and dead space ventilation and since only 5% of each tidal pulsation does useful ventilation in HFJV as compared with 66% in conventionally delivered tidal volumes, it is not surprising that this could be a considerable problem. Small changes in dead space would be expected to have a profound effect on alveolar ventilation. Additionally, the high convective velocity of the gas favors maldistribution of the tidal breath in favor of the lower lobes and leaves the upper lobes relatively underventilated. Two potential approaches to alleviate this problem have been attempted, and both have been successful. Using frequency at or near the resonant frequency of the lung (5 Hz) results in a reduction in pulmonary impedance and thus allows deeper penetration of each pulsation of gas into the lung, effectively reducing the physiologic dead space. This technique will be discussed in a separate section in this chapter. A second technique involves the use of bidirectional jet ventilation such that exhalation becomes active and carbon dioxide elimination can be enhanced. Similar in style to oscillators where exhalation is always active, this jet ventilation technique can result in normalization of the CO_2 levels by controlling the amount of activity during the expiratory phase.

As seen in Figure 6–26, the primary solenoid valve drives the jet nozzle, which is placed in the proximal portion of the endotracheal tube and is used to insufflate fresh gases into the patient, whereas the secondary solenoid valve is placed more distally in the endotracheal tube and controls the expiratory phase by creating a venturi-like effect essentially sucking the air out of the trachea. In effect, placement of the second jet nozzle within the endotracheal tube effectively reduces the anatomic dead space of the lung as well. More effective washing out of the CO_2 from the proximal airways will also create a larger gradient between the alveolus and the large airways and improve the conditions for CO_2 diffusion. Animal data have demonstrated that this form of HFJV usually results from a hyperinflated state caused by the short expiratory times of the pulsations of gas. The secondary nozzle could result in a reduction in FRC and therefore impair oxygenation when elastic recoil of the lung is high such as in patients with ARDS.

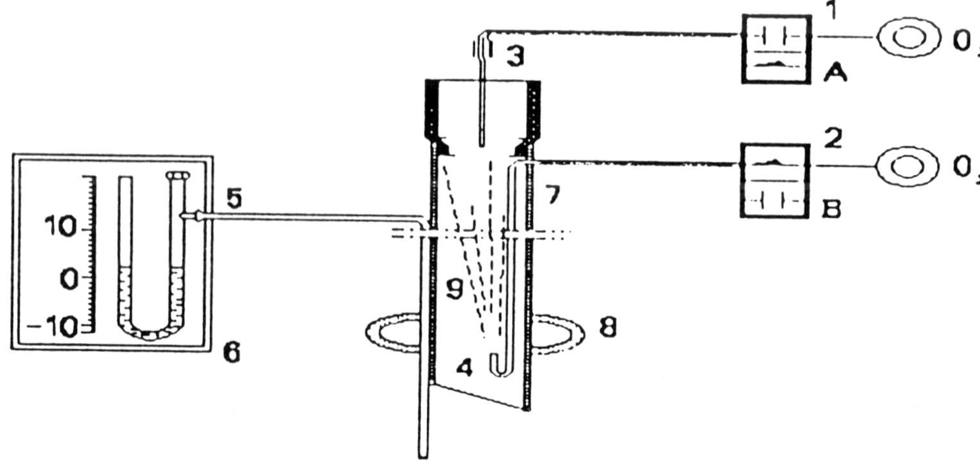

FIG 6–26
Gas flow through the breathing circuit of a bidirectional high-frequency jet ventilator. (From *Crit Care Med* 1992; 20:421. Used by permission.)

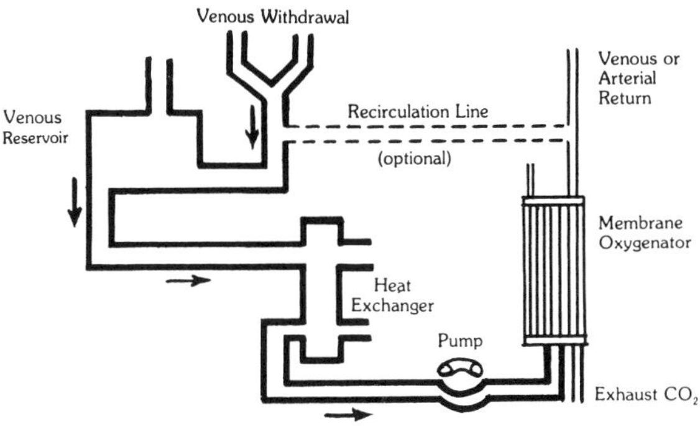

FIG 6–27
Schematic rendering of a typical extracorporeal membrane oxygenator (ECMO) device. Blood flow is indicated by *arrows*. (From McDowell JR Jr: *Michigan Soc Respir Care* Winter 1980; 14:11. Used by permission.)

EXTRACORPOREAL MEMBRANE OXYGENATION

Extracorporeal membrane oxygenation (ECMO) (Fig 6–27) has been available for 25 to 30 years in the United States. It forms the mainstay of support for patients undergoing cardiovascular surgery in which cardiopulmonary bypass is necessary. In this device, blood is removed from the right side of circulation and pumped through a machine with a membrane oxygenator, at which point oxygen is added to the system and carbon dioxide is removed, and then the blood is pumped back into the arterial side of the patient with sufficient force to propel the blood through all the major blood vessels and finally to all the end organs. In patients with acute respiratory failure (ARF), bypass or ECMO can reduce the right-to-left shunt sufficiently to reduce the ventilatory support and inspired concentrations of oxygen required. It was hoped that this reduction in F_{IO_2} and ventilator support would provide more favorable conditions and allow the lung to recuperate while the organs were adequately oxygenated. However, as will be seen later in this section, bypass is a much more complex and difficult procedure to perform than mechanical ventilation since it requires the expenditure of large amounts of manpower, time, and resources of the hospital; therefore is not widely accepted at the present time as a form of routine support for patients with severe lung injury.

The major experience with ECMO for the support of patients with ARF was achieved in the early 1970s anecdotally from 150 patients suffering from acute lung injury of varying causes and severity. These patients had undergone ECMO and had achieved a survival rate of 10% to 15%. However, because of the nonrandomized nature of the study and tremendous disparity of lung injury to which it was applied, the true survival rate that could be attributed to the use of ECMO could not be determined.[44]

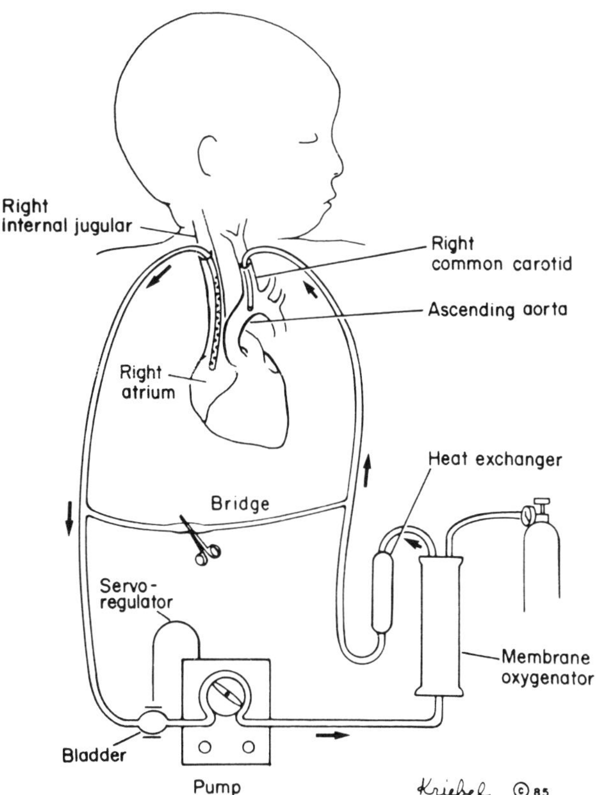

FIG 6–28
Diagram showing components of and direction of blood flow in a venoarterial ECMO circuit. (From O'Rourke PP: *Respiratory Care* 1991; 36:684. Used by permission.)

Bypass therapy can be done in many different ways. Presently in the United States there are at least six different types of venoarterial partial bypass systems available. All of them, however, rely on similar mechanisms of removing venous blood by using a roller pump, controlling its temperature, and then pushing the blood through a membrane oxygenator and returning the blood to the systemic circulation (Fig 6–28). Patients must be fully anticoagulated to prevent the blood from coagulating within the membrane oxygenator. The bypass flow can be regulated to achieve any desired cardiac output that is necessary. The tubing that is used is usually (silicon) rubber and is usually treated by flushing it with deionized water and then steam autoclaving. A 10-ft drainage line brings the blood to the cart from the patient, where it passes through an oximeter that continuously displays the oxygen saturation of the inflow blood. Blood is then collected in a venous reservoir bag that is monitored to prevent accidental exsanguination of the patient. This bag contains a switch that can stop the pump if drainage is impaired. From the reservoir a roller pump propels the blood through the membrane oxygenator. The circuit has a "Y" connection that allows the addition of a second membrane for rapid replacement of a failing membrane. Pressure transducers continuously monitor the gradient across the membrane. A silicone rubber bubble trap and an outflow oximeter attached to a 10-ft return line complete the circuit. There are a number of Luer-lock connectors so that venous access channels are available for sampling blood and adding additional medications or blood products. The circuit requires a priming volume of approximately 900 mL and is assembled by using sterile technique while the cannulation of the patient is underway. The cannulation of the patient can be done in two ways. Initially in the early 1970s, direct insertion of a catheter into the right ventricle was done to promote complete bypass of the pulmonary circuit. As an alternative, cannulation of a large venous access such as the inferior vena cava can be used when only partial bypass is necessary. The priming of the system is usually done with albumin, blood, and lactated Ringer's solution along with the associated necessity of heparin to prevent coagulation. Theoretically, ECMO could be done with a venovenous perfusion system such that venous blood taken out of the inferior vena cava could be returned to the inferior vena cava at a different site after it has been oxygenated and had the CO_2 removed (Fig 6–29). Insertion of the cannulas is usually done either in the operating room or in the intensive care unit (ICU) with the patient under local anesthesia except in circumstances where the catheter is to be placed in the right ventricle. Venovenous perfusion is obviously technically easier and safer and usually affords adequate oxygenation; however, under certain circumstances where the lung is severely damaged and virtually all of the cardiac output is required to be oxygenated and have CO_2 removed, venoarterial perfusion must be undertaken (Fig 6–30). This would also be necessary if there is a concomitant injury to the heart. Oxygenated blood must be returned, however, to the arch of the aorta in order to ensure that the coronary and cerebral circulation will be adequately oxygenated. Once the patient has improved significantly, he or she can be gradually removed from the bypass by decreasing the amount of blood removed from either the right ventricle or the inferior vena cava and gradually returning the circulation back to the patient's own pulmonary arterial circulation.

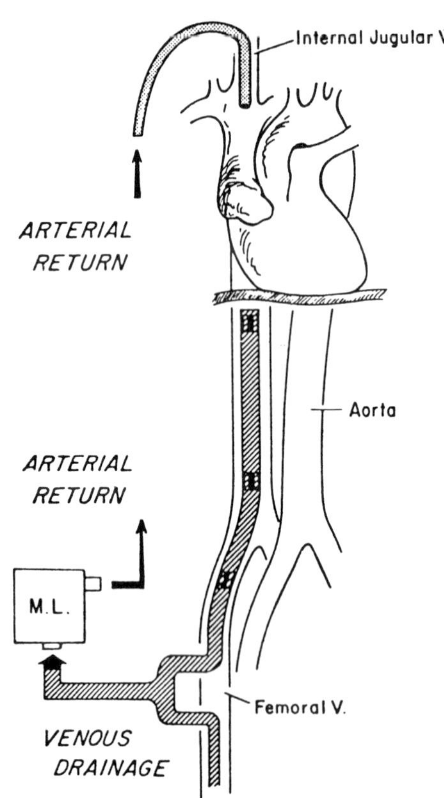

FIG 6–29
Diagram of the venovenous perfusion route. *M.L.* = membrane lung.

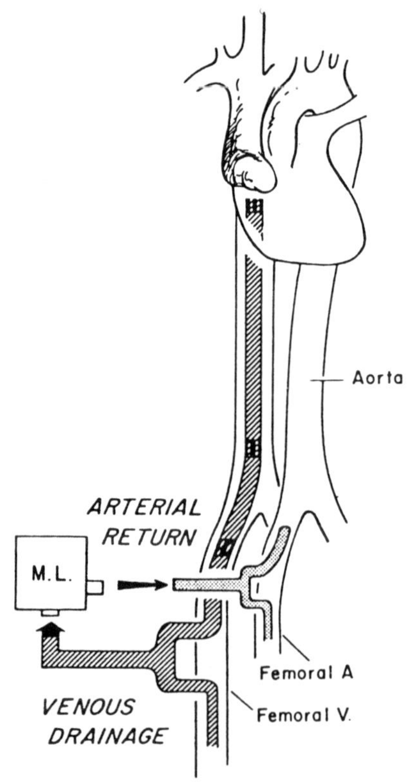

FIG 6–30
Diagram of the venoarterial perfusion route with femoral artery cannulation and distal aortic return (also see Fig 6–31). *M.L.* = membrane lung. (From Zapol WM, Ovist J, Pontoppidan H, et al: *Journal of Thoracic and Cardiovascular Surgery* 1975; 69:3.)

In the first study done and presented in the *Journal of the American Medical Association* in 1979,[44] patients were entered from multiple institutions in a prospective randomized nature. The criteria for entry, however, were so severe that the expected survival rate without ECMO was less than 5%. Entrance criteria included an arterial Po_2 that had to be less than 50 mm Hg for more than 2 hours when the inspired oxygen concentration that the patient was receiving was a 1.0 (rapid-entry criteria). Patients could also be included if the arterial Po_2 was less than 50 for more than 12 hours when the Fio_2 was greater than 0.6 and PEEP was higher than 5 cm H_2O if the right-to-left shunt was at least 30% of the cardiac output (slow-entry criteria). A total of 90 patients were studied in this manner. Forty-eight patients received conventional therapy, and 42 patients received ECMO therapy. About half the patients were entered by the rapid-entry criteria for oxygenation and the other half by the slow-entry criteria. The survival rate of the ECMO-treated group was 9.5%, whereas in the conventionally treated it was 8.3%, but this was not statistically significantly different. Thus, for the population in general, there did not appear to be any significant benefit in using ECMO for ARF. One cannot reach any conclusions for individual cases. Of interest is that bypass did not increase the risk of septicemia or decrease the incidence of pneumothorax. Bypass was associated with a reduction in platelet count and white blood cell concentrations, and there was an increase in the mean blood and plasma infusion rates from 1,000 to 2,500 mL/day. Bypass did seem to prolong life for a short period. The number of bypass patients surviving the first 11 days of the study was significantly greater than the number lasting that long while receiving conventional therapy. Thus, if there was a reversible component, bypass might "buy" the patient significant amount of time for this reversible component to be treated. The patients in the bypass group had significantly higher Po_2 and lower Pco_2 values, and the Fio_2 was significantly lower during bypass than during the conventional treatment. The conclusions reached in this study were that ECMO was a modality of therapy that could prolong the life of patients with severe lung injury over the short term but that the limiting factor in survivorship in this subgroup of patients with severe lung injury was not the method of support but the underlying process itself. In 1988, Dr. Egan[45] and others reported their 10-year experience with ECMO and severe respiratory failure. In this study, they used primarily venovenous bypass and studied patients with varying diagnoses, including aspiration pneumonia, chest trauma, and legionnaire's disease. The ages of the patients included in their study were from 13 to 49 years, with a mean duration of 151 hours of bypass time. The group included only 17 patients, however, and of those 17, only 3 were alive and well at the time that they reported the results. A fourth patient had been weaned from ECMO and went to lung transplantation but died of complications of the lung transplant about 68 days after ECMO had been discontinued.

Complications

The complications associated with ECMO included technical failures, although these seem to be fairly uncommon at the present time, immunologic difficulties, and anticoagulation-associated sequelae resulting in significant bleeding complications. Significant thrombocytopenia developed in virtually all patients. Several of the patients had platelet counts of less than 10,000 (normal, 350,000). Many patients required massive transfusions for gastrointestinal bleeding and retroperitoneal bleeding, and several patients were reported to have had intracerebral bleeding. Deep venous thrombosis at the site of the cannulation was a significant problem, as was the development of aneurysmal dilatation of the blood vessels that had been cannulated for the procedure. Sepsis is a very common complication of ARF, and it is difficult to determine whether patients who are receiving ECMO or perfusion have a greater risk for sepsis or a poor survival since there is not a large enough patient population to make this determination. Renal failure is also commonly associated with patients with this severe type of lung injury. Therefore, to determine whether renal failure is more common in these patients is very difficult. It was initially felt that nonpulsatile blood flow to the renal arteries would result in some acute renal impairment.

Summary

In summary, instituting ECMO requires a tremendous commitment with respect to personnel and ancillary hospital services and should only be undertaken when there is a reversible lung process. The factors that most limit the usefulness of ECMO are really not technical but relate to the ability of the lung to recover from its underlying insult. One could make a case for long-term use of ECMO where it is feasible in somebody who has a reasonable chance of recovery but has not responded to conventional therapy. An example is neonates with specific respiratory conditions such as respiratory distress syndrome, meconium aspiration syndrome, persistent fetal circulation, congenital diaphragmatic hernia, and neonatal pneumonia.[46]

INTRAVASCULAR OXYGENATION

Introduction and History

During the late 1970s and 1980s most intensive care physicians recognized the unacceptably high morbidity and mortality rates of patients with advanced, potentially reversible ARF. As a consequence, a search began for new or better ways to augment the deficient blood gas transfer that threatened the life of these patients with ARDS. Simply turning up the F_{IO_2}, flow rates, or ventilatory gas pressures delivered by the positive-pressure mechanical ventilator often failed to correct the hypoxemia or hypercarbia, which at times was accompanied by pneumothorax, mediastinal and/or subcutaneous emphysema (barotrauma), depressed hemodynamics (inadequate venous return to the right heart), rapid progression of the pulmonary pathologic lesions, and/or development of refractory multiorgan failure. A plethora of innovative techniques were developed for improving the efficacy and decreasing the adverse sequelae of mechanical ventilator assistance of sick natural lungs. At the same time (1970 to 1980), significant advances were occurring in mechanical blood gas transfer membrane technology. Substitution of a membrane oxygenator for the blood gas transfer function of natural lungs, in the form of cardiopulmonary bypass for cardiac surgery, was a well-established procedure routinely and successfully carried out for up to 8 hours on a daily basis throughout [1]the world. Prolonged (up to 2 weeks) extrapulmonary augmentation of deficient blood gas transfer by extracorporeal perfusion of blood through a pump-oxygenator system (ECMO), as was previously discussed, had been demonstrated to be an effective means for salvaging infants in life-threatening ARF, and the frequency and effectiveness of its use were expanding.

By making logical modifications in the design, materials, and functional characteristics of the existing hollow-fiber membrane oxygenator technology, Mortensen and associates in 1982[47, 48] developed an oxygenator that could be inserted into a subject's venae cavae and, under properly controlled circumstances, could transfer oxygen into and carbon dioxide out of circulating venous blood without the use of pumps or reservoirs and without involving the natural lungs.* Thus, intravenous administration of oxygen and removal of carbon dioxide became feasible. Between 1982 and 1985, further fundamental research and development activities by this group of scientists produced the IVOX device and demonstrated its safety and efficacy in laboratory animal experiments. Significant limitations existed in the volume of gas (O_2 and CO_2) that this device could exchange with normally circulating blood and in the time period that it could remain functional while indwelling in the venae cavae.[49, 50] Nevertheless, by 1989 the IVOX device had been shown to be sufficiently safe and effective in awake, standing sheep (both normal and with induced ARF) that clinical trials were authorized by the FDA in selected patients whose hypoxemia and hypercarbia were refractory to intensive mechanical ventilator support.[51] These clinical trials are currently in progress in 29 international respiratory intensive care centers with the objective of determining the risks, hazards, and clinical effectiveness of this method for temporary augmentation of gas exchange in patients with acute, potentially reversible respiratory failure.[52–58]

Conceptual and Design Features of the Intravascular Oxygenator

The IVOX device is a small, elongated, gas-on-the-inside/blood-on-the-outside, hollow-fiber membrane oxygenator (Fig 6–31) designed to lie within the venae cavae where venous blood en route to the right heart and lungs flows over and around the hollow fibers of the IVOX (Fig 6–32). Gas exchange takes place between the venous blood outside the hollow fibers and the gas within the lumina of the hollow fibers. This O_2 and CO_2 transfer takes place across the gas (but not liquid) permeable walls of the hollow fibers. Each hollow fiber thus resembles the respiratory bronchiole-alveolus-pulmonary capillary bed complex of the natural lung and accomplishes gas transfer between venous blood and an airway across a gas-permeable/liquid-impermeable membrane (Fig 6–33). The intraluminal gas within the IVOX hollow fibers is then exhausted into the atmosphere through the gas exit conduit. Blood flows by natural hemodynamic forces over and around this artificial alveolar-capillary membrane interposed in the venae cavae and results in prepulmonary blood gas exchange that can augment the gas transfer being achieved through the natural lungs. These fundamental design, material, and functional concepts of the IVOX device are summarized as follows:

- The IVOX is a small-diameter, elongated, hollow-fiber membrane oxygenator without an external case.
- The IVOX is placed into the subject's venae cavae through a peripheral venotomy.
- Oxygen is introduced into the hollow-fiber lumina via a small-diameter gas inlet conduit that is the central limb of a double-lumen gas transport tube.

*The authors wish to thank Dr. Mortensen for his contribution to this section of the chapter. Dr. Mortensen is the founder, Senior Medical Advisor, Chief Technical Officer, and a member of the board of directors of Cardiopulmonics, Salt Lake City, Utah.

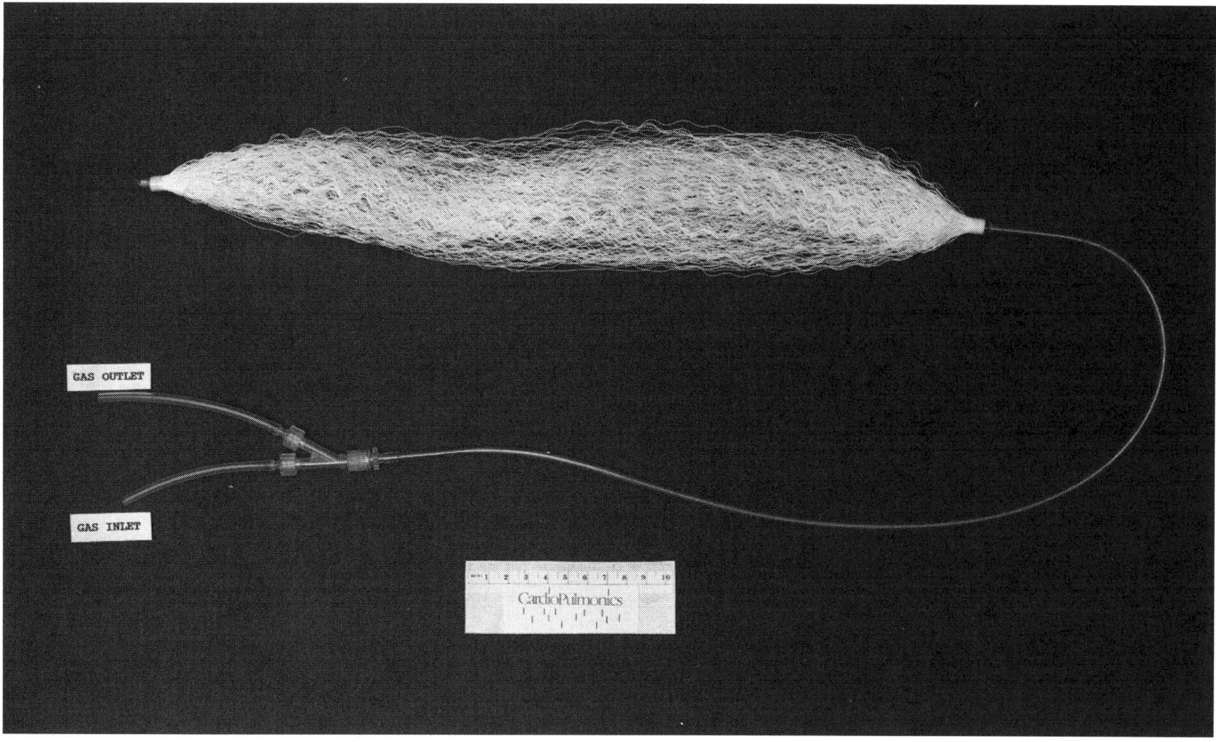

FIG 6–31
Photograph of the intravascular blood gas exchanger (IVOX). Crimped hollow fibers (approximately 1,000) lie free in the blood flowing in the superior and inferior venae cavae and right atrium en route to the right ventricle and lungs. Oxygen enters the inlet limb of a double-lumen gas conduit at atmospheric pressure. It is carried in the central gas conduit to the distal potting where it is distributed into the lumina of the hollow fibers. Gas exchange occurs with the blood outside each hollow fiber through the walls of the hollow fibers. Gas remaining in the hollow-fiber lumina exits the body via the outer portion of the double-lumen gas conduit, being pulled through the device by suction applied to the gas outlet limb of the double-lumen gas conduit.

- Venous blood en route to the right heart flows over and around the external surfaces of each hollow fiber.
- Blood gas exchange (O_2 into the blood and CO_2 from the blood) takes place across the walls of the hollow fibers.
- Carbon dioxide–rich gas exits the body via the outer gas outlet limb of the double-lumen gas transport conduit.

In order for the IVOX device, lying freely in the venae cavae, to transfer clinically significant quantities of O_2/CO_2 into/out of venous blood and to remain functional for several days, significant modifications in the design, materials, and functional properties of the usual hollow-fiber membrane oxygenator were necessary[48–50, 59]:

- Coat the microporous hollow fibers with an ultrathin, continuous, pinhole-free, gas-permeable siloxane coating.
- Arrange the hollow fibers within the venae cavae to produce a distributed blood flow pattern over and around each hollow fiber (Bellhouse principle).
- Develop a mechanism to furl the fibers into a small-diameter bundle for peripheral vein entry and then unfurl the fibers to achieve optimum deployment and filling of the vena caval lumen.
- Coat each hollow fiber and the entire intravascular device with an effective, covalently bonded thromboresistant coating.
- Use subatmospheric pressure (vacuum) on the gas outlet to achieve optimum gas flow through the IVOX device at low (negative) intraluminal gas pressures.

For example, a method had to be developed for furling (compressing) the hollow fibers into a compact bundle with a cross-sectional diameter small enough to enter a peripheral access vein and then unfurling (deploying) the fibers into a configuration that would fill the cross-sectional diameter of the larger venae cavae. The blood flow pattern of venous blood over and around the external surface of each hollow fiber needed to be

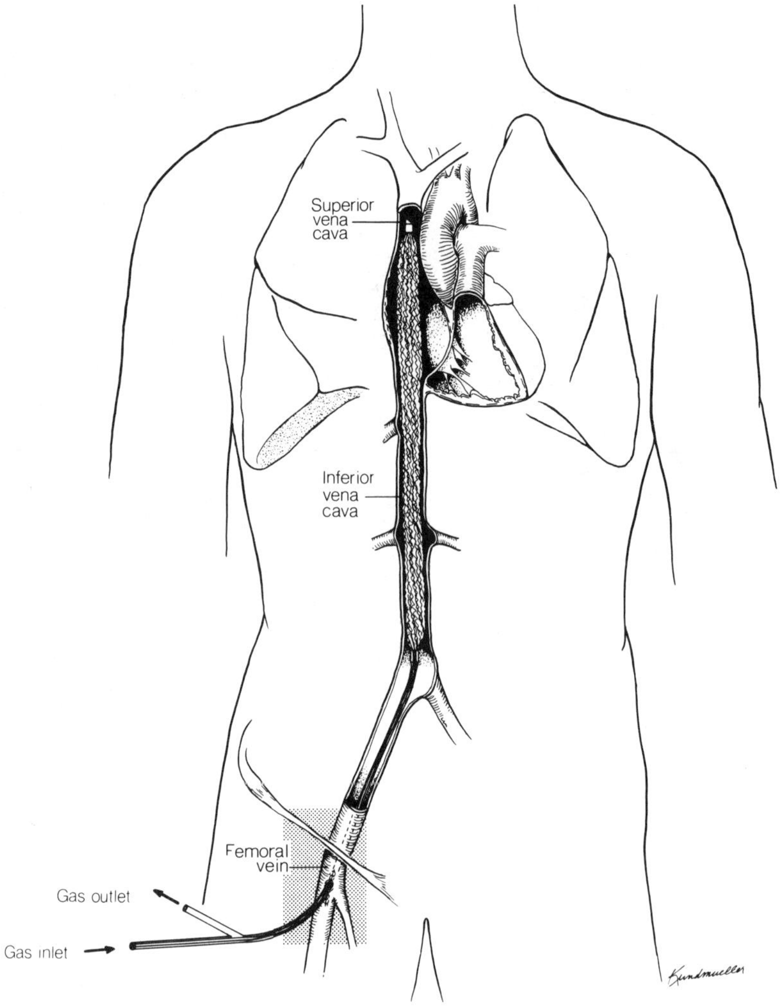

FIG 6–32
Diagram of an IVOX device in its intra–vena caval position in a human patient. An IVOX device has been introduced into the body through a venotomy in the right common femoral vein, then advanced up the iliac vein and inferior vena cava, through the lateral aspect of the right atrium, and up the superior vena cava, with its tip lying in the superior vena cava. The crimped hollow fibers lie free in the vena caval bloodstream. The double-lumen gas conduit connects to the potted manifolds at the ends of the hollow fibers. The inner *(inlet)* gas conduit is connected to an oxygen source; the outer *(outlet)* gas conduit is connected to a vacuum pump that pulls the gas through the hollow fibers at controlled subatmospheric pressures. The IVOX device can remain functional in the venae cavae for up to 19 days; then (or whenever it is no longer needed) the IVOX is removed and the access venotomy repaired surgically.

altered to produce good mixing of the blood rather than permitting laminar flow along the hollow fibers. Specific disadvantages of microporous hollow fibers (such as roughness of their outer surface, filling of the mural micropores with fluid, and serum leakage from the blood into the gas phase of the oxygenator) needed to be overcome if the IVOX device (in the event that the hollow fibers, the gas transfer membrane, or the gas conduits were damaged and/or leaked) were to be successful. Finally, it was necessary to significantly reduce the thrombogenicity of the IVOX device lying in the vena caval bloodstream.

Characterization of Intravascular Oxygenator Performance

Engineering/Mechanical Characterization

Results of engineering bench assessments of IVOX gas pressures, flow rates, various dimensional specifications, and the mechanical and functional characteristics of the IVOX device have been summarized in Table 6–13. The device is manufactured in four sizes: 7, 8, 9, 10; the size corresponds to the nominal cross-sectional OD (in millimeters) of the furled fiber bundle, the distal tip, and the proximal potting. As received by an IVOX user, the IVOX kit contains the IVOX device per se and a collection of ancillary components used in the preparation of the device for implantation, including a tubular hydration chamber, a furler, stiffener stylet, guidewire, insertional sheath, and gas inlet and outlet conduits, all of which are sterile and disposable (Fig 6–34). In addition, IVOX utilization requires use of a permanent gas controller that connects to an electrical source and to a source of compressed oxygen (Fig 6–35). Contained within the gas controller unit are a small electrical vacuum pump, gas flowmeter, gas reassurance gauges, and manual control knob. Operation of an indwelling IVOX device is simple and requires only occasional adjustment of the vacuum applied to the IVOX gas outlet, assurance of a supply of oxygen flowing into the device, monitoring of the CO_2

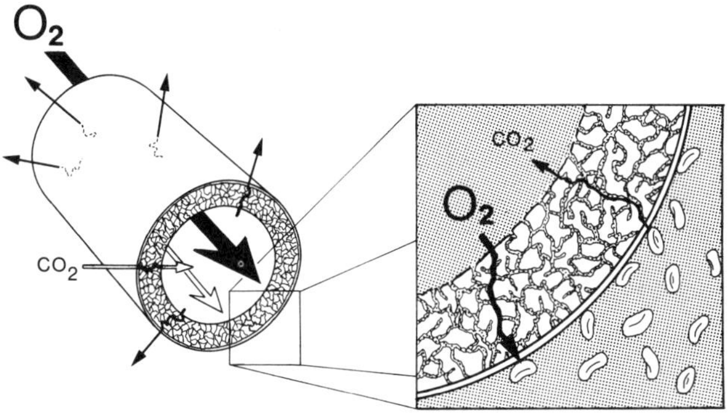

FIG 6–33
Diagram of the IVOX hollow-fiber gas transfer membrane. The microporous wall of the hollow fiber acts as a skeleton or framework supporting the ultrathin siloxane gas transfer membrane and permits gas on the inside of each hollow fiber to make contact with the siloxane membrane separating the gas from the blood outside the hollow fiber. Oxygen and carbon dioxide permeate through the gas-permeable, but fluid-impermeable siloxane membrane in response to partial pressure differences (gradient) between the gas inside the hollow fiber and blood outside the hollow fiber, as shown in the *inset.* The composition of gas entering and flowing inside the hollow fibers of the IVOX is 100% oxygen; gas flowing out of the hollow fibers and exhausted into the atmosphere contains carbon dioxide and residual oxygen. The inside diameter of each IVOX hollow fiber is 190 μm, the microporous hollow fiber wall is 30 μm thick, and the continuous siloxane gas transfer membrane is 1 μm thick. The similarities in dimensions and function between the hollow-fiber component of IVOX and the natural pulmonary alveolar-capillary membrane complex is apparent.

content of the IVOX exit gas by continuous capnometry, and adjustment of systemic heparin administration to produce moderate systemic anticoagulation (activated clotting time [ACT] of approximately 180 seconds).

Laboratory Animal Assessments

Safety and efficacy testing in normal animals. The primary performance characterization of the IVOX device is related to the risks and hazards associated with its utilization. Data from a series of standing, awake, highly instrumented but otherwise normal sheep with a functioning IVOX in the venae cavae were compared with data from similarly prepared and managed control sheep without an IVOX for up to 10 days of observation in the animal ICU. Extensive blood gas, hemodynamic, hematologic, blood chemistry, bacteriologic, and vital function testing was carried out to compare the IVOX-implanted with normal control animals. All the animals were then euthanized, and necropsy findings in the two groups were compared. Results of these experiments demonstrated no significant difference between the IVOX-implanted and control animals. Utilization of the IVOX device appeared to be free from significant risks and hazards, and the device was found to exchange significant quantities of O_2 and CO_2 into and out of circulating venous blood (Table 6–14).[51]

Quantification of gas transfer by intravenous oxygenation. Ex vivo and in vivo animal experiments indicated that the quantity of gas transferred by an IVOX

TABLE 6–13
Intravascular Oxygenator Mechanical/Engineering Specifications/Characteristics

	IVOX* Size			
Dimensional/Mechanical Specifications	7	8	9	10
Number of hollow fibers	589	703	894	1107
Length of each fiber (cm)	38	41	45	50
Length of crimped fiber bundle (cm)	30	33	37	40
Surface area of siloxane gas transfer membrane (m^2)	0.21	0.32	0.41	0.52
OD* of furled fiber bundle (mm)	11.1	12.0	13.5	14.6
OD of insertional sheath (mm)	12.6	13.5	15.0	15.8
Nominal gas flow into and out of functioning IVOX device (cc/min)	2,500	2,700	3,300	3,400

Nominal Gas Pressure at Various Sites in a Functioning IVOX Device	All Sizes of IVOX
O_2 inlet to gas conduit	+5 mm Hg
O_2 inlet to hollow fiber	−110 mm Hg
Gas outlet from hollow fibers	−210 mm Hg
Gas outlet at Y connector	−295 mm Hg
Vacuum delivered to gas outlet conduit	−355 mm Hg
ID* of each hollow fiber	0.190 mm
OD of each hollow fiber	0.236 mm
Thickness of siloxane coating on each hollow fiber	.001 mm

*IVOX = intravascular oxygenator; OD = outside diameter; ID = inside diameter.

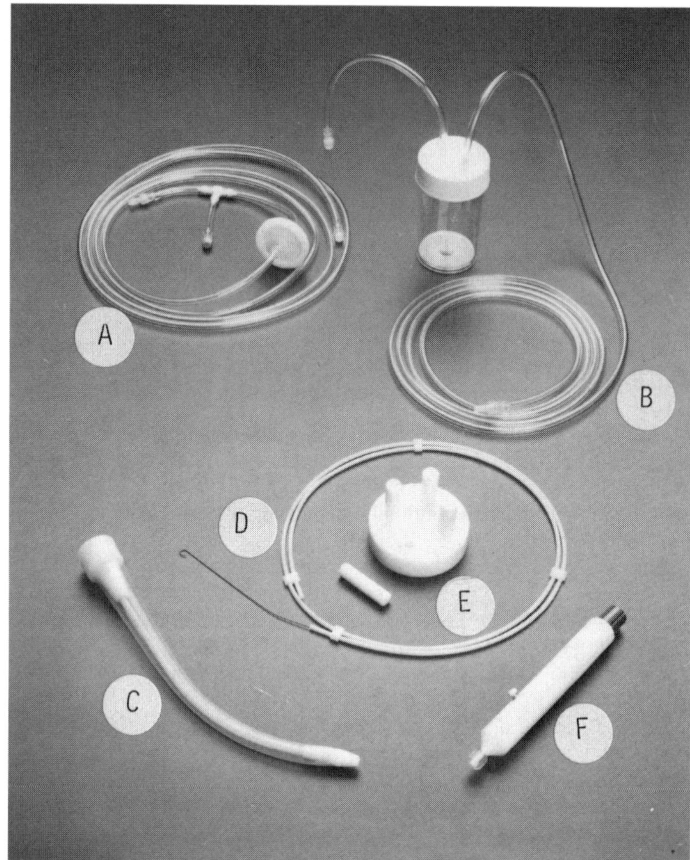

FIG 6–34
Photograph of IVOX ancillary devices. **A,** the O_2 inlet line from the gas controller to the IVOX device is 10 ft in length with a bacterial filter included. **B,** the CO_2 outlet line from the IVOX device to the gas controller is 10 ft in length with a water vapor condensation trap included. **C,** insertional cannula through which the IVOX device is inserted into the access vein. **D,** guidewire over which the IVOX is inserted. **E,** access vein sizer to determine the diameter of the access vein. **F,** furler for furling the IVOX fiber bundle into a small cross-sectional dimension for insertion.

device was variable, depending upon the following factors (listed roughly in order of decreasing influence on the gas transfer rate)[49, 50, 59]:

1. Size of the IVOX device (surface area of the gas transfer membrane exposed to blood)
2. Flow rate of blood over the IVOX hollow fibers (cardiac output/venous return of the subject with an indwelling IVOX)
3. Blood flow pattern around the IVOX hollow fibers (proper deployment of crimped hollow fibers, ratio of hollow-fiber volume to blood volume within the venae cavae, extent of mixing of blood flowing over the IVOX device)
4. P_{CO_2} and P_{O_2} in the blood exposed to IVOX (CO_2 and O_2 partial pressure gradients across the IVOX membrane)
5. Rate of gas flow through (into/out of) the IVOX device
6. Intraluminal pressure (vacuum) of gas within IVOX hollow fibers
7. Composition of gas delivered to the IVOX device
8. Hemoglobin content of circulating blood exposed to the IVOX device

These IVOX gas transfer experiments also demonstrated that quantification of CO_2 removal by the IVOX device could be accomplished accurately and easily by simply reading the flow rate of gas through the IVOX device and noting the carbon dioxide content of the exhaust gas coming out of the IVOX. Placing an accurate flowmeter in the IVOX gas conduit and routing IVOX exit gas through a continuous-reading capnometer produces the necessary data to calculate the quantity of CO_2 removed from blood flowing over the IVOX. Since 100% oxygen is delivered to the IVOX device (the CO_2 content of the IVOX inflow gas is zero), the percent CO_2 in the IVOX outflow gas multiplied by the gas flow rate through the IVOX device (in milliliters per minute) gives the rate of CO_2 removal from the blood by IVOX (in milliliters per minute). This simple method of quantifying the CO_2 transfer rate can be applied whether the IVOX is indwelling in the subject's venae cavae or whether blood flow passes over an extracorporeal IVOX device in an ex vivo perfusion experiment.

On the other hand, accurate assessment of the rate of O_2 transfer into blood through an IVOX device lying in the venae cavae presents formidable problems. Determination of the O_2 content of gas flowing into and out of an

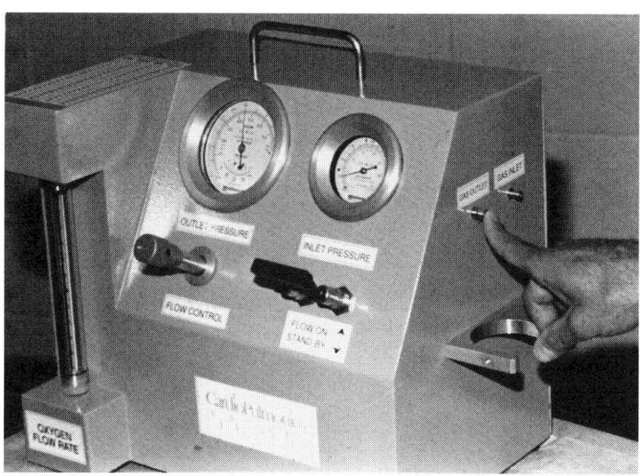

FIG 6–35
Photograph of an IVOX gas controller. This permanent component of the IVOX system connects to (1) a source of AC electrical power, (2) a continuous source of oxygen, (3) the IVOX gas inlet line, and (4) the IVOX gas outlet line. The gas controller contains a control knob to adjust the vacuum applied to the IVOX gas outlet line and gas inlet and outlet pressure gauges; a gas flowmeter is also included.

IVOX device to the degree of accuracy necessary requires rather sophisticated techniques (such as mass spectrometry) not readily applicable or available in the operating room or the ICU. Corrections for the accumulation of nitrogen, CO_2, and water vapor in the IVOX outlet gas must also be considered. Attempts to calculate the O_2 transfer rate by assessing the O_2 content of blood coming to the IVOX in the venae cavae require a meaningful sample of pre-IVOX blood to compare with the readily available post-IVOX (pulmonary arterial) blood. Because of differences in the O_2 content of renal, hepatic, coronary sinus, azygos, subclavian, and jugular veins (all of this blood being exposed to IVOX), no truly representative pre-IVOX mixed venous blood sample can be obtained in vivo.

An estimated O_2 transfer rate by means of an IVOX device indwelling in the venae cavae can be arrived at by comparing (1) the O_2 content of pulmonary artery blood sampled with an IVOX device indwelling in the venae cavae but with no flow of gas into or out of the IVOX and (2) the O_2 content of pulmonary artery blood collected after oxygen flow through the IVOX has been established for 5 minutes. In order to be meaningful, the IVOX-on and IVOX-off samples of pulmonary artery blood must be taken in as little time as possible (allowing at least 5 minutes for equilibration between sampling). Also, the subject's cardiac output, O_2 transfer through the natural lungs, and metabolic gas utilization/production must be stable during the IVOX-on and IVOX-off time periods to permit the calculation of an estimated rate of O_2 transfer through the IVOX device. Unfortunately, as a consequence of the difficulty in maintaining physiologic stability during the IVOX-on/IVOX-off time periods, this method of estimating O_2 delivery through an IVOX device in the venae cavae may produce erratic, variable, and rather inaccurate results.

Because of these difficulties in quantifying O_2 transfer through an IVOX device lying in the venae cavae, an ex vivo experimental model has been utilized to accurately assess the gas transfer performance of the IVOX device. In these ex vivo experiments, venovenous bypass of blood from an anesthetized animal (sheep or dog) was pumped through a test chamber approximately the size and configuration of the venae cavae in which an IVOX device is deployed. In such experiments, simultaneous samples of blood entering and exiting the test chamber can be obtained for an analysis of the O_2 content; the flow rate of blood over and around the IVOX device can be varied at will and can be accurately measured; and gas pressures, flow rates, and samples for analysis can be readily obtained. Data thus produced permit accurate, reliable quantification of both the O_2 and O_2/CO_2 transfer performance of an IVOX device under conditions that simulate but are not identical with the in vivo conditions where the IVOX device lies in the venae cavae.

A summary of the quantitative gas transfer performance of various-sized IVOX devices as determined by

TABLE 6–14
Quantitative Gas Transfer Achieved by Means of Intravascular Oxygenation

	Average O_2 Transfer (cc/min)			Average CO_2 Transfer (cc/min)		
IVOX Size (mm OD)*	Animal, Ex Vivo	Animal, In Vivo	Human, In Vivo (ARF*)	Animal, Ex Vivo	Animal, In Vivo	Human, In Vivo (ARF)
5 (experimental)	15.4	18.0	–	20.5	13.8	–
6 (experimental)	22.8	35.5	–	33.2	24.8	–
7 (clinically available)	28.5	66.7	52.4	44.8	39.8	48.2
8 (clinically available)	34.9	97.5	66.3	53.2	48.6	70.5
9 (clinically available)	45.9	115.7	73.2	66.8	60.4	72.8
10 (clinically available)	52.9	133.0	104.7	80.7	72.2	74.3

* OD = outside diameter; ARF = acute respiratory failure.

TABLE 6–15

Changes in Blood Gases in Pulmonary Artery Blood Related to Turning Indwelling IVOX On and Off*

Parameter	IVOX On	IVOX Off
Gas flow rate into IVOX (mL/min)	2,640	0
CO_2 content of IVOX exhaust gas (%)	3.03	0
Cardiac output (L/min)	6.1	6.1
Pulmonary artery blood		
po_2 (mm Hg)	43.9	40.2
pco_2 (mm Hg)	47.3	54.4
pH	7.365	7.326
Hemoglobin (g/dL)	11.8	11.8
O_2 saturation (mm Hg)	55.1	48.4
O_2 content (mL/dL)	9.3	8.2

O_2 transfer by IVOX = (9.3 − 8.2) × 6.1 × 10 = 67.1 mL/min
CO_2 transfer by IVOX = 2,640 × 0.0303 = 79.99 mL/min.
Sheep no. 279
Sheep body wt = 88 kg
IVOX size = 10

*Sheep made mildly hypoxic and hypercarbic by hypoventilation.

animal ex vivo and animal in vivo experiments and in the first few human clinical trials of IVOX is recorded in Table 6–14.

Intravascular oxygenator gas transfer efficacy in experimental animals with induced acute respiratory failure. The performance characterization of the IVOX device was investigated by its performance in hypoxemic, hypercarbic laboratory animals. Again, sheep were used. ARF was simulated in anesthetized, curarized animals by controlled hypoventilation during acute experiments. For chronic experiments in awake, standing animals, ARF was induced by applying various methods that simulate the pathophysiology of human ARDS. IVOX performed well in all these experiments; it removed significant quantities of CO_2 from hypercarbic blood and added similar amounts of oxygen to hypoxemic blood.

The changes in blood gases during IVOX utilization in sheep made hypoxemic and hypercarbic by hypoventilation-induced ARF are summarized in Tables 6–15 and 6–16. The quantity of O_2/CO_2 transferred by IVOX to/from the animal's circulating blood is also shown in Tables 6–15 and 6–16. More than 40 acute hypoventilation experiments of this type have been carried out, all demonstrating similar findings. Studies in lung-traumatized animals are presented in Tables 6–17 and 6–18.

Acute respiratory insufficiency was induced in an otherwise normal, mature, 71-kg sheep by the Kolobow

TABLE 6–16

Changes in Pulmonary Artery Blood Gases With IVOX On and Off*

Parameter	IVOX Off	IVOX On
Gas flow into IVOX (mL/min)	0	2,730 ml/min
CO_2 content of IVOX exhaust gas (%)	0	4.9
Cardiac output (L/min)	4.93	4.93
PA blood		
po_2 (mm Hg)	20.2	38.8
pco_2 (mm Hg)	97.9	90.1
pH	7.119	7.127
Hemoglobin (g/dL)	20.3	32.6
O_2 saturation (%)	20.3	32.6
O_2 content (mL/dL)	4.8	6.9

CO_2 transfer by IVOX = 2,370 × 4.9% = 116.1 mL/min
O_2 transfer by IVOX = (4.93 × 10) × (6.9 − 4.8) = 103.5 ml/min
Sheep no. 279 (body wt = 88 kg; IVOX size = 10)

*Sheep made severely hypoxemic and hypercarbic by hypoventilation.

TABLE 6–17

Effects of IVOX on Arterial Blood Gases of a Sheep With Acute, Severe, Ventilator-Dependent Respiratory Failure (Kolobow Barotrauma Model)

Event	Ventilator Parameter				Arterial Blood Gases			
	F_{IO_2} (mm Hg)	Min Vol (mL)	PIP* (cm H_2O)	PEEP* (cm H_2O)	pa_{O_2} (mm Hg)	pa_{CO_2} (mm Hg)	O_2 Sat. (%)	O_2 (mL/dL)
Baseline, preinjury	0.21	7000	23	0	88.4	31.9	100.0	–
ARF* w/normal ventilatory assist	0.21	8400	23	0	24.2	58.4	30.3	–
ARF w/intensive ventilatory assist	1.0	8400	50	13	50.7	53.0	73.4	–
Ventilatory assist and IVOX* for 30 min	0.70	8400	45	10	55.9	38.0	85.6	18.3
Ventilatory assist and IVOX for 2 hr	0.60	8400	36	3	90.7	35.8	96.7	19.8
Ventilatory assist and IVOX for 24 hr	0.35	8400	33	0	70.1	40.3	89.6	16.6
Ventilatory assist and IVOX for 48 hr	0.30	8400	29	0	75.7	34.3	93.6	21.4

* PIP = peak inspiratory pressure; PEEP = positive end-expiratory pressure; ARF = acute respiratory failure; IVOX = intravascular oxygenation.

airway barotrauma method. After 40 hours of mechanical ventilation with peak inspiratory pressures of 50 cm H_2O and a minute volume of 8.4 L/min, the Pa_{O_2} was 50.7 mm Hg, Pa_{CO_2} was 53.0 mm Hg, pH was 7.179, pulmonary artery p O_2 was 42.7, CO_2 was 57.8 mm Hg, and cardiac output was 7 L/min (Tables 6–17 and 6–18). These findings remain essentially unchanged during 6 hours of intensive mechanical ventilator support. At this point, a size 7 IVOX device was inserted into the venae cavae through the right jugular vein, and oxygen was pulled through the IVOX at 2 L/min. Within a half hour of IVOX assistance, Pa_{O_2} had increased to 55.9 mm Hg, whereas the ventilator F_{IO_2} was reduced to 0.70 (Table 6–17). Similar but more striking changes were seen in Pa_{CO_2}. Normal ventilation in the barotraumatized animal resulted in hypercarbia, with a Pa_{CO_2} of 58.4 mm Hg and a pH of 7.179. Intensive ventilator support reduced the Pa_{CO_2} only slightly, to 53 mm Hg. However, after 30 minutes of IVOX assistance, the Pa_{CO_2} was down to 38 mm Hg, and it remained in the normal range for 48 hours, even though mechanical ventilator assistance was reduced markedly (Table 6–17). The relationship between F_{IO_2} in the ventilator to the animal's Pa_{O_2} before and after implementation of IVOX assistance is illustrated by Figure 6–36. There was a significant increase in oxygenation of the blood with IVOX assistance, even though the concentration of oxygen delivered to the injured natural lungs by the ventilator was progressively reduced. The effect of IVOX on the pulmonary arterial blood p_{CO_2} of a hypercarbic, ventilator-supported animal was favorable and showed a return to normal levels within 2 hours after IVOX support was begun (Fig 6–37). The gas pressures produced in the animal's airways by the mechanical ventilator before and during IVOX utilization showed a favorable course (Fig 6–38). A significant decrease in both PEEP and peak inspiratory pressure was achieved during IVOX assistance. The quantity of oxygen delivered to the sheep's circulating blood by the IVOX device during this exper-

TABLE 6–18

Oxygen Transfer Through IVOX in Experimental Barotrauma Sheep With Adult Respiratory Distress Syndrome

	Oxygen Content of PA* Blood						Cardiac Output		
Time After IVOX* Implantation	IVOX On	–	IVOX Off	=	On-Off Difference	×	L/min × 10	=	O_2 Transfer by IVOX (cc/min)
30 min	18.3		16.0		2.3		60		138
2 hr	19.8		18.2		1.6		71		114
24 hr	16.6		14.8		1.8		65		117
48 hr	21.4		18.0		3.4		45		153

*IVOX = intravascular oxygenation; PA = pulmonary artery.

Note: Data points referring to the pH, pulmonary artery pressure (mixed venous), are not shown in Tables 6–17 and 6–18 in order to keep the tables as simple as possible.

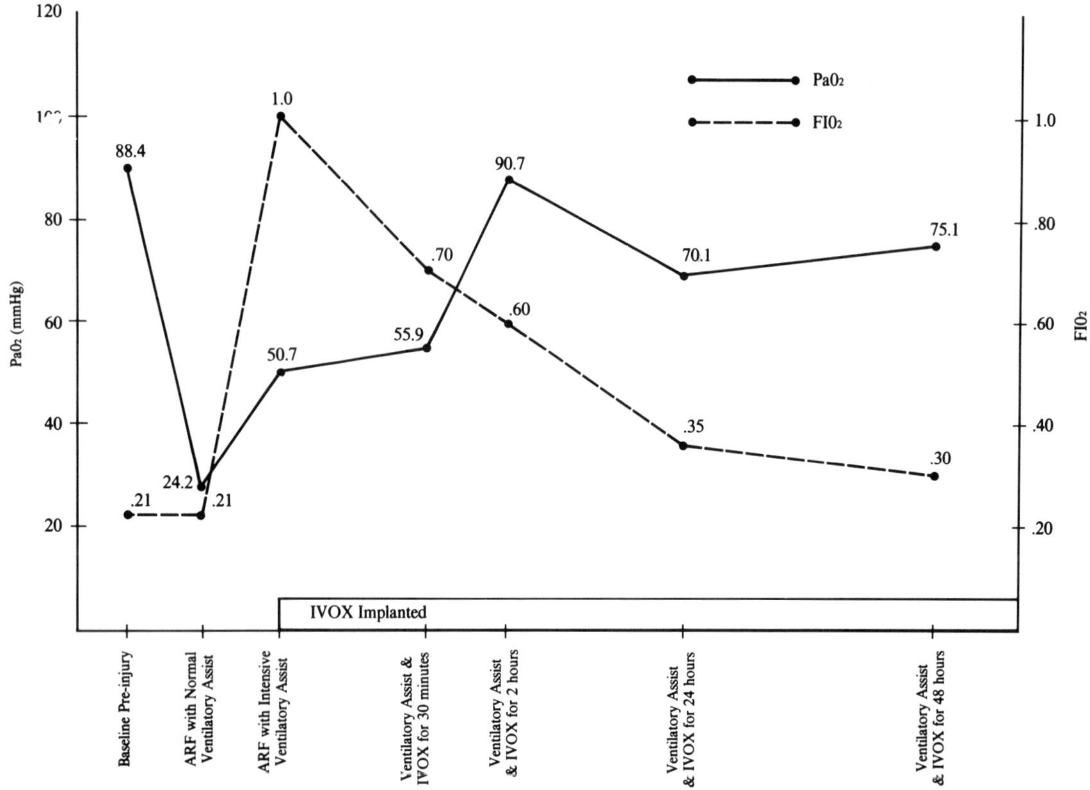

FIG 6–36
Relationship between ventilator F_{IO_2} and Pa_{O_2} in ventilator-dependent animal in acute respiratory failure (ARF) with and without IVOX support.

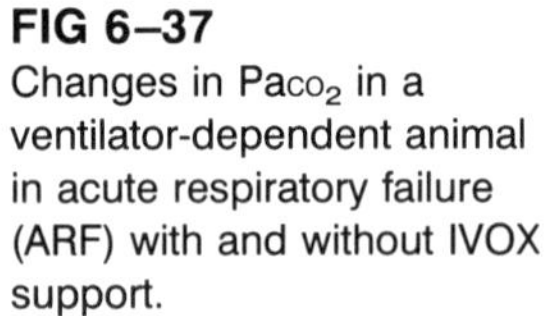
FIG 6–37
Changes in Pa_{CO_2} in a ventilator-dependent animal in acute respiratory failure (ARF) with and without IVOX support.

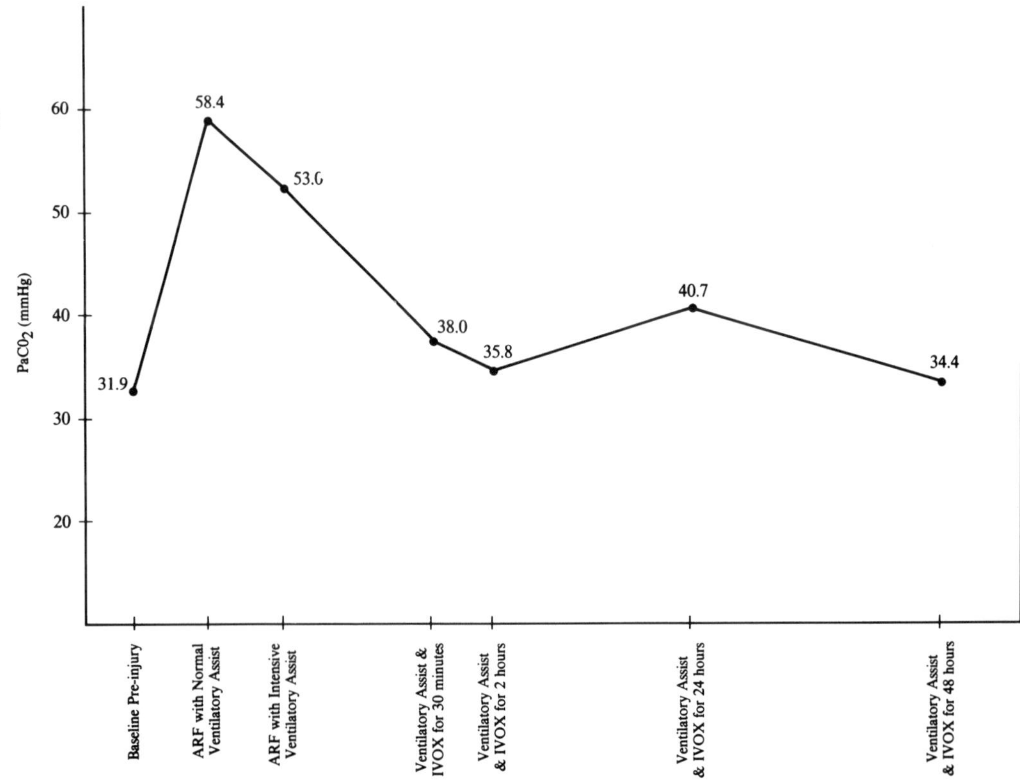

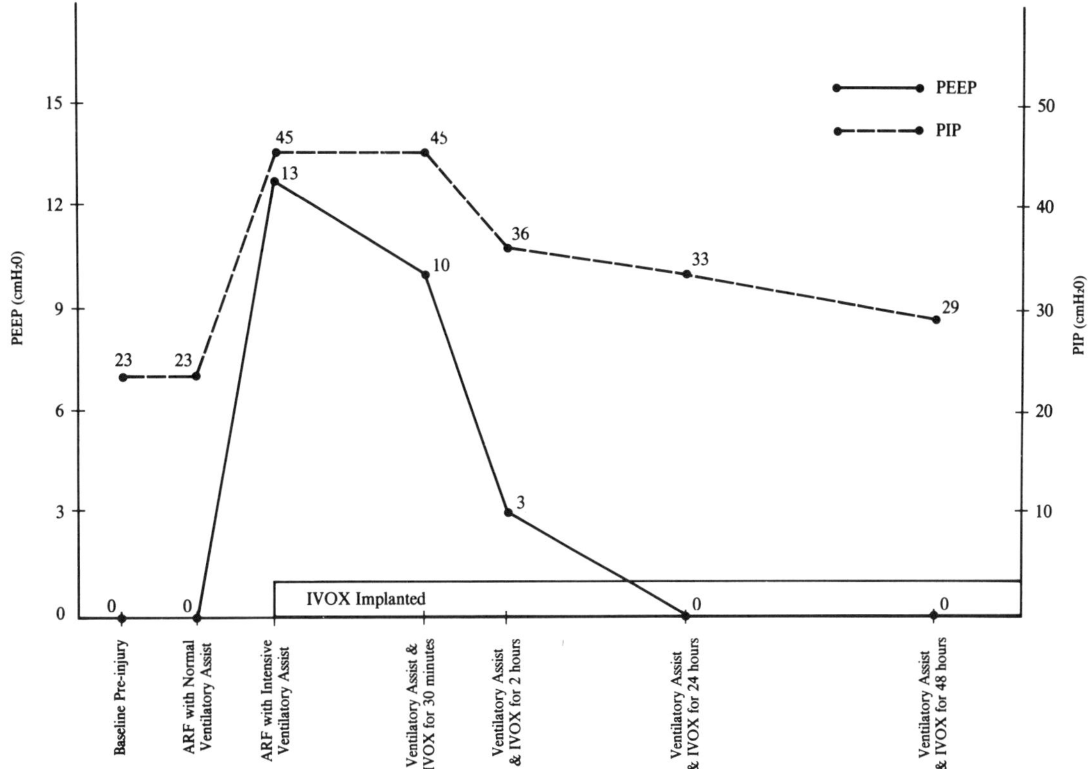

FIG 6–38
Ventilator pressures in a ventilator-dependent animal in acute respiratory failure (ARF) with and without IVOX support.

iment was estimated by the difference in O_2 content of the pulmonary artery blood when the IVOX device was turned off as compared with the content when it was turned on, multiplied by the cardiac output. As shown in Table 6–18, between 114 and 153 mL of O_2 was delivered by IVOX during this experiment. The amount of CO_2 transferred out of the animal's venous blood by the IVOX in its venae cavae during this experiment varied from 41 to 76 mL/min (Table 6–19).

Similar experiments have been carried out that demonstrate the efficacy of IVOX in augmenting O_2/CO_2 transfer to/from the venous blood of experimental animals with simulated ARF induced by smoke inhalation[55] and by intravenous injection of Placidyl®.

Current Status of Intravenous Oxygenation

Preliminary Results of Phase I (Safety Assessment) Early Human Clinical Trials of Intravascular Oxygenation

Between February 1990 and April 1991, a limited number of human patients with advanced ARDS received IVOX implantation to augment blood gas exchange as phase I of the FDA-supervised IVOX clinical trials. The objective of these initial IVOX implantation trials was to determine the risks and hazards of IVOX utilization. Detailed protocols were followed, under FDA surveillance, to obtain data relative to the safety of IVOX utilization. By means of these clinical trials of IVOX, considerable preliminary data relative to its risks and

TABLE 6–19
CO_2 Transfer Through IVOX in Barotrauma-induced Sheep With Experimental Adult Respiratory Distress Syndrome

Time	CO_2 (%) in IVOX Outlet Gas (Capnograph)	Pa_{CO_2} (mm Hg)	Gas Flow Rate Through IVOX (cc/min)	CO_2 Removal by IVOX (cc/min)
Immediately after IVOX turned on	3.8	53.0	2.000	76
30 min after IVOX implantation	2.3	38.0	2.000	46
2 hr after IVOX implantation	2.8	35.5	1.600	44
24 hr after IVOX implantation	3.4	40.3	2.000	68
48 hr after IVOX implantation	3.4	34.8	1.200	41

hazards are available for consideration. The efficacy of IVOX in supporting patients in potentially reversible ARF is currently under investigation as phase II of the ongoing clinical trials of this device.

A summary of the safety data from the first 18 patients entering phase I of the clinical trials of IVOX is recorded in Table 6–20 and Figures 6–39 to 6–42. The major safety concerns were considered to be possible IVOX-related causes of death, pulmonary thromboembolism, introduction of gas into the circulation, obstruction of venous return to the heart, bleeding, injury to the venae cavae, and infection. These concerns were assessed by pathologists at necropsy of the first 10 patients dying during or after IVOX utilization. IVOX utilization did not result in necropsy evidence that any of these major concerns actually occurred. Similarly, clinical observations by the attending physicians during IVOX utilization (Table 6–20) indicated that the major clinical or clinical laboratory concerns (such as febrile response, hemodynamic derangements, hematologic abnormalities, blood chemistry alterations, etc.) were not associated with the utilization of IVOX.

At necropsy, several incidental findings were recorded (Table 6–20), none of which the pathologist analyzing the cases considered to have clinical significance. These incidental findings were all related to the access veins utilized for IVOX insertion or to the venae cavae in which the IVOX device was indwelling. Some bleeding was noted during IVOX insertion (Table 6–20), utilization, and removal in 35% of the phase I clinical trial cases. However, this blood loss was relatively minor in amount and did not constitute a major risk or hazard in these patients. Hematologic changes observed during IVOX utilization were infrequent. The platelet count decreased in 58% of the cases, but the decrease was mild and of no clinical significance and did not require treatment. In only one case did the platelet count decrease to less than 100,000. It is possible that the transient changes in platelet counts were related to heparin administration rather than to the IVOX device per se. The white blood cell count, hemoglobin, and hematocrit were not altered by IVOX implantation. Significant hemolysis of red blood cells was not noted during IVOX utilization. The fibrinogen decreases noted were small in amount and appeared not to have clinical significance. Fibrin degradation products, such as D-dimer, and complement appeared not to be altered by IVOX utilization.

During phase I of the clinical trials, an occasional patient was noted to experience a transient decrease in arterial pressure and a decrease in cardiac output during IVOX implantation. Spontaneous return to the pre-IVOX levels occurred within a few minutes in all cases.

Noteworthy favorable hemodynamic changes during

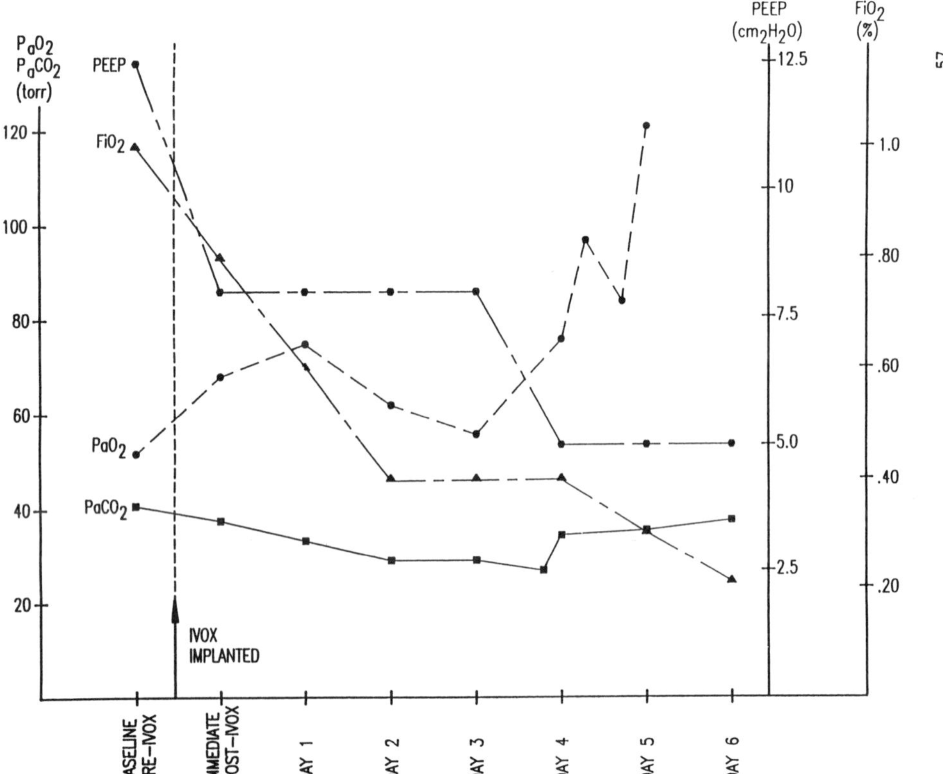

FIG 6–39
Case 1. Note the rapid decrease in the PEEP and FiO_2 delivered by the mechanical ventilator following insertion of the IVOX device. This was accompanied by recovery from hypoxemia and hypercarbia along with the patient's acute respiratory failure. The patient made a complete recovery.

TABLE 6–20

Preliminary Observations From Initial IVOX Phase I Clinical Trials

Major IVOX* Safety Concerns	Incidence
Necropsy findings	
IVOX-related *primary* cause of death	0/10
IVOX-related *contributing* cause of death	0/10
Grossly recognized thromboemboli in right heart/pulmonary arterial tree	0/10
Grossly recognized pulmonary infarction	0/10
Histopathologic evidence of IVOX-related thromboemboli/pulmonary infarction	0/10
Gross or microscopic gas, bubbles, or foam in venae cavae, right heart, or pulmonary vessels	0/10
Evidence of IVOX-related obstruction or interference to blood flow to right heart	0/10
Laceration, perforation, disruption, or bleeding from venae cavae	0/10
IVOX-related sepsis, bacteremia, or localized infection	0/10
Clinical observations relative to risks and hazards	
Clinical evidence of toxic/allergic/rejection responses to IVOX	0/14
Febrile response to IVOX	0/14
Edema/color change upstream to venotomy in	
Right leg	3/10
Right side of head/neck	0/14
Infection	
Systemic	0/14
At venotomy site	0/14
Remote	0/14
Clinical evidence of pulmonary thromboembolism	0/14
Cliical evidence of pulmonary infarction	0/14
Incidental IVOX-Related Findings at Necropsy	
Hematoma, IVOX insertion site	30%
Thrombus in repaired access vein	
Nonocclusive	33.3%
Occlusive	16.7%
Ligation of entry vein	
Jugular	100%
Femoral	16.7%
Thrombus on vena caval intima	
Minor (1–3 patches < 1 cm in diameter)	40%
Moderate (1 or more patches > 1 cm in diameter)	0
Extensive (nonocclusive thrombus involving 50% or more of caval diameter)	0
Occlusive (thrombotic material occluding venae cavae)	0
Inflammatory changes in vena caval intima/subintima	30%
Bleeding Related to IVOX Utilization	
No significant bleeding	65%
Blood loss at insertion/explantation	
50–100 mL	14.3%
>100 mL	21.4%
Postinsertion oozing at entry site	
Mild—no sequelae	14.3%
Moderate—required nonsurgical therapy	14.3%
Severe—required surgical correction	0
Bleeding at remote sites	
Mild—no clinical sequelae	7.1%
Moderate—required transfusions but no other clinical sequelae	14.3%
Severe—required transfusions, surgical intervention	0

*IVOX = intravascular oxygenation.

IVOX utilization included a decrease in pulmonary artery pressure in 71% of the cases and decreased pulmonary wedge and right atrial pressures in most of the patients in whom signs of congestive heart failure were present before the IVOX device was inserted. It is particularly gratifying to note that of those patients who needed intensive inotropic support for depressed cardiac function before the IVOX device was inserted, 67% experienced improvement in hemodynamics with a decrease or withdrawal of inotropic medication during IVOX utiliza-

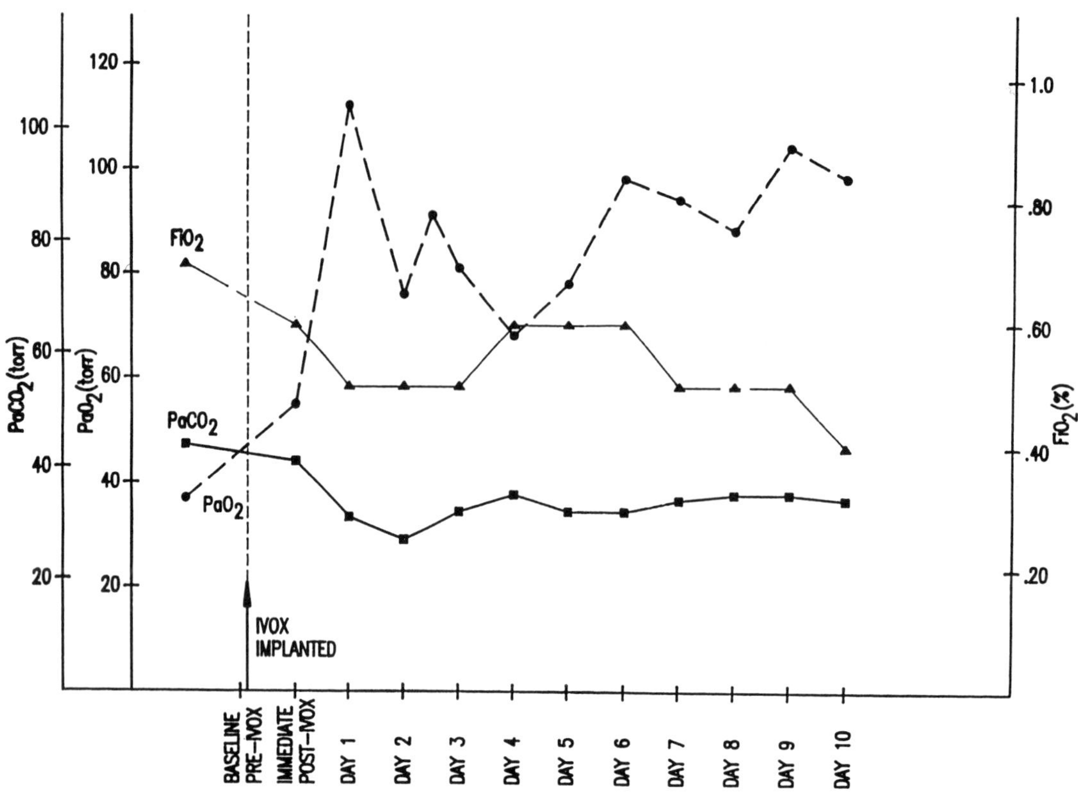

FIG 6–40

Case 2. Note the improvement in Pa_{O_2} and Pa_{CO_2} while the F_{IO_2} decreased significantly. This patient's lung dysfunction was being overcome nicely following augmentation of blood gas transfer by means of IVOX. However, death occurred a few days later from causes unrelated to his ARDS or to the IVOX utilization.

tion. It is suspected that the decreased airway pressure (PEEP, peak inspiratory pressure, and mean arterial pressure) required during IVOX utilization and the associated increase in arterial p_{O_2} were likely causes for the improved hemodynamic status.

The objective of these first clinical trials (phase I) was to assess the risks and hazards (safety) of IVOX utilization. Most of the data collected therefore pertained to this subject. Nevertheless, some information was obtained from these early phase I trials relative to the efficacy of the device or to any possible benefits its utilization may have had for the patient. For example, measurable quantities of O_2 and CO_2 were transferred into and out of circulating venous blood in all phase I patients receiving IVOX implantation. Quantitative O_2 and CO_2 transfer by means of the implanted IVOX device in these first clinical trials indicates that the devices performed as expected: transferring significant quantities of O_2 into and CO_2 out of the circulating blood of these patients with ARF. Other evidence of clinical benefit from IVOX utilization in these initial phase I IVOX clinical trials included improved blood gas parameters and decreased intensity of mechanical ventilator support during IVOX utilization in most patients receiving the device. Lung dysfunction decreased, bronchopleural air leaks sealed or decreased, and inotropic lung support for depressed hemodynamic status was discontinued or decreased in a number of patients receiving an IVOX device.

Phase II (Efficacy Assessment) of the Intravenous Oxygenator Clinical Trials: Selected Case Reports

As a result of the favorable risk/benefit ratio noted in phase I of the IVOX clinical trials, the FDA approved entrance into phase II (more definitive efficacy assessment), which commenced in May 1991. To date (November 1992), 135 patients with advanced and progressive ARF have received IVOX implantations in 29 international clinical trial centers. While detailed data analysis has not yet been completed and the final report of the finding has not yet been submitted to the FDA, the following general observations are apparent from preliminary review of the phase II findings:

1. IVOX utilization is relatively easy to institute and carry out.

2. Complications from IVOX utilization are infrequent and are of relatively minor significance.

3. IVOX transfers measurable quantities of oxygen into and carbon dioxide out of circulating venous blood for up to 29 days in patients with ARF who are receiving mild to moderate systemic anticoagulation.

4. A decrease in intensity of mechanical ventilator support accompanied by improved arterial blood gas profiles is observed during IVOX utilization in the majority of patients with ARF in whom this new method for augmenting gas exchange has been tried.

Potential Clinical Application of Intravascular Oxygenation

Objectives of Intravascular Oxygenator Utilization

From experience with IVOX in the experimental animal laboratory and from current human intensive care practices in respiratory ICUs it would seem reasonable to consider the intended clinical application of IVOX to be temporary augmentation of deficient blood gas exchange of patients with moderate to moderately severe, potentially reversible ARF in the ICU setting. With this application in mind, specific objectives for utilization of IVOX in patients with ARF in different stages of lung dysfunction (severity of ARF) have been suggested:

I. In severe reversible ARF
   A. Augment inadequate mechanical ventilator support to
      1. Gain additional time for recovery of natural lungs
      2. Possibly avoid extracorporeal perfusion
   B. Reduce the intensity of mechanical ventilator support:
      1. Decrease the F_{IO_2}
      2. Lower the PEEP, peak inspiratory pressure, and mean arterial pressure
      3. Decrease the minute volume
      4. Decrease the danger of barotrauma/oxygen toxicity

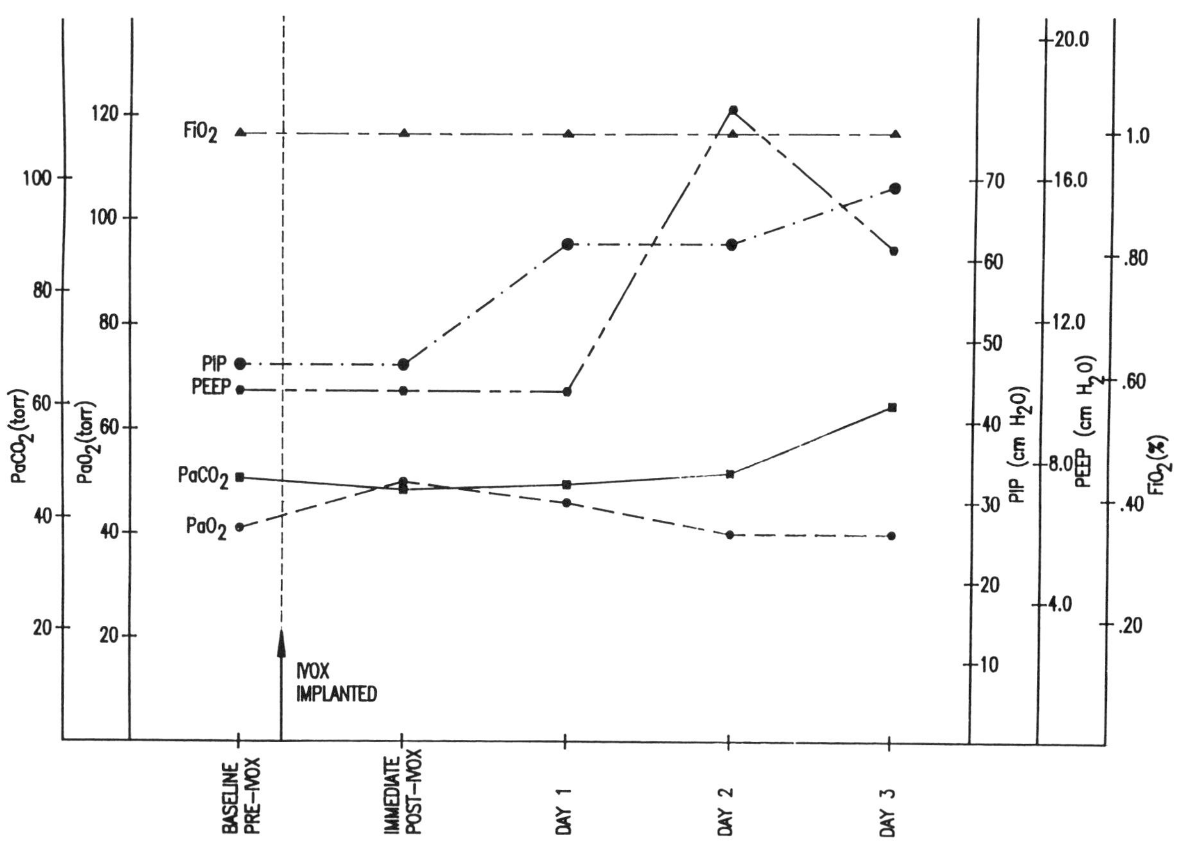

FIG 6–41
Case 3. Note that the F_{IO_2} delivered by the mechanical ventilator remained at 1.00. Also, the airway pressures (PEEP and PIP) had to be increased significantly on the second day after the IVOX device was implanted. Despite all this augmentation of blood gas transfer, the hypoxemia and hypercarbia were refractory. The patient died on the third day of IVOX utilization, with complete respiratory failure, sepsis syndrome, and hemodynamic failure.

II. In moderate reversible ARF
   A. Decrease the time that ventilator support is required:
      1. Hasten discontinuation of ventilation
      2. Facilitate weaning from the ventilator
      3. Shorten the stay in the ICU
      4. Decrease the danger of barotrauma/oxygen toxicity
III. In early reversible ARF
   A. Adequately augment the deficient blood gas exchange while at the same time
      1. Avoiding endotracheal intubation
      2. Avoiding utilization of closed-system positive-pressure mechanical ventilator support

In patients who have severe (advanced stages) ARF, including ARDS, and are hypoxemic and/or hypercarbic while receiving maximum support by means of mechanical ventilation, IVOX could be utilized to augment deficient, life-threatening blood gas exchange, thus supporting the patient a few days longer to permit some resolution of the natural lung dysfunction.

In less ill patients who are in moderate to moderately severe ARF and in whom acceptable Po_2 and/or pco_2 can be maintained with mechanical ventilator support at rather high, potentially damaging levels (Fio_2 between 0.60 and 0.80, with PEEP greater than 10, peak inspiratory pressure greater than 45, mean arterial pressure greater than 30, and/or minute volume greater than 150 mL/min/kg body weight), IVOX could be utilized to permit maintenance of acceptable blood gas values while the intensity of mechanical ventilator assistance is reduced to harmless levels (Fio_2 less than 0.50, PEEP less than 10, peak inspiratory pressure less than 45, mean arterial pressure less than 30, minute volume less than 150 mL/min/kg). Continued use of IVOX in this manner could shorten the time of tracheal intubation, and mechanical ventilation might also be avoided.

Contraindications for Intravascular Oxygenator Utilization

As a result of experience with the IVOX device in the experimental animal laboratory, coupled with observations during its early clinical trials, IVOX utilization is probably contraindicated in a number of clinical situations, including the following:

1. The likelihood that long-term intensive respiratory assistance will be required (longer than 3 weeks)
2. Recent major surgery or trauma in which systemic anticoagulation could cause bleeding
3. Uncontrolled sepsis (active infection, bacteremia)
4. Major venous or vena caval thrombi that could embolize
5. No usable right femoral or right internal jugular access vein and/or diminutive or truncated venae cavae
6. Advanced multiorgan failure
7. Significantly depressed cardiac output unresponsive to inotropes/fluids
8. No adequately trained personnel available for IVOX insertion and operation
9. Adequate gas transfer and anticoagulation monitoring capability not available

In general, these contraindications have to do with pre-existing conditions that could result in dislodging thrombotic material within the venae cavae or access veins, the likelihood of bleeding from the moderate systemic heparinization required during IVOX utilization, the threat of infection in or around patients who are unlikely to recover because of nonrespiratory problems, or the time limits currently imposed on IVOX utilization.

Limitations of Intravascular Oxygenation

The small surface area of the IVOX gas transfer membrane that can be inserted into the venae cavae effectively limits the quantity of O_2 and CO_2 that the device can transfer into/out of circulating venous blood. Also, the relatively short time that the current model of IVOX device can safely remain indwelling in the venae cavae constitutes a significant limitation to its use in patients with ARF. The large venotomy (requiring an open surgical procedure for introduction and for explanation of the IVOX device) likewise limits its clinical application. The necessity for systemic anticoagulation during IVOX utilization imposes significant limitations on its application to some patients. The recognized limitation of IVOX, as it currently exists and can be used, is therefore that current models can only provide approximately a third to a half of the metabolic O_2 and CO_2 gas transfer requirements of most adult patients with ARF (70 to 150 cc of O_2 or CO_2 per minute).

Future Potential, Development, Plans

It appears clear that the limited quantity of gas transfer achievable by means of the IVOX device as it is currently constituted and used significantly interferes with the full benefit it could provide if more oxygen could be delivered and more CO_2 removed by an optimized device. Indeed, the developers and manufacturers of this device have been working intensively to optimize its performance capabilities without producing more adverse effects or complicating its insertion and operation. A number of design, material, and performance modifications have been developed and are in the bench and animal testing stages, so a more effective, equally safe, easy-to-operate, second-generation IVOX device may be forthcoming in the foreseeable future.

Equally intriguing is the potential for the unique siloxane-covered, hollow-fiber, gas transfer membrane technology that makes the IVOX device perform as well as it does to be applied to other types of membrane gas transfer devices and systems. A series of pumpless membrane intracorporeal and extracorporeal membrane gas transfer devices and systems have been designed and fabricated and are in bench and animal testing programs. If successful, this emerging technological advancement could usher in a new era of clinically applicable membrane blood gas exchanger applications and potentially lead to a permanent intrathoracic, implantable prosthetic lung for use in patients with chronic, irreversible, end-stage lung disease.

PROLONGED EXTRACORPOREAL CARBON DIOXIDE REMOVAL

ECCO2R is an invasive procedure that uses a modified ECMO as described by Gattinoni et al.[60] to remove CO_2 from venous blood and reduce the required support by mechanical ventilation.

It differs from the IVOX device described earlier in that a mechanical pump must be used in the system to withdraw blood from the body, circulate it through the membrane lung, and return it to the body.

Development of Extracorporeal Carbon Dioxide Removal

The use of an extracorporeal device to provide gas exchange to a patient in ARF was first reported by Hill et al.[61] in 1972. Subsequently, from 1974 to 1976, the National Heart, Lung and Blood Institute suggested a nationwide multicentered trial[62] of patients with ARF to compare extracorporeal venous-arterial plus conventional continuous positive-pressure ventilation (CPPV) with CPPV alone. There was no improvement noted in survival with ECMO. These results greatly restricted the clinical use of extracorporeal systems for life support in ARF for years to come.[63] In 1979, Luciano Gattinoni and colleagues began investigation of an extracorporeal support device for ARF that was conceptually different from ECMO.[63] He named the technique low-frequency positive-pressure ventilation with extracorporeal CO_2 removed ($ECCO_2R$).

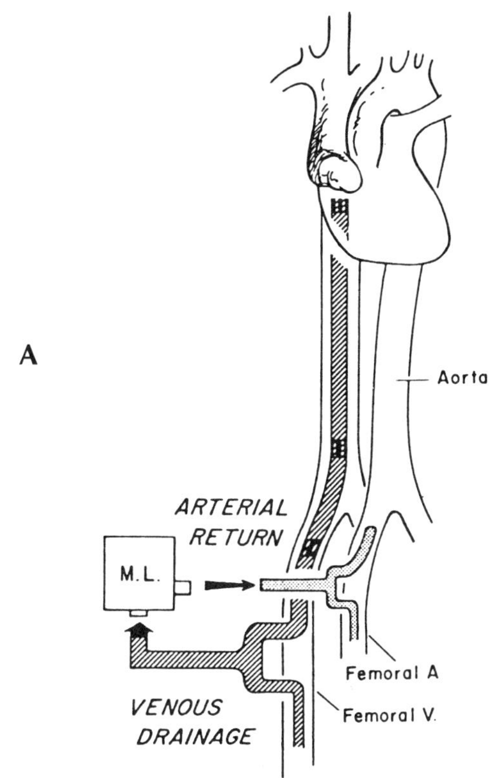

FIG 6–42
A, Routes for venovenous bypass.

Approaches to Establishing Venovenous Bypass

Two approaches have been recently reported by Gattinoni et al.[60] for establishing a venovenous bypass: a femoral-jugular route and a saphena-saphenous route (Fig 6–42, A and B). In Figure 6–42, a cannula is inserted into the right and left saphenous veins and positioned for maximum blood flow. Each cannula is attached via connecting tubes to either the inflow or outflow side of the pump oxygenator to form a complete blood circuit (Fig 6–43).

The latter approach is more desirable because it requires only superficial surgery as compared with the femoral-jugular route, which involves the surgical exposure of larger and deeper vessels and does not require drainage of the distal vein. The membrane lung used two circuits, one to carry blood and the other to provide air and oxygen.

Blood Circuit

The drainage line *(1)* (Fig 6–43) originates at the patient's venous drainage catheter and terminates at the reservoir inlet *(2)*. The reservoir bag *(A)* empties via the reservoir outlet line *(3)*, which is connected to the pump

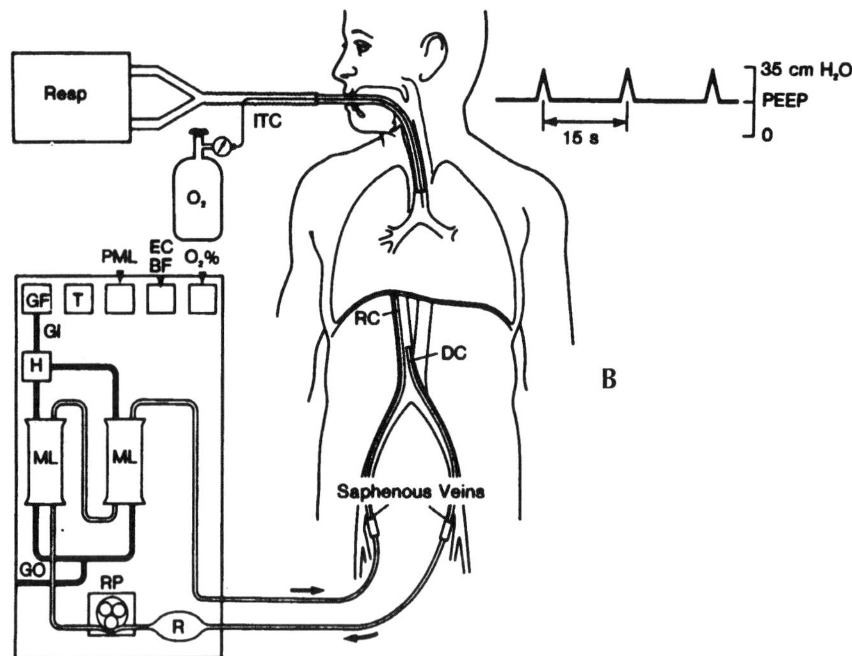

FIG 6–42
B, Cannulation and perfusion circuit. *DC* indicates blood drainage catheter; *EC BF,* extracorporeal blood flow; *GF,* gas flow monitor; *GI,* gas inlet; *GO,* gas outlet; *H,* humidifier; *ITC,* intratracheal catheter; *ML,* membrane lung; O_2% venous drainage blood oxygen monitor; *PML,* membrane lung pressure, in-out; *R,* venous resevoir; *RC,* blood return catheter; *Resp,* respirator; *RP,* roller pump; *PEEP,* positive end-expiratory pressure; and *T,* ambient temperature control.

"boot" *(5)* at its inlet *(4)*. The pump "boot" passes through the roller pump *(B)* and is attached to membrane lung no. 1 inlet *(7)* at the pump "boot" outlet *(6)*. Membrane lung no. 1 outlet *(8)* connects to membrane lung no. 2 inlet *(8)* by way of the midlung line. Blood returns from the outlet of membrane lung no. 2 to the patient through the venous return line *(9)*. Sideports *d, e,* and *f* are used to measure pressure in the blood phase at the inlet to membrane lung no. 1, the midlung, and the outlet of membrane lung no. 2, respectively. Port *a* provides access for heparin infusion, whereas port *b* is reserved for the addition of blood and blood products to the circuits. Samples for circuit blood gas analysis are drawn from port *c*. Sideport *g* is exclusively for blood cultures. Sideports *h* to *j* may be used for other drug infusions or additions. As blood is removed from the body and circulated through the membrane lungs, it becomes exposed to oxygen and air sources, which enables CO_2 and O_2 exchanges to occur. A typical gas circuit is explained below (Fig 6–44).

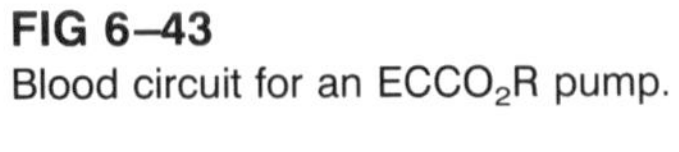

FIG 6–43
Blood circuit for an $ECCO_2R$ pump.

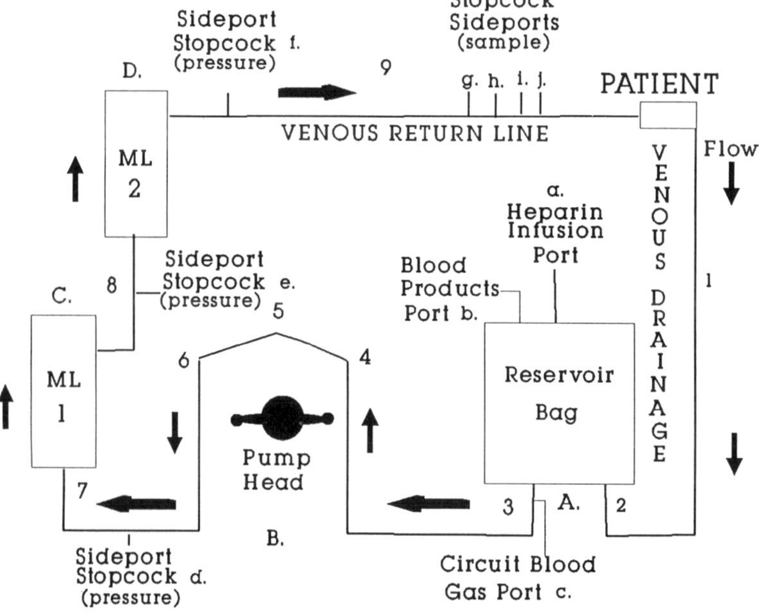

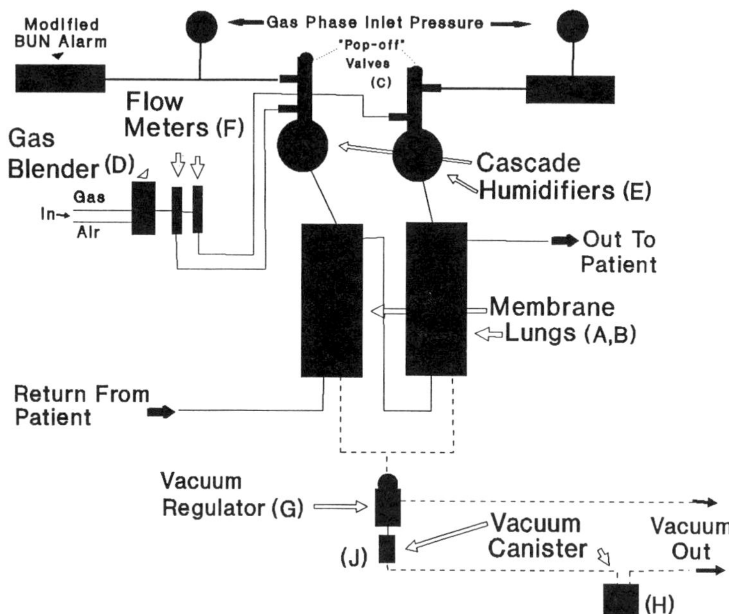

FIG 6–44
Gas circuit for an $ECCO_2R$ pump.

Gas Circuit

Oxygen and air sources are connected to a gas blender *(D),* which provides the selected FIO_2. The minute ventilation of the membrane lungs *(A, B)* is set by the flowmeters *(F).* The gas flows from the flowmeters to the cascade humidifiers *(E),* where it is heated and humidified before entering the membrane lungs. "Pop-off" valves together with modified BUNN alarms *(C)* monitor the input pressure of the gas admixture to prevent inadvertent high pressure from reaching the membrane lungs. The pressure of the gas entering the lungs is measured by pressure gauges *(I).* Gas phase pressures are maintained below those in the blood phase by the application of vacuum to the gas outlet of each lung. Vacuum is provided from a wall outlet through a vacuum regulator *(G)* and vacuum canister *(J).* A large vacuum canister *(H)* (with a separate suction connection) provides the means to empty the smaller canister *(J)* without disturbing the system's operation.

Monitoring the Pump System

Blood Pressure Measurements

The blood pressure monitoring system (Fig 6–45) displays pressures in the blood phase for the $ECCO_2R$ circuit. Pressures are measured at three points: at the inlet to the first membrane lung, at a point midway between the two lungs, and at the outlet of the second membrane lung. Each pressure is relayed from a sideport through a transducer to a gauge. Readings are in millimeters of Hg. Blood-phase pressure is maintained such that it is always higher than that in the gas phase. This is to ensure that in the event of a membrane lung rupture, gas emboli will not form in the blood. Blood-phase pressures are above ambient pressure. Gas-phase pressures are below ambient pressure. A flow-resistive pressure drop across the system causes the blood pressure to be highest at the inlet to the first lung, lower between the two, and lowest at the outlet of lung no. 2.

Patient Monitoring

Patients receiving $ECCO_2R$ require the same careful monitoring of physiologic values as would be required of any critical care patient on a mechanical ventilator. As described by Gattinoni et al., oxygen uptake and carbon dioxide removal were accomplished separately: oxygenation through apneic oxygenation (lungs at rest)[60, 64] and

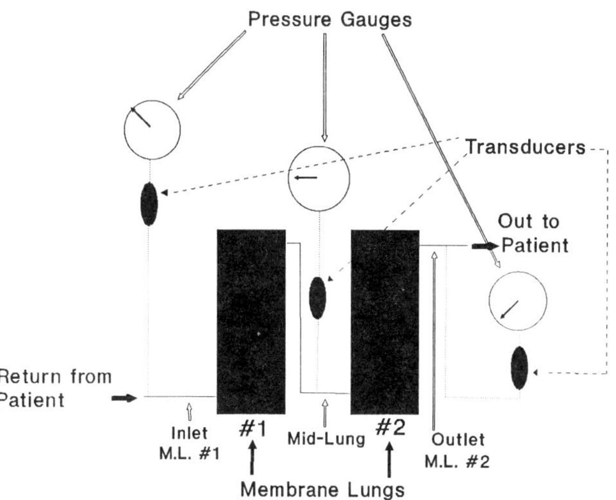

FIG 6–45
Blood pressure measurements during $ECCO_2R$.

CO_2 removal via the $ECCO_2R$ device. Forty-three patients with ARF were treated by using this technique, with 21 (48.8%) surviving for discharge. In over 8,000 hours of $ECCO_2R$ utilization, no major accidents occurred, and the overall survival rate of 51.2%[60] was much higher than in the previously cited ECMO multicentered trials, which reported mortality rates of 91.93%.[44, 65] This study encouraged a renewed interest into the use of $ECCO_2R$ as an alternative to the exclusive use of mechanical ventilation for the treatment of ARF.

Clinical Conditions Treated With Extracorporeal Carbon Dioxide Removal

ARDS with refractory hypoxia and hypercarbia that cannot be treated by using conventional mechanical ventilators appears to be the primary indication for the application of $ECCO_2R$. This patient population includes those with septic syndrome, aspiration of gastric contents, multiple transfusions, or pulmonary contusion.[66, 67] The estimated annual incidence of ARDS is 1.5 to 3.5/100,000,[68] and the mortality rate ranges from 28% to 90% as reported by nine different centers.[69] The high mortality reported from ARDS may be somewhat misleading because death is usually caused by multiple organ system failure[70] and is not limited to just pulmonary failure.

Potential Hazards

Pesenti et al. have logged more than 11,000 patient hours on bypass over the past decade with no major technical accident or interruption of procedure because of equipment failure.[71] Problems reported with the use of $ECCO_2R$ include the following:

1. Bleeding as a result of systemic anticoagulation
2. Limited blood flow through the saphena-saphenous cannulation
3. Disseminated intravascular coagulation (DIC) syndrome
4. Untimely wear of pump tubing inserts
5. Multiorgan failure in patients who do not recover
6. Pneumothoraces

Use of Extracorporeal Carbon Dioxide Removal With Low-Frequency Positive-Pressure Ventilation

One benefit of $ECCO_2R$ is that the level of mechanical ventilation (V, f, F_{IO_2}) can be reduced, thus enabling the lung to heal. This is accomplished in three steps, with equilibration achieved in each step before progressing to the next step.

Step 1.–The patient is intubated and placed on controlled mechanical ventilation at an F_{IO_2} of 1.0. The patient is connected to membrane lung bypass, and the blood temperature is maintained at 37°C. Extracorporeal blood flow is raised 200 to 300 mL/min until it reaches 20% to 30% of the normal cardiac output. Mechanical ventilation is lowered to adjust the Pa_{CO_2} for CO_2 that is removed by the membrane lungs. PEEP levels of 15 to 25 cm H_2O may be maintained or increased in order to maintain the main airway pressure at levels to prevent acute pulmonary edema (35 to 45 cm H_2O).

As the respiratory rate was slowed to less than 5 breaths per minute, Gattinoni et al.[60] introduced a low flow of 100% humidified oxygen (1 to 2 L/min) into the trachea through a small sideport in the endotracheal tube.

Step 2.–After the patient is stable on step 1, the goal is to provide for maximum gas exchange at the lowest possible F_{IO_2} and airway pressure. F_{IO_2} and PEEP levels are reduced in the ventilator whenever the P_{AO_2} is greater than 80 mm Hg at an F_{IO_2} of 0.40.

Step 3.–The third step involves weaning of the patient from $ECCO_2R$. The criteria used by Gattinoni et al.[63] included

a. A Pa_{O_2} consistently above 80 mm Hg (10.7 kPa) on an F_{IO_2} of 0.40.
b. A total static lung compliance of greater than 30 mL/cm H_2O (0.306 L/Pa).
c. Cleaning of the lung fields on chest radiographs.
d. A gradual reduction of gas flow to the membrane lungs until the patient is able to maintain adequate ventilation on a ventilator with an F_{IO_2} of 0.40 and a PEEP of 10 to 15 cm H_2O (0.1 to 1.5 kPa) or at low-frequency IMV for at least 6 hours without use of the membrane lungs.

DIAPHRAGMATIC PACING

Patients with respiratory hypoventilation or high cervical lesions resulting from trauma, stroke, or surgery have an intact respiratory system despite the loss of the primary neurologic drive. If the phrenic nerves have not undergone degeneration, an electrical impulse can be applied to them and may restore adequate alveolar ventilation. Under these circumstances, diaphragmatic pacemaking can make a major contribution.

Worldwide there have been over 1,000 phrenic nerve implants in patients ranging in age from a few months to 80 years of age. Many of these patients have been successfully supported on diaphragm pacing for more than 10 years. They experience fewer respiratory tract infections than those on mechanical ventilators, enjoy close to normal speech, and can often live at home and eliminate the high cost of chronic hospitalization. Diaphragm pacing is indicated for patients who have damage to the respiratory control centers and pathways in the brain stem or in the spinal cord. It is contraindicated for use in patients who have inadequate phrenic nerve, lung, or diaphragm function to accommodate electrical stimulation.

Respiratory Pacing System

The respiratory pacer activates the patient's natural mechanisms of breathing, nerve activity, and muscle contraction. The pacing equipment produces impulses that stimulate the phrenic nerve to activate the diaphragm for inspiration. The system (Fig 6–46) is composed of an external transmitter and antenna and an implanted electrode and receiver. The transmitter produces impulses that are delivered via the external antenna loop. This loop is taped to the skin over the implanted receiver site. The receiver relays the impulse through the implanted electrode, which is positioned under the phrenic nerve. This stimulation of the phrenic nerve causes contraction of the diaphragm and results in inspiration. When the signals cease, the diaphragm relaxes and causes expiration. The repetition of stimulation and nonstimulation cycles produces near-normal breathing.

NOTE: There are two electrode models available for diaphragm pacing: the unipolar electrode, used in most cases, and the bipolar electrode, used in patients already implanted with electrical stimulation devices such as a demand cardiac pacemaker.

Recent work with the new system indicates that adjusting the pulse duration can substantially increase tidal volumes, at least in some quadriplegics, probably by recruiting small fibers with longer chronaxie times. Similarly, computerized optimization of the inspiratory time may alleviate upper airway problems, particularly in sleep apneic children, and computerized threshold/ramp adjustment can result in larger tidal volumes and more comfortable diaphragm contractions.

Equipment Summary

The antenna system provides for transmission of the electrical signal to send an impulse to the phrenic nerve without the necessity of transcutaneous wires. The

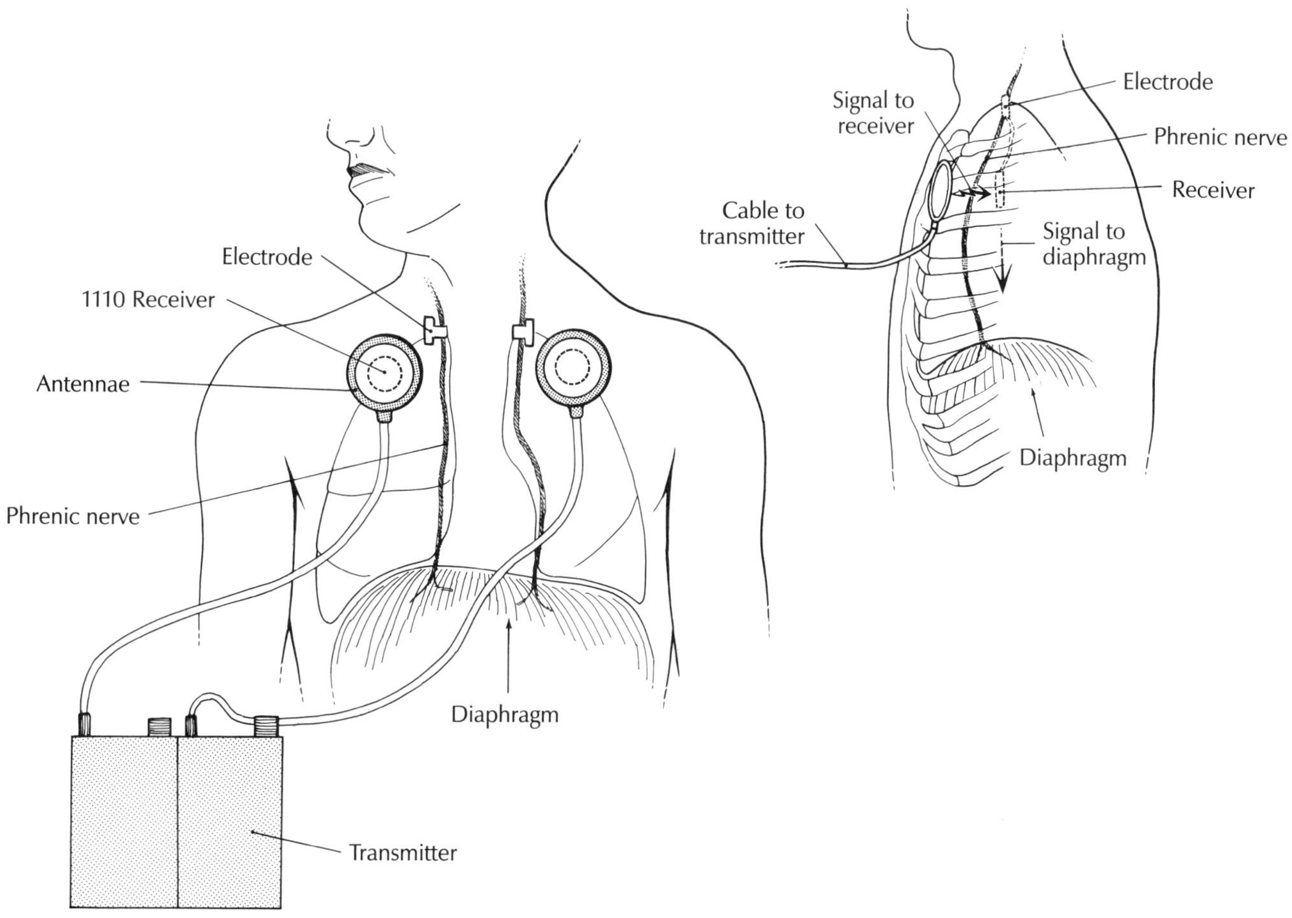

FIG 6–46
Diaphragmatic pacer showing the electronic module pacer leads and placement.

receiver is expected to have a life expectancy of greater than 10 years, whereas the transmitter may require replacement at 5-year intervals. In the event of transmitter battery failure, the patient will note a gradual reduction in tidal volume over a several-day time period. With the new computer-"optimized" signal selection, more neural fibers are activated, which results in more comfortable breathing patterns. The intensity and the duration as well as the frequency of the pulsations can be altered to allow patients the flexibility to match respiratory demands to the current activity level.

Trans-Telephonic Monitoring (TTM) allows for routine follow-up of all neurostimulation equipment via standard telephone lines.

Preoperative Evaluation of Diaphragm Function and Phrenic Nerve Viability

Before surgery, different screening tests have been used to test the function of the phrenic nerve and diaphragm. Tests include one or more of the following:

1. Voluntary movement of the diaphragm under fluoroscopy
2. Diaphragm response through transcutaneous stimulation of the phrenic nerves in the neck (electromyography [EMG], fluoroscopy)
3. Phrenic nerve conduction time (PNCT)
4. Transdiaphragmatic pressure monitoring.

However, the tests are fickle and may produce many "false negatives," especially if the EMG laboratory has limited experience. For example, many sleep apneics have been reported as "negative." Physicians are chagrined when it is pointed out that the phrenic nerve must be viable since the patient is able to breathe when awake. In quadriplegics, the nerve may conduct, but little or no diaphragm movement may be observed. Months of stimulation may be required before diaphragm function returns. *The most unequivocal test is to expose the nerve in the neck and stimulate it directly.*

The simplest method of predicting nerve viability and diaphragm function is transcutaneous phrenic nerve stimulation in the neck with simultaneous fluoroscopy of the diaphragm as well as measurement of the PNCT. The phrenic nerve is stimulated transcutaneously with a hand-held cathode (covered with saline or electrode jelly) pressed against the skin overlying the anterior scalene muscle above the clavicle and behind the lateral-posterior border of the sternocleidomastoid muscle. The anode is usually strapped over the subclavicular area. The stimulator is set to deliver square wave pulses of 500- to 100-μs duration at the frequency of 1 pulse per second and a current level of 20 to 100 mA. Using airflowmetry and fluoroscopy, a tidal volume of more than 100 mL and a diaphragmatic movement in excess of 3.0 cm are considered desirable in patients with no voluntary movement of the diaphragm. However, the lower limits are uncertain, particularly with patients who have been ventilator dependent for long periods. When measuring PNCT, two surface electrodes are placed at the costal margin in the anteroposterior auxiliary line in the eighth or ninth intercostal space, and a ground electrode is placed on the xiphoid process. The conduction time from the site of phrenic nerve stimulation in the neck to the diaphragm action potential is recorded on a storage oscilloscope.

The normal PNCT is between 6 and 9 ms (shorter in children). A prolonged PNCT of more than 11-ms latency may suggest damage to the phrenic nerve, but the clinical significance of this is uncertain. Recent work suggests that large-diameter fibers may be preferentially destroyed in many patients (especially victims of cervical trauma). The residual population of smaller, slower-conducting fibers require very different stimulus parameters to be effectively excited. Consequently, many patients who were previously considered unsuitable for stimulation may be candidates after computerized stimulus optimization. In turn, some of these patients may require custom modifications of external transmitters to produce the appropriate stimulus train.

Surgical Procedure

All implanted components are autoclaved at the time of surgery. The phrenic nerve electrode can be implanted either in the thoracic or in the cervical region. We recommend that patients be implanted in the neck whenever possible in order to avoid the risk and morbidity associated with thoracotomies. Nerve viability is confirmed intraoperatively by using a nerve test probe (see above).

Cervical Approach

This approach is preferred because of its simplicity and low morbidity. If necessary, such implants can be done on an outpatient basis with local anesthesia. However, implantation is usually performed bilaterally in one session with general anesthesia. Muscle relaxants must be avoided, and antibiotics are given prophylactically for 24 to 48 hours. In order to keep the operative field clean, the tracheal cannula is temporarily removed and the patient intubated endotracheally.

Thoracic Approach

This approach is used as a second alternative in adults and as a standard procedure in infants. The thoracic approach has been recommended because the presence of an accessory phrenic nerve from the fifth cervical root to the main trunk in the mediastinum may optimize electrophrenic stimulation, but this has not been clearly established. Bilateral implants can be made in the same session. The procedure requires the insertion of chest tubes. A 5- to 7-cm transverse incision is made over the second or third costal cartilage and rib from the sternal border. The incision is extended down to the costal cartilage and rib surface. The second costal cartilage is sometimes resected, and the pleural space is entered. A small pediatric retractor is placed into the wound. Ventilation is achieved by the indwelling tracheostomy tube. The lung is packed off with two pads, both superiorly and inferiorly. Traction sutures are placed above the phrenic bundle, approximately 1 cm inferior to the sternal edge. These are elevated and attached to hemostats, and the pericardium is lifted superiorly. The phrenic nerve can be easily identified along the anterior surface of the pericardium. It is isolated high, well above the heart to avoid ventricular fibrillation by the repetitive stimuli. On the right side, the ideal site for implantation is just inferior to the junction of the superior vena cava with the right atrium. On the left side, the site of implantation is approximately at the level of the left main pulmonary artery as it crosses out from the pericardial reflection.

Once the phrenic nerve is identified, two parallel incisions are made on each side of the phrenic nerve. The entire phrenic nerve bundle, consisting of artery, nerve, and vein, is gently lifted off with a right-angle Gemini clamp. A unipolar phrenic nerve electrode is inserted, with the toe of the electrode coming from below so that the entire phrenic bundle lies within the U-shaped monopolar phrenic nerve electrode. The electrode is affixed to the pericardium with ligatures. At the lateral portion of the thoracic incision, a subcutaneous pocket is created in the prepectoral plane to implant the radio receiver unit and excess wire.

Complications

Phrenic nerve pacing is an effective means of achieving ventilation, but it is not without certain risks. The complications reported by Weese-Mayer et al. in a study that covered 192 system years' experience in pediatric patients represent the most frequently encountered problems with this device[72]:

1. Receiver failure (26 instances)
2. Electrode wire or wire insulation breakage (6 cases)
3. Infection causing removal of the pacer (3 cases)
4. Mechanical nerve injury (2 cases)

Miller and associates, in a more recent study of phrenic nerve pacing in adult patients, reported this procedure to be a success in freeing quadriplegic patients from ventilator dependency with only minor complications.[73]

Summary

Diaphragmatic (phrenic) nerve pacing is still another alternative to mechanical ventilation in specific patient populations that may require long-term ventilation because of quadriplegia or other conditions that prevent normal nervous system control of the diaphragm. Studies have been reported for over 20 years for both adult and pediatric patients with varying degrees of success.

As the technology evolves, modified receiver design, stronger electrodes, and better surgical techniques will make this procedure an even more acceptable alternative to mechanical ventilation in certain long-term ventilator patients.

REFERENCES

1. Froese AB, Bryan A: State of the art—high frequency ventilation. *Am Rev Respir Dis* 1987; 135:1363–1374.
2. Civetta JM: Does ventilatory support affect outcome in ICU patients? *Respir Care* 1987; 32:594–604.
3. Weissman IM, Riraldo JE, Rogers RM: Positive end-expiratory pressure in adult respiratory failure. *N Engl J Med* 1982; 307:1381–1384.
4. McCarthy EF, Dillard JE III: AANA Journal Course: New technologies in anesthesia: Update for nurse anesthetist—high frequency ventilation. *J Assoc Nurse Anesthetists* 1990; 56:478–484.
5. Simon BA, Mitzner W: Design and calibration of a high frequency oscillatory ventilator. *IEE Trans Biomed Eng* 1991; 38:214–218.
6. Emerson JH (inventor): Apparatus for vibrating portions of the patients' airway. *US Patent* 1959; 2:917–918.
7. Butler WJ, et al: Ventilation by high frequency ventilation in humans. *Anesth Analg* 1980; 59:577–584.
8. Sjöstrand UH, Erickson IA: High rates and low volumes in mechanical ventilation—not just a matter of ventilatory frequency. *Anesth Analg* 1980; 59:567–576.
9. Carlon GC, Miodownik S, Ray E, et al: Technical aspects and clinical implications of high-frequency jet ventilation with a solenoid valve. *Crit Care Med* 1980; 9:47–50.
10. Carlon GC, Havland WS, Ray D, et al: High frequency jet ventilation: A prospective randomized evaluation. *Chest* 1983; 84:551–559.

11. Hurst JM, Branson RD, Davis K Jr, et al: Comparison of conventional mechanical ventilation and high frequency ventilation—a prospective, randomized trial in patients with respiratory failure. *Ann Surg* 1990; 211:486–491.
12. OCTAVE Study Group: Multicenter randomized controlled trial of high against low frequency positive pressure ventilation. *Arch Dis Child* 1991; 66:770–775.
13. Weber KR, Asselin JM: High frequency oscillatory ventilation: New technology for the neonatal intensive care unit. *Neonatal Intensive Care* May/June 1990; 20–23.
14. Butler WJ, et al: Ventilation by high frequency oscillation in humans. *Anesth Analg* 1980; 59:577–584.
15. Crawford M, Rehder K: High frequency small volume ventilation in anesthetized humans. *Anesthesiology* 1984; 62:298–304.
16. Marchak BE, Thompson WK, Duffy P: Treatment of RDS by high frequency oscillatory ventilation: A preliminary report. *J Pediatr* 1983; 99:287–288.
17. Frantz IO, Werhammer J, Stark AR: HFV in premature infants with lung disease: Adequate gas exchange at low tracheal pressure. *J Pediatr* 1983; 71:483–488.
18. Jaeger MJ, Kurzweg UH, Banner MJ: Transport of gases in high frequency ventilation. *Crit Care Med* 1984; 12:1209.
19. Klocke RA, Saltzman AR, Grant JB, et al: Role of molecular diffusion in conventional and high frequency ventilation. *Am Rev Respir Dis* 1990; 142:802–806.
20. Lehr JL, Butler JP, Westerman PA, et al: Photographic measurement of pleural surface motion during lung oscillation. *J Appl Physiol* 1985; 59:623–33.
21. Taylor G: The dispersion of matter in turbulent flow through a pipe. *Proc R Soc Lond* 1954; 223:446–453.
22. Hazelton FR, Sherer PW: Bronchial bifurcations and respiratory mass transport. *Science* 1980; 208:69–71.
23. Banner MJ: Technical aspects of high frequency ventilation. *Curr Rev Respir Ther* 1985; 7:91–95.
24. Fredberg JJ: Augmented diffusion in the airways can support pulmonary gas exchange. *J Appl Physiol* 1980; 49:232–238.
25. Slutsky AS, Drazen JM, Kamm RD: Alveolar ventilation at high frequencies using tidal volumes less than anatomic dead space, in Engel LA, Paica M, Lenfant C (eds): *Lung Biology in Health Care Disease.* New York, Marcel Dakker, 1984, pp 137–176.
26. McCulloch P, Forkert P, Froese A: Lung volume maintenance prevents lung injury during high frequency ventilation in surfactant deficient rabbits. *Am Rev Respir Dis* 1988; 137:1185–1192.
27. Maunder RJ: Clinical prediction of the adult respiratory distress syndrome. *Clin Chest Med* 1985; 6:413–426.
28. Shoemaker NJ: *Textbook of Critical Care.* Philadelphia, WB Saunders, 1984.
29. Civetta JM, Taylor RW, Kirby RR (eds): *Textbook of Critical Care.* Philadelphia, JB Lippincott, 1988.
30. Hundson L: Respiratory failure: Etiology and mortality. *Respir Care* 1987; 2:584–593.
31. Calkins JM: High-frequency ventilation. *Curr Rev Respir Ther* 1984; 6:139–143.
32. Freitag K, Schroer M, Bremme J: High frequency oscillator with adjustable wave forms: Practical aspects. *Br J Anaesth* 1989; 63:385–435.
33. Chang HK, Weber ME, King M: Mucus transport by high frequency nonsymmetrical oscillatory airflow. *J Appl Physiol* 1988; 65:1203–1209.
34. Borg UR, Stoklosa JC, Șiegel JH, et al: Prospective evaluation of combined high frequency ventilation in post-traumatic patients with adult respiratory distress syndrome refractory to optimized conventional ventilatory management. *Crit Care Med* 1989; 17:1129–1142.
35. Cioffi WG, Graves TA, McManus WF, et al: High-frequency percussive ventilation in patients with inhalation injury. *J Trauma* 1989; 29:350–354.
36. Gallagher TJ, Boysen PG, Davidson DD, et al: High frequency percussive ventilation compared with conventional mechanical ventilation. *Crit Care Med* 1989; 17:364–366.
37. Thomas SHL, Langford JA, Gengi JD, et al: Aerosol deposition in the human lung: Effect of high frequency oscillation on the deposition characteristics of an inhaled nebulized aerosol. *Clin Sci* 1988; 75:535–542.
38. Cioffi WG Jr, Rue LW III, Graves TA, et al: Prophylactic use of high-frequency percussive ventilation in patients with inhalation injury. *Ann Surg* 1991; 213:575–580.
39. Carlon G, Kahn D, Hawland W, et al: Clinical experience with high-frequency jet ventilation. *Crit Care Med* 1981; 9:1–6.
40. Schuster D, Klain M, Snyder J: Comparison of high frequency ventilation during severe acute respiratory failure in humans. *Crit Care Med* 1982; 10:625–630.
41. Turnbull AD, Carolon G, Howland WS, et al: High-frequency ventilation in major airway or pulmonary disruption. *Ann Thorac Surg* 1981; 32:468–474.
42. Orlando R, Gluck E, Chohn M, et al: Ultra-high frequency jet ventilation in a broncho-pleural fistula model. *Arch Surg* 1988; 123:591–593.
43. Ritz R, Benson M, Bishop MJ: Measuring gas leakage from broncho-pleural fistula during high-frequency jet ventilation. *Crit Care Med* 1984; 12:836–837.
44. Zapol WM, Snider MT, Hill JD, et al: Extracorporeal membrane oxygenation in severe acute respiratory failure. *JAMA* 1979; 242:2193–2196.
45. Egan TM, Duffin J, Glynn MF, et al: Ten-year experience with extracorporeal membrane oxygenation for severe respiratory failure. *Chest* 1988; 94:681–687.
46. Hopkins S, Cowell R: Making sense of neonatal ECMO. *Nurs Times* 1991; 87:36–37.
47. Mortensen JD: An intravenacaval blood gas exchange (IVCBGE) device. Preliminary report. *Trans Am Soc Artif Intern Organs* 1987; 31:570–573.
48. Mortensen JD, Berry G: Conceptual and design features of a practical, clinically effective intravenous mechanical blood oxygen/carbon dioxide exchange device (IVOX). *Int J Artif Organs* 1989; 12:384–389.
49. Mortensen JD: Extracorporeal respiratory assistance in adults, in *Update in Cardiac Surgery Anaesthesia and Intensive Care.* Ghent, Belgium, 1991, pp 29–35.

50. Mortensen JD: Augmentation of blood gas transfer by means of an intravascular blood gas exchanger (IVOX), in Vincent JL, Marini J (eds): *Update in Intensive Care and Emergency Medicine,* vol 15. *Ventilatory Failure.* Berlin, Springer-Verlag, 1991, pp 318–346.
51. Mortensen JD: Laboratory studies relative to IVOX safety and efficacy (report to FDA). Salt Lake City, CardioPulmonics, 1989.
52. Morioka T: A method for intravenous blood gas exchange. *Clin Anesth* 1990; 4:49–56 (Japanese).
53. Kallis P, Al-Saady NM, Bennett D, et al: Clinical use of intravascular oxygenation. *Lancet* 1991; 1:549.
54. Zwischenberger JB, Cox CS: A new intravascular membrane oxygenator to augment blood gas transfer in patients w/acute respiratory failure. *Tex Med* 1991; 87:60–63.
55. Cox CS Jr, Zwischenberger JB, Traber LD, et al: Use of an intravascular oxygenator/carbon dioxide removal device in an ovine smoke inhalation injury model. *Trans Am Soc Artif Intern Organs* 1991; 37:411–413.
56. Imai H, Yoshimura H, Ishihara A, et al: Preliminary clinical experience in use of intravascular blood gas exchanger (IVOX). *Kokyu To Junkan* 1992; 40:461–465 (Japanese).
57. Jurmann MJ, et al: Intravascular oxygenation for advanced respiratory failure. *Trans Am Soc Artif Intern Organs* 1992; 38(2):120–124.
58. Von Segesser LK, Schaffner A, Stocker R, et al: Extended (29 days) use of intravascular gas exchanger. *Lancet* 1992; 1:1536.
59. Mortensen JD: Intravascular oxygenator (IVOX): A new, alternative method for augmenting blood gas transfer in patients with acute respiratory failure. *Artif Organs* 1992; 1:75–82.
60. Gattinoni L, Pesenti A, Daniele M, et al: Low frequency positive-pressure ventilation with extracorporeal CO_2 removal in severe acute respiratory failure. *JAMA* 1986; 256:881–886.
61. Hill JD, O'Brien TG, Murray JT: Prolonged extracorporeal oxygenation for acute post-traumatic respiratory failure (shock-lung syndrome). *N Engl J Med* 1972; 286:629–634.
62. *Protocol for Extracorporeal Support for Respiratory Insufficiency.* Bethesda, Md, National Heart, Lung, and Blood Institute, 1974.
63. Gattinoni L, Kolobow T, Damia G, et al: Extracorporeal carbon dioxide removal ($ECCO_2R$): A new form of respiratory assistance. *Int J Artif Organs* 1979; 2:183–185.
64. Frumin MJ, Epstein RM, Cohen G: Apneic oxygenation in man. *Anesthesiology* 1959; 20:789–798.
65. Greene R, Zapol W, Snider MT, et al: Early bedside detection of pulmonary vascular occlusion during acute respiratory failure. *Am Rev Respir Dis* 1981; 124:593–601.
66. Fowler AA, Hamman RF, Zerve GO, et al: Adult respiratory distress syndrome: Prognosis after onset. *Am Rev Respir Dis* 1985; 132:472–478.
67. Petty TL: Indicators of risk, course and prognosis in adult respiratory distress syndrome (ARDS) (editorial). *Am Rev Respir Dis* 1985; 132:471.
68. Villar J, Slutsky AS: The incidence of the adult respiratory distress syndrome. *Am Rev Respir Dis* 1989; 141:659–665.
69. Durvin CG Jr: Intravenous oxygenation and CO_2 removal device: IVOX. *Respir Care* 1992; 37:147–153.
70. Montgomery AB, Stager MA, Carrico CJ, et al: Causes of mortality in patients with adult respiratory distress syndrome. *Am Rev Respir Dis* 1985; 132:485–489.
71. Pesenti A, Gattinoni L, Cugno M: *Problems in Long-Term Veno-Venous Bypass* (reprinted from Gillie JP (ed): *Neonatal and Adult Respiratory Failure Mechanisms and Treatment*). Paris, Elsevier, 1989, pp 173–177.
72. Weese-Mayer D, Morrow A, Brouillette R, et al: Diaphragm pacing in infants and children. A life-table analysis of implanted components. *Am Rev Respir Dis* 1989; 139:974–979.
73. Miller J, Farmer J, Stuart W, et al: Phrenic nerve pacing of the quadriplegic patient. *J Thorac Cardiovasc Surg* 1990; 99:35–39.

SUGGESTED READING

Bagley B, Bagley A, Henrie J, et al: Quantitative gas transfer into and out of circulating venous blood by means of an intravenacaval oxygenator (IVOX). *Trans Am Soc Artif Intern Organs* 1991; 37:413–415.

Cox CS, Zwischenberger JB, Kurusz M: Development and current status of a new intracorporeal membrane oxygenator (IVOX). *Perfusion* 1991; 6:291–296.

Durbin CG: Intravenous oxygenation and CO_2 removal. *Respir Care* 1992; 37:147.

High KM, Snider MT, Richard R, et al: Clinical trials of an intravenous oxygenator in patients with adult respiratory distress syndrome. *Anesthesiology* 1992; 77:856–863.

Kallis P, Al-Saady NM, Bennett ED, et al: Intravascular oxygenation with the IVOX. *Br J Hosp Med* 1992; 47:824–828.

Kallis P, Treasure T: Intravascular oxygenation (IVOX). *Surgery* 1991.

Lanigan CJ, Withington PS: Support when gas exchange fails—ECMO, $ECCO_2R$, and IVOX. *Clin Intensive Care* 1991; 2:210–216.

Mortensen JD: Progress in the ICU management of the adult patient with advanced acute respiratory failure. *Intensive Crit Care Dig* 1991; 10:27–28.

Mortensen JD, Talbot S, Burkart JA: Cross sectional internal diameters of human cervical and femoral blood vessels: Relationship to subject's sex, age, body size. *Anat Rec* 1990; 225:115–124.

Von Segesser LK, Weiss BM, Pasic M, et al: Temporary lung support using an intravascular gas exchanger. *Thorac Cardiovasc Surg* 1992; 40:121–125.

Zapol WM: Volotrauma and the intravenous oxygenator in patients with adult respiratory distress syndrome. *Anesthesiology* 1992; 77:847–849.

Zwischenberger JB, Cox CS Jr, Graves D, et al: Intravascular membrane oxygenation and carbon dioxide removal—A new application for permissive hypercapnia? *Thorac Cardiovasc Surg* 1992, 40(3):115–120.

7

Cardiopulmonary Bedside Monitoring

ROBERT FALLAT, M.D.
MICHAEL SNOW, R.P.F.T., R.R.T.

OBJECTIVES

- Explain the value of monitoring the patient at the bedside.
- Differentiate between the various methods for measuring the patient's lung volumes and gas flow rates at the bedside.
- Describe the techniques for continually monitoring the spontaneously breathing patient using minimally invasive techniques.
- Discuss the gas laws that may be applied to monitoring lung volume, compliance and PEEP.
- Point out how esophageal pressure measures can be used to determine intrathoracic pressure.
- Contrast various automated ventilator monitoring systems discussed in this chapter.
- Discuss the indications for measurement of compliance and resistance in mechanically ventilated patients.
- Compare various techniques and instruments used to perform indirect calorimetry.
- Compare equipment and non-invasive techniques available to assess arterial blood gasses (ABG).
- Discuss the techniques and applications of capnography.
- Describe the methods of measuring cardiovascular system pressures.
- Appraise the value and limitations of invasive cardiovascular monitors.

Bedside monitoring covers a wide range of technologies. A knowledgeable and caring nurse or respiratory care practitioner (RCP) observing the mannerisms, speech, skin color, temperature, and pulse of a patient is the time-honored and best form of monitoring that technology must strive to equal. Unfortunately, cost considerations are reducing the time that experienced personnel can spend with patients. Moreover, certain events are too acute and critical to wait for the watchful human eye. Cardiovascular events in particular can be acutely fatal; the noninvasive electrocardiogram (ECG), ideal in cost, safety, and efficiency, was appropriately the first of the technological monitors. Cardiopulmonary resuscitation (CPR) is an emergency response to an ECG alarm that is commonly successful.

Unfortunately, many survivors later suffer severe morbidity and mortality from respiratory or multiorgan failure. This has led to the recognition that the lungs and other organs of the body need equal attention to detect events earlier and achieve a better quality-of-life outcome. Indeed, many of the "cardiac events" may well have their origin in respiratory perturbations, particularly in hospitalized patients taking many medications and artificially ventilated. Zwillich et al.[1] reported 400 complications in 354 consecutive patients who were mechanically ventilated and continuously monitored. Although it is the patient who is mechanically ventilated in the intensive care unit (ICU) who has received the most attention regarding monitoring, technologies are available today for monitoring patients at all levels of care, even in the home, as will be discussed.

This chapter will be divided into three sections: ventilatory monitoring, which will focus on spirometry, respiratory mechanics, and the adequacy of ventilation; a gas exchange section focusing on noninvasive monitoring and metabolic assessment; and a section on hemodynamics focusing on heart-lung interactions and the adequacy of tissue perfusion. This chapter will emphasize the technological methods of monitoring while recognizing the importance of all levels of monitoring. In fact, validation of the efficacy of even the most advanced monitors will usually depend on fundamental clinical observations. Cardiopulmonary monitoring can complement but cannot replace a competent bedside observer.

VENTILATORY MONITORING

Ventilatory monitoring is clearly dependent on clinical conditions. A spontaneously breathing patient outside intensive care is usually limited to intermittent monitoring at the bedside with spirometers, peak flowmeters and mouth pressure measurements. However, the respiratory rate (f), tidal volume (V_T), minute volume (V_E), and respiratory mechanics, including measurement of resistance (R) and compliance (C), can be measured intermittently in a spontaneously breathing patient since this equipment is now portable enough to be brought to the bedside.

Mechanically ventilated patients lend themselves to much more sophisticated and continuous monitoring with a variety of pressure and flow as well as inspired and expired gas sensors. Many of these monitors are included in the design of newer ventilators. In this section we will emphasize the basic technologies used to monitor pulmonary mechanics with examples of free-standing systems as well as those included within mechanical ventilators.

Intermittent Monitoring of Spontaneously Breathing Patients

With the availability of small portable electronic systems, bedside spirometry can be as sophisticated as that done in the pulmonary function laboratory. More commonly used is less expensive equipment that can be left at the bedside with the patient. This includes peak flowmeters and incentive spirometers. Peak flowmeters have long been used for monitoring obstructive airways disease (OAD) and are currently strongly emphasized as a necessary modality in the optimum management of asthma. These devices have much less value in patients with severe chronic obstructive pulmonary disease (COPD) where peak flow may reflect the compression volume of the large airways and not the severity of diffuse airway obstruction. In these instances, an accurate measurement of the forced expiratory volume in 1 second (FEV_1) and vital capacity requires spirometry. In patients with restrictive lung disease (RLD), ventilatory capacity can be monitored as well as therapeutically sustained by the use of incentive spirometers, but a more precise monitoring of the degree of restriction and response to treatment will depend on spirometry.

Bedside Spirometry

A wide variety of inexpensive spirometers is available for office or bedside use. The oldest, least complicated, and perhaps most reliable is the standard volume displacement spirometer for obtaining a volume-time tracing from which the FEV_1, forced vital capacity (FVC), and other measures of flow can be hand-calculated. Originally, the displacement device was a metal bell floating in a water seal and was not easily brought to the bedside. Most models now have rolling plastic seals and can be bounced in and out of elevators without spilling water or losing calibration. If equipped with electrical transducers proportional to volume, these electronic volume signals can be differentiated by using a potentiometer on a moving drum, to obtain flow and then used to derive flow-volume loops. However, these volume displacement devices are relatively large and cumbersome and have generally been displaced by smaller units using pneumotachographs. A more complete review of spirometry and spirometers is available in Chapter 8.

Several pneumotachograph-based bedside spirometers are available to make spirometric measurements as well as flow-volume curves. These systems generally meet the American Thoracic Society (ATS) guidelines for spirometry and usually have independent confirmation of compliance with the recommendations.[2] Spirometers that use laptop computers, such as the Koko spirometer from Pulmonary Data Services Instrumentation, can provide the same quality of testing and configurability of reports as the systems described in Chapter 8. The Koko spirometer, shown in Figure 7–1, uses a bacteria filter to protect the pneumotachograph resistance element. Small microprocessor-based spirometers sacrifice some of the software flexibility but can be carried in a coat pocket. The Puritan-Bennett Renaissance spirometer, shown in Figure 7–2, uses a disposable flow sensor and provides extensive coaching instructions as part of the standard software. The limitation in features is offset by a significantly lower price.

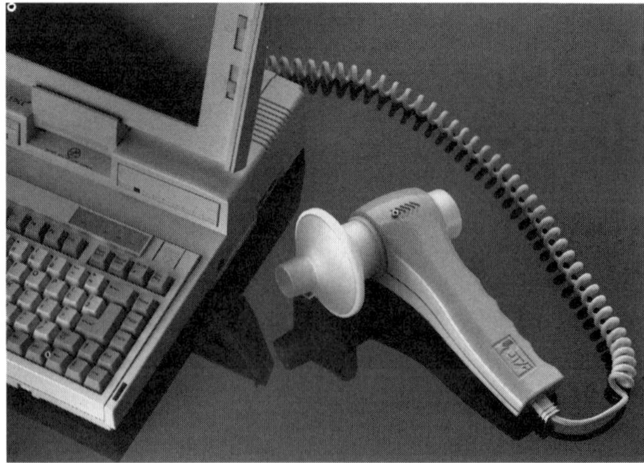

FIG 7–1
A Koko spirometer provided by Pulmonary Data Services is a convenient spirometer that can be used for bedside testing. It has a lightweight pneumotachograph resistance element and provides full flow-volume analysis via its built-in microprocessor. (Courtesy of Pulmonary Data Service, Inc, Louisville, Colo.)

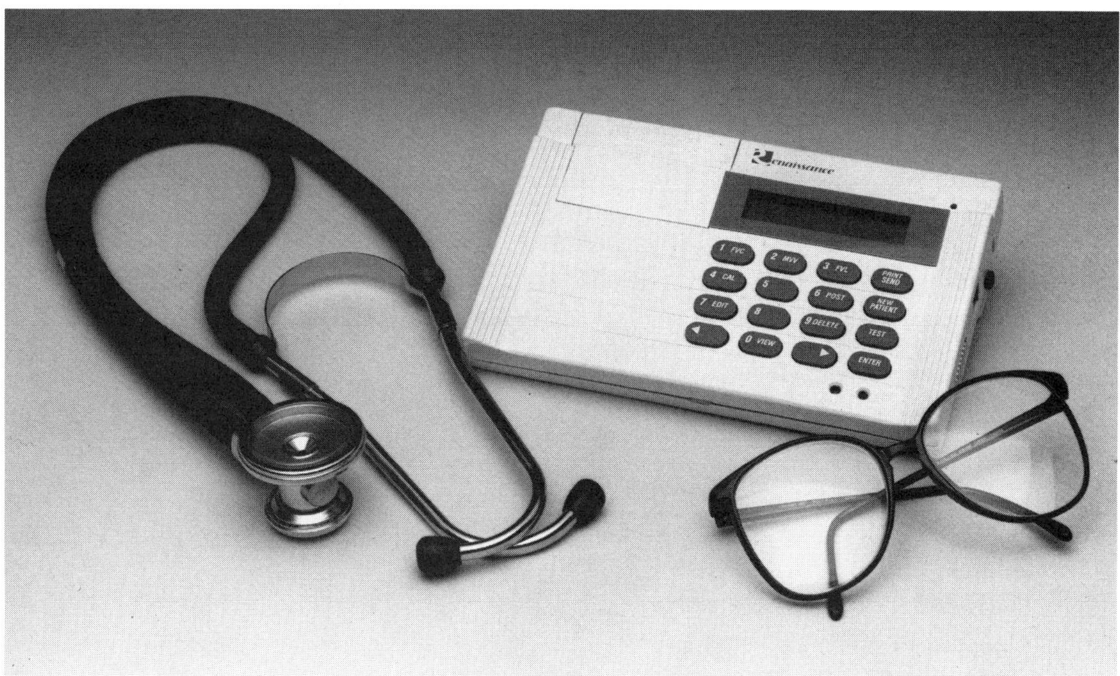

FIG 7–2
A Puritan-Bennett Renaissance spirometer is provided with a disposable flow sensor and has extensive coaching instructions for ease of use. (Courtesy of Puritan-Bennett Corp, Carlsbad, Calif.)

Clinical applications and limitations of bedside spirometry. The objective assessment of OAD is best done with simple spirometry. If the FVC maneuver is done properly and the instrument is properly calibrated, the FEV_1 and FVC should be reliably measured to within 5% or 100 mL, whichever is larger, the ATS criteria for adequate spirometry.[2] However, in performing the test on ill patients at the bedside, there are difficulties that will decrease this accuracy. Most difficulty is encountered in obtaining a reproducible FVC because of either incomplete inhalation or exhalation. Many systems measure only exhalation and require the patient to sustain a full inflation before connecting to the mouthpiece; sick patients will find this difficult. With severe OAD, the time to exhale fully to residual volume (RV) may require more than 15 seconds, and many patients are too dyspneic to sustain such long exhalations. Therefore, it is best to rely on the FEV_1 and not the FVC, which may be underestimated, or the FEV_1/FVC ratio, which may be overestimated because of the low FVC.

Perhaps the most limiting aspect of bedside spirometry is the intermittent nature of the assessment. In addition, the test requires considerable time and effort by a qualified RCP. For that reason, peak flowmeters for OAD and incentive spirometers for RLD are the more common methods of assessing ventilatory capacity at the bedside.

Peak Flowmeters

In 1991[3] the National Institutes of Health (NIH) and the Department of Health, Education, and Welfare (DHEW), in response to the rising concern about the incidence of asthma and asthma deaths, made a major effort to improve the management of asthma. It has been recognized that patients with declining or volatile fluctuations in spirometry are most prone to the development of acute and even life-threatening episodes. The peak flowmeter is considered a simple objective method to detect these airway problems earlier and optimally prevent more serious events.

There are a wide variety of peak flowmeters available at low cost, so each patient can have his or her own at home or at the bedside. Patients learn to correlate their peak expiratory flow (PEF) values to the severity of disease and the need for further treatment. Typical peak flowmeters are shown in Figure 7–3, A to C. After full inhalation, the patient exhales as rapidly as possible into the device, which has a spring-loaded or other resistance element that moves in proportion to the peak flow generated. Normal values vary with age, sex, and size; reliable predictive nomograms and tables are available.[4, 5]

In adults, values below 300 L/min are generally abnormal, and values below 200 L/min are a risk zone. Many patients with severe COPD will never be above 200, and the value of small changes in PEF in these patients is

FIG 7–3
Three examples of peak flowmeters. **A,** the original Wright peak flowmeter shown is heavier, sturdier, but costly and made for permanent use in a pulmonary laboratory. **B,** first of two examples of personal peak flowmeters that are inexpensive enough to be given to a patient for home use. (**A** and **B,** courtesy of Ferraris Medical, Inc, Holland, NY)

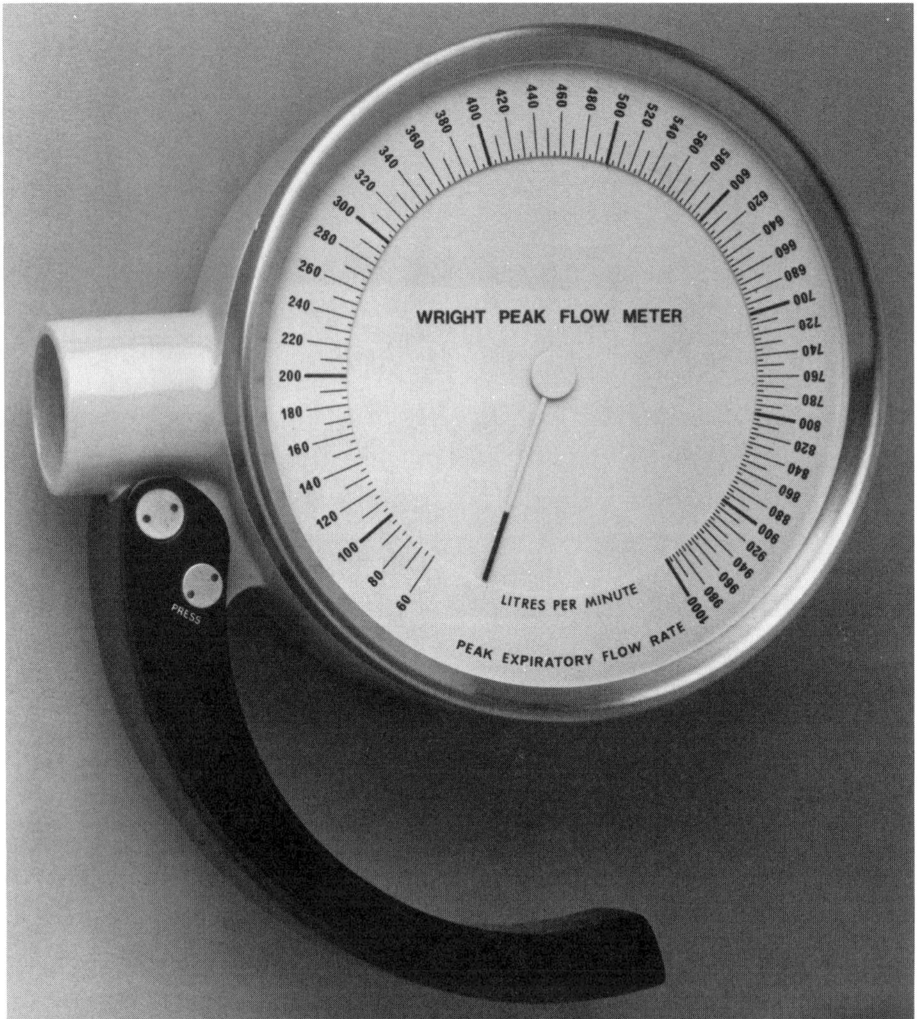

A

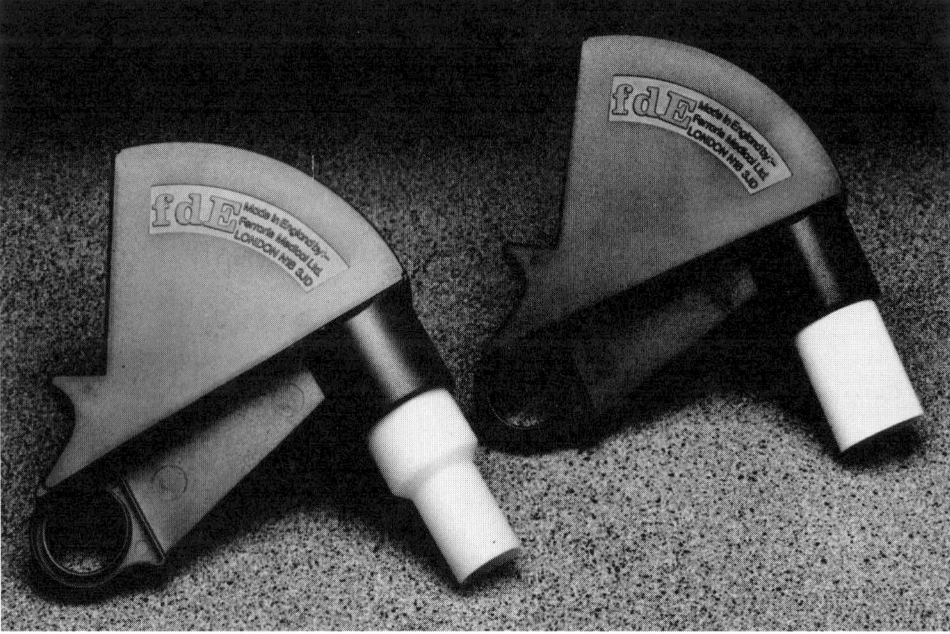

B

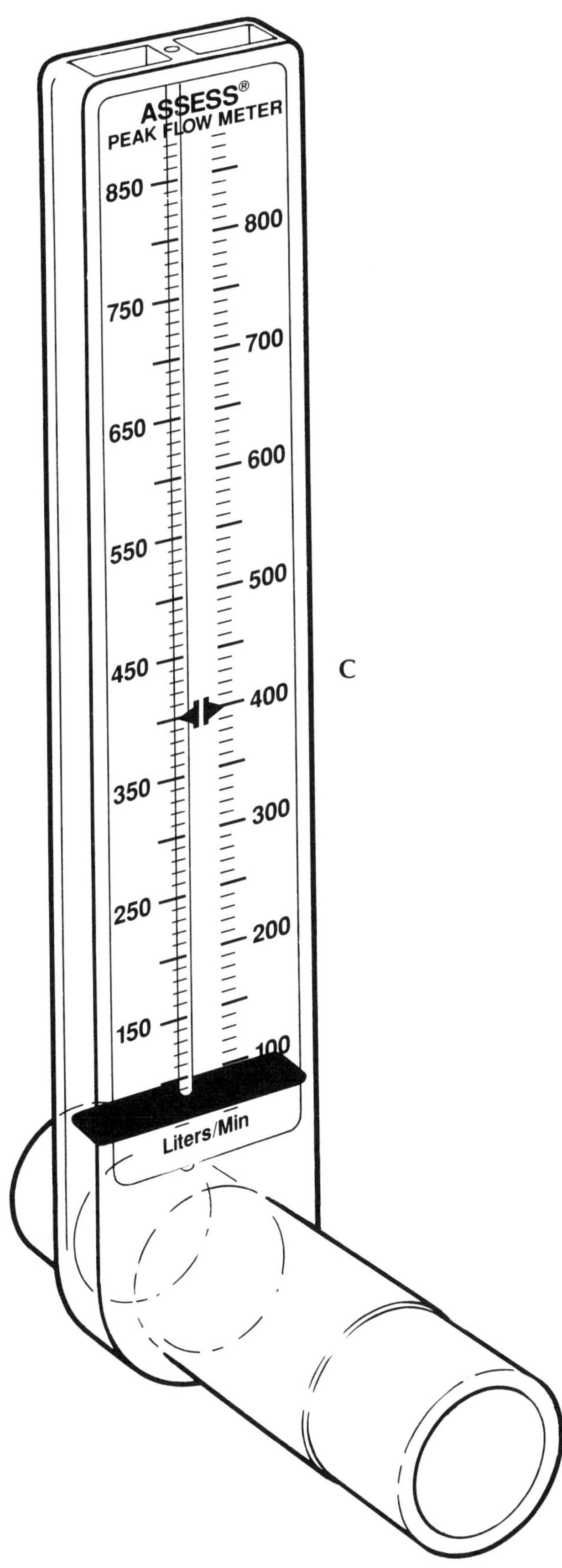

FIG 7–3 (cont.)
Three examples of peak flowmeters. **C,** second of two examples of personal peak flowmeters that are inexpensive enough to be given to a patient for home use. (**C,** courtesy of Healthscan Products, Cedar Grove, NJ.)

not as established as the wide fluctuations seen in asthmatics or a patient with reversible OAD. In patients with severe COPD, peak flows are persistently low and represent collapsing large airways. In these patients, spirometry, mouth pressure measurements, oximetry, and arterial blood gas (ABG) measurements are more frequently necessary to assess the response to treatment.

Incentive Spirometers

While standard spirometry and peak flowmeters depend primarily on exhalation, incentive spirometers require a forced inhalation. Perhaps the original "incentive spirometer" was introduced following surgery and used a surgical glove. Patients are encouraged to blow up the glove like a balloon; as the glove expands, the patient must exert a greater expiratory pressure, which can only be done as they inhale deeper. However, patients with upper abdominal or chest pain learn that they can continue to splint the chest, not take deep breaths, and yet still blow up the glove or balloon with pressure generated by the cheek and mouth muscles. There are devices that measure the degree of inflation by using a variety of visual feedback displays to encourage the patient to inhale further. An example of an incentive spirometer is shown in Figure 7–4.

Clinical applications and limitations. The most frequent application of incentive spirometry is in the postoperative patient, particularly after thoracic or upper abdominal surgery when atelectasis is so common. Incentive spirometry may be beneficial for any condition associated with atelectasis such as pneumonia, congestive heart failure (CHF), and pulmonary emboli and anyone with chest wall pain or limitation of chest movement such as those with neuromuscular disease. Some devices have a good correlation with the measured vital capacity, whereas others are primarily for visual stimulation of inhalation. A more accurate assessment of ventilatory capacity and respiratory muscle strength can be made by using mouth or esophageal pressure measurements.

Mouth Pressure Measurements

Combining pneumotachographs and pressure transducers permits monitoring of adult and pediatric/neonatal patients for maximal pressures as well as spirometry. The systems calculate spirometric values and, with a measurement of functional residual capacity (FRC),

How to use your VOLDYNE® Volumetric Incentive Deep Breathing Exerciser

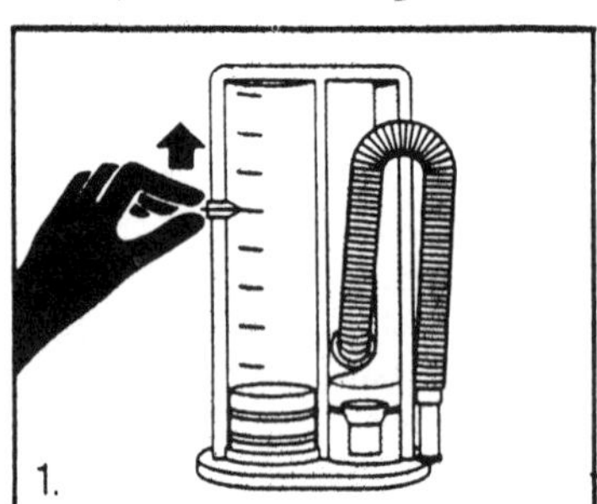

Slide the pointer of unit to prescribed volume level. Hold or stand exerciser in an upright position.

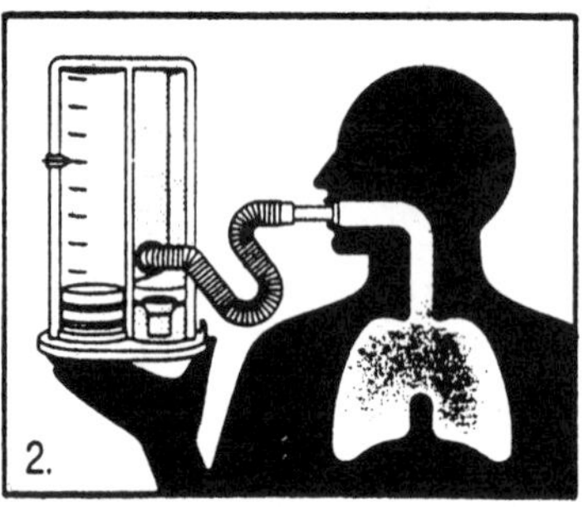

Exhale normally. Then place lips tightly around mouthpiece.

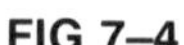

FIG 7–4
An inexpensive incentive spirometer that the patient keeps at the bedside or takes home with him or her. This type of incentive spirometer can give a rough estimate of vital capacity. The elevation of the marker is roughly proportional to the vital capacity of the patient. (Courtesy of Sherwood Medical, St Louis.)

can correlate maximal inspiratory/expiratory pressures with absolute lung volume. Adding pneumatic directional control valves provides the ability to assess occlusion pressure ($P_{0.1}$). A detailed description of a pediatric system (SensorMedics 2600) is given in Chapter 8. A system for monitoring spontaneously breathing adults (MedGraphics RPM) is shown in Figure 7–5.

More commonly, an inexpensive, handheld aneroid or spring-loaded pressure gauge is used to measure maximum inspiratory pressure (MIP) and maximum expiratory pressure (MEP) at the mouth as a measure of the adequacy of respiratory muscle strength and the need for ventilatory support.

A typical maximum pressure setup is shown in Figure 7–6.[6] These are simple spring-loaded pressure gauges that are occluded except for a pinhole opening so that as patients try to generate maximum inspiratory or expiratory pressures, they must do so by maintaining that pressure with a volume of air from the lung rather than being able to artifactually increase the pressure by sucking or compressing the air within the mouth with the cheek muscles. Aneroid gauges, being small and easily

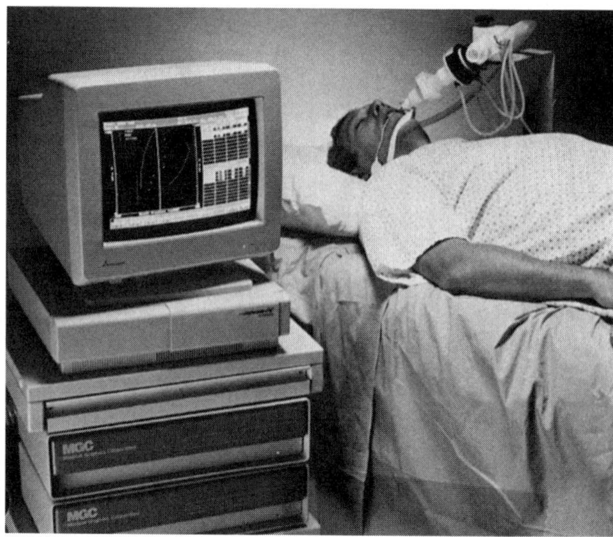

FIG 7–5
The MedGraphics Corporation RPM unit is shown. This cart is designed for use in a laboratory but can be taken to the bedside for monitoring respiratory mechanics. (Courtesy of MedGraphics Corp, St Paul, Minn.)

dropped, may lose accuracy and should be regularly calibrated against a pressure manometer.

Clinical applications and limitations. Respiratory muscle strength is assessed by measuring the MIP and MEP. Starlings' law states that the force generated by a muscle will increase as it is stretched; consequently, MIP and MEP will vary greatly depending on the volume at which it is measured (see Fig 7–7.)[7] Normal values reported vary widely.[8, 9] This may in part be due to the differences in the equipment assembly but perhaps more due to a lack of control over the volume at which the measurement is made. Maximal inspiratory forces (MIP) would occur at RV and expiratory forces at total lung capacity (TLC), both of which are difficult to maintain and require good patient cooperation. Measurements from the resting position at the end of a tidal breath (FRC) are most reproducibly done but are not truly maximal. In clinically normal men, MIP is generally greater than 90 cm H_2O and MEP is greater than 140 cm H_2O. Values are 25% lower in females and will decline 20% in the elderly.[10]

Maximum pressure can be useful in predicting or suggesting the onset of ventilatory failure or hypercapnia. In patients with neuromuscular disease, hypercapnia is likely to develop when the MIP falls to a third of the predicted value.[11] In patients with COPD, Pa_{CO_2} may increase at higher MIP values, 50% of predicted or approximately 50 cm H_2O.[12]

A commonly used method to measure MIP that has been shown to give reasonably reproducible results, even in critically ill patients, is to connect the pressure gauge

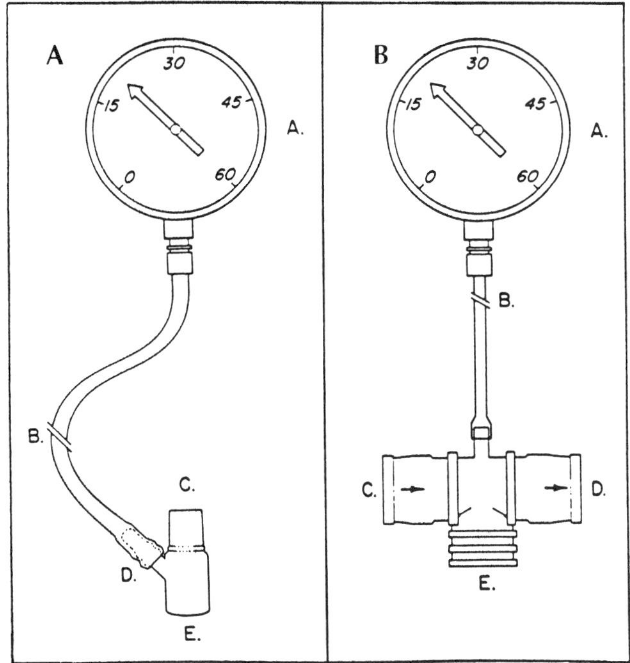

FIG 7–6
Methods for monitoring spontaneously breathing results. **A,** simple occlusion method: manometer *(A),* connecting tubing *(B),* port for thumb occlusion *(C),* port for attachment of tubing *(D),* and a 22-mm–inner diameter port for attachment to an artificial airway *(E).* The adapter represented by *C, D,* and *E* is an Artec Tee. **B,** one-way valve method: manometer *(A),* connecting tubing *(B),* inspiratory one-way valve with a port for thumb occlusion *(C),* expiratory one-way port *(D),* and a 22-mm–inner diameter port for attachment to an artificial airway *(E).* The adapter represented by *C, D,* and *E* is an Airlife U-Adapit. (From Kacmarek RM, Cycyk-Chapman MC, Young-Palazzo PJ, et al: *Respir Care* 1989; 34:868. Used by permission.)

to a one-way expiratory port (Fig 7–6) and have the patient maintain the effort for a 20-second period. As the patient exhales to a lower volume because he cannot inhale, the inspiratory force would increase to some maximal value.[13] This is a standard measurement used to predict weaning. One study suggests that an MIP of -30 cm H_2O will predict success whereas an MIP of only -20 cm H_2O would predict failure.[13] Others have disputed such clear cutoff points.[14] This may be due to the fact that mouth pressure readings fail to account for the differences in lung and thoracic compliance; a stiff lung will require higher MIP to sustain ventilation. On the other hand, an overdistended thoracic cage with a compliant, emphysematous lung may not be able to generate -30 cm H_2O but may still sustain ventilation, albeit probably at a high Pa_{CO_2}.

Additionally, as discussed above, MIP measurements are sensitive to changes in lung volume. Without accounting for the actual FRC, a hyperinflated patient may be erroneously classified as having reduced force when the MIP is in fact perfectly normal for the elevated lung volume. Simply treating the airway obstruction and reducing the hyperinflation can restore normal maximal pressures.

When a continuous pressure waveform is available, the pressure generated 100 ms after occluding the airway (P-100) can be obtained as a measure of respiratory drive. Brief airway occlusion can be randomly and repeatedly done every 10 to 30 seconds without patient awareness or discomfort. A low P-100 indicates a reduced ventilatory drive. Surprisingly, three studies with high values of P-100, indicating a strong central respiratory drive, were

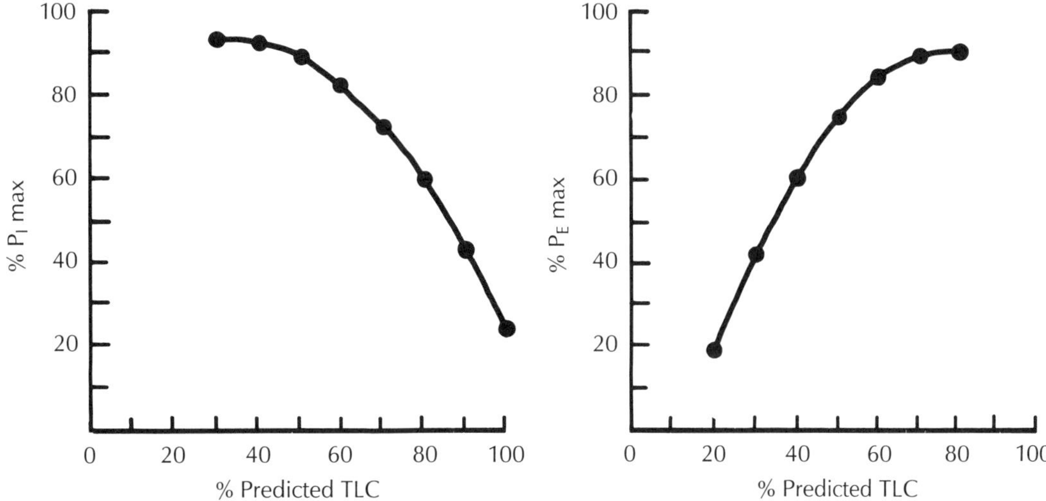

FIG 7–7
Variability of maximum inspiratory and expiratory pressures with lung volumes. Note that the maximum values for MIP are at RV whereas the maximum values for MEP are at total lung capacity *(TLC).* Variations in lung volume at which the measurement is made will obviously greatly affect the value obtained. (From Black LF, Hyatt RE: *Am Rev Respir Dis* 1971; 103:641–650. Used by permission.)

predictive of weaning failure.[15–17] This is presumably due to the patient's drive to maintain a level of ventilation greater than the respiratory muscles can support. Others have failed to confirm this observation.[18] The respiratory drive should increase if the patient is exposed to stimuli such as increased levels of F_{ICO_2} hypoxia, or pharmacologic stimuli such as caffeine. Assessing these responses can provide additional documentation of the patient's ability to maintain ventilation without mechanical support.

Continuous Monitoring of Spontaneously Breathing Patients

Spontaneously breathing patients can be monitored continuously with minimal invasiveness in several ways. The ECG and oximetry are the most common methods. When nasal O_2 is already being delivered, the nasal catheter can also be used to monitor the respiratory rate (RR) and even obtain an approximation of Pa_{CO_2} by using the end tidal CO_2 (P_{ETCO_2}). In critically ill neonates and infants, transcutaneous O_2 and CO_2 are frequently monitored. These modalities will all be considered in the next section on gas exchange. There are a number of methodologies that have attempted to quantitate ventilation by using some device around the torso, including bellows pneumography, differential linear transducers, circumferential inductive transducers, magnetometers, and mercury Silastic strain gauge belts.[19] These methods are used primarily in sleep laboratories for monitoring ventilatory effort. Precise quantitation of V_T and V_E has been difficult in long-term monitoring.

The most readily available and most common form of RR monitoring of a spontaneously breathing patient uses the ECG leads to monitor chest impedance changes as the lung inflates and deflates. The most effective quantitative ventilatory monitors in spontaneously breathing patients are respiratory inductive plethysmographs (RIPs) placed around the chest and abdomen. These systems allow monitoring of V_T, RR, and V_E. Finally, an esophageal balloon can be used to continuously monitor lung mechanics, although it is more invasive and usually limited to special study units, critically ill patients, or mechanically ventilated patients.

Impedance Pneumography

The principle that electrical conductivity through the chest would decrease as the lung inflates was recognized early in this century but not developed until stimulated by monitoring in aerospace.[20, 21] Theoretically, transthoracic electrical impedance could be used to monitor RR, V_T, FRC, and even changes in lung H_2O. If properly placed over the heart, impedance changes have been used to monitor stroke volume and cardiac output.[22]

Clinical applications and limitations. Because many intrathoracic compartments affect transthoracic impedance and because of the artifacts introduced by chest wall contraction and movement, this method has found common use only as a monitor of RR and detection of apnea with two standard ECG leads. It is available as a module on most ECG monitoring systems. Impedance pneumography (IP) has real value in timing the respiratory cycle to allow identification of heart-lung interactions, as explained below in the hemodynamics monitoring section.

Respiratory Inductive Plethysmography

This method is based on the demonstration by Konno and Mead[23] that respiratory movement behaves as two simple physical systems, the rib cage and abdomen (Fig 7–8). During normal inspiration, the chest expands, and as the diaphragm descends, so does the abdomen. They used magnetometers, but current systems use two inductance coil belts or vests to produce signals from the rib cage and abdomen to approximate V_T (Fig 7–9).[24] The method requires a difficult calibration procedure; the subject must do inspiratory and expiratory efforts during voluntary closure of the glottis or airway occlusion (i.e., isovolume maneuvers) in order to set the rib cage and abdomen signals to equal each other. With improved

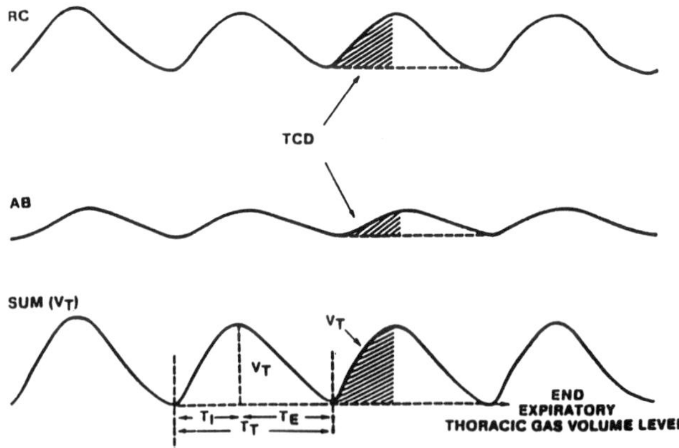

FIG 7–8
Respiratory inductive plethysmographic tracings showing rib cage *(RC)* and abdomen *(AB)* waveforms; the electrical sum of RC + AB = V_T. Total compartmental displacement *(TCD)* is the absolute sum of the area during inspiration (T_I) of the RC + AB *(shaded areas),* irrespective of sign. When the RC and AB compartments are in synchrony (as depicted here), the TCD will equal the sum (V_T), and the TCD/V_T ratio will equal unity (1.00). The end-expiratory thoracic gas volume (or FRC level) is shown, as well as timing components (T_E = expiratory time; T_T = total respiratory cycle time). (From Krieger BP: *Respir Care* 1990; 35:700. Used by permission.)

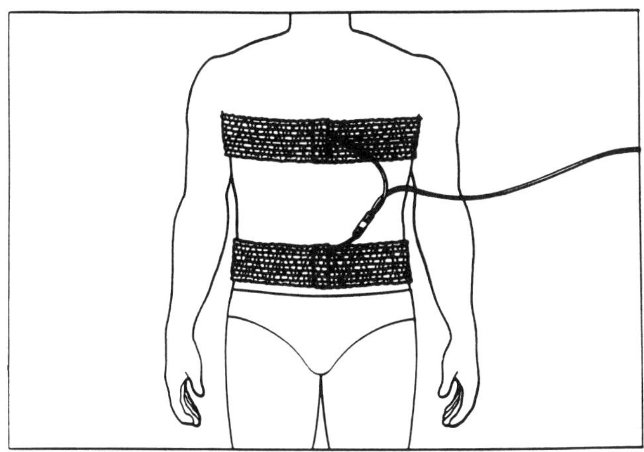

FIG 7–9
Respiratory inductance plethysmography. Two inductance coils fitted around the chest and abdomen can be used to monitor spontaneously breathing patients. Proper placement of RIP transducer bands, which are connected by snaps to the oscillator module, is shown. The rib cage band is placed on the upper portion of the chest above the breasts in female subjects or at the nipple level in male subjects, and the abdomen band is placed at the level of the umbilicus. (From Krieger BP: *Respir Care* 1990; 35:700. Used by permission.)

engineering and simplification of calibration, the best results report V_T to be measured within 20% of spirometric values, even with positional changes.[24]

Clinical applications and limitations. Clinical application is proposed for sleep laboratories, for critical care units, and possibly on home monitors. The major use of RIP has been in sleep laboratories where detection and quantification of ventilation is so necessary to diagnose obstructive sleep apnea. However, even in sleep laboratories, the much simpler mercury Silastic strain gauge belts or IP are often preferred because precise quantification is so difficult and not necessary. Obstructive apnea can be determined by noting the presence of chest movement associated with the absence of nasal CO_2 or air temperature changes (Fig 7–10).[24] However, errors can be made if chest and abdominal wall measurements are not precise (Fig 7–11).

In critical care, RIP can be used to monitor V_E, V_T, and the breathing pattern. The detection of paradoxical movement of the abdomen or respiratory cage has been associated with either respiratory muscle fatigue[25, 26] or increased respiratory load.[27] However, as suggested by McIntyre,[28] the abdominal paradox can readily be seen by an astute RCP. However, the RCP cannot be present for prolonged periods, particularly during sleep when abnormalities such as paradoxical breathing or upper airway obstruction may occur and trigger a major pulmonary event such as severe hypoxemia that can then lead to a major cardiac event such as tachyrhythmia or infarction.

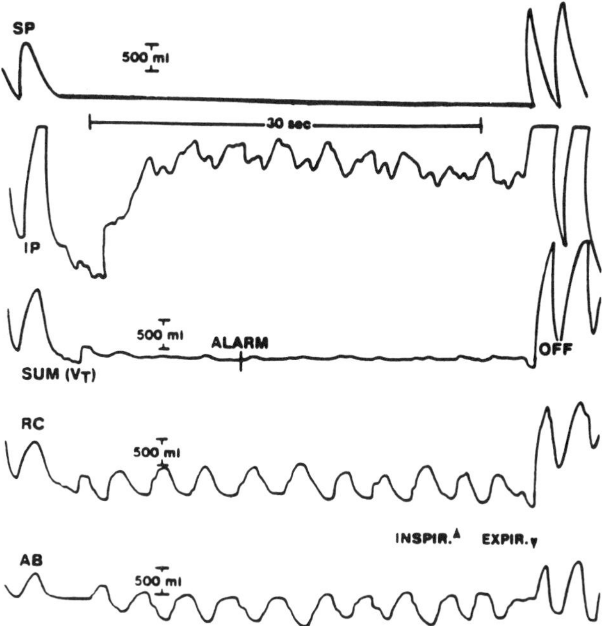

FIG 7–10
During a simulated obstructive apnea (as evidenced by respiratory inductive plethysmography [RIP] signals showing rib cage *[RC]* and abdominal *[AB]* movements in opposite directions resulting in a flat sum [V_T] signal and no volume measured by simultaneous spirometry *[SP]*), the signal from an impedance pneumograph *(IP)* continues to show motion because of RC movement. Because RIP calibration is based on two degrees of freedom, it appropriately senses an apnea and sounds an alarm, whereas the IP fails to sound an alarm because it falsely interprets RC movement as a breath. (From Krieger BP: *Respir Care* 1990; 35:698. Used by permission.)

Demonstrating that such sophisticated ventilatory monitoring can save lives and be cost-effective is needed before recommending use. Home monitoring remains a controversial and unsettled issue. At the present time, no home monitoring device has been shown to be reliable in quantitatively monitoring ventilation.

Monitoring Mechanically Ventilated Patients

In spontaneously breathing patients, monitoring ventilation is predominantly intermittent. When a patient is on a mechanical ventilator, continuous measurements of not only V_E, RR, and V_T but also airway pressures (P_{aw}) are readily done; with these measurements it is possible to define the mechanics of the respiratory system. The physiologic management of a patient on mechanical ventilation requires an understanding of the practical application of respiratory mechanics. This is essentially being done by the RCP every time he looks at the pressure gauges on a ventilator and, at the same time, notes the tidal volume. Since these measurements are available

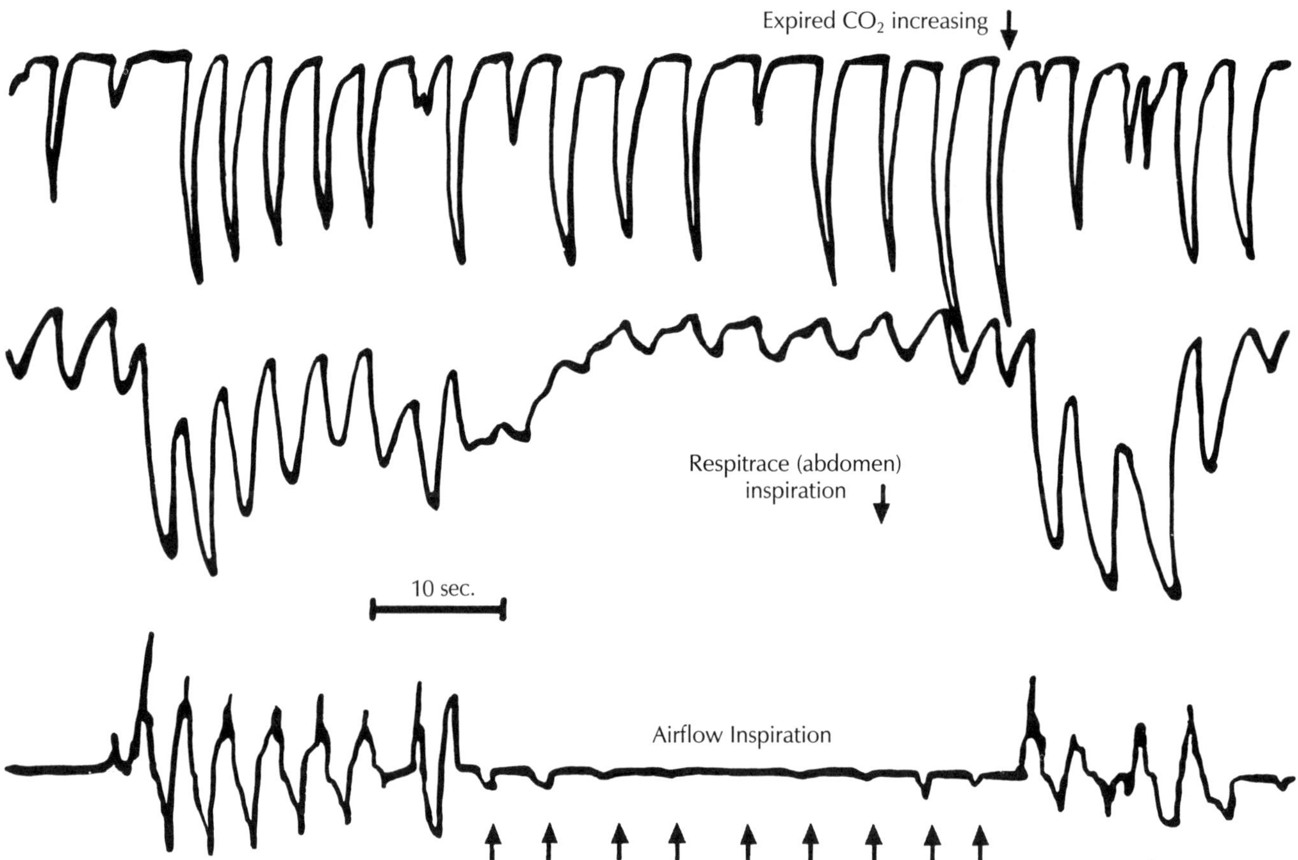

FIG 7–11
An example of the limitations of noninvasive airflow detection. *Top trace,* airflow detected by a carbon dioxide analyzer. *Middle trace,* respiratory inductance plethysmography (RIP). *Bottom trace,* airflow measured with a pneumotachograph. With each apnea-related expiratory deflection documented by the pneumotachograph (*arrows* in the bottom trace), there is a sustained shift in the baseline of the RIP. This suggests an incremental decrease in functional residual capacity resulting from absent inspirations with continued small expiratory puffs. If only the top two traces were available, then this would have been mistakenly called hypoventilation or hypopnea when it is clearly total occlusion on inspiration. (From West P, Kryger MH: *Clin Chest Med* 1985; 6:706. Used by permission.)

continuously with each breath when mechanical ventilators are being used, they readily lends itself to continuous monitoring.

Historically, such measurements were considered too technically difficult and costly to be practical. Although many physiologic experiments in the 1950s and 1960s were done with continuous monitoring of compliance and resistance, it was seldom if ever implemented in humans in the ICU because too much technical expertise was required to monitor the monitors, which were cumbersome and unstable. In the late 1960s, Dr. John Osborn and colleagues in conjunction with International Business Machines (IBM) and NIH funding developed an effective continuous monitoring system for both respiratory mechanics and gas exchange.[29] The system was costly, used a main frame computer that filled a 15 × 20-ft room, and therefore was not practical for general hospital use. IBM chose not to continue the development. Subsequently, microcomputer technology has developed to the point where it is possible to house similar technology within the space of a modern ventilator or a portable monitoring system, as will be described in this section. First, however, we will describe the theory and physiology of continuous mechanics measurements.

Theory and Definitions

Although simple and sometimes inaccurate in the real world, the ideal gas law (Boyle's and Charles' laws) $PV = nRT$ is helpful to understand the concept that the product of the pressure and volume of a gas is constant if the temperature is constant since n and R in the ideal gas law are also constants. As temperature increases, either pressure or volume must increase. So too, a simple mechanical model of the lung consisting of a resistance element, the airway (R_{aw}), and a compliance element, the lung or alveolar sacs, C_l, can practically describe the pressure and volume characteristics of ventilation as shown in Figure 7–12. If esophageal or intrapleural pressure is not measured, as it usually is not, then the compliance of the chest wall (C_{cw}) must be added to the C_l. The sum of the two, $C_l + C_{cw}$, is generally referred to as the compliance of the respiratory system (C_{rs}). At any time, the mouth pressure (P_m) will be a sum of the pressure required to overcome the resistance to flow (P_R) and the pressure required to overcome the compliance of elastic recoil of the lung and chest wall, P_C:

$$P_T = P_R + P_C. \quad (1)$$

If the starting point of inspiration is not at zero pressure, such as would occur when positive end-expiratory pressure (PEEP) is present, then it is necessary to add a PEEP term to the equation. Therefore

$$P_T = P_R + P_C + PEEP. \quad (2)$$

The pressure resulting from the airway resistance elements, P_R, is defined as

$$P_R = \text{Flow} \times \text{Resistance} = \dot{V} \times R_{aw}. \quad (3)$$

Similarly, the pressure, P_C, to overcome compliance of the respiratory system (C_{rs}) is

$$P_C = V_T/C_{rs}. \quad (4)$$

Combining Equations 2, 3, and 4,

$$P_T = \dot{V}\, R_{aw} + V_T/C + PEEP. \quad (5)$$

This simple, single-compartment model of the lung can be mathematically developed to give very good simulations of model lungs[30] as well as a clinically useful description of the mechanics of the respiratory system even in diseased patients.[31] The reader is referred to the references cited for the details of how such mathematical models have been used to allow an on-line computer system to continuously monitor C_{rs} and R_{aw} from the continuous measurements of pressure and flow. First we describe how to manually perform the measurements since such manual calculations are invaluable to verify the automated computer outputs.

Figure 7–13[32] shows characteristic flow, volume, and pressure curves of a patient on a ventilator. Maximum inspiratory airway pressure ($P_{aw}max$), static or plateau pressures (P_{st}), and PEEP may all be readily measured manually by using the pressure gauges on the ventilator. These pressures in combination with tidal volume (V_T) may be used to calculate compliance of the lung and chest wall. Two parameters are most commonly measured—static compliance (C_{st}) and dynamic "characteristic" (C_{dyn}):

$$C_{st} = V_T/(P_{st} - PEEP) \quad (6)$$

$$C_{dyn} = V_T/(P_{aw}max - PEEP) \quad (7)$$

It should be understood that these compliance measurements may differ significantly from measurements of *lung* compliance measured by using the esophageal balloon (or some other estimate of pleural pressure) because of the inclusion of compliance of the chest wall. Any active contracture of respiratory musculature (chest wall and diaphragm) may affect these measurements. Meaningful and reproducible measurement of lung mechanics on ventilator patients without

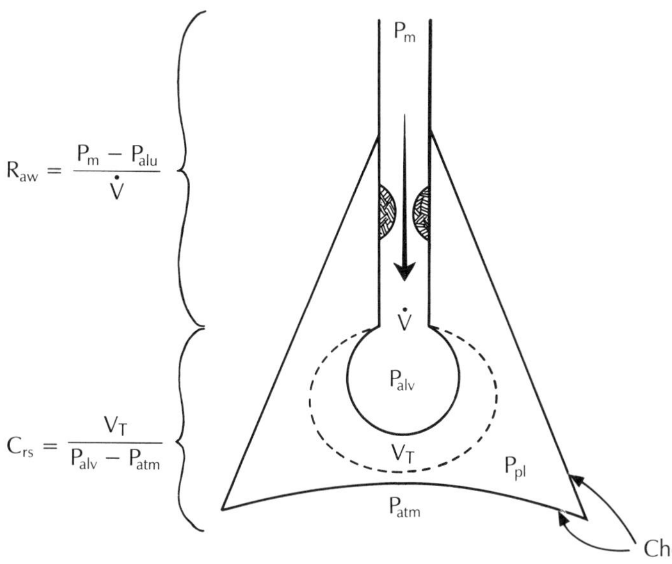

FIG 7–12
(Equation A), A simple schematic model of the lung consisting of a single airway resistance element,

$$R_{aw} = P_m - P_{alv}/V_T = P_R/V_T \quad \text{(Equation A)},$$

and two compliance elements, the lung, $C_l = V_T/P_{alv} - P_{pl} = V_T/P_1$, and the chest wall, $C_{cw} = V_T/(P_{atm} - P_{pl}) = V_T/P_{C_{cw}}$, which can be combined to give the compliance of the respiratory system:

$$C_{rs} = (V_T/P_{alv} - P_{atm}) = V_T/(P_1 + P_{cw}) \quad \text{(Equation B)}.$$

As described in the text, the overall pressure requirements with positive-pressure ventilation can be described by combining Equation A and equation B:

$$P_m = P_t = P_R + P_C = R_{aw} \cdot V_t + V_T/C_{rs}.$$

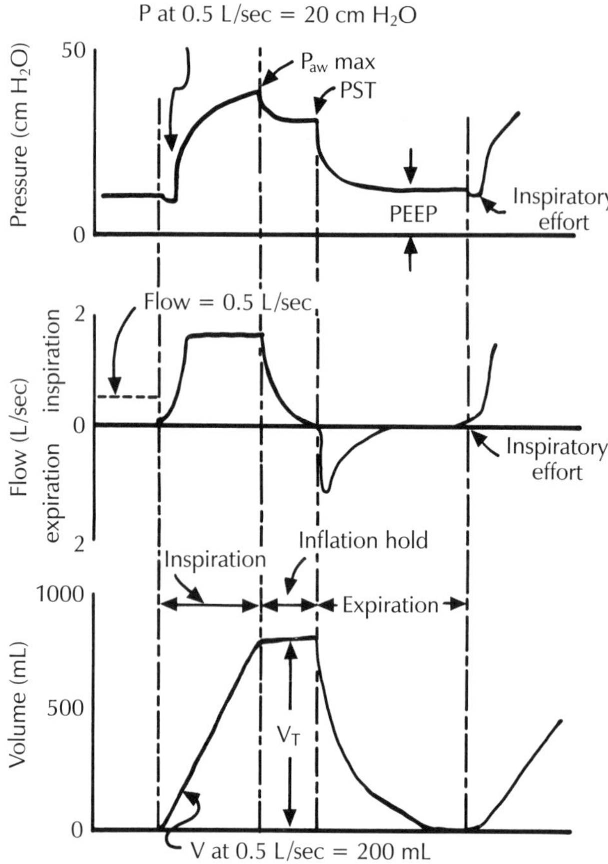

FIG 7–13
Airway pressure is measured in the airway close to the patient's endotracheal tube. A small inspiratory effort is seen and initiates inspiratory flow. The flow is of the square-wave type, very quickly reaching a plateau. There is a period of inflationary hold and flow falls to zero, but the lungs are maintained inflated; during this time a static airway pressure (P_{st}) is obtained before exhalation. Pressure returns to some predetermined positive end-expiratory pressure *(PEEP)* level. Flows are not readily obtained except from flow measuring devices such as the pneumotachograph. Pressure readings may be readily obtained from the pressure gauge on the ventilator. Tidal volume (VT) can also be measured from a spirometer placed in the exhalation line. (From Clausen JL (ed): *Pulmonary Function Testing Guidelines and Controversies.* London, Grune & Stratton, 1984, pp 293–310. Used by permission.)

using an esophageal balloon requires the patient to be passive, not "fighting" the ventilator during the measurement.[33] A short period of negative pressure that initiates inspiration, as shown in Figure 7–13,[32] can be present without seriously affecting the results.

The dynamic characteristic (C_{dyn}), as measured in the ICU setting and commonly referred to as dynamic compliance, is not a true compliance since the P_{aw}max is measured under conditions of flow and therefore includes the pressure required to overcome resistance elements. The difference between P_{aw}max and P_{st} is one measure of R_{aw}:

$$R_{aw} = (P_{aw}max - P_{st})/\dot{V}max, \quad (8)$$

where flow is the flow at end-inspiration, the time of the P_{aw}max measurement. In Figure 7–13, P_{aw}max = 37.5, P_{st} = 30, and flow = 1.5, so

$$R_{aw} = (37.5 - 30)/1.5 = 5 \text{ cm } H_2O/L/sec.$$

Alternatively, R_{aw} can be calculated at any other point during inspiration by using the flow at that point and the pressure corrected for the component resulting from static compliance factor. A flow of 0.5 L/sec is commonly used for R_{aw} measurement. For example, from Figure 7–13, at a flow of 0.5 L/sec and a volume of 200 mL where P_{st} = 30 cm H_2O, PEEP = 10 cm H_2O, and VT = 800 mL,

$$C_{st} = 800/(30 - 10) = 40 \text{ mL/cm } H_2O.$$

Assuming a constant C_{st}, the pressure resulting from compliance (P_C) at V = 200 is

$$P_C = V/C_{st} = 200/40 = 5 \text{ cm } H_2O.$$

R_{aw} at 0.5 L/sec then is

$$R_{aw} = (P \text{ at } 0.5 - PEEP - P_C)/Flow = (20 - 10 - 5)/0.5 = 5/0.5 = 10 \text{ cm } H_2O/L/sec.$$

Note that the R_{aw} at 0.5 L/sec is twice that calculated at end inspiration from Equation 8. Such large and variable R_{aw} measurements can be expected in ventilator patients because of the large flow-dependent resistances found in the endotracheal tube and the expansion of airways that occurs during inflation. Manual measurement of P_{st}, C, and R_{aw} are not easily or routinely done because they depend on the visualization of a single point during a brief inspiratory hold time where true equilibrated P_{st} may not be reached. Because automated systems use all the pressure and flow data throughout the breathing cycle, more precise information about ventilatory mechanics is possible.

In addition to measuring compliance and resistance, automated systems may calculate the work of breathing (WOB). When only P_{aw} is available, the WOB measured is primarily that done by the ventilator. If there is a measure of intrathoracic P, it is possible to measure the WOB done by the patient (WOB_p). Esophageal balloons provide such a capability.

Esophageal Pressure Measurements (Intrathoracic Pressure)

In patients who are spontaneously breathing, airway pressure is not available for monitoring mechanics and can only be done if intrathoracic pressure measurements are made. In addition, chest wall and abdominal muscle movements introduce errors in measuring C_{rs}. Accurate measurement of the compliance of the lung (C_l) requires a measurement of the intrathoracic or pleural pressures to separate the lung from the chest wall. Chest tubes are frequently already in patients in the intensive care setting and could be used to monitor pleural pressures. This is not commonly done because chest tubes are usually sterile systems attached to negative pressure for suctioning air and fluid out; therefore, intrathoracic or pleural pressure measurements are not possible.

However, measuring the pressure in the esophagus by using esophageal balloons allows an estimate of pleural pressure at the bedside. Nasogastric tubes are available that have an intrathoracic balloon attached to allow such measurements without additional invasion in those patients who already require nasogastric suction. The major problem with the measurement of esophageal pressure is that patients are usually supine and the gravity effects of the mediastinal organs, in particular the heart, can cause variation in the pressure readings, particularly as the patient changes positions. In addition, balloon inflation and position are critical and difficult to maintain for continuous monitoring. With careful attention to all these details, accurate measurements can be made of esophageal or intrapleural pressure. At least two commercial systems (BICORE, MedGraphics) that use esophageal measurements can be brought to the bedside for intermittent or continuous monitoring. These systems and the continuous monitoring systems in ventilators will be described.

Automated Ventilatory Monitoring Systems

BICORE CP-100 Pulmonary Monitor

The CP-100 pulmonary monitor uses sophisticated microcomputer technology to automate the measurement of ventilation, pulmonary mechanics, WOB, and respiratory drive. Continuous pulmonary monitoring is available for patients who require mechanical ventilation or those who are capable of spontaneous, unassisted ventilation because of the use of esophageal pressure (P_{es}).

BICORE's VarFlex flow transducers are disposable bidirectional flow measuring devices that use a variable area, flexible obstruction for measuring flow as a function of the pressure differential generated by the obstruction (Fig 7–14).[34] They weigh only 22 g, have 9.6 cc of dead space, and can measure flow from 0.02 to 3.0 L/sec with ±3% accuracy. The pressure drop of the transducer is 3.6 cm H_2O at 3 L/sec. Pressure is measured at the transducer over a range from −60 to +120 cm H_2O.

BICORE's esophageal catheter is a multifunction balloon catheter that when placed in the patient's esophagus acts as the transducer to monitor heart rate, respiratory pressures, and core temperature. A triple-lumen catheter allows gastric suctioning or internal feeding. The P_{es} allows a more direct and accurate measure of intrinsic PEEP ($PEEP_i$) since it is defined as the presence of positive intrapleural pressure at the start of inhalation.

WOB is the PV product over time. When P_{aw} and VT are measured during mechanical ventilation, the area under the pressure versus volume curves represents the work of the ventilator (WOB_v). During spontaneous breathing, the area under the P_{es}- and VT-versus-time curves measures the work of the patient. Measures of this type allow analysis of the patient effort required during various modes of ventilation and may produce strategies for optimizing ventilator use.[34] Figure 7–15[34] shows the combined patient and ventilator WOB that can be measured by using a combination of P_{aw} and P_{es} and VT-versus-time curves.

MedGraphics CCM/RPM System

The CCM/RPM system provides computer-assisted measurement of spirometry, ventilation, static and dynamic compliance, WOB, and respiratory drive (occlusion pressure). Designed for discrete measurements in the cardiopulmonary laboratory, the CCM/RPM can be brought to the bedside for intermittent use but will not support continuous monitoring or pediatric/neonatal measurements.

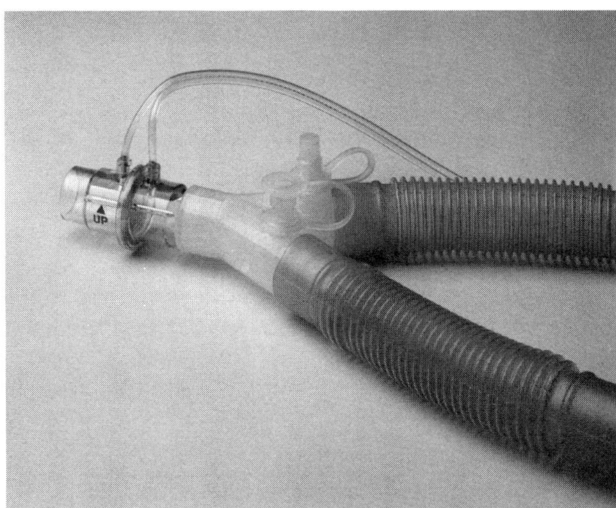

FIG 7–14
VarFlex flow transducers are disposable bidirectional flow measuring devices that use a variable-area, flexible obstruction for measuring flow as a function of the pressure differential generated by the obstruction. (Courtesy of BICORE, Irvine, Calif.)

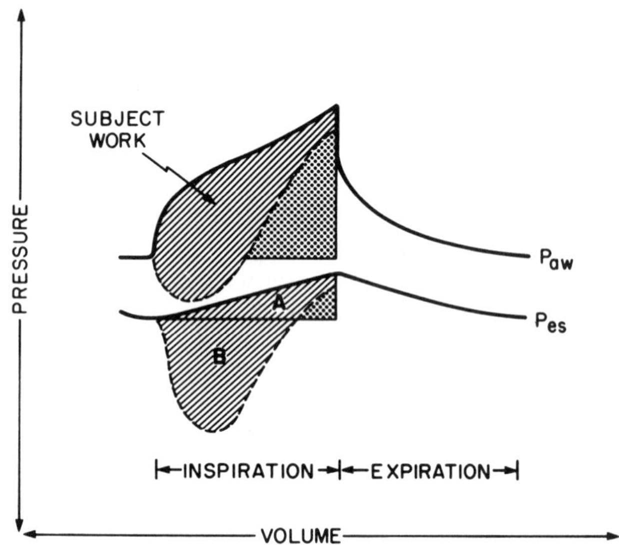

FIG 7–15
Patient work (W_p) during triggered breathing can be quantified by subtracting the planimetered area under the airway pressure tracing (P_{aw}) of a triggered breath from that of a controlled mechanical breath, provided that equal flow and volume are delivered. Alternatively, W_p can be quantified from differences in panimetered areas between triggered and controlled esophageal pressure-volume plots, provided that equal flows and volumes are delivered. *Solid lines* represent a controlled breath, and *dashed lines* represent an assisted triggered breath. Area *A* represents work performed by the patient in expanding the chest wall. Area *B* represents the work performed by the patient in expanding the lungs and moving volume against resistance. When P_{aw} is used to compute W_p, triggered and controlled breaths must have equivalent inspiratory resistance. (From Marini JJ: *Clin Chest Med* 1988; 9:73–100. Used by permission.)

MedGraphics uses a screen-type pneumotachograph as described in Chapter 8. Pneumatically driven balloon valves provide directional control and occlusion of airflow. The pneumotachograph and balloon valve can be detached from the system by using an umbilical to facilitate measurements on mechanically ventilated patients.

Maximal pressures measurements are performed in association with a spirographic tracing that permits assessment of the volume:pressure relationship by occluding the shutter at various known lung volumes. The mechanics software supports the use of esophageal balloons or airway pressure signals from the ventilator. A balloon placement program provides visual assurance of appropriate placement of the esophageal balloon. Occlusion pressures include three modes of testing that permit measurement of baseline values and response to stimuli such as increased CO_2, lowered O_2, or caffeine. The WOB program measures elastic, resistive, and total work. Additionally, the integration algorithm can be changed to integrate from zero pressure or the end-expiratory pressure.

In-Ventilator Monitor Systems

Puritan-Bennett 7200 ventilator and monitor. The Puritan-Bennett 7200 monitoring system provides the capability of performing intermittent maneuvers to measure vital capacity (Vc), MIP, and static compliance. The Vc is measured by asking the patient to perform a maximal inspiratory effort after a Vc activation mode is started. The ventilator waits 10 seconds for the patient to initiate the breath; if the breath is not initiated, the ventilator returns to preset ventilatory modes. The exhalation phase lasts for a maximum of 15 seconds and records only the exhaled volume; it is not a forced Vc maneuver, therefore flows and FEV_1 are not calculated.

Similarly, the MIP is measured by asking the patient to do a maximal inspiratory effort after activating the test. If the patient reduces the P_{aw} to below the PEEP minus the sensitivity settings within 10 seconds, the inspiratory and expiratory valves remain closed for 3 more seconds and record the MIP as the negative pressure produced plus the PEEP pressure, which was also overcome by the patient's inhalation effort.

The static mechanics maneuver initiates a 0.5- to 2.0-second closure of the exhalation valve while a plateau pressure is recorded. C_{rs} and R_{aw} are calculated as described in the manual calculation above.

Continuous "dynamic mechanics" monitoring is also done during any ventilator-initiated breath by using a model slightly more complicated than the single C_{rs} and R_{aw} described above. This model attempts to separately measure the compliance and resistance of the "patient service system" (C_{pss} and R_{pss}) running in parallel and series respectively with the patient's C_{rs} and R_{aw}. The C_{pss} and R_{pss} are measured independently before connecting the system to the patient.

The dynamic measurements are based on P_{aw} and flow and volume measurements taken every 20 ms during the mandatory breath. A P_{aw} is calculated from the model equation by using an estimate of the R_{aw} and C_{rs}. The R_{aw} and C_{rs} chosen are those that give the best fit between the calculated P_{aw} and measured P_{aw} based on minimizing the sum of the square of the differences. A running average for R_{aw} and C_{rs} is obtained over eight breaths. A new value for R_{aw} and C_{rs} must fall within 20% of the running average to be included. This eliminates many of the errors introduced by patient effort or erratic breathing patterns. Because the resistance and compliance are not truly constant during inspiratory maneuvers, measurement of the static resistance and compliance may not agree with these dynamic continuous measurements, but there is good correlation over time.

Siemens 300C. The Siemens 300C system is shown in Figure 7–16. Shortly after the gas inlet (I), the galvanic O_2 fuel cell monitors the *dry* inspired gas. The pressure of the gas stored in the bellows is monitored and displayed by a manometer, with a safety valve pop-off at 120 cm H_2O.

There are two flow transducers, one on the inspiratory side and one on the expiratory side; note that these are housed in the ventilator and therefore leaks in or out of the tubing leading to and from the patient may be detected by the difference between the two flows; the expansion volume of the tubing is included in the V_T measurement, and therefore the tubing is part of the C_{rs} measured. The flow transducers are from a sidestream system shown and described in Figure 7–17.

There are also two pressure transducers, one on the inspiratory and one on the expiratory sides of the circuit within the ventilator. A strain gauge similar to that used in the flow transducer is used. Again, pressure drop in the patient circuit is included in the estimate of the R_{aw} and C_{rs} measurements reported.

The $PEEP_i$ measurement is made by occluding both the inspiratory and expiratory valves before inhalation and measuring the pressure at the pressure transducer. The expansion volume in the tubing will therefore reduce the $PEEP_i$ measurement and result in a falsely low measurement by a magnitude determined by the Pmax during inspiration.

Clinical Applications and Limitations

The measurements of Pmax, P_{st}, $\dot{V}$, V_E, and V_T are routinely done on all mechanically ventilated patients with a frequency determined by the patient's status. The usefulness and indications for automated systems that continuously monitor respiratory mechanics is assumed but not well established. Respiratory mechanics measurements are of most importance in critically ill patients requiring high airway pressures or high F_{IO_2} to maintain oxygenation. Usually this means the use of a modern volume ventilator that depends on respiratory mechanics for the ventilator to function; therefore, mechanics measurements are available. If such a ventilator is not available but the patient has the conditions described in

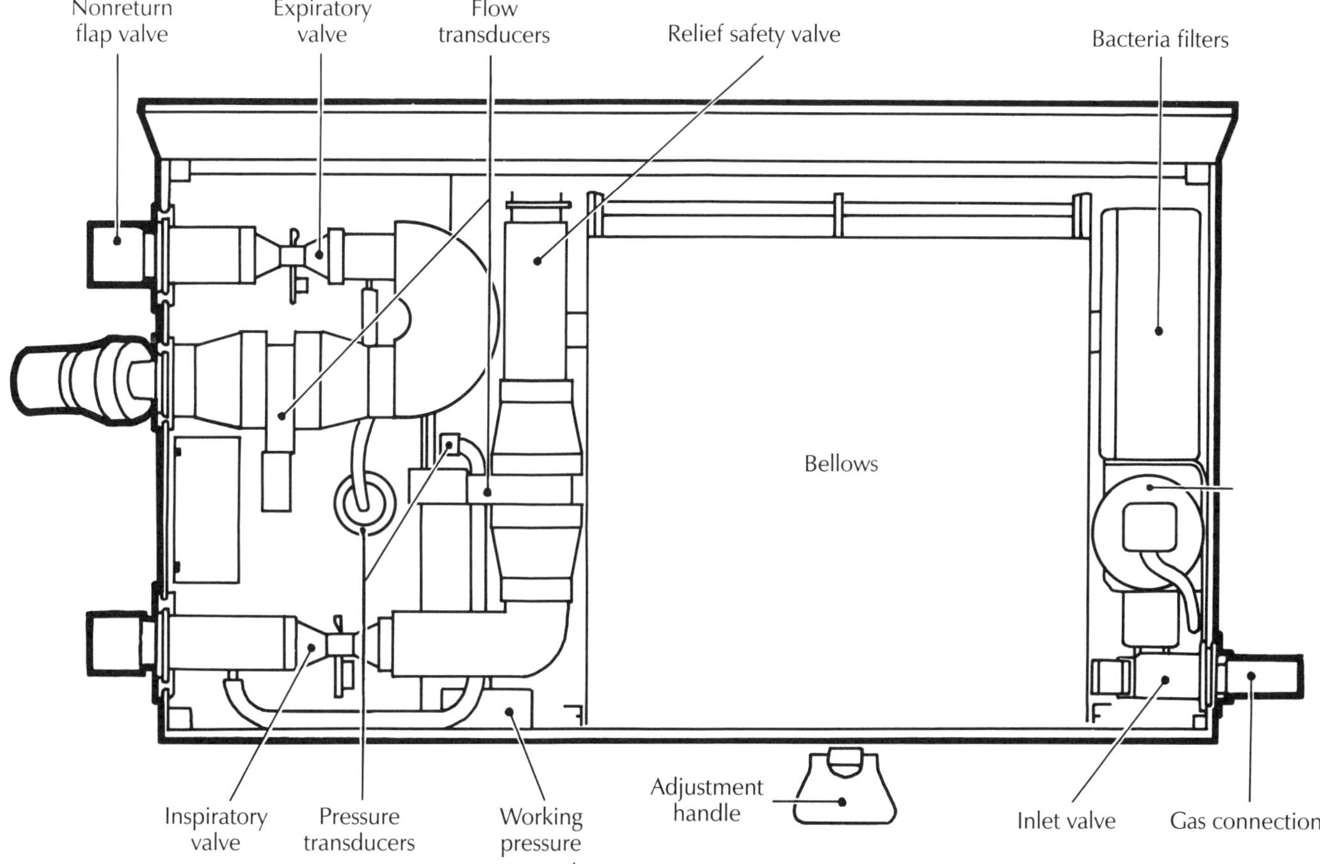

FIG 7–16
Schematic of the Siemens 300c system. Note the presence of the oxygen cell on the dry inspiratory side of the system. Note also the two flow and two pressure transducers monitoring both the inspiratory and expiratory sides of the patient's circuit. (Courtesy of Siemens-Elema Ventilatory Systems, Schaumberg, Ill.)

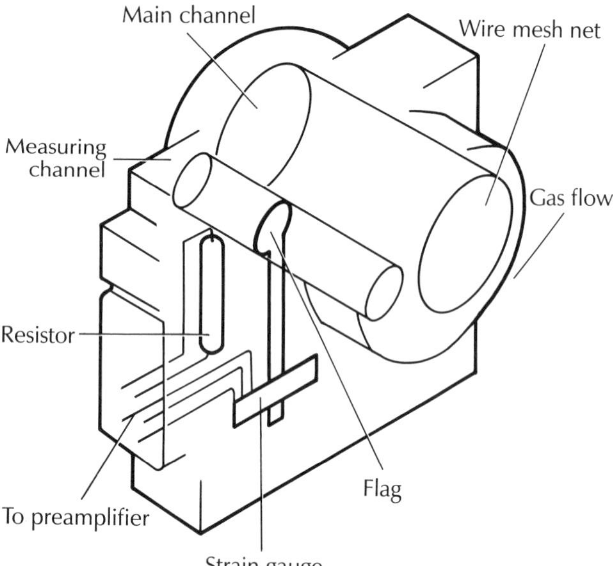

FIG 7–17
The flow transducer used in the Siemens ventilators is shown. The gas flows through the flow transducers in two parallel channels: a large main channel and a small measuring channel. The main channel has a wire mesh net that causes a certain proportion of the gas to flow through a parallel measuring channel. The flow-through and the differential pressure across the measuring channel act on a small metal disk ("flag") that presses on a small semiconductor strain gauge via a metal pin. (Courtesy of Siemens-Elema Ventilatory Systems, Schaumberg, Ill.)

Table 7–1, a free-standing monitor such as those described above (Bicure CP100 and medgraphics CCM/RPM) may be used.

As mechanical ventilators become more automated with a wide variety of modes of ventilation, manual bedside monitoring becomes more difficult. Current ventilator support involves intermittent, spontaneous breaths or ventilator modes that may shift from constant-volume ventilation to partial-pressure support ventilation with variable VT. The ability of volume ventilators to do partial pressure support depends on the use of respiratory mechanics to be able to guide the pressure support required. The ability to perform these new ventilator modes depends on the adequacy of the respiratory mechanics model used. The adequacy of computer algorithms within ventilators to monitor respiratory mechanics should not be blithely assumed; manual measurements to verify the ventilator monitors are always necessary. An independent system measuring P_{aw} or even P_{es} proximal to the patient may add useful information. These issues are discussed further below and in other chapters specific to mechanical ventilation.

Regardless of the mode of ventilation, it should be reemphasized that measurements of R_{aw} and C_{rs} provide a means for differentiating between potential sources of

TABLE 7–1
Indications for Measurement of Compliance and Resistance in Mechanically Ventilated Patients

High airway pressures (P_{st} > 40 cm H_2O, Pmax > 50 cm H_2O
High PEEP (>10 cm H_2O)
Rapidly changing pressures or volumes
Severe hypoxemia (Pa_{O_2} < 60 mm Hg with F_{IO_2} > 0.50)
Unstable hemodynamics
Progressive or prolonged disease

pressure requirements of a mechanically ventilated patient. A rise in R_{aw} indicates airway problems such as bronchospasm or secretions, whereas a rise in C_{rs} points toward lung parenchymal problems such as atelectasis, consolidation, or pulmonary edema. Stated another way, if the peak airway pressure rises without a rise in the static pressure while flow and VT are constant, this indicates a rise in the pressure requirements under flow conditions and, therefore, an increase in the resistance properties of the system. Conversely, if the rise in the static or plateau pressure is equal to or greater than the rise in peak airway pressures, then one needs to look for problems in the compliance of the lung or the chest wall. A third way of conceptualizing this is shown in Figure 7–18.[35] The concept of dynamic compliance C_{dyn} based on peak airway pressure as opposed to C_{st} based on static pressure measurements will help to differentiate the source of the rise in the pressure requirements.

A major caveat in all of these measurements is the potential for error introduced by a patient who is not

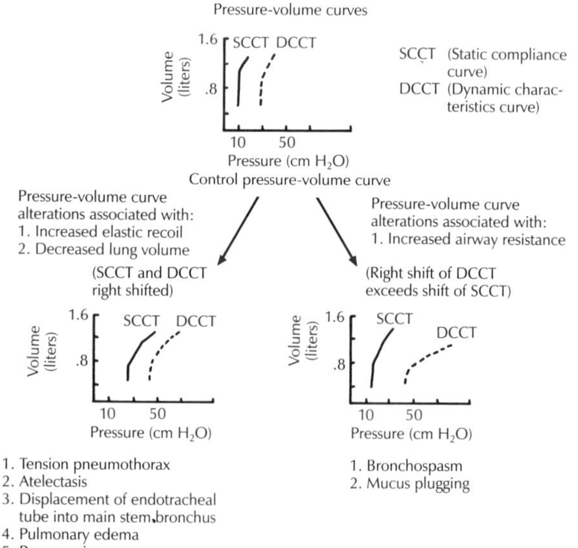

FIG 7–18
Pressure-volume curves using peak airway pressure *(dotted line)* or static or plateau pressure *(solid line)*. See the text for further explanation. (From Bone R: *Crit Care Med* 1976; 4:148. Used by permission.)

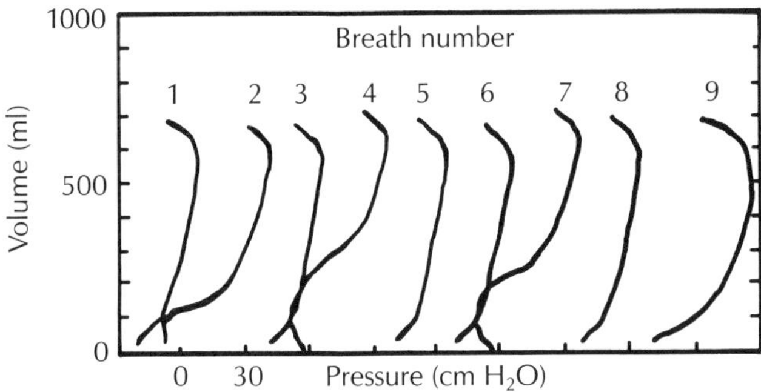

FIG 7–19
Volume-vs.-pressure curves for each of nine breaths during a 30-second monitoring period are shown. During breaths 1, 3, 5, 6, and 8 the patient was relaxed and allowed the ventilator to inflate the lung without interference from active movements by the patient. The patient is on 10 cm H_2O PEEP, pressures reach a maximum of approximately 30 cm H_2O at a volume of 600 mL, and the pressures decline to approximately 20 cm H_2O during the inflationary hold. During breaths 2, 4, and 7 the patient had a strong inspiratory effort that produced negative airway pressures. The patient subsequently relaxed and allowed airway pressures to reach the usual maximum level of approximately 30 cm H_2O. Breath 9 was taken with partially occlusion of the airway tubing to produce a high airway resistance. The peak airway pressure in this case rose to almost 60 cm H_2O and then fell all the way back to 20 cm H_2O during the inflationary hold. Such marked bowing of the volume-pressure curve is characteristic of increased airway pressure. (From Fallat RJ: *Clin Chest Med* 1982; 3:181. Used by permission.)

relaxed and whose muscular contractions of the chest wall and diaphragm introduce artifacts in the measurement of C_{rs} and R_{aw} because the model does not account for patient effort. Figure 7–19[33] shows how prolonged patient respiratory effort can spuriously alter the C_{rs} measurements. Esophageal or pleural pressure measurements are needed to detect and correct for these effects. Leaks in the system will obviously introduce error. Leaks are detected in ventilator monitors by the difference between upstream and downstream VT. The errors introduced by patient effort and leaks may also be detected by the inability to obtain reproducible values. Automated systems have the advantage of maintaining internal quality control by detecting increased or unacceptable variability in the measurement. The inability to get reproducible estimates of C_{rs} or R_{aw} usually indicates errors in the measurement.

When VT is measured in the ventilator or downstream in the exhalation line, another error in C_{rs} is introduced that is due to the compliance of the ventilator tubing. Volume expansion of the ventilator tubing during inflation is added to the VT even though it has never entered the patient's lung. This leads to an error in the estimate of C_{rs} and adds to ventilatory dead space. A rough approximation of the expansion volume is to assume a 3–mL/cm H_2O airway pressure, but this will vary depending on the tubing and the ventilator used. In patients with very stiff lungs, such as occurs in acute respiratory distress syndrome (ARDS) where Pmax may be 80 cm H_2O, there will be an error of $80 \times 3 = 240$ mL, or almost 50% if the VT is only 500 mL. Bedside systems with bidirectional pneumotachographs placed at the patient's tracheostomy or endotracheal tube can measure the VT going directly into the patient and will detect leaks around the endotracheal tube or out chest tubes by the reduction in VT out of the patient.

There are other problems in the monitor systems within ventilators. Since the pressure sensors are within the ventilators and not at the airway, errors occur due to pressure loss in downstream tubing. The Siemens 900C, which uses an airflow interrupter technique, was found to have a −18% and 26% error of resistance and compliance, respectively; still the authors concluded that the errors were sufficiently low to allow useful clinical monitoring.[36]

Yet another important physiologic factor that is not readily measured even by automated systems is the detection of overinflation or increasing FRC. Measurements of lung overinflation at the bedside are difficult, but one aspect of such barotrauma is that of dynamic pulmonary hyperinflation or intrinsic PEEP (PEEPi) which is the spontaneous development of increased alveolar pressure at end expiration resulting from insufficient time to allow for exhalation. This has been shown to be quite common in mechanically ventilated patients with COPD[37]; it is also not uncommon in other mechanically ventilated patients inasmuch as 24 of 62 patients had increased $PEEP_i$ and only 5 of those had COPD.[38] Recently the same phenomenon has been shown in spontaneously breathing patients with COPD.[39]

$PEEP_i$ is best measured by monitoring P_{es} but can also be suspected when flow fails to fall to zero when the next breath is initiated. It can be measured without P_{es} by occluding the expiratory port at end expiration and allowing the pressure in the system to rise as the exhalation continues. However, errors of 2 to 9 cm H_2O underestimation of $PEEP_i$ occur in the Siemens Servo 300 because of inclusion of the expansion volume from ventilator tubing in the equilibration volume.[40] $PEEP_i$ can be measured accurately only if the patient is relatively sedated or paralyzed and does not initiate inspiration when the ventilator breath is delayed.

GAS EXCHANGE

The monitoring of gas-phase O_2 and CO_2 is critical in respiratory care and has the advantage of being the least invasive but also the most removed from the adequacy of organ perfusion. Measuring inspired O_2 is frequently critical in patient management. Fortunately, a variety of monitors are available and will be discussed first. Analysis of arterial blood for O_2, CO_2, and pH, commonly referred to as ABG analysis, has been the touchstone and mainstay of pulmonary and critical care monitoring. The standard electrodes measuring oxygen, CO_2, and pH, as well as point-of-service instruments using the same technology, are discussed in Chapter 8. In this chapter the focus is on noninvasive methods for monitoring arterial O_2 and CO_2 with an emphasis on oximetry since that has become so widely used and accepted. Transcutaneous methods are also available and particularly in use in the neonatal and infant populations; transcutaneous CO_2 and capnography monitoring airway CO_2 are applicable to adults. Newer intravascular catheters that can measure ABGs and even electrolytes continuously are now available and will also be discussed in this chapter.

Gas Monitors

Monitoring airway gas is the least invasive technique but furthest removed from tissue respiration. In anesthesia, there is a need to monitor multiple anesthetic gases; sophisticated and costly mass spectrometry, gas chromatographs, and more recently, Raman spectroscopy give that capability.[41] For most pulmonary–critical care situations, it is O_2 that is necessary and essential to monitor. Monitoring CO_2 via capnography is discussed in the context of noninvasive ABG monitoring since end-tidal CO_2 is a way to monitor $Paco_2$. This section will focus on monitoring airway O_2.

There are a variety of O_2 monitors currently in use. Paramagnetic monitors are based on the magnetic affinity of O_2. In the earlier designs, O_2 would cause rotation in metal dumbbells suspended between magnets. These instruments were bulky and had a slow response time; they have been replaced by differential-pressure paramagnetic sensors that have a rapid response time of 200 ms and are also used in the DeltaTrac metabolic cart.

Other O_2 analyzers are based on thermal conductivity. When a wire is cooled, electrical resistance is reduced and current increases. The ability of a gas to cool a heated wire is proportional to its mass and thermal conductivity properties; O_2 has a higher mass and affects thermal conductivity more than N_2. The differential current between a reference wire exposed to air and another exposed to an unknown O_2 sample will be proportional to the percentage of O_2. Water vapor and CO_2 introduce similar or even greater effects and therefore must be absorbed out before entering the sample chamber. Because of the confounding effects of other gases and

A

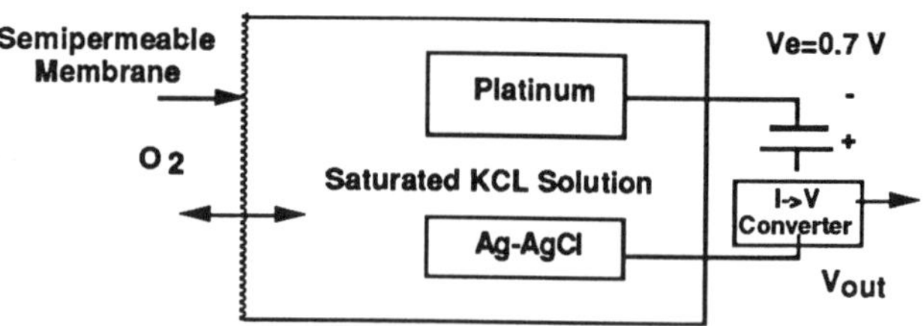

B

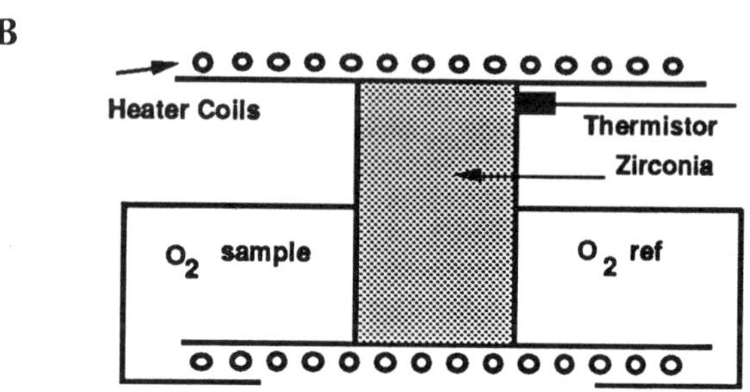

C

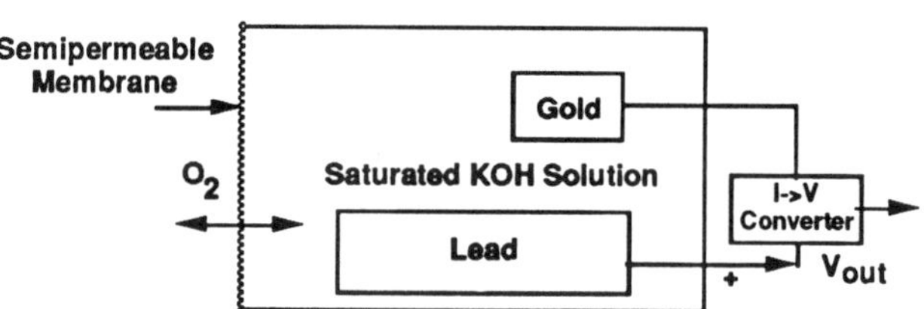

FIG 7–20
Oxygen sensors that depend on chemical reactions. **A,** Clark-type polarographic oxygen electrode. **B,** solid electrolyte oxygen electrode. **C,** fuel-cell oxygen electrode. (From East TD: *Respir Care* 1990; 35:500. Used by permission.)

vapors, these instruments have gone out of use in favor of electrochemical instruments more specific to O_2, i.e., polarographic electrodes and fuel cells.

The polarographic principle is that used in the Clark electrode for measuring arterial po_2, as described in the ABG section of Chapter 8 and shown schematically in Figure 7–20, A.[41] High-temperature zirconia crystal fuel cells have a rapid response and are used for monitoring in exercise and metabolic monitoring instruments (Fig 7–20, B). The most common O_2 monitor is the low-temperature fuel cell, or galvanic cell (Fig 7–20,C), which is used now in most ventilators to monitor O_2 delivery and is available in small, inexpensive portable devices for bedside, office, or clinic use.

Principle of Fuel Cells

The fuel cell is essentially a battery with a lead anode and gold cathode electrodes immersed in a saturated KOH solution (Fig 7–20,C). As O_2 diffuses through the semipermeable membrane, two reactions occur:

Cathode: $O_2 + 2\ H_2O + 4e^- \rightarrow$
$2\ H_2O_2 + 4e^- \rightarrow 4\ OH^-$

Anode: $2\ Pb + 6\ OH^- \rightarrow 2\ PbO_2H^- + 2\ H_2O + 4e^-$

The oxidation of lead (Pb) at the anode generates the electrons (e^-) necessary for O_2 reduction at the cathode. Like any battery, these devices have a limited life because of the consumption of Pb and OH^-. This may take as long as 15 months with low O_2, i.e., room air exposure, but as little as 3 months when exposed to 100% O_2.

These sensors are proportional to the partial pressure of O_2 since that determines diffusion through the membrane. When used under pressure, e.g., in ventilator circuits, there can be a falsely high reading, e.g., at 100 cm H_2O, which is 0.11 atm, there will be an 11% overreading of the O_2 concentration.

Humidity will reduce O_2 measurement by dilution, e.g., in an 80% O_2 mixture that is humidified to room temperature, the percentage of O_2 will be reduced to 77.5. More important, H_2O condensation on the sensor will change the diffusion characteristics of the membrane and give falsely low readings. These instruments are best used and placed on the dry side of breathing circuits, as shown in Fig 7-16.

Temperature will also affect the calibration. Most instruments have temperature sensors that will adjust the calibration over operational temperature ranges from 0 to 40°C.

Clinical Applications and Limitations

Because of the marginal accuracy and slow response time, galvanic fuel cells should be used only as gross monitors of airway O_2. When the above error factors are considered, the measurement can be made to within 2.0%. The proper clinical assessment of $Pa{O_2}$ can only be done if it is related to the $F{IO_2}$. This is frequently done by using the alveolar-arterial O_2 gradient ($P{AO_2} - Pa{O_2}$), which requires the following calculation of $P{AO_2}$:

$$P{AO_2} = (P_B - P_{H_2O}) \times F{IO_2} - Pa{CO_2}/R.$$

Frequently R, the respiratory exchange ratio or $\dot{V}CO_2/\dot{V}O_2$, and pCO_2 are not known. In addition, the normal values for this gradient increase from 10 to 20 mm Hg on room air to 50 mm Hg or more on 100% O_2 and may vary unpredictably with $F{IO_2}$. The $Pa{O_2}/P{AO_2}$ ratio may be preferable since it is more stable with $F{IO_2}$ and normal values are close to unity.[42, 43] The ratio of the two direct measurements $Pa{O_2}/F{IO_2}$ may be the simplest and best way to relate the adequacy of $Pa{O_2}$ at a given $F{IO_2}$.[44, 45]

These electrodes are essential to monitor the adequacy of O_2 from mechanical ventilators. As mentioned, for operative purposes it is best to have the monitor in a dry, unheated port of the circuit as it is on the Siemens ventilator (see Fig 7–16). However, leaks into the system or into the patient circuit downstream would not be detected. Sensors located at the airway or downstream in the exhalation circuit should be used when hypoxemia is critically low or unexplained.

Metabolic Carts

Normal metabolism is dependent on the cellular availability of adequate high-energy compounds such as adenosine triphosphate (ATP) and creatinine phosphate (CP). The replenishment of ATP is accomplished by the oxidation of carbohydrates, fat, and to a lesser extent, protein. When this expenditure is matched by appropriate caloric intake, the patient is said to be in energy balance. If caloric intake is insufficient (negative energy balance) or exceeds these needs (positive energy balance), the result is a shift in the utilization of nutritional substrates. This energy balance relationship is shown in Table 7–2.

The choice of one substrate over another has implications for the respiratory system since the different substrates require varying amounts of available oxygen to oxidize and the oxidation produces different amounts of CO_2 that must be excreted. Beyond limited buffering capacity, the CO_2 must be removed by ventilation. The relationship of carbon dioxide produced to oxygen consumed during oxidation is termed the respiratory quotient (RQ). The RQ of various oxidative and ventilatory patterns is shown in Table 7–3.

It should be stressed that the RQ resulting from substrate utilization is not the same as the respiratory exchange ratio (RER) measured during gas exchange. RQ reflects substrate utilization during steady-state conditions. The RER reflects dynamic gas exchange and reflects non–steady-state conditions such as hyperventilation as

TABLE 7–2
Energy Balance Relationship

Balanced:	Intake = Expenditure →	Energy requirements met by caloric intake
Catabolism:	Intake < Expenditure →	Endogenous fats and proteins consumed, nitrogen lost
Anabolism:	Intake > Expenditure →	Lipogenesis; increase in endogenous fats, carbon dioxide produced

TABLE 7–3
Respiratory Quotient of Substrate Oxidation

Substrate	RQ
Carbohydrate	1.00
Fat	0.71
Protein	0.82
Ethanol	0.67
Mixed substrate utilization	0.87
Starvation	0.65–0.70
Lipogenesis	1.0–1.2
Hyperventilation	1.0–1.5

well as substrate utilization. The RER has a narrow physiologic range of 0.65 to 1.5.

Negative energy balance causes depletion of energy stores, primarily glycogen stored in the liver. Endogenous sources of glucose are limited and cannot be redistributed. Muscle glycogen cannot be shifted to other organs and can only be used by the muscles. Once available glycogen stores are depleted, glucose must be produced from other endogenous sources. Decreased plasma insulin levels stimulate the catabolism of protein in skeletal muscle, result in nitrogen loss, and increase the utilization of free fatty acids from fat stores. Positive energy balance causes an increase in energy stores and lipogenesis, or the laying down of fat. Lipogenesis is associated with an RQ of 6 to 10, depending on the lipid produced.[46] Even after ventilatory buffering, respiratory changes induced by the large glucose loads of total parenteral nutrition (TPN) can produce measured RERs of 1.0 to 1.2.[47, 48] This increased RER results in increased ventilatory demands because of the increased carbon dioxide production.[49]

The components of resting energy expenditure (REE) include maintenance of cellular metabolism, dietary thermogenesis, and activity. REE typically accounts for approximately 70% of the total energy expenditure (TEE) for a healthy individual over a 24-hour period. In hospitalized patients, several factors can profoundly increase the energy expenditure. Stress such as major surgery, sepsis, and burns all increase energy expenditure unpredictably. Additionally, cancer and chronic illness are also accompanied by an increased metabolic rate. Increases in body temperature elevate energy demand as much as 100 kcal/°C. When combined with reduced caloric intake, these stress factors can quickly cause malnutrition. The effects of malnutrition can lead to significant impairment in ventilatory function, immune response, wound healing, tissue repair, and surfactant.

Optimal patient management requires that adequate nutrition be provided that matches the clinical goal of maintenance, repletion, or depletion of the patient's energy reserves. The effect of malnutrition on respiratory function can be observed directly. In critically ill patients, the hypermetabolism is accompanied by increases in oxygen uptake, carbon dioxide output, minute ventilation, and cardiac output. With a negative energy balance, these increased ventilatory demands are accompanied by numerous other effects that impair the respiratory system's ability to provide increased ventilation. Reductions in cell-mediated immunity increase the risk of respiratory infection, and decreased surfactant production results in decreased lung compliance and atelectasis. In addition, the response to hypoxia and hypercabia is blunted in malnourished patients.

During prolonged mechanical ventilation, the respiratory muscles atrophy and, like other somatic muscles, are cannibalized to meet nutritional requirements. Decreased circulating serum albumin leads to decreased plasma oncotic pressures. This decreases the ability of the pulmonary vasculature to reabsorb fluids. The increase in hydrostatic pressures may in turn contribute to the formation of pulmonary edema. In patients prone to increased capillary permeability or patients with CHF, edema formation is even more probable.

The combination of respiratory failure and inappropriate nutrition is even more complex. Positive energy balance conditions create increased ventilatory demands to remove the additional CO_2 generated by lipogenesis. The effect of predominantly feeding carbohydrate also increases the CO_2 output as compared with fat or protein utilization. In patients with impaired respiratory function, this additional demand can make successful weaning from mechanical ventilation more difficult. Conversely, this increased demand can contribute to respiratory failure in a compromised patient who is unable to match the increased ventilatory demand.

Predicting Resting Energy Expenditure

Assessing the adequacy of nutrition can be made by noting progressive weight change and measurement of skin fold thickness and through laboratory tests such as total protein, albumin, transferrin levels, and total lymphocytes. These measurements provide retrospective confirmation of energy balance assumptions and do not provide timely information for adjusting TPN. REE is commonly estimated on the basis of height, weight, age, and sex by using the Harris-Benedict equation. This value is further adjusted for stress factors such as disease or treatment-specific influences.[50, 51] However, this combination of estimates can be significantly in error.[52]

Several factors contribute to this error. Increased fluid retention will increase body weight and surface area but will not increase metabolism, therefore leading to an overestimation of REE. Sedation tends to reduce motion and muscle activity, which can also lead to overestimation. Muscle paralysis reduces oxygen uptake significantly since skeletal muscle contributes 30% to 40% of the total $\dot{V}O_2$, which will result in substantial overestimation of REE. In general, the predictive equations are less accurate in acutely ill patients. Most of the predictive formulas and stress factor adjustments are based on healthy subjects and mean responses to specific stress factors. The coefficient of variation for these adjustments is high. Weissman et al.[53] calculated a mean difference of 3.8% between measured and predicted REE in 45 mechanically ventilated postoperative patients. However, the range of measured to predicted REE for individual patients was as low as 70% and as high as 140%. Hunker et al.[54] observed that eight of ten heavily sedated or paralyzed patients had measured REE below that predicted.

Measurement of Indirect Calorimetry

Measurement of gas exchange, specifically $\dot{V}O_2$, provides a noninvasive method for assessing actual metabolic requirements. In conjunction with $\dot{V}CO_2$ and calculation of the RER, it is possible to assess the substrate utilization pattern. This method can be performed on spontaneously breathing patients as well as those receiving ventilatory support. Measurements of gas exchange in the critical care area are an offshoot of the systems used for exercise testing. In fact, many of the available systems perform both functions. A more complete explanation of gas exchange measurements is provided in Chapter 8. Only adaptations specific to indirect calorimetry will be discussed in this chapter.

Gas Exchange Measurement During Mechanical Ventilation

Reliable gas exchange measurement using the classic open-circuit method during mechanical ventilation requires a leak-free system and direct connections to the patient. To accurately measure ventilation, all exhaled volume must pass through the sensor. Ventilator circuits have many potential sources of leaks, both volume leaks from the circuit and gas leaks into the system. A loss of gas from the endotracheal tube, either through an uncuffed tube or an inadequate seal, can render the results unreliable.

Effect of Inspired Oxygen Changes

One aspect of most systems that must be understood when making indirect calorimetry assessments on ventilators is the Haldane transformation. The Haldane transformation assumes that there is no net shift in nitrogen and that the only gases exchanged are oxygen and carbon dioxide. Therefore, the fractional concentrations for nitrogen can be calculated as

$$F_{EN_2} = 1 - F_{EO_2} - F_{ECO_2}$$

and

$$F_{IN_2} = 1 - F_{IO_2} - F_{ICO_2};$$

therefore

$$\dot{V}_I = (F_{EN_2}/F_{IN_2})\dot{V}_E.$$

Including this correction in the general equation for $\dot{V}O_2$ results in

$$\dot{V}O_2 = \dot{V}_E\left(\frac{(1 - F_{EO_2} - F_{ECO_2})}{(1 - F_{IO_2} - F_{ICO_2})}(F_{IO_2} - F_{EO_2})\right)$$

and

$$\dot{V}CO_2 = \dot{V}_E\,(F_{ECO_2} - F_{ICO_2}).$$

Difficulties develop with this correction as the inspired oxygen concentration approaches 100% since the numerator and denominator in the transformation approach zero. Small errors in F_{ECO_2}, F_{EO_2}, and F_{IO_2} cause large errors in calculated $\dot{V}O_2$. An analysis error of 0.1% oxygen on both inspired and expired concentrations can lead to over 100% errors at 80% oxygen depending on the direction of the measurement error. Since some measurement error is unavoidable in the gas analysis and the calculation error grows hyperbolically, the results rapidly become clinically meaningless at F_{IO_2} values greater than 0.65.

An additional difficulty with elevated levels of inspired oxygen is the assumption that there is no net change in nitrogen concentration. With large changes in inspired oxygen there is an acute shift in nitrogen concentration in the FRC of the patient until the gas concentrations equilibrate. This will result in a washout of nitrogen from the lungs, and until equilibration is reached, the expired nitrogen levels will be higher than the inspired concentration. This will obviously introduce significant errors into the calculation of $\dot{V}O_2$. The duration of this washout is unpredictable since it is dependent on the dynamic distribution of ventilation but will be several minutes.

This problem is not limited to deliberate changes in ventilator F_{IO_2} settings. Most mechanical ventilators use a blender to combine room air and 100% oxygen to provide higher levels of inspired oxygen. The efficiency of this blender varies dramatically from machine to machine and even breath to breath.[55] Small changes (less than 2%) in inspired oxygen levels may not create clinical problems for the patient but will totally invalidate the measurement of gas exchange when an assumed inspired oxygen concentration is used.

This problem is compounded when the patient assists or fights the ventilator and when aerosolized bronchodilators are delivered with the ventilator. These fluctuations with each breath are smaller versions of the washout described earlier. All metabolic systems are sensitive to these errors to some degree. Systems that reference a single F_{IO_2} value are most susceptible. Breath-by-breath systems measure F_{IO_2} as well as F_{EO_2} and are therefore not as affected but will still report spurious readings until the FRC nitrogen concentrations stabilize.

One solution is to use a ventilator with good inspired oxygen characteristics. However, it may not always be possible to predict which patients will require metabolic assessment and changing the ventilator after initiation of mechanical ventilation is not desirable. Another approach is to power the ventilator's oxygen supply from a controlled, known source.

Airway Pressure Effects

Another problem common to mechanically ventilated patients is the effect of varying airway pressure on the gas analyzers. Many gas analyzers are sensitive to pressure changes since they measure concentration as partial pressure. Zirconia cells, for example, are exquisitely sensitive to pressure changes, with increased pressure resulting in an apparent increase in oxygen concentration. Varying techniques are used to overcome this problem. Most commonly, this involves using pressure transducers to correct for pressure-induced changes, maintaining the analyzers at a different pressure to minimize the effect, or isolating the gas analyzer from the airway pressure.

Gas Analyzers

For use in metabolic applications, a sealed reference chamber is desirable to minimize the effect of background gases on the analysis. Other gases have absorption characteristics similar to CO. Nitrous oxide (N_2O) and carbon dioxide (CO_2) have overlapping wavelengths. High levels of ambient oxygen can also affect the reading. If these gases are present in the room atmosphere and therefore the reference chamber, an erroneous determination will result. A sealed reference permits use of the analyzer in a wider range of clinical settings.

Canopy (Flow-Through Systems)

Canopy systems offer the advantage of no direct contact with the patient (Fig 7–21). Rather than a mouthpiece or face mask, the canopy envelops the patient's head. Thus, measurements can be made for an extended period of time, and alterations in REE related to patient response to the mouthpiece are reduced.

The classic canopy system was described by Kinney et al.[56] This system consisted of a cubic transparent box approximately 40 L in volume that worked as a mixing chamber. A fan or blower was used to flush the chamber with 40 L/min. The CO_2 inside the canopy was equal to the CO_2 production times the flow. Modern canopy designs are designed to reduce the volume of the canopy so as to minimize F_{ICO_2} levels. Exhaled gas is diluted and carried out by this bias *flow*. With appropriate gas sampling, the technique can be used on both spontaneously breathing and mechanically ventilated patients.

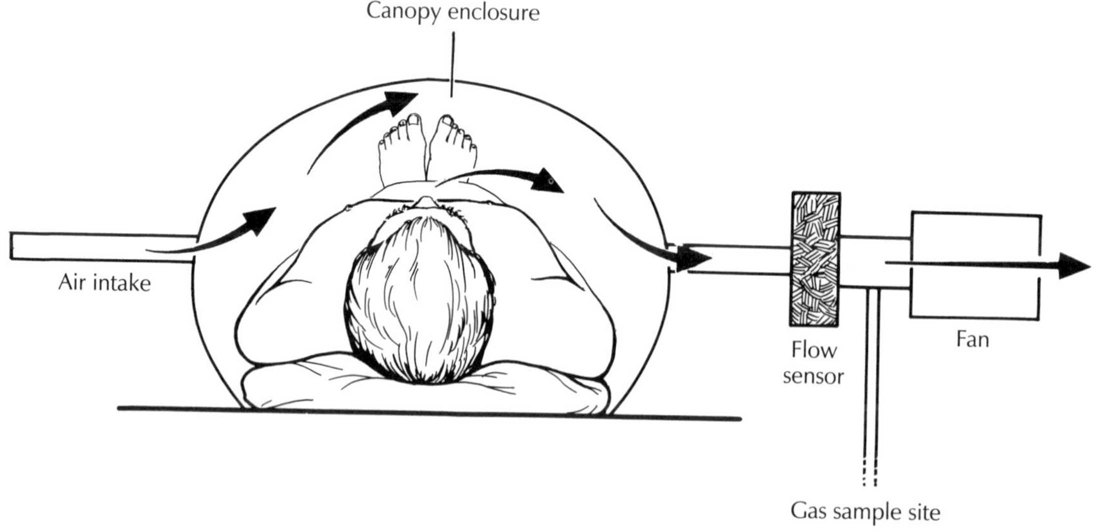

FIG 7–21
A fan pulls air through the canopy enclosure across the patient's face. All non–room air oxygen and carbon dioxide come from the patient. The concentrations measured at the sample site downstream are diluted by the fan bias flow, but the volume of CO_2 and O_2 in the mixed gas represents the patient's ventilation.

Since the desired measurements are the *volumes* of oxygen uptake and carbon dioxide output, measurement of the patient's exhaled volume is not necessary as long as the output from the canopy includes all of the exhaled gas. The concentration of these gases reflects their relative contribution to the total volume.

For example, in a classic Douglas bag collection, exhaled volume is measured as 5 L during a 1-minute collection. The resulting averaged CO_2 concentration in the bag is 5%. Therefore, the $\dot{V}CO_2$ will be 250 mL/min (5 × 0.05). In a canopy collection, the blower flow is fixed at a predetermined rate that substantially exceeds the patient's minute ventilation. This rate is set high enough to ensure adequate flushing of the circuit and capture of all CO_2 but not so high as to dilute the sample beyond the measurement range. If the rate was set to 50 L/min, the patient's 5 L/min would be entrained with this flow, and the CO_2 would be diluted by an extra 45 L of air containing no CO_2. The resulting CO_2 concentration would be 0.5%. At the output, the system would calculate the $\dot{V}CO_2$ as 250 mL/min (50 L × 0.005).

As long as the gas concentrations entering the canopy are known and the gas concentrations leaving the canopy can be measured, $\dot{V}O_2$ and $\dot{V}CO_2$ can be calculated. The only limitations are the precision with which the gas concentrations can be measured and the accuracy of assumptions regarding the gas concentrations made available for the patient. Obviously, gas analyzer performance is critical since the gas concentration changes are far smaller.

Examples of Metabolic Carts

MedGraphics CCM. Medical Graphics Critical Care Monitor (CCM) is a cart-based system that uses a disposable flow sensor, zirconia cell oxygen analyzer, and infrared carbon dioxide analyzer. The CCM can use either a canopy mode or expired gas collection. The system provides breath-by-breath measurements in both modes with selectable averaging techniques. This system is identical to the CPX exercise system described in Chapter 8 except for the canopy adaptation.

For the canopy mode, a centrifugal fan is added to the flow module, and a disposable plastic collector is mounted within an acrylic, transparent canopy. The canopy is a spherical hinged bubble that opens for access to the patient. Unlike competitive systems, results are displayed breath by breath but may be averaged over any time interval desired. This permits easy access to the patient without invalidating results or requiring restarting the collection. The data interruption is only for two breaths after reestablishing the collector.

Functionally, the canopy is placed around the patient's head and the collector adjusted to match the patient's nose and mouth contours. The bias flow fan is individually adjusted to the patient by maximizing the CO_2 waveshape. Inadequate bias flow will result in blunted waveshapes and elevated F_ICO_2 since all CO_2 within the canopy will not be entrained. High bias flows will blunt the waveshape and reduce the $P_{ET}CO_2$. Essentially, the fan is adjusted until the waveshape is optimized.

For pediatric applications, the disposable collector can be used without the canopy. The operator simply holds the collector over the child's face and adjusts the bias flow. The primary function of the canopy is to hold the collector in position and prevent cross-drafts. It does not function as a mixing chamber.

Using CO_2 changes as the breath detector, the system calculates $\dot{V}O_2$, $\dot{V}CO_2$, and REE breath by breath. Additionally, end-tidal readings of oxygen and carbon dioxide are also provided. Interfacing with other devices such as oximeters, ECG monitors, and indwelling blood gas monitors can be made with updates triggered on each breath. Calculation of cardiac output can be made breath by breath by using the Fick equation if continuous arterial-venous differences are provided. The CCM system is shown in Figure 7–22.

SensorMedics Metabolic Measurement Cart 2900MMC. The SensorMedics Metabolic Measurement Cart (MMC) is the same system used for gas exchange measurement in the exercise application. Using a hot-wire anemometer for flow, a zirconia cell oxygen analyzer, and an infrared carbon dioxide analyzer, the MMC supports both mixing chamber, dilution (flow-through), and breath-by-breath applications, although in the nutritional assessment mode the system uses the mixing chamber. The 2900 uses a hot-wire anemometer for flow sensing, a zirconia cell for oxygen analysis, and infrared for carbon dioxide analysis. This system is described in more detail in Chapter 8. The 2900MMC is shown in Figure 7–23.

SensorMedics DeltaTrac metabolic monitor. The DeltaTrac system uses a modification of the flow-through canopy air-dilution method described by Kinney et al. The canopy shape is designed to reduce the F_ICO_2 levels within the canopy by more effective flushing. Gas analysis is made by using an infrared carbon dioxide analyzer and a paramagnetic oxygen analyzer. The principles of operation of the analyzers are described in Chapter 8.

Measurement of $\dot{V}O_2$ and $\dot{V}CO_2$ for spontaneously breathing patients is calculated from gas concentration differences measured between upstream and downstream flows at a constant flow. For measurements on mechanically ventilated patients, additional gas sampling

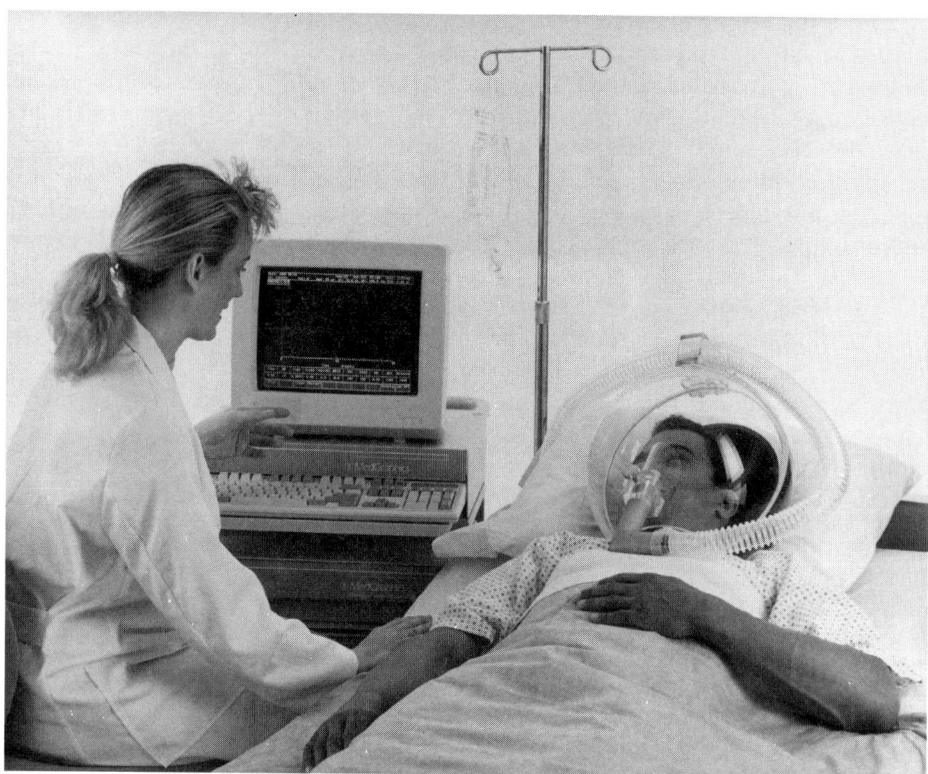

FIG 7–22
The MedGraphics CCM Metabolic Cart System. (Courtesy of Med-Graphics Corp, St Paul, Minn.)

ports are used to provide measurement of inspiratory and mixed expiratory oxygen and carbon dioxide in addition to the diluted CO_2-air mixture. During measurements on mechanically ventilated patients,the O_2 and CO_2 baselines are automatically checked periodically with room air.

Cybermedic Metascope metabolic monitor. The Cybermedic Metascope (Fig 7–24) is a stand-alone portable indirect calorimeter that uses the open circuit technique with a 3-L mixing chamber. Cybermedic uses a heated Fleisch-type pneumotachometer for flow, a direct paramagnetic analyzer for oxygen, and an infrared analyzer for carbon dioxide. The system is capable of performing studies on patients on ventilators on all modalities including but not limited to intermittent mandatory ventilation (IMV), continuous positive airway pressure (CPAP), flow-by, PEEP, and high frequency.

When measuring oxygen consumption by any open circuit system, a stable FIO_2 is mandatory. The Metascope allows monitoring of the FIO_2 before, during, and after the study. Before actual collection of data the Metascope will provide to the user the oxygen sensitivity resulting from fluctuation of the FIO_2. Oxygen sensitivity is the confidence of accuracy expressed as a percent.

A unique system feature is the graphic touch screen for patient data entry, system operation, and display of results. During patient setup the graphic display gives the technician a picture of the hookup technique that should be used with different ventilators.

The system can also perform measurements by mask, mouthpiece, or hood. The hood is a flow-through canopy using the air-dilution method. During testing, the flow of the hood is automatically controlled by the Metascope by monitoring the carbon dioxide percentage.

The data are stored after collection, and results for up to 60 patients can be retained. The technician enters into the system the calories and protein that the patient is receiving and, if available, the 24-hour urine urea nitrogen. The Metascope will provide the patient's caloric requirements and a substrate analysis of the amount of fat, carbohydrate, and protein expressed in grams, calories, and percentage that the patient is using. The data can be displayed, printed directly, or downloaded to an external computer.

Noninvasive Assessment of Arterial Blood Gases—Introduction and History

Analysis of arterial blood was introduced in the 1960s and was rapidly accepted and so widely used that it became a major medical care cost issue in the 1980s when it was estimated that over $1 billion a year was being spent on ABG measurements in the United States. Alternatives to this invasive, intermittent, and costly method were eagerly sought. Ear oximetry using one or two wavelengths of infrared spectrophotometry was developed in the 1930s but was cumbersome and unstable and needed frequent calibrations with arterial blood measurements.[57] An eight-wavelength oximeter combined with a complex computer fit of an eight exponential equation that was developed by Hewlett Packard in the late 1970s provided the first clinically practical ear oximeter. Although this device is still used in limited situations such as during exercise evaluations, its production was discontinued in the mid-1980s because it could not compete with the less costly and more manageable pulse oximeters.

Pulse oximeters use the fact that the pulse in tissues is produced by oxygenated arterial blood; by measuring the pulsatile absorption of infrared light, it is possible to obtain measurements of oxygen saturation with only two wavelengths of infrared light. The development of ultrabright, light-emitting diodes (LEDs) and the use of powerful compact microprocessors allowed the design of small, easily applied and rapidly responding instruments for continuously monitoring oxygen saturation (Spo_2). Although only introduced in the mid-1980s, they are currently widely used and have been referred to as the "fifth vital sign." The devices are not without pitfalls, however, as will be discussed.

About the same time that the Hewlett Packard oximeter was developed, there was a concurrent development of transcutaneous methods for measuring O_2 and CO_2 ($Ptco_2$, $Ptcco_2$). Each measurement is simply an adaptation of the ABG electrodes applied to the skin. The problems encountered in adults are multiple, and their successful clinical use has been largely limited to neonates and infants where the skin gradients are minimized. $Ptcco_2$, however, can be monitored successfully in adults by using either the Stowe-Severinghaus electrode or an infrared system discussed below. Transcutaneous devices are more cumbersome and time-consuming and therefore do not have the widespread use that pulse oximetry has achieved, but they still play a role, particularly in neonatal and infant populations and where estimates of Pao_2 rather than Spo_2 are

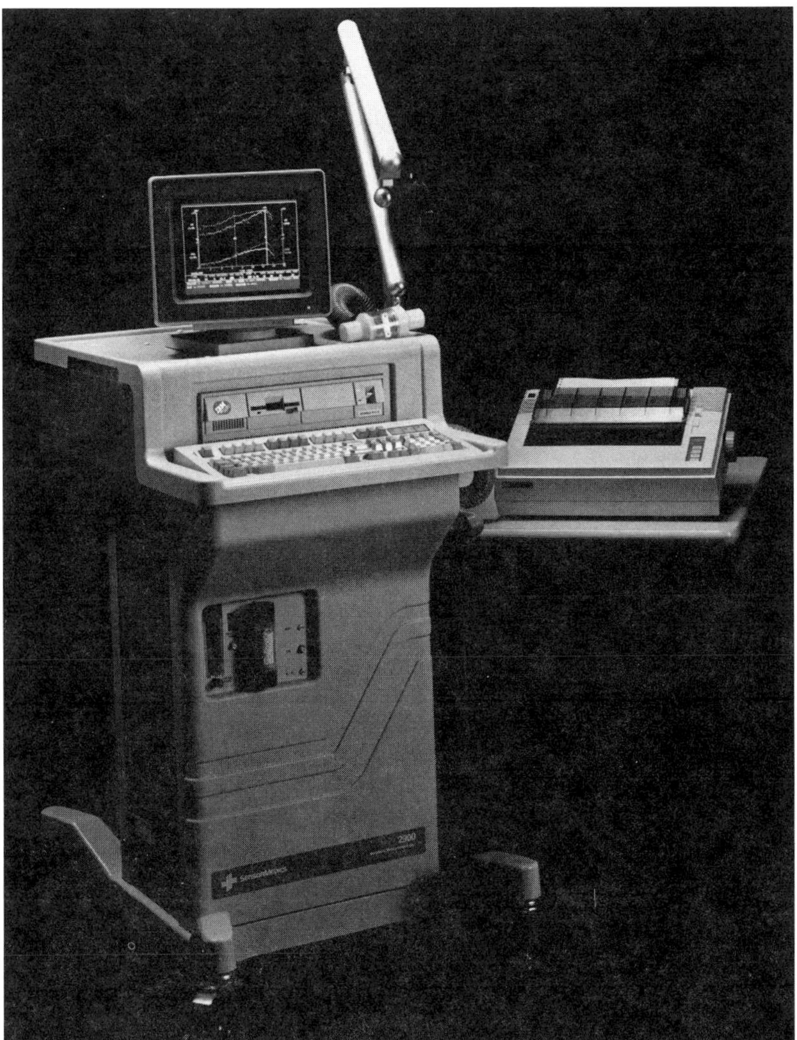

FIG 7–23
The SensorMedics 2900 Metabolic Cart System. (Courtesy of SensorMedics Corp, Yorba Linda, Calif.)

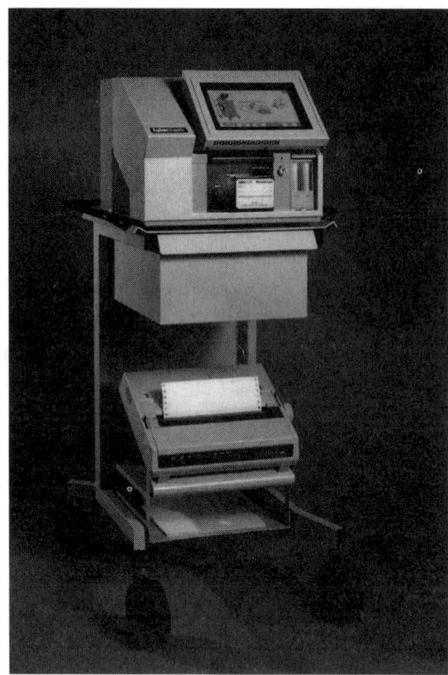

FIG 7–24
The Cybermedic Metascope Metabolic Monitor. (Courtesy of Cybermedics Corp, Boulder, Colo.)

frequently necessary to detect serious toxicity from high Pa_{O_2}.

Oximetry—Principles of Measurement

Infrared spectroscopy uses the Beer-Lambert law, which defines the relationship between the concentration of a substance and the absorption of infrared light passing through the substance:

$$I_{out} = I_{in}e^{-alc} \text{ or } I_{out}/I_{in} = e^{-alc} = A,$$

where **I** is the intensity of the light going in (I_{in}) and coming out (I_{out}), ***a*** is the absorption coefficient, ***l*** is the path length and ***c*** is the concentration of the substance that results in an absorption fraction **A**. The law assumes that all light passes through the solution without scatter and the solution is homogenous, neither of which is true of light transmitted through tissue or even pure blood since hemoglobin is concentrated within light-scattering red blood cells (RBCs).

If measurements of **A** are made at two different wavelengths through the same path ***l***, then

$$A1/A2 = e^{alc}/e^{alc}$$

Since ***l*** is constant and ***a*** is known, measurement of A***1*** and A***2*** at two appropriate wavelengths allows an estimation of the concentration of the unknown ***c***.

Infrared oximetry uses two infrared waves that emit narrow-band light at approximately 660 and 930 nm. The absorption coefficients for infrared light of different wavelengths by the various hemoglobins in the blood are shown in Figure 7–25.[58] The 660-nm wavelength is largely absorbed by deoxyhemoglobin (Hgb), whereas the 930-nm light has very little absorbency by Hgb. This difference allows an estimate of the fraction of Hgb as compared with the other hemoglobins (oxyhemoglobin [HbO_2], carboxyhemoglobin [HbCO], or methemoglobin [HbMet]) since there is little difference in their absorption at the two wavelengths. The HbO_2 saturation (Sa_{O_2}) reported is therefore roughly equivalent to the sum of HbO_2 plus HbCO and HbMet. When the latter two are in high concentration, there will be a significant difference between the SpO_2 and the Sa_{O_2} calculated from the Pa_{O_2} or arterial blood measured in a co-oximeter, which measures the concentration of each component of Hgb.

Since there are multiple substances in tissue that absorb these two infrared beams, it would be necessary to independently measure HbO_2 by arterial blood sampling in order to calibrate the oximeter for each specific person or set of measurements. This invasive and tedious procedure was necessary with the early oximeters, which made them unacceptable for routine use. Hewlett Packard overcame this problem by empirically choosing eight different wavelengths to account for most of the absorbing substances in the ear. By heating the ear to 39.5°C, blood is arterialized, and then by making 50 estimates per second of absorption fraction **A** for each of the eight wavelengths, a microcomputer is able to solve an eight-component differential equation to estimate the HbO_2 component.[59]

Pulse oximetry was made possible by a Japanese engineer who made the observation in 1974 that absorp-

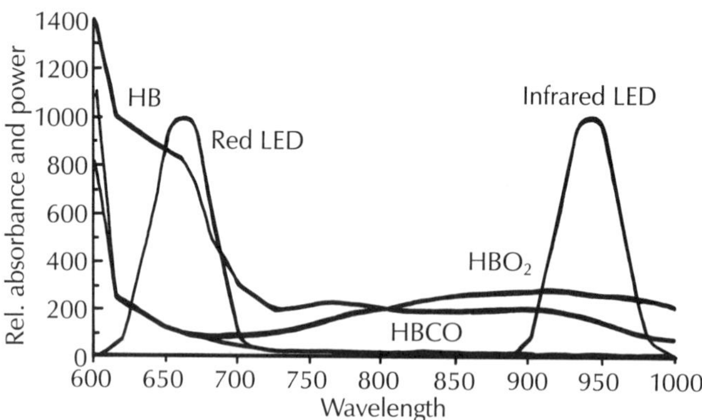

FIG 7–25
Infrared absorption curves and light-emitting diode *(LED)* power spectrum. The power spectrum of the ultrabright infrared LED (930 nm) and the high-power red LED (660 nm) in relationship to the absorbance spectrum of *Hb, HbO_2,* and *HbCO.* (From Clark JS, et al: *Am Rev Respir Dis* 1992; 145:220–232. Used by permission.)

tion of infrared light in a pulsatile organ consisted of a nonpulsating or constant absorption (A_c) due to tissue and venous and capillary blood and a much smaller, pulsating absorption component (A_p) due to arterial blood.[59] Measurement of arterial HbO_2 was theoretically possible by observing this pulsatile signal. Similar to the Hewlett Packard device, it was necessary to develop empirical calibration curves to account for the many assumptions necessary in such indirect observations that deviate from the ideal Beers-Lambert law of absorption of purely transmitted light, not light that is scattered and reflected and now pulsatile.

Modern pulse oximetry was made possible by the development of small, powerful narrow-beam LEDs that could be placed on the finger, ear, or bridge of the nose. Some are even placed on flat skin surfaces such as the forehead and use reflected infrared light instead of transmitted light. Each manufacturer has developed its own algorithms based on empirical observations to allow an estimation of $Sa{O_2}$. The disposable LEDs have unique calibration factors determined by the manufacturer and then used in the specific computer algorithm in order to optimize accuracy. With so many "unknowns" within the black box that are unique to each of the now multiple manufacturers of pulse oximeters, one can readily understand the need to be cautious in the interpretation and use of pulse oximetry $Sa{O_2}$ data. These inherent problems of the variability in manufacturing of LEDs and of the variability of the spectral characteristics of LEDs with temperature have been minimized with careful quality control, calibration by the manufacturer, and the use of temperature probes adjacent to the LED.

The most significant error with pulse oximetry, as with all noninvasive methods, occurs when blood flow diminishes and causes a decrease in the pulse as well as a decrease in $Sp{O_2}$ because of tissue metabolism. These instruments are inaccurate below 60% saturation and have dubious meaning as $Sp{O_2}$ approaches 70% since the empirically derived algorithms fail in these extremes of oxygenation.

The measurement is also dependent on corrections from pure transmitted signals vs. scattered reflected light. These characteristics may vary considerably when RBC geometry changes such as in sickle cell anemia or thalassemia. Fortunately, fetal hemoglobin does not differ from adult hemoglobin in its spectral and reflective characteristics, so pulse oximetry is effective in neonates. The use of dyes such as methylene blue can cause marked decreases in $Sa{O_2}$ as the dye absorbs infrared light.

Another major problem encountered with pulse oximetry is noise artifacts. If one squeezes the finger 60 to 90 times per minute, it is possible to induce a "venous pulsation" that can be spuriously seen as an arterial pulse. Such artifacts may occur as a result of repetitive motion such as a tremor or with exercise and indicate a spuriously low $Sa{O_2}$. One method to overcome this problem has been to lock the ECG signal to the infrared absorption pulse and not accept pulsations that do not coincide with the ECG beat.

The site of application is generally the finger or ear. Note that the time delay from the lung to the ear is 20 to 30 seconds and approximately 12 seconds more to the finger. These times may be even greater with low cardiac output. Hyperventilation or a change in $Fi{O_2}$ adds the additional delay of lung washout before the changes are detected. The use of different monitoring sites and maneuvers such as hyperventilation or changing $Fi{O_2}$ values that alter $Sp{O_2}$ is helpful to document the response characteristics and clinical accuracy of the device.

Transcutaneous Oxygen

These devices are modifications of the Clark electrode used for arterial blood oxygen measurements but are designed to be sealed on the skin and allow heating of the skin and subcutaneous tissues sufficient to "arterialize" the tissue. Gradients across the skin epidermis may be minimized in adults by abrasion or the use of cellophane tape as described for the CO_2 device, but this is not necessary in neonates and infants. A greater problem is the dependence of skin surface $p{O_2}$ on cutaneous blood flow and metabolism, the sensitivity of the $p{O_2}$ to the low solubility of the oxygen, and the resultant wide arteriovenous gradient of oxygen.[60]

These latter two characteristics make the $Ptc{O_2}$ measurement much less reliable than the $Ptcc{O_2}$ measurement. Even with increasing the skin temperature to 42 to 44°C, skin blood flow, particularly in an adult, will be variable and result in variable measurements of $Ptc{O_2}$ that do not coincide with the $Pa{O_2}$. The sensitivity to skin blood flow has been used as an indicator of perfusion rather than $Pa{O_2}$.[61] The setup time for $Ptc{O_2}$ is several minutes. First, the skin must be prepared for application of the device in a sealed manner, and then time is necessary for the skin and subcutaneous tissues to be heated to a higher temperature. The response time of the Clark electrode itself is prolonged to several minutes because of the time for diffusion of oxygen through the tissue. The rapidly changing $Pa{O_2}$ characteristics, therefore, cannot be measured as they can be with pulse oximetry or an indwelling catheter.

The need to heat the skin causes first- or second-degree burns, which necessitates changing the electrode site every 4 to 6 hours. Electrodes have been developed to fit in the conjunctiva of the eye, where heating is unnecessary, or inside the mouth on the buccal mucosa, where temperatures of 44°C are well tolerated indefinitely, but neither of these devices has been successfully marketed.

Transcutaneous CO_2 ($Ptcco_2$)

It was demonstrated two centuries ago that CO_2 passes through the skin,[58] but only in the last decade has CO_2 been successfully measured by using either the Stowe-Severinghaus electrode[62] or an infrared detector.[63] The Stowe-Severinghaus electrode is discussed under the ABG section of Chapter 8. Essentially, the same electrode is used, but adapted to have a sealed application to the skin surface, and as with $Ptco_2$, a collar for heating the skin surface is used. Currently, most units combine both electrodes (see Fig 7–26).[64]

In contrast, the infrared CO_2 electrode developed by Hewlett Packard consists of a 50-mL sealed chamber with a quartz window through which the infrared beam passes (Fig 7–27, A and B).[63] The CO_2 that has diffused through the skin into the chamber can then be measured. The 50-mL volume of the chamber is the smallest size capable of infrared technology. This chamber is large when compared with the chamber of the Stowe-Severinghaus electrode and results in a 30- to 45-minute start-up time to allow diffusion of the tissue CO_2 into the chamber. The diffusion is facilitated by prior preparation of the skin surface by repeated application of a strong adhesive tape to remove the stratum corneum. The same unit may be fitted on a chamber that fits in line with the airway to monitor airway CO_2 (Fig 7–27,C).

Unlike $Ptco_2$, $Ptcco_2$ can be successfully monitored in adults because of the 20-fold greater solubility of CO_2 vs. O_2. This reduces the influence of the cutaneous perfusion/metabolism ratio on the $Ptcco_2$. The increased CO_2 solubility also accounts for the narrow arterial-venous difference of only 6 to 10 mm Hg as compared with 40 to 60 mm Hg for O_2; this narrower band between arterial and venous blood in turn gives a narrower absolute error for $Ptcco_2$, but the percent error can be even larger than with $Ptco_2$.

Another advantage of transcutaneous CO_2 monitoring over O_2 monitoring is it can be successfully done without the high temperatures necessary for $Ptco_2$. The Stowe-Severinghaus electrode characteristically operates at 42°C, whereas the infrared Hewlett Packard unit operates at 39.5°C due in part to the skin preparation procedure. It is possible that the Stowe-Severinghaus electrode could also operate at a lower temperature given similar skin preparation, but that has not been reported. The time constant for blood in the Stowe-Severinghaus electrode has been reported to be between 7 and 26 seconds. The time constant for the transcutaneous Stowe-Severinghaus electrode for in vivo operation is 40 to 65 seconds. With the infrared instrument, there is virtually no time delay for the measurement of CO_2 in the chamber, but because of the large size of the chamber and

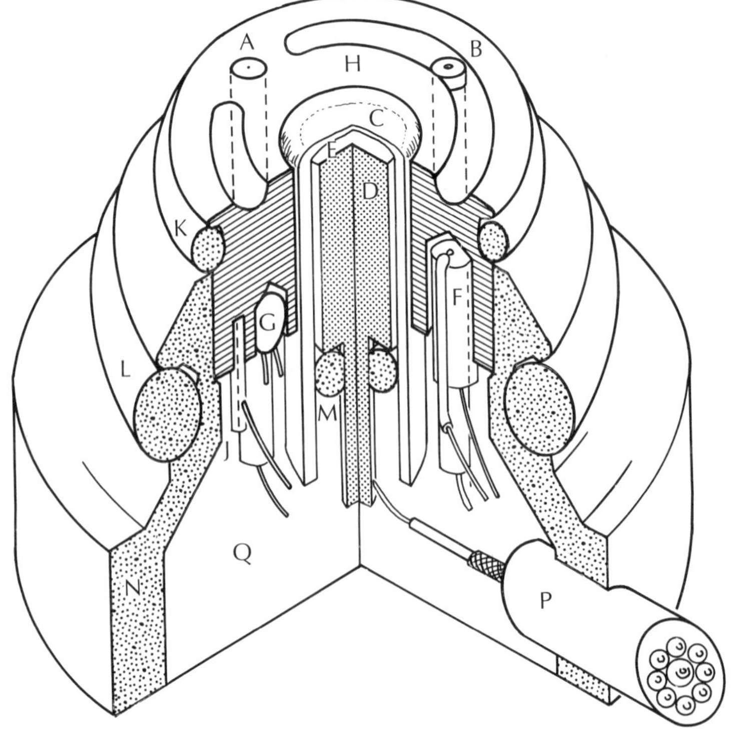

FIG 7–26
Construction of silver Po_2-Pco_2 electrode. Cathode *A* and anode *B* are platinum. The glass pH electrode *C* is nearly filled with its silver internal reference *D.* Electrolyte *E* is buffered to pH 6.5, and a Zener diode *F* heats the body *H* to a constant temperature as measured by the thermistor *G.* Electrical connection to the silver body is made through the brass pin *J. K, L,* and *M* are neoprene O-rings (no. 10, 100, and 001, respectively). The housing *N* of Lexan is filled with epoxy WQ after cable *P* connections are made. A semiannular groove increases electrolyte volume for long-term stability. (From Severinghaus JW: *J Appl Physiol* 1981; 51:1027–1032. Used by permission.)

A

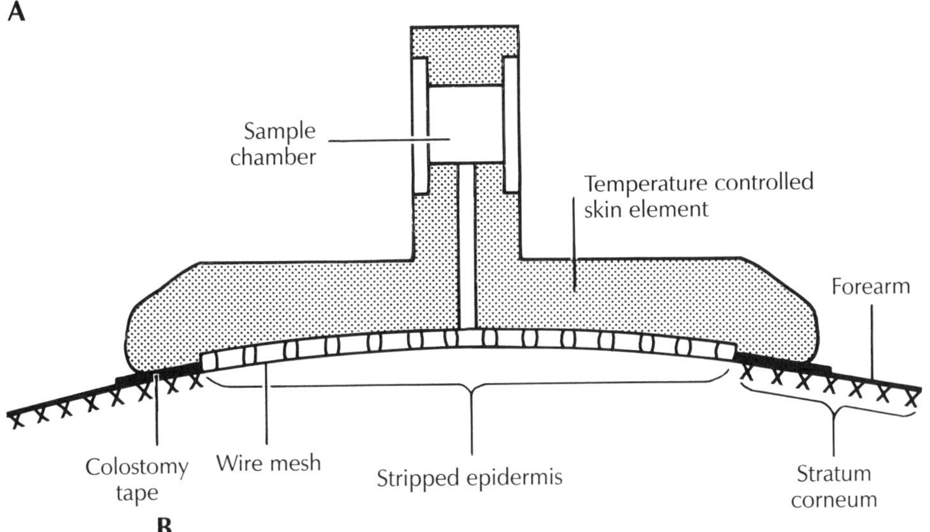

B

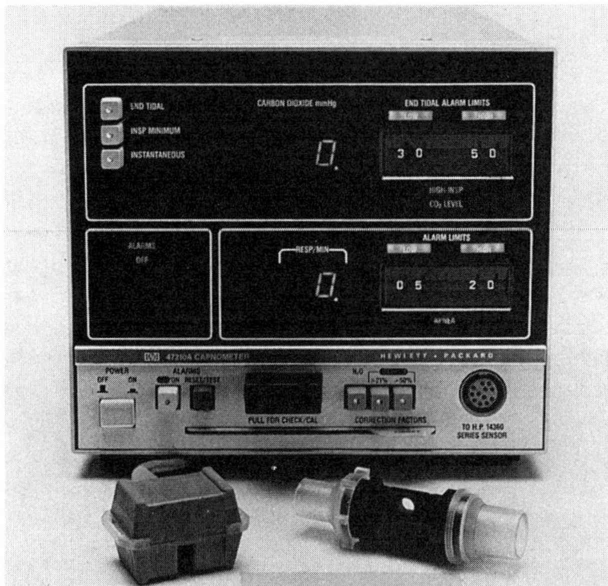

FIG 7–27
A, Skin element. The wire mesh that separates the stripped epidermal area from the base of the element serves as a collection manifold that allows CO_2 released from all of the stripped areas to reach the hole leading to the sample chamber. It is important to keep the overall volume of this manifold as small as possible because the time constant of the measurement depends upon the ratio of stripped surface to the volume of the sample chamber and manifold. (From Eletr S, Jinison H, Ream AK, et al: *Acta Anaesthesiol Scand Suppl* 1978; 68:123–127. Used by permission.) **B,** infrared CO_2 sensor with an airway chamber. (Courtesy of Hewlett-Packard, Andover, Mass.)

the time for diffusion into the chamber, an in vivo time constant of 2.2 to 3 minutes has been reported.[65] This longer time constant may also be in part due to the lower temperature used.

The higher temperature used with both instruments increases the pco_2 by 4.5% per degree centigrade. In addition, the Stowe-Severinghaus electrode increases its sensitivity 4% per degree centigrade. The net result is that the $Ptcco_2$ is 30% to 60% higher just from these temperature effects; many models incorporate a temperature correction factor based on analysis of a large population. When the cardiac output is normal, the $Ptcco_2$ is 23 ± 11 mm Hg higher than the $Paco_2$ with a regression coefficient of $r = .8$. When the cardiac index is low (<1.5 L/min, m^2), the $Ptcco_2$, like the $Ptco_2$, no longer accurately reflects arterial values.

Such large correction factors are not present in the infrared system since the temperature is only 39.5°C and the instrument is not temperature sensitive. Characteristically, the $(Ptc - Pa)co_2$ gradient is 6 to 20 mm Hg and must be determined by a $Paco_2$ measurement. The gradient is stable for up to 24 hours as long as the monitor is tightly adherent and tissue perfusion is stable.

Description of Transcutaneous Devices

The most common transcutaneous device now used in neonatal care is a combined CO_2 and O_2 monitor shown in Figure 7–26, B. Both O_2 and CO_2 diffuse through a single membrane into the electrolyte solution. The O_2 diffuses to the platinum cathode where it is reduced and generates four electrons and a current that is measured against the reference silver anode electrode—a standard Clarke electrode. The $Ptcco_2$ is a miniaturized Stowe-Severinghaus electrode. Heating elements and temperature devices are essential, as described above, for accurate calibration of the output signal. Safety alarms to detect temperatures over 46°C or excessive energy consumption to maintain temperature are employed to avoid skin burns. Alarms occur if the temperature deviates more than 0.3°C from the preset value.

Manufacturers' stated range for po_2 is 0 to 800 mm Hg with an accuracy of ±1.0 mm Hg, or 0.1%, whereas for po_2 there is a range of 5 to 200 mm Hg and an accuracy of ±1 mm Hg, or 1.0%. However, clinical trend monitoring is stated to be limited to 40 to 100 mm Hg for po_2 and 30 to 80 mm Hg for CO_2. The pco_2 is corrected to 37°C by using the following formula:

$$Ptcco_2\ (37°C) = Ptcco_2 \times 10^{-0.021\ (T - 37) - K},$$

where K is a metabolism correction factor for that particular patient application.

After application of the membrane, electrodes must be checked with a zero solution and the CO_2 electrode sloped with 5% and 10% CO_2 gas. Electrodes are also calibrated in 5% CO_2 and 20.9% O_2 before application to the skin or if a reading error is suspected. The 90% response time for $Ptco_2$ is approximately 20 seconds, and that for $Ptcco_2$ is approximately 50 seconds; both are said to have a drift in calibration of <1 mm Hg/hr. However, a number of "troubleshooting" causes for losing calibration and excess drift are listed and include improper application, interference from patient movement, nearby equipment, use of halothane anesthesia, and most commonly, poor perfusion or an unfavorable or changing skin blood flow/metabolism ratio, as discussed.

Monitoring Airway CO_2 (Capnography)

Airway CO_2 is a very accessible, noninvasive means to monitor ventilation. Arterial CO_2 ($Paco_2$) is in equilibrium with alveolar CO_2 (P_{ACO_2}) and is directly related to alveolar ventilation (V_A) and CO_2 production (Vco_2):

$$Vco_2 = V_A \times F_{ACO_2} = V_A \times P_{ACO_2}/P_B - 47$$
$$= V_A \times Paco_2/P_B - 47,$$

where P_B is barometric pressure and 47 is the water vapor pressure at 37°C. Since $V_E = V_A + V_D$ and if the Vco_2 and V_D are constant as they would be in a resting patient, then V_E is inversely proportional to P_{ACO_2} or $Paco_2$. Expired CO_2 curves are shown in Figure 7–28. In a normal subject, the CO_2 at the end of a tidal breath (P_{ETCO_2}) will approximate the P_{ACO_2} within 2 to 5 mm Hg.[66, 67] Changes in P_{ETCO_2} will vary inversely to changes in V_E unless Vco_2 or V_D changes.

Unfortunately, in disease there can be marked maldistributions of ventilation resulting in increased physiologic V_D. V_D may vary with V_T, patient position, and changes in pathophysiology. A change in V_D will change the $(P_{ET} - Pa)co_2$ gradient, and changes in P_{ETCO_2} may either be reflecting true changes in $Paco_2$ or a variation in the $(Pa - P_{ET})co_2$ gradient as discussed below.

Capnography instrumentation. Airway CO_2 is usually measured by near-infrared spectroscopy. Mass spectroscopy can also be used, but because of the expense, it is usually limited to monitoring during anesthesia when multiple anesthetic gases are simultaneously monitored. More recently, Ramen spectroscopy, which can also monitor multiple gases, has become available for monitoring during anesthesia. These expensive instruments are set up to monitor several operating rooms with one unit. A less expensive infrared capnograph as a backup is also available to each anesthesiologist for monitoring end-tidal CO_2 and therefore ventilation. Some instruments are now made with combined pulse oximetry and capnography since both are useful in the operating room and ICU. Units are inexpensive enough that they can be dedicated to a single patient.

The airway gas can be looked at directly with a miniaturized assembly that fits in the airway (Fig 7–27, B), or air can be sampled and pumped through a bedside monitor. Instead of using two or more wavelengths, only one wavelength at 4.26 μm where CO_2 has the highest absorption of infrared light is used. The instruments incorporate a chopper wheel that contains two reference cells, one with known CO_2 and another with only nitrogen. The difference between the absorption through the two cells allows for calibration. The chopper also provides a dark, zero light period that is used to eliminate zero drift and noise signals from thermal or outside light sources. Some mainstream, in-line sensors use the zero CO_2 during inspiration as the reference cell. Such devices will be erroneous if CO_2 is in the inspired air.

To provide accurate measurements, the capnometer should be calibrated before use and at regular intervals (every 12 to 24 hours) by using a known (approximately 5%) CO_2 mixture. Accuracy should be within 12%, or 4 mm Hg.

The frequency response of the sensor is capable of providing an accurate replication of the capnogram. However, sidestream sampling devices may distort the capnogram if the tubing is too long or the air sampling rate too slow. Also, with sidestream sampling, H_2O and secretions must be removed before entering the analysis cell. This is done by heating sampling lines and using filters and H_2O traps. Some systems use a reverse flow to purge the water and secretions, but this is not desirable for infection control reasons.

Analysis of the CO_2 waveform. Although the P_{ETCO_2} measurement is the most useful to monitor V_E and

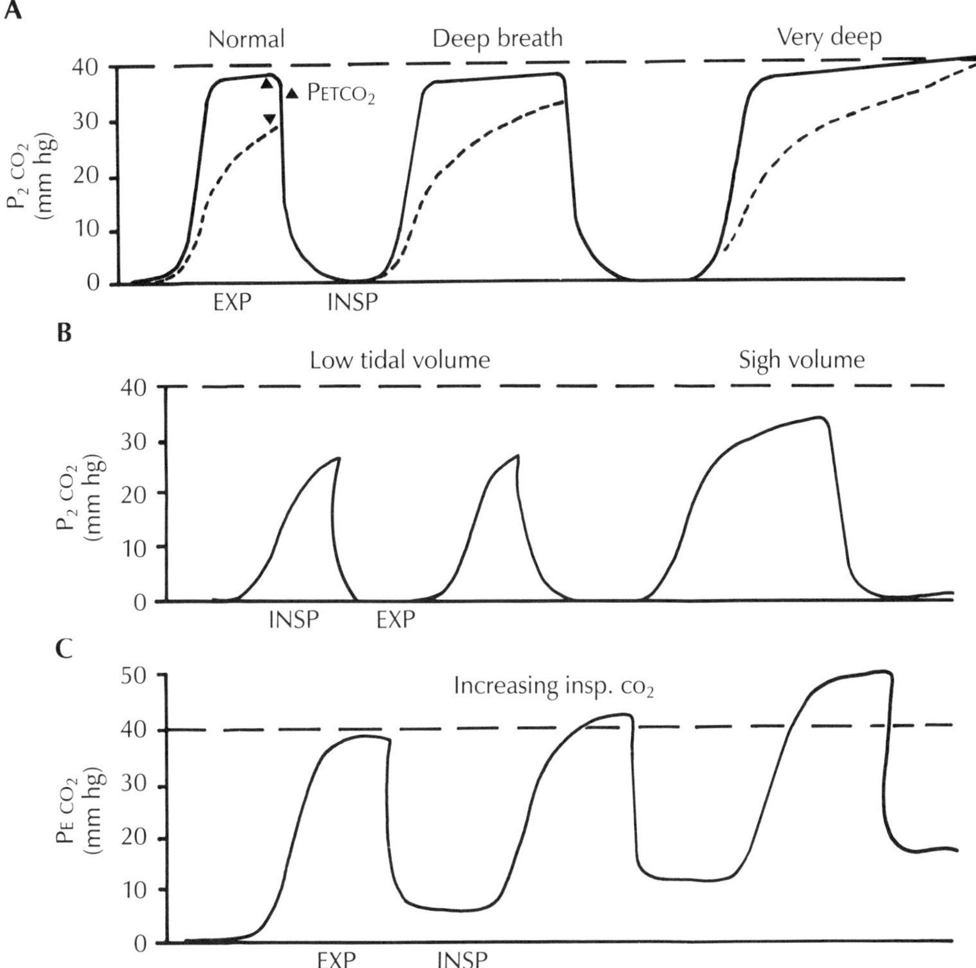

FIG 7–28
Examples of expired CO_2 curves. **A,** a normal expired CO_2 curve rises rapidly to a plateau 1 to 5 mm Hg below Pa_{CO_2} = 40 mm Hg (dashed line). For a patient with increased dead space or maldistribution of ventilation. The PET_{CO_2} is much lower. With a deeper breath the PET_{CO_2} may increase toward the Pa_{CO_2} and with prolonged exhalation can even exceed Pa_{O_2}. **B,** a normal sharp rise of the CO_2 but no plateau because of shallow, rapid breathing with failure to clear the dead space or show a true alveolar CO_2. Note that on the third breath, with the more prolonged exhalation, the end-tidal CO_2 approaches the arterial CO_2. **C,** if the external dead space is increased or CO_2 is inspired because of malfunction of the exhalation valve or depletion of CO_2 absorber, the CO_2 will not fall to 0 on exhalation and the P_{ETCO_2} will rise.

Pa_{CO_2}, the variability of the $(Pa - P_{ET})_{CO_2}$ gradient and errors in selecting the end-tidal value must be recognized and avoided by examination of the capnogram over several breaths and with special maneuvers.

Figure 7–28 shows several expired CO_2 curves. A normal subject will have a clear CO_2 plateau and a well-defined P_{ETCO_2} 2 to 5 mmHg below Pa_{CO_2} (Fig 7-27, A). A patient with COPD and severe maldistribution of ventilation will show a steep CO_2 exhalation curve (Fig 7–28, A), and the P_{ETCO_2} may be 10 or more below Pa_{CO_2}. If the patient is asked to do a forced, prolonged exhalation, the P_{ETCO_2} will more closely approximate Pa_{CO_2} and could even exceed Pa_{CO_2} if exhalation is prolonged because of the emptying of low ventilation units as well as Pa_{CO_2} equilibrating with $P\bar{v}_{CO_2}$. Tidal volumes vary even on ventilators. A low tidal volume that does not clear the dead space will obviously give a low P_{ETCO_2} (Fig 7–28, B). This will frequently occur when a patient is being weaned from mechanical ventilation, and the V_T will decrease significantly. The low P_{ETCO_2} could be seriously misleading if it is taken as representative of Pa_{CO_2}, which in fact is probably increasing because of the low V_T.

If there is excessive dead space tubing downstream from the capnogram or a malfunctioning exhalation valve or if there is depletion of the CO_2 absorbent in a rebreather circuit, there will be increased CO_2 during inspiration that may cause a rise in the P_{ETCO_2} (Fig 7–28,C). Physiologic dead space as occurs in any diseased lung will also lower P_{ETCO_2} and increase the $(P_{ET} - Pa)_{CO_2}$ gradient. Finally, P_{ETCO_2} may be useful to monitor the adequacy of pulmonary blood flow during CPR or a severe shock state (Fig 7–29).[68]

Clearly, many factors can affect the P_{ETCO_2}, but analysis of curves over time, deep inhalation and exhalation maneuvers, and recognition of the precise physiologic relationship of P_{ETCO_2} with Pa_{CO_2}, $\dot{V}_{CO_2}$, $\dot{V}_A$, $\dot{V}_E$, and V_D will allow optimum use of the capnogram.

Remember:

$$P_{ETCO_2} \sim P_{ACO_2} = Pa_{CO_2}$$
$$P_{ACO_2} = \dot{V}_{CO_2}/\dot{V}_A - V_D$$
$$\dot{V}_E = \dot{V}_A + V_D$$

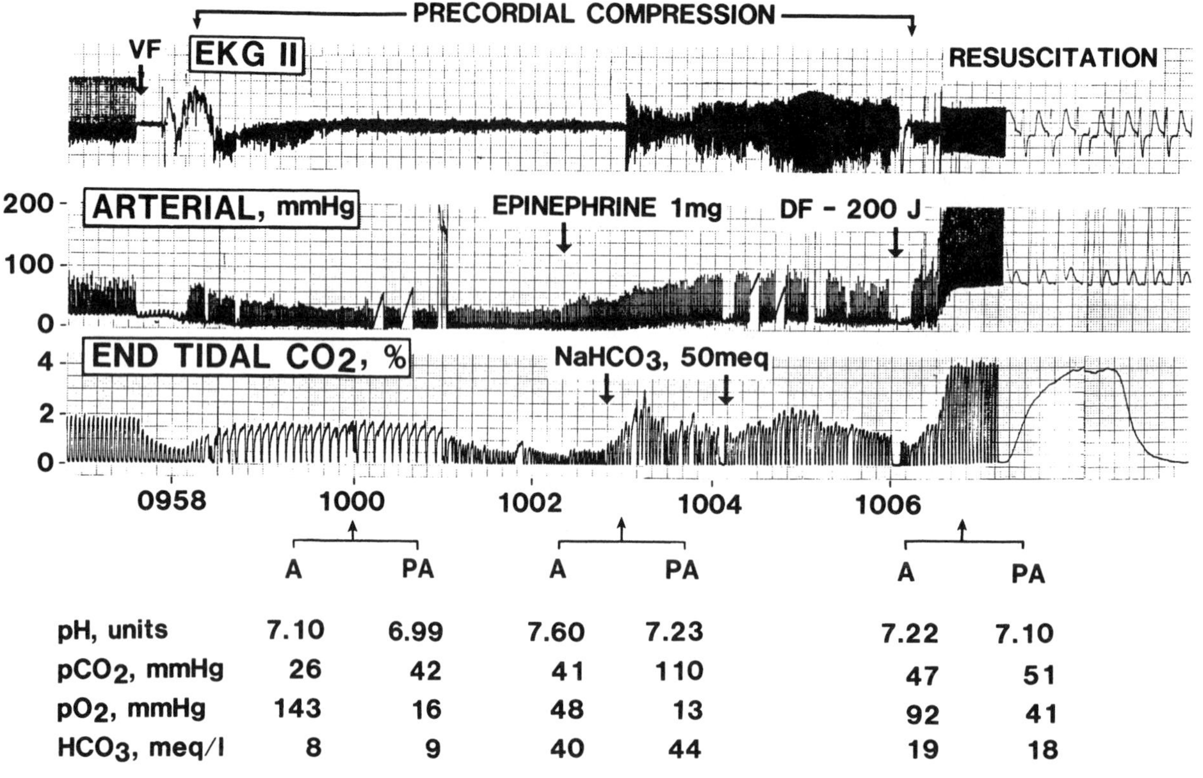

FIG 7–29
Serial changes in the end-tidal CO_2 concentration (ET_{CO_2}) and arterial *(A)* and mixed venous *(PA)* blood gases in a representative patient before and immediately after cardiac arrest, during precordial compression, and after defibrillation *(DF)* and resuscitation. The transient increase in the ET_{CO_2} after the administration of sodium bicarbonate *($NaHCO_3$)* is also demonstrated. (From Falk JL, Rackow EC, Weil MH: *N Engl J Med* 1988; 318:707–711. Reprinted with permission from *The New England Journal of Medicine*, vol. 318, page 610, 1988.)

Clinical Applications and Limitations of Noninvasive Oxygen Monitoring

Table 7–4 indicates the recommendations regarding the use of noninvasive techniques in various clinical subspecialties as adapted but changed from the recent state-of-the-art review article.[58] The most widespread and accepted use of noninvasive measurements is pulse oximetry (Sp_{O_2}). The rationale for these recommendations will be summarized here, but the reader is referred to the cited references for more details.

Exercise. Noninvasive exercise studies using the Hewlett Packard ear oximeter have long been popular, and currently, pulse oximetry is gradually replacing this no-longer–produced instrument. However, there are limitations in the use of Sp_{O_2}. The Sp_{O_2} is insensitive in detecting changes in Pa_{O_2} in the 60– to 100–mm Hg area since that is in the flat portion of the oxyhemoglobin dissociation curve. Since clinically significant hypoxemia during exercise would generally be considered below 60 mm Hg, this is not a major concern. More important are the potential high and low errors reported in the Sp_{O_2}, as large as 5% at rest and 13% to 14% during exercise.[69]

TABLE 7–4
Recommendations for Clinical Use of Noninvasive Techniques

	Sp_{O_2}	Ptc_{O_2}	P_{ETCO_2}	$Ptcc_{O_2}$
Exercise	+ + +	+/−	+ + +	+/−
Sleep	+ + +	+/−	+ +	+
Critical Care				
Adult	+ + +	−	+ +	+
Pediatric	+ + +	−	+ +	+ +
Neonate	+ +	+ + +	+	+ +
Anesthesia	+ + +	+/−	+ + +	+/−

Studies reporting these errors are generally from small groups of patients and with earlier models of pulse oximeters.[69–71] Exercise studies using the Hewlett Packard ear oximeter have shown more satisfactory results, perhaps because careful attention has been paid to ear preparation and motion artifacts.[72] Further studies are needed to validate pulse oximetry measurements during exercise. If findings are not consistent with clinical or physiologic observations, ABG measurements may be necessary.

Anesthesia. In anethesia, Sp_{O_2} is now virtually indispensable. In October 1989, the American Society of

Anesthesiologists mandated Spo_2 during all types of anesthesia.[73] Use of dyes and radiofrequency electrocautery may have a spurious effect, as can certain high-intensity ambient lighting used in the operating room. Shielding the Spo_2 electrode with aluminum foil can avoid the problem of ambient lighting. Vasoconstriction during surgery with diminished arterial pulsation is the most serious limitation, particularly with finger probes. Use of ear or bridge-of-the-nose sensors may offer some improvement over the finger, but this has not been well documented. Differences in the pulse rate, as noted by the pulse oximeter vs. that obtained simultaneously from the ECG, may indicate an erroneous Spo_2.

Sleep. Sleep studies were enhanced in the 1970s with the use of the Hewlett Packard ear oximeter. The frequency and severity of hypoxemia during sleep apnea was for the first time readily documented. Pulse oximeters with their simplified, nonheated probes have now replaced the Hewlett Packard ear oximeters. Spo_2 agrees to within 6% of arterial blood measurements when the saturation is in excess of 75%. However, as the Spo_2 falls below 75%, the accuracy deteriorates, and precise correlation with Pao_2 is not possible.

Clinical practice. Pulse oximetry has become a very common method for monitoring oxygen therapy in the home, medical office, and hospital practice. Routine use of oxygen in hospital patients can now be titrated to suit the needs of an individual patient without repeated arterial punctures. Patients receiving oxygen are routinely monitored daily or more frequently if oxygen needs are high (>4 L/min) or the clinical condition is variable. It is useful to determine Spo_2 on room air first and then titer the oxygen via the nasal catheter or mask until the desired Spo_2 is achieved. Generally, an Spo_2 greater than 92% would be desirable, but patients with carbon dioxide retention may be titrated to 86% to 90%. ABG measurements can then be made to validate the Spo_2 as well as to measure the Pco_2 and pH when that is of concern.

Errors in Spo_2 may occur in both directions in the clinical setting, but the frequency and extent of such errors have not been systematically studied or reported. Low estimates of Spo_2 are quite common in critically ill patients who frequently have low or poor peripheral perfusion. Motion artifacts and loss of signal from electrode movement are not uncommon reasons for spurious alarms. Inaccurate pulse readings or the absence of an appropriate response with hyperventilation or changing Fio_2 values are useful to verify the Spo_2.

Long-term oxygen therapy for home care of patients with chronic hypoxemia is now universally recognized as effective in reducing cor pulmonale and prolonging life.[74] The initial guidelines for the use of oxygen was a Pao_2 of less than 55 mm Hg since the studies in the early 1980s used that for selecting treatment with oxygen. As Spo_2 measurements replaced ABGs, initial medicare guidelines suggested an Spo_2 of less than 85% as equivalent to a Pao_2 of 55 mm Hg. Studies subsequently showed that as many as 40% of patients would be erroneously judged to not need oxygen if the criterion Spo_2 of 85% is used.[75] This led to the recommendation that 88% be used as the cutoff point rather than 85%.[76] Monitoring patients during exercise or sleep gives further insight into the need for oxygen therapy even when resting values are normal or greater than 90% saturation at rest.

Neonatal and pediatric practice. Monitoring oxygen in neonatal critical care units and in small infants requires special attention to the Pao_2. High Pao_2 values in neonates and young infants may lead to retrolental fibroplasia and blindness. Since the Spo_2 may be reading at 98% to 100% when the Pao_2 is in excess of 150 mm Hg, ABG measurements or transcutaneous oxygen monitoring is needed to detect the high Pao_2. Fortunately, $Ptco_2$ provides acceptable accuracy in neonates and young infants.[77–79] The direction and degree of change also generally correlate well with Pao_2. Correlations are poor in older children and may even be poor in older infants.[80–83]

Pulse oximetry is increasingly preferred in neonatal and infant care because of the ease of application, the avoidance of skin burns, and the faster response times when compared with $Ptco_2$. Despite the inaccuracy of Spo_2 vs. Pao_2 as Spo_2 exceeds 95% because of the flat shape of the oxyhemoglobin dissociation curve, hypoxemia can still be effectively monitored. ABG measurements are needed if the Spo_2 appears to be spuriously low or rises to greater than 95% saturation, in which case toxic levels of po_2 may be of concern.[84,85]

Noninvasive Monitoring For CO_2

Noninvasive monitoring of carbon dioxide is less successful than that of oxygen. In part, this is because the need to monitor CO_2 is less critical than for oxygen. Hypoxemia is common and can occur rapidly in clinical situations, which makes continuous monitoring more desirable if not essential. Monitoring CO_2 is also important since it reflects the adequacy of ventilation and possible acid-base disturbances. Gas-phase monitoring of CO_2 has been available for half a century, whereas transcutaneous monitoring of CO_2 has only been available for the past decade. Current technology allows CO_2 monitoring to be done in routine clinical situations, but studies documenting the usefulness of such monitoring are more limited and give mixed reviews, as will be discussed for each clinical application.

Clinical Applications and Limitations of Noninvasive CO_2 Monitoring

Exercise. Expired gas CO_2 is essential in any metabolic or exercise study, whether it be an invasive study using an indwelling arterial catheter or a noninvasive study as has been described in the metabolic monitoring section of this chapter. Use of the end-tidal CO_2 as a surrogate for Pa_{CO_2} has problems. Even in normal subjects at rest, there is a variability in the $(Pa - P_{ET})_{CO_2}$ gradient of 2 to 5 mm Hg. As one introduces abnormal distribution of ventilation in diseased subjects or during exercise in normal subjects, the gradients will increase. In diseased subjects, the $(Pa - P_{ET})_{CO_2}$ gradient can increase to over 20 mm Hg, but this may be decreased if one uses the maximum expiratory maneuver, as discussed in the previous section (see Figure 7-27).

During exercise, however, there is the added variable of the rising venous CO_2, which may introduce P_{ETCO_2} values higher than Pa_{CO_2}.[86] At peak exercise, the average CO_2 gradient was negative, −4.1 mm Hg (range, +1 to −14), in 77 middle-aged, sedentary men without a clinical history of lung disease.[87] Despite these large differences and the potential overestimate of arterial CO_2 by the end-tidal CO_2, the measurement of end-tidal CO_2 remains a useful monitor during exercise testing. The level of the P_{ETCO_2} at rest can confirm the adequacy and stability of the ventilation observed.

Decreases in P_{ETCO_2} occur at the onset of lactic acidosis and are valuable in determining the lactate threshold. Hyperventilation provoked by anxiety or other causes than the lactate threshold can also cause a decrease in P_{ETCO_2} as well as an increase in CO_2 production and an increase in the RER as occurs at the lactate threshold. In most instances it is difficult for a patient to maintain a spurious, anxiety-related degree of hyperventilation at an exercise level at which lactate threshold tends to occur; therefore, the two should not be commonly confused. V_D/V_T calculated by using P_{ETCO_2} should be interpreted with caution since errors of ±10% from observed Pa_{CO_2} values can occur.

It should also be noted that the transcutaneous CO_2 electrode has a time constant of over 2 minutes, thus making it impractical for use during exercise unless a steady-state exercise protocol is used with stages lasting longer than 2 minutes.

Sleep. CO_2 during sleep studies is measured via a nasal catheter and, in some cases, the transcutaneous CO_2 device as well. The accuracy of the P_{ETCO_2} from a nasal catheter is poor because of the absence of a closed system, but it can be used to effectively monitor the respiratory rate and at least affords some estimate of potential changes in arterial CO_2.

Transcutaneous CO_2 can be used and is especially applicable in those subjects with known elevated P_{ACO_2}. In these situations, the effect of the use of nocturnal supplemental oxygen or the use of nasal CPAP may be deleterious to ventilation, which may be detected by using transcutaneous monitors. Because of the wide and sometimes variable nature of $(Ptc - Pa)_{CO_2}$ gradients, one or more ABG determinations are generally needed during sleep monitoring. The need for such arterial blood sampling, difficulties in the application of the monitors, and the slow time constants have limited the use of Ptc_{CO_2} in sleep laboratories.

Anesthesia. During anesthesia, P_{ETCO_2} has been generally accepted as a valuable method for monitoring the adequacy of ventilation. Ptc_{CO_2} has found only limited use because of its slow time response and the setup time required. In addition, ABGs are usually more readily available under anesthesia where indwelling catheters are already being used.

Clinical practice. In the clinical setting, P_{ETCO_2} has had its widest acceptance in the ICU for monitoring of patients who are mechanically ventilated, as discussed previously.

Although there are a number of studies indicating the validity of Ptc_{CO_2} measurements in hemodynamically stable critical care patients, the wide variations in the $(Ptc - Pa)_{CO_2}$ gradients necessitate ABG determinations. When Ptc_{CO_2} measurements are made within 4 hours of a calibrating blood gas measurement, there is excellent correlation between Pa_{CO_2} and Ptc_{CO_2} (r = .94).[88] When Pa_{CO_2} changes are greater than 5 mm Hg, they were uniformly detected by the Ptc_{CO_2} monitor.[89] Others have reported lower correlations (r = .84) and high CO_2 gradients of 20 ± 5.2 mm Hg.[90] Gradients are less with the low-temperature infrared devices, with mean differences of 4 mm Hg[91] and 5.2 mm Hg[63] reported. Because of the acceptance of arterial punctures and arterial lines in adult patients, the transcutaneous devices have not been as widely used as they are in neonates and infants.

Neonates and infants. In neonates, transcutaneous electrodes usually combine both the O_2 and the CO_2 sensors. In a review of nine studies[88] including 210 neonates, correlation between Pa_{CO_2} and Ptc_{CO_2} ranged from .85 to .99, with most studies having an r of greater than .94, thus demonstrating the acceptability of this measurement in neonatology. Transcutaneous CO_2 provides an ideal way of monitoring an infant who may have acute and critical changes in ventilation in the ICU setting.

HEMODYNAMIC MONITORING AND ORGAN PERFUSION

Introduction

Ventilation and gas exchange are the major concerns of the RCP, but without attention to the cardiovascular system, the ultimate goal of tissue and organ respiration will not be achieved. It is the heart that needs the most critical monitoring, both temporally and quantitatively. Temporal monitoring is readily available via the ECG. Of the approximately 75,000 adults and pediatric ICU beds, virtually all have ECG monitoring capability. This chapter will not cover ECG technology but will rather focus on quantification of the work of the heart: cardiac output (Q_T) and the pressures needed for effective organ perfusion.

In this section, we will first describe the methods for measuring systemic pressures. The traditional cuff application to the upper portion of the arm is readily automated, as demonstrated in the many automated blood pressure devices in shopping malls. That technology will be discussed as used at the bedside. The majority of ICU beds today are capable of continuously monitoring vascular pressures by using intravascular catheters. Arterial catheters, which came into use at the same time as ABG measurements, provide a ready source of blood for ABG analysis as well as for monitoring systemic pressures. Basic rules of setup, use, and interpretation of arterial pressure waveforms are an essential part of critical care monitoring.

The next historical development in hemodynamic monitoring was the pulmonary artery catheter. The initial demonstration that such measurements were possible was by Forstmann in 1939, who inserted the catheter into himself. Development of this technique by Forstmann in Germany and Drs. Cournand and Richards in New York led to classic studies and awarding of the Nobel Prize to the three of them. Such catheters were limited to transient use in cardiac catheterization laboratories until 1970 when Swan et al. introduced the idea of inserting more flexible catheters at the bedside to enable clinicians to use the same physiologic information for the management of critically ill patients.[92]

With the development of the pulmonary artery catheter, it was an easy step to measure the cardiac output by using the concepts of indicator dye dilution as used in the catheterization laboratory for measuring cardiac output, but with substitution of cold water as the indicator "dye." The use and abuse of this method and the importance of recognition of basic waveforms will be discussed. Next, cardiac output methodologies using the pulmonary artery catheter will be reviewed. Continuous monitoring of mixed venous saturation ($S\bar{v}O_2$) by using fiber-optic catheters and the intra-arterial catheters capable of continuous monitoring are now available. A bedside metabolic system allows continuous measurements of $\dot{V}O_2$ and $\dot{V}CO_2$. Finally, coordination of all the measurements, pressures, $\dot{V}O_2$, Q_T, and $(Ca - C\bar{v})O_2$ to monitor the adequacy of tissue perfusion by using integrative physiologic principles will be discussed.

To show the overwhelming importance of using the fundamental Fick equation of O_2 mass balance (i.e., the O_2 absorbed by the lungs, $\dot{V}O_2$, must in steady-state conditions equal the O_2 used by the tissues, $Q_T \times (Ca - C\bar{v})O_2$) $(a - \bar{v})O_2d$ will be emphasized by using the measurements of each of these variables in the ICU. Unfortunately, recent literature has been controversial, to a large extent because of inadequate attention to errors in measurements, as will be discussed in the final section of this chapter on tissue perfusion.

Arterial Pressure Monitoring

The typical arterial pressure waveform and simultaneous ECG in proximal and peripheral arteries is shown in Figure 7–30.[93] Characteristically, there is a rapid rise in pressure to a sharp peak, or systolic pressure, following the QRS component of the ECG. As the ventricle relaxes, there is a rapid fall in pressure to the diastolic level. Note that the systolic pressure is higher and the diastolic pressure lower in the peripheral, radial artery than in the proximal, subclavian artery because of the resonance characteristics of the vascular system.[93]

Noninvasive Arterial Pressure Monitoring

There are three methods to measure arterial pressure. The first is the classic method for detection of flow distal

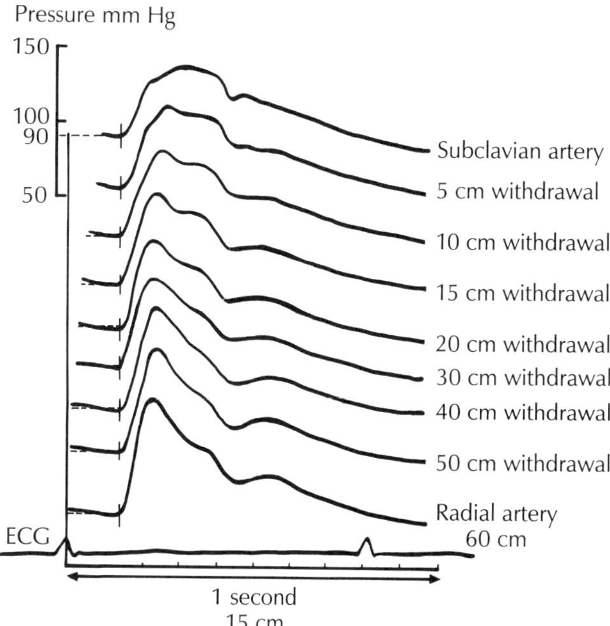

FIG 7–30
Arterial pressure waveform changes due to resonance as a catheter is withdrawn from the central aorta into a peripheral artery. (From Marshall HW, Helmholz HF, Woods EH: Physiological consequences of congenital heart disease, in Hamilton WF, Dow P (eds): *Handbook of Physiology,* vol 1. Washington, DC, American Physiological Society, 1962, p 417. Used by permission.)

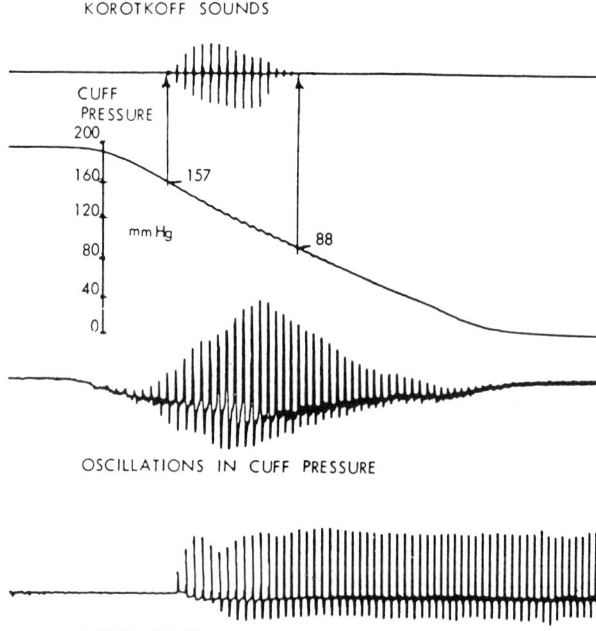

FIG 7–31
Simultaneous recording of return to flow (arterial line), cuff oscillations, and Korotkoff sounds during cuff deflation. Maximum oscillations occur at mean arterial pressure. (From Geddes LA: *The Direct and Indirect Measurement of Blood Pressure.* St Louis, Mosby–Year Book, 1970. Used by permission.)

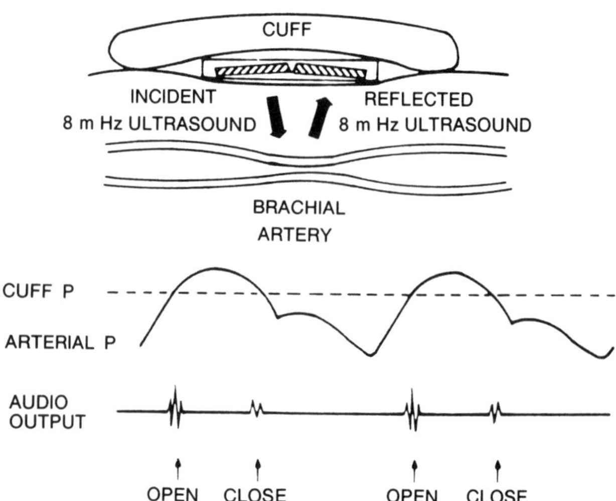

FIG 7–32
The method of using ultrasound to "hear" vessel wall movements during automatic cuff deflation (Arteriosonde). (From Geddes LA: *The Direct and Indirect Measurement of Blood Pressure.* St Louis, Mosby–Year Book, 1970. Used by permission.)

to an occlusive cuff. This method uses the stethoscope to detect the Korotkoff sounds as shown in Figure 7–31. The sound starts as flow begins to pass the cuff and stops as the vessel becomes less distorted and flow is more uniform. Common errors are a cuff that is either too large or too small and causes, respectively, a low or high estimate of blood pressure. Cuff width should be 1 to 1.5 times the diameter of the extremity.

Systolic pressure can be determined by any system that detects the onset of pulsations as the cuff pressure is reduced manually. Using an ultrasound Doppler probe beneath the cuff allows the detection of arterial wall movement, which will produce the oscillations shown in Figure 7–31, and allows a determination of systolic and diastolic pressures. The patient must be quite still; this method is most applicable in anesthetized or sedated patients. An example of this type of unit is the Arteriosonde produced by Kontron, which is schematically shown in Figure 7–32.[94]

The second noninvasive method is use of the oscillometer, which is the basis for most current automatic cuff blood pressure devices. Detection of the oscillations in the cuff pressure allows an estimation of systolic blood pressure (start of oscillation) and diastolic blood pressure (end of oscillation), and it has been shown that the mean blood pressure correlates with the peak oscillations.[95] These systems are also sensitive to monitor artifacts. The cycle time can be quite long when arrhythmias are present, and awake patients complain of pain from repeated inflation of the cuff. Accuracy is good for normal and low systolic blood pressure, underestimated for high blood pressure, and erratic for diastolic blood pressure.

A third method is one that uses infrared detection of the change in arterial volume of a finger when plethysmograph occlusion occurs (Fig 7–33).[96] This method can provide a continuous arterial pulse waveform that approximates but is slightly lower than an intra-arterial catheter measurement.[97] Continuous use can cause venous occlusion and ischemia.[98]

Catheter Monitoring System

A block diagram showing the components of a common computer-processed arterial monitor is shown in Figure 7–34,[99] and a schematic visualization of the bedside components is shown in Figure 7–35.[99] The "plumbing system" is characteristically under the care and supervision of the ICU nurse, but not infrequently, the RCP is called upon to manipulate the system. In fact, every time an arterial blood sample is drawn, there is the potential to introduce changes in the response characteristics of this "plumbing system." For example, the introduction of air bubbles into the tubing will cause an overshoot of the systolic pressure and give a falsely high measurement.

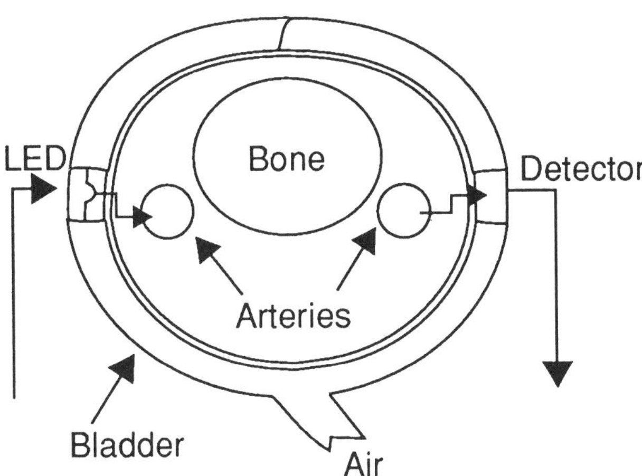

FIG 7–33
Peñaz method of measuring finger blood pressure: cross section of a finger with the cuff and photodetector positioned. A servo-controlled device applies pressure to the bladder to maintain constant output from the detector. The pressure required to maintain a light path of constant length is the arterial pressure waveform. (From Boehmer RD: *J Clin Monit* 1987; 3:23. Used by permission.)

Transducers

The measuring element for vascular pressure is the same as that for airway pressures. The early transducers had large electrical drifts and zero offsets that required frequent, difficult calibrations. Current designs incorporate solid-state piezoelectric crystals with more stable output proportional to pressure.

Today, most transducers are disposable and limited to a single patient use. Most have integrated and automated flush devices that can be used to check the dynamic response of the system by suddenly introducing a high pressure from the flush system. The disposable transducers are cost-effective, ensure sterility, are precalibrated, and have smaller volume displacement, which ensures better dynamic response characteristics. For more details on the methods to properly set up, calibrate, and correct for overdamped and underdamped systems and methods of general "troubleshooting," the reader is referred to work by Gardner and Chapman.[99]

The electronic/computer components of the monitor system have low-pass filters that are used to eliminate artifacts in the waveform but may prevent accurate assessment of the dynamic characteristics of the system. Algorithms in the microprocessor vary widely and can give different results with the same patient waveform. Computer digital outputs carry a ring of truth that may be misleading. One study found that errors of 5 to 10 mm Hg were frequent and errors as large as 30 to 40 mm Hg were not uncommon.[100] General precautions for all catheter monitoring systems have been proposed and should be rigorously followed.[101] These precautions are listed in Table 7–5.

Pulmonary Artery Pressure Monitoring

Since the introduction of the flexible pulmonary artery catheter in 1970 by Swan et al.,[92] hemodynamic monitoring in the ICU has become a sophisticated but complicated reality. Although there continues to be controversy over the safety and cost-effectiveness of such monitoring,[102] there is no doubt that it allows for effective physiologic measurements of cardiac function and pulmonary vascular resistance and, from mixed venous

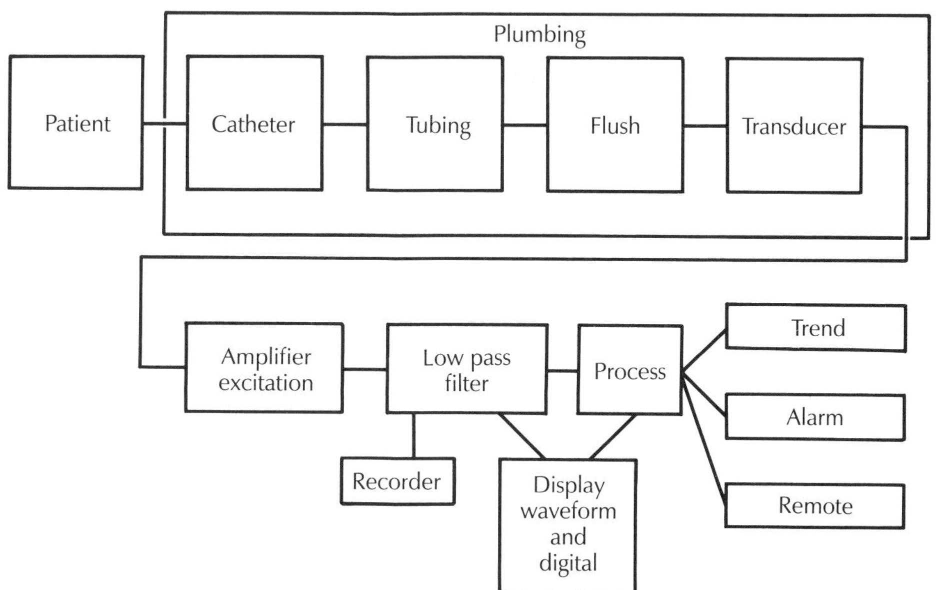

FIG 7–34
Block diagram of a pressure-monitoring system showing the components that affect the accuracy of the results. The *upper part* shows the patient and attached plumbing system, and the *lower part* shows components of the pressure-monitoring system usually contained in the bedside monitor. (From Gardner RM, Chapman RH: Troubleshooting pressure monitoring systems: When do the numbers lie? In Fallat RJ, Luce JM (eds): *Cardiopulmonary Critical Care Management.* New York, Churchill Livingstone, 1988, p 145. Used by permission.)

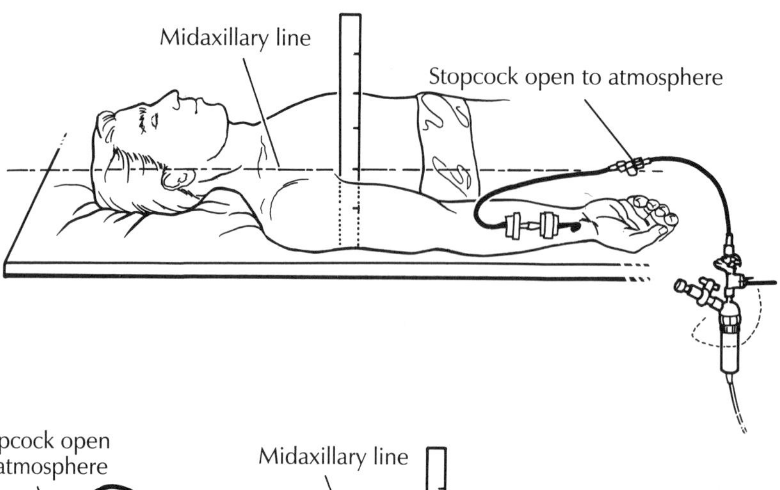

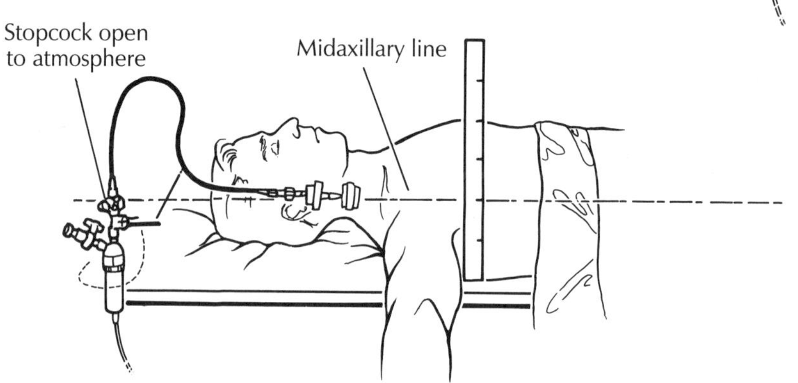

FIG 7–35
Two methods of zeroing a pressure transducer. Note that the place at which the water-air interface occurs must always be at the midaxillary line when zeroing. The stopcock is placed near the transducer at the midaxillary line **(A).** The stopcock near the catheter is placed at the midaxillary line **(B).** (From Gardner RM, Chapman RH. Troubleshooting pressure monitoring systems: When do the numbers lie? In Fallat RJ, Luce JM (eds): *Cardiopulmonary Critical Care Management.* New York, Churchill Livingstone, 1988, p 145. Used by permission.)

sampling, a means of globally assessing tissue perfusion. This section will emphasize the importance of assessing the validity of pulmonary artery pressure (PAP) measurements.

The pulmonary artery waveform shown in Figure 7–36[103] has characteristics similar to but lower in magnitude than the systemic artery pressure waveform. The figure also shows the typical central venous or right atrial waveform, which is quite different in shape and magnitude because of atrial contractions coinciding with the P wave in the ECG. Note that there is a sudden rise in pressure as the right ventricle is entered and the diastolic pressure falls to 0. As the pulmonic valve is passed, the PAP waveform takes on the appearance of the systemic waveform with a diastolic pressure that should approximate the wedge pressure (PAW) obtained when the balloon is inflated, as shown in Figure 7–36.

TABLE 7–5
General Precautions With All Catheters

Never flush air into the system.
Left atrial, aortic, or carotid catheters should not be used for blood sampling because of the danger of cerebral air embolism.
Avoid the use of sharp instruments when removing dressings around the catheter.
Unless specifically directed, never administer drugs in an arterial catheter.

Figure 7–37[104] shows several pulmonary artery waveforms under different ventilatory conditions. It is here that knowledge of heart-lung interactions is so important in recognizing potential errors in the computerized output of the PAP and PAW. Note the large negative pressure swings that can occur with spontaneous ventilation in a patient with low compliance or high airway resistance (Fig 7–37, D and E). The proper reading of the PAW should occur during the resting end-tidal breath period of the ventilatory cycle. The computer algorithm may calculate the mean pressures during the entire cycle and result in a falsely low reading. Conversely, high positive airway pressures from mechanical ventilators can result in falsely high computer readings (Fig 7–37, B and C). Newer systems simultaneously monitor respiration by using impedance pneumography, as previously described. Algorithms can then incorporate this information and allow the computer to choose only those pressures measured during end-tidal breathing when intrathoracic pressures are minimized.

Cardiac Output Measurements

The measurement of organ blood flow is physiologically more important than the pressure measurements just

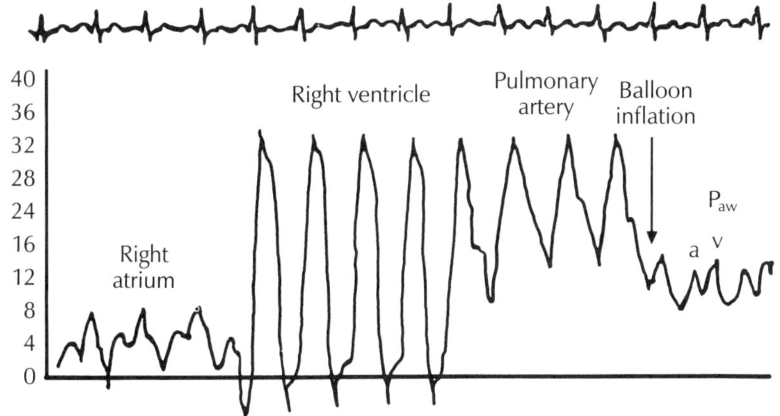

FIG 7–36
Pressure waveforms during Swan-Ganz insertion. See the text. (From Fallat RJ: Hemodynamic monitoring, in Clausen JL, Zarins LP (eds): *Pulmonary Function Testing Guidelines and Controversies.* New York, Academic Press, 1982, p 311. Used by permission.)

discussed. QT is a global view of total organ perfusion. In pulmonary and critical care, monitoring QT is particularly important since many respiratory maneuvers that improve oxygenation may adversely affect QT and therefore organ perfusion.

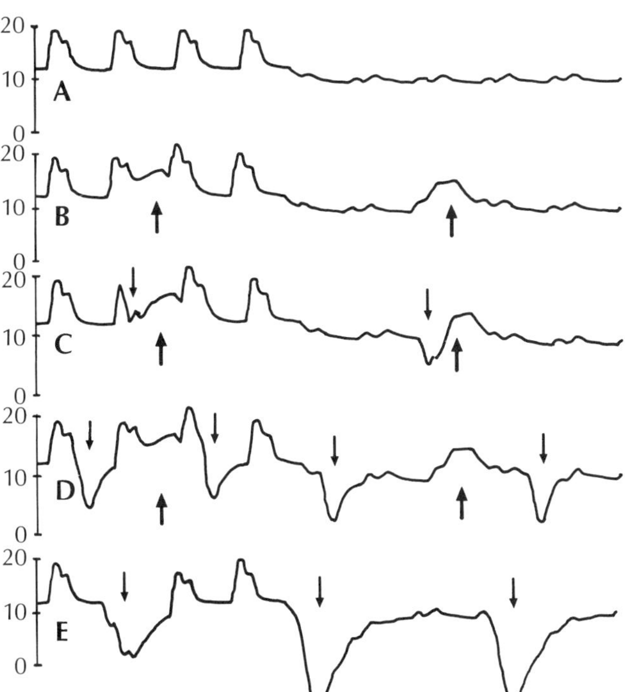

FIG 7–37
The pulmonary artery pressure tracing before and after balloon occlusion as it would appear during apnea **(A)** and four respiratory patterns: controlled mechanical ventilation **(B)**, assisted mechanical ventilation **(C)**, intermittent mandatory ventilation **(D)**, and spontaneous ventilation **(E)**. *Downward arrows* indicate spontaneous inspiration, and *bold upward arrows* show ventilator breaths. (From Culver BH: Hemodynamic monitoring: Physiological problems in interpretation, in Fallat RJ, Luce JM (eds): *Cardiopulmonary Critical Care Management.* New York, Churchill Livingstone, 1988, p 165. Used by permission.)

Noninvasive Measurement of QT

Electrical impedance,[105] Doppler flow,[106] and CO_2 rebreathing methods[107–110] have been described to monitor QT. Although successful in controlled situations, they have not been suitable for bedside or critical care use and will not be discussed further here.

Invasive Measurement of QT

The introduction of the pulmonary artery catheter allows two direct methods to measure QT based on mass balance or the Fick principle: what goes in must equal what goes out in the steady state. Measuring the O_2 going to the body, Ca × QT, less the O_2 coming back from the body, Cv × QT, must equal the O_2 consumed, Vo_2:

$$Vo_2 = (Ca - Cv)o_2 \times QT \text{ (Fick equation)},$$

where Vo_2 can be measured in the expired gas. Another mass balance can be derived from dilution of an indicator dye or cold H_2O injected into the right atrium and the concentration measured downstream at the tip of the catheter. Here the dilution of the indicator as measured downstream is proportional to the volume per unit time or flow of blood into which the indicator was injected. Each method has assumptions, errors, and limitations.

The mass balance methods can be erroneous in several ways. The most important assumption is that steady-state conditions exist with no leaks into or out of the system, i.e., that there is no change in the total indicator (O_2, dye, or cold H_2O) in the system. If, for example, some of the dye injected in the right atrium goes into the left atrium via a patent foramen ovale, then the total dye in the pulmonary artery system has not been conserved. Similarly, if the O_2 is leaking out of a chest tube or from around the tracheostomy tube, the estimate of Vo_2 will be erroneously low.

The dye or thermal dilution methods assume that there is "perfect" mixing at the downstream site, i.e., that there is no streaming of the indicator past the sensor. The injection is made in the right atrium, and it is hoped that passage through two valves and the right atrium results in good mixing and that flow is uniform to all the pulmonary vascular bed including the one in which the pulmonary artery catheter is placed. Typically, three cold water injections are made 1 to 2 minutes apart, and agreement within 10% is expected between the three independent measurements of Q_T. Any change in the activity of the patient will result in a change in Q_T, so the three injections should be done when the patient is stable.

The simultaneous measurement of the arteriovenous O_2 difference $(Ca - Cv)o_2$ allows for a cross-check of the thermodilution method by using the Fick equation described above. If the three Q_T determinations by thermal dilution are done before and after sampling of arterial and pulmonary artery blood, they can be used to verify the measurement if an independent Vo_2 measurement is available from a metabolic cart described above. Even if Vo_2 is not available, when serial measurements are made, then Q_T should vary inversely with $(Ca - Cv)o_2$, i.e., if Q_T rises, $(Ca - Cv)o_2$ must decrease if the Vo_2 has not changed between the two times.

Unfortunately, in most critical care situations where pulmonary artery lines are in place, the patients frequently are hemodynamically and metabolically unstable, with changes occurring in temperature and physical activity. It is then necessary to have an independent measure of Vo_2 to accurately assess the hemodynamic changes. This is particularly true because of the inherent errors in the measurements of Q_T, Ca and Cv, e.g., the Q_T by thermal dilution has known errors of as much as 10% to 20%,[111] even in stable patients. Similarly, as pointed out in the ABG section of Chapter 8, there can be a 10% error in Ca and Cv. Should all these errors be present, they would be additive in calculating the Vo_2 or O_2 delivery (Do_2) and result in a 30% to 40% change that may all be due to inherent errors in the method and not due to physiologic responses. Changing O_2 demands and simultaneous errors in Q_T and $(Ca - Cv)o_2$ can lead to serious misjudgments concerning the basic physiologic mechanisms.

Continuous Monitoring of Hemodynamics and Gas Exchange

The application of infrared reflectance technology using three wavelengths in a pulmonary artery catheter allows continuous measurement of Cvo_2. Pulse oximetry or intravascular ABG analysis allows continuous measurement of Cao_2. Metabolic carts are now available that allow bedside continuous measure of Vo_2 and Vco_2. Integration of all these measurements can facilitate recognition of errors and changes from steady-state conditions. Medical Graphics markets a variant of their metabolic cart that is configured to accept the signal from an Oximetrics catheter and provide continuous measurements of cardiac output by using the Fick equation. No system is currently marketed that completely integrates all of these devices, but a description of each follows.

Intra-arterial, Continuous Arterial Blood Gas Analysis

ABG measurements and pH are essential to decision making in critical care situations. The usefulness of ABGs is limited by the time of the analysis and the intermittent nature of the measurements. ABG values reflect dynamic processes that can change on a minute-by-minute basis. The number of measurements that can be made is limited by the fact that discrete amounts of blood must be withdrawn for each determination. One of the most common sources of error is the collection and transport of discrete samples. Intra-arterial monitoring eliminates this potential source of error. New technologies permit continuous monitoring of ABGs and pH by placing electrodes or other sensors within a catheter without requiring removal of blood.[112]

There are basically four technologies that permit continuous monitoring of ABGs. Miniaturization of traditional Clark blood gas electrodes provides one technique.[112] Infrared reflectance, similar to that used for oximeters, is the second. Optical sensors, called optodes, that use light absorbance or fluorescence represent the other technologies.[113, 114] Some systems use mixtures of these technologies.[115]

Optical absorbance involves measuring changes in the intensity of light transmitted through a dye that modifies its optical properties according to the concentration of the analyte, e.g., O_2, CO_2, or hydrogen ions. Typically, sensing is accomplished by monitoring the light that is able to pass through the cell and into a separate optical fiber. Specific wavelength light is attenuated by absorption, scattering, or reflection because of the presence of analytes at the electrode tip reducing the intensity but not the wavelength. The return light must therefore travel through a separate fiber. A schematic example of an absorbance-type sensor is shown in Figure 7–38, B and is used in the Optex BioSentry. In practice, a system for monitoring Pco_2, Po_2, and pH by this technique would require three optical fibers for transmission and three additional fibers for optical return. The resulting six-fiber bundle imposes minimum size constraints on the catheter and limits the application in pediatric patients and neonates.

Another technology is based on chemical fluorescence.[116] Fluorescent dyes sensitive to oxygen, carbon dioxide, and pH are applied to the tip of an optic fiber. The dye absorbs light at short, high-energy wavelengths,

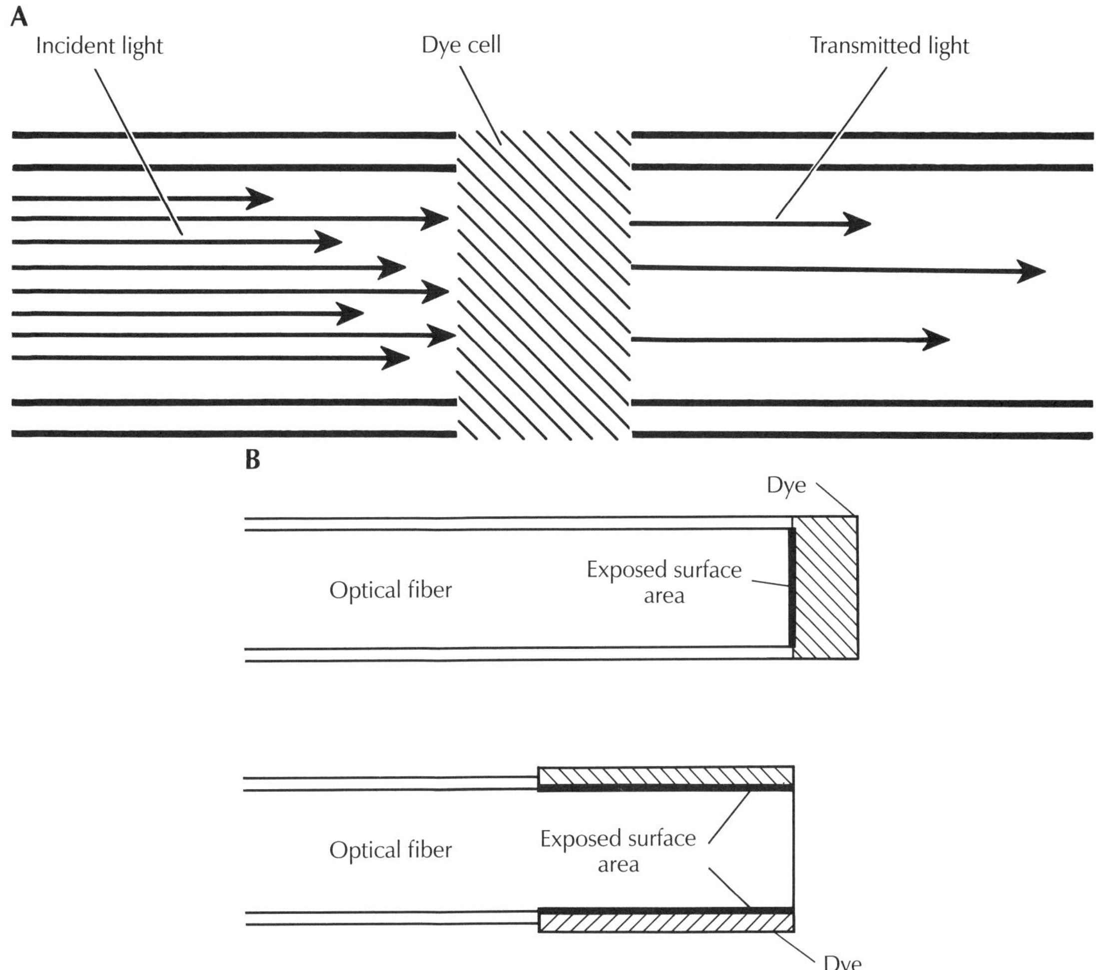

FIG 7–38

A, in absorbance-based sensors, the dye absorbs incident light, depending on the analyte concentration. The intensity of the returned, unabsorbed light is then measured. **B,** this illustration compares the conventional *(top)* configuration with dye immobilized on the fiber end and the Buckless configuration *(bottom)* with dye immobilized on the outer surface of the fiber. In the Buckless configuration, a larger surface area of dye is exposed to excitation light. (From Puritan Bennett Progress Notes/Spring 92. Used by permission.)

such as ultraviolet or violet. The light energy absorbed by the dye is emitted as a fluorescent signal at a lower energy level in the visible range (Fig 7–39, A). Since the excitation and emitted light have different wavelengths and intensities, the emitted light can return in the same fiber.[112] The intensity of the fluorescence is a measure of the concentration of the analyte. Another technique for oxygen monitoring uses a fluorescent dye that quenches in the presence of O_2. The degree of quenching therefore reflects the concentration. Since the fluorescence is a different wavelength than the excitation light, a single optical fiber can be used for each signal (Fig 7–39, C).

Oximetrix 3 SO_2/CO System

This is a three-wavelength spectrophotomatic pulmonary artery catheter system based on reflectance of infrared light and is shown in Figure 7–40. The use of three wavelengths has allowed for better compensation of reflectance of light from RBCs and vascular walls. Three narrow-bandwidth LEDs, one in visible light and two in the near infrared are used. Every second 244 sets of readings of the reflected light are obtained and used to compute O_2 saturation from a 5-second running average. The manufacturer states that a 90% response time for a step change is 5 seconds with an accuracy of ±2% over a 40% to 100% range for So_2.

Cardiac output can be measured by thermal dilution using H_2O from 0 to 25°C measured by a universal temperature probe connected to the computer system. The Q_T measurement range is 0.5 to 20 L/min with an accuracy of ±2% based on an electronic simulated test signal. The system can be used to monitor either arterial or venous O_2 and most commonly is used as a pulmonary artery catheter system.

Each catheter system used must be individually calibrated before insertion with a standard optical refer-

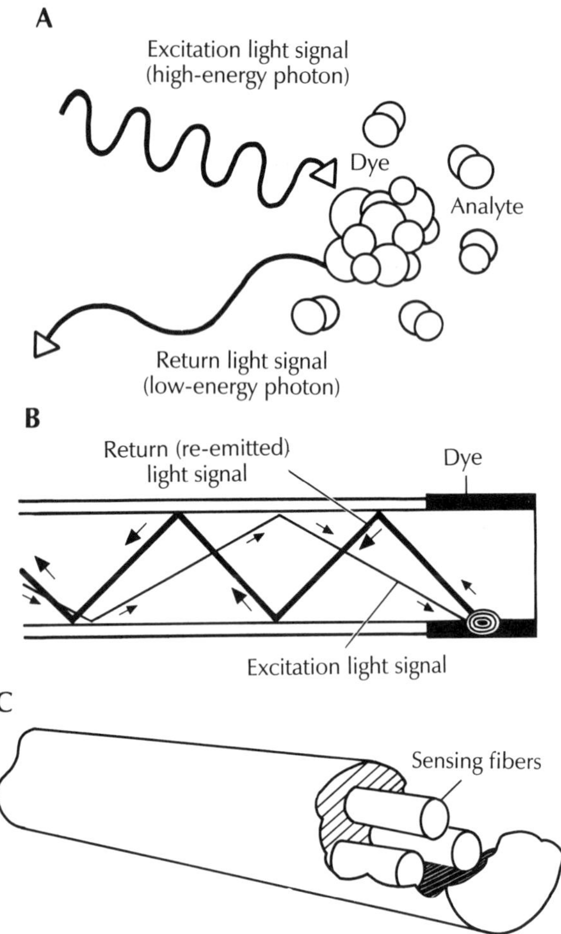

FIG 7–39
A, in a fluorescence-based system, the dye molecules in the sensor tip absorb the excitation light and then emit a fluorescent signal, depending on the concentration of the analyte. **B,** in a fluorescence-based sensor, excitation light is sent down the fiber. The dye at the tip reacts to the excitation light and analyte concentration by fluorescing. The fluorescent signal then returns in the same fiber to the monitor, which measures the intensity of the signal. **C,** this illustration shows an example of a fluorescence-based intra-arterial blood gas sensor. It contains three fibers: one each for pH, Pco_2, and Po_2. (From Puritan-Bennett Progress Notes/Spring 92. Used by permission.)

ence module. In vivo calibrations are possible by using blood sampled from the vessel when the patient is in a stable condition and a stable signal is obtained from the catheter. Drift is said to be only ±2% over a period of 24 hours, but calibration should be checked if readings are not consistent with clinical or physiologic assessment.

Two-hour time displays of So_2 are presented, and high- and low-So_2 alarms can be set. Three error signals are built into the system. "High Intensity" indicates that a catheter tip may be against the vessel wall. "Damped Intensity" may indicate clot formation in the optic tip. "Erratic Intensity" may also indicate clot formation or that the catheter is in the wedge position with occlusion of good flow past the tip, which is necessary for accurate readings.

Puritan-Bennett 3300 Intra-arterial Blood Gas Monitor

This system uses a single 20-gauge catheter with three optic fibers with optically fluorescent dyes sensitive to pH, Pco_2, and Po_2. The dyes are physically separated from the blood by a permeable barrier. The dye is immobilized on the outer surface of the fiber near the tip rather than simply plugging the tip. The effect of this approach is to provide more surface area of the dye, which in turn results in a stronger signal. Additionally, a thermistor is embedded at the catheter tip to measure temperature. A single calibration is required, and continuous blood results are displayed and trended for up to 72 hours. The microsensors are transportable between instruments for patient transfer. The PB-3300 is shown in Figure 7–41.

Optex Biosentry

The BioSentry incorporates two fluorescent sensors for pH and Pco_2 and an absorbance sensor for Po_2 within a 20-gauge catheter.

Clinical Indications and Limitations of Hemodynamic Monitoring

ECG monitoring, as mentioned, is universally used in the critical care setting and needs no elaboration.

An arterial line is indicated when ABG values are severely abnormal or are changing rapidly and require frequent sampling. With a small, 23- to 25-gauge needle, three to five arterial punctures a day are not too traumatic for the patient or the artery. If more than five punctures a day are needed or if several days of monitoring are anticipated, an arterial line is indicated. Even when ABGs are stable and not grossly abnormal, an arterial line may be indicated because of hemodynamic instability. Blood pressure fluctuations are often pronounced, particularly in patients with ARDS who require mechanical ventilation.

Monitoring of the pulse pressures on the arterial pressure trace may give an indication of adverse effects of positive-pressure breathing. As the lung inflates and increases intrathoracic pressure and compresses the heart, a paradoxical pulse or narrowing of the pulse pressure may be seen (Fig 7–42).[117]

Cardiac complications rather than pulmonary disease are usually the indications for a pulmonary artery catheter. Two possible exceptions to this are when pulmonary hypertension or right heart failure is suspected or for the differential diagnosis of pulmonary edema. If pulmonary emboli or pulmonary hypertension is found, continuous monitoring with a pulmonary artery line is necessary to ensure adequate filling of the left ventricle as measured by the P_{aw}. When arterial and pulmonary artery lines are present, it is possible to use the pressure and arteriovenous O_2 differences, $(Ca - Cv)O_2$, to help in the differential diagnosis of the pathophysiology and the cause of the pulmonary edema and hypoxemia.[118] An algorithmic scheme for such analysis is shown in Figure 7–43.[118]

The drop in QT that occurs with positive-pressure breathing, particularly when PEEP is used, is well recognized. Although levels of PEEP, VT, and P_{st} can be initially optimized by using mechanical measurements,[119] the ultimate decision regarding proper ventilation must rest with adequate oxygenation to the tissues. An improvement in PaO_2 may be associated with an even greater fall in QT and result in a fall in the net O_2 delivery and a fall in SvO_2 and QT. Both arterial and pulmonary artery catheters are useful in unstable patients requiring high FIO_2, high airway pressures, and cardiotropic drugs. It is in this situation that serial measurements of QT, Ca, and Cv can be made to optimize O_2 delivery ($DO_2 = CaO_2 \times$ QT) and tissue perfusion. Although QT and CaO_2 may be normal or adequate, the tissue or organ perfusion can still be inadequate, perhaps indicated by a low SvO_2.

Unfortunately, the SvO_2 can be misleadingly high. Causes of an unexplained increase in SvO_2 are a left-to-right intracardiac shunt, severe mitral regurgitation, or the spurious sampling of blood when the catheter is in the wedged position.[120] A not uncommon critical clinical situation, septic shock, occurs when peripheral utilization of O_2 is decreased because of either peripheral arteriovenous shunting of blood or a reduction in O_2 consumption resulting from cytotoxicity.[121] This situation can usually be recognized because of the simultaneous presence of a metabolic lactic acidosis. Clinically patients demonstrate cold, blue hands and feet because of poor

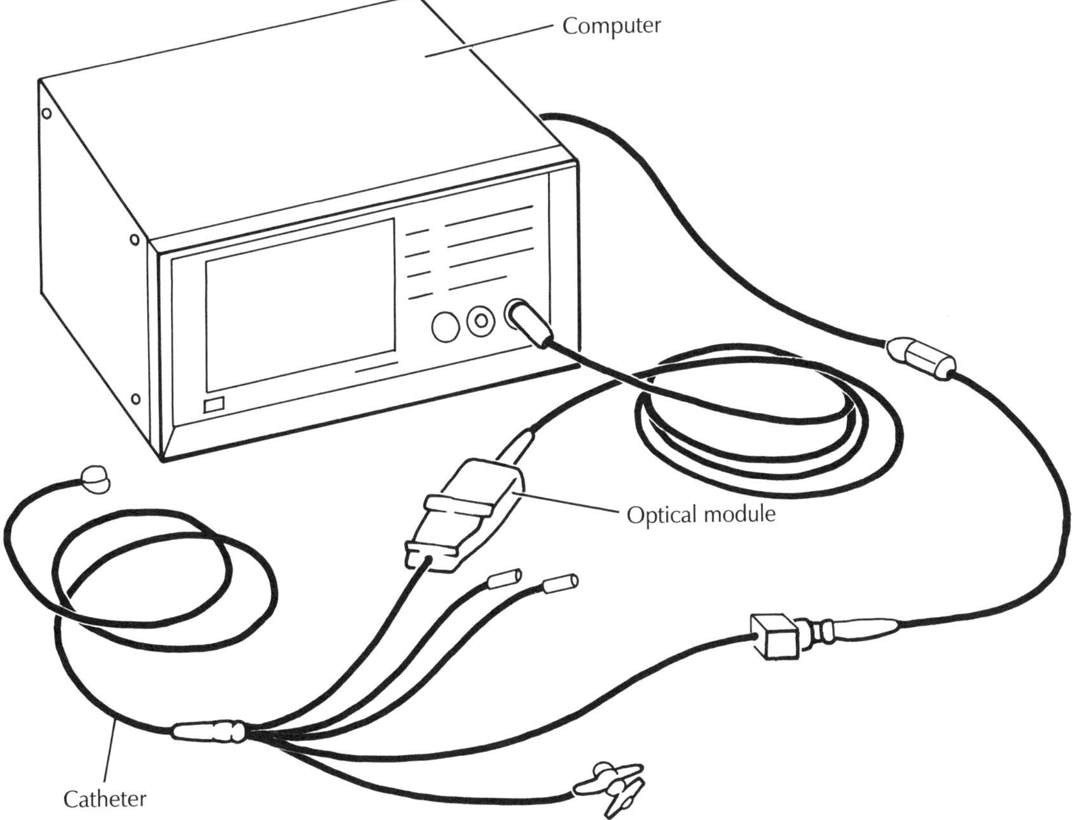

FIG 7–40
The Oximetric 3 system consists of three basic components: (1) various Opticath catheters, each including fiber optics for light transmission, a distal port lumen for conventional catheter uses, and a disposable optical reference packaged with the catheter; (2) an Optimetrix optical module containing three light-emitting diodes, a photodetector, and associated electronics; and (3) an Oximetrix 3 SO_2/CO computer equipped with two groups of control keys and a screen for display of oxygen saturation, thermodilution curves, calculated values, alarm status, and operating instructions for selected functions. (Courtesy of Abbott Laboratories, Mountainview, Calif.)

perfusion of the extremities. Measurements of Spo_2 or $Ptcco_2$ are now inaccurate, and the Svo_2 may be misleadingly high. Thus, monitoring must depend on observing organ function, adequate blood pressure and normal ABGs, urine output, central nervous system responsiveness, liver function tests, etc.

There is currently controversy regarding treatment of multiorgan failure by maximizing the Do_2 with high Fio_2 and high PEEP and maximizing $\dot{Q}_T$ by using cardiotropic drugs.[122–124] Such therapy is reasonable when there is increased blood lactate, increased glycolysis, and metabolic acidosis. The concept that there is abnormal delivery-dependent O_2 consumption is based on the controversial observations that Vo_2 seems to continuously increase in patients with ARDS and sepsis as the delivery of O_2 is increased.[125] These findings are in part due to the lack of steady-state conditions and also to the lack of measurements of Vo_2, independent of $\dot{Q}_T$. When that is done, the Vo_2 is found to be independent of Do_2, except when the Do_2 is critically low and acidosis or elevated blood lactate levels are present.[126–128] If unphysiologic high levels of Sao_2 and $\dot{Q}_T$ are to be used, they should be justified by demonstrating reduced acidosis or better organ perfusion and function and, if available, an independent metabolic cart measurement of improved Vo_2.

Having argued the case for the use of the pulmonary artery catheter and the metabolic cart, it must be added that there are as yet no definitive studies that document benefit from their use. Serious complications directly related to the pulmonary artery catheter have been documented to occur in 3% to 4% of all patients.[129] This has led to a call for a large-scale clinical trial to provide a more precise definition of which patients would most benefit from such intervention.[130]

The development of newer, less invasive modalities for assessing the adequacy of organ perfusion such as

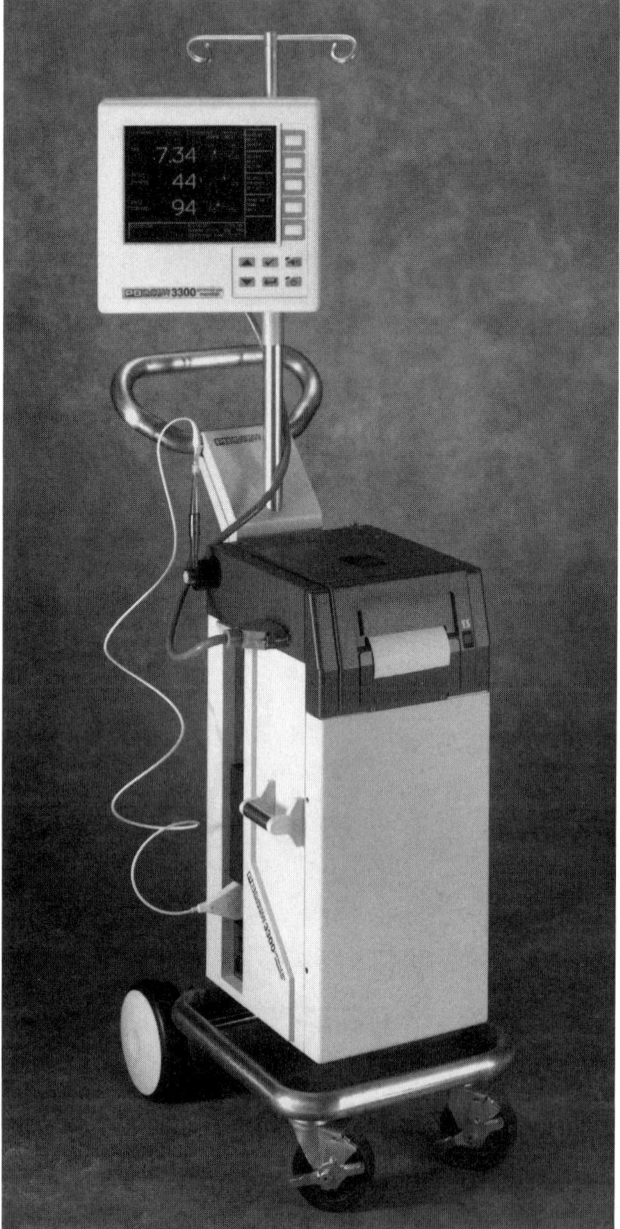

FIG 7–41
The PB-3300 intra-arterial blood gas monitoring system provides continuous blood gas data. Note that the catheter is housed in a sterile calibrating solution on the portable cart. (Courtesy of Puritan-Bennett Corp, Carlsbad, Calif.)

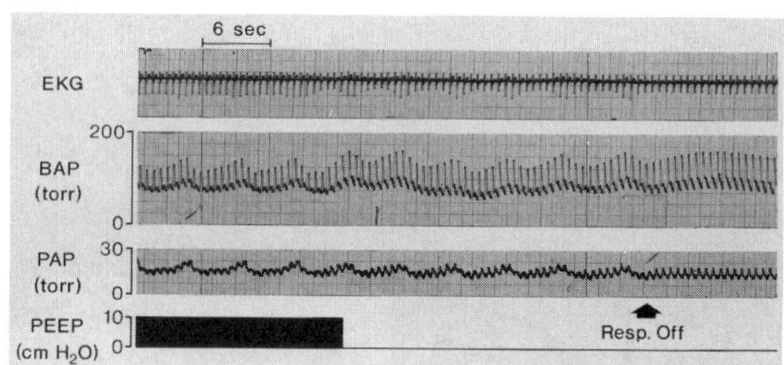

FIG 7–42
Effect of ventilation and airway pressure on hemodynamics. Variation in pulmonary artery pressure *(PAP)* and brachial artery pressures *(BAP)* with ventilation and positive end-expiratory pressure *(PEEP)* is shown in a patient with severely stiff lungs that required high ventilatory pressures. When PEEP is stopped, there is a rise in the pulse pressure and less of a sinusoidal variation or "swing" with each inspiration in both the PAP and BAP. When the ventilator is turned off, there is a further rise in the pulse pressure and complete loss of the "swing." Note that even the ECG shows a "swing" resulting from position change of the heart with each inspiration, thus changing the electrical axis; this is not an indication of conduction abnormalities in the heart. (From Fallat RJ, Osborn JJ: Patient monitoring techniques, in Burton GG (ed): *Respiratory Care: A Guide to Clinical Practice.* Philadelphia, JB Lippincott, 1977. Used by permission.)

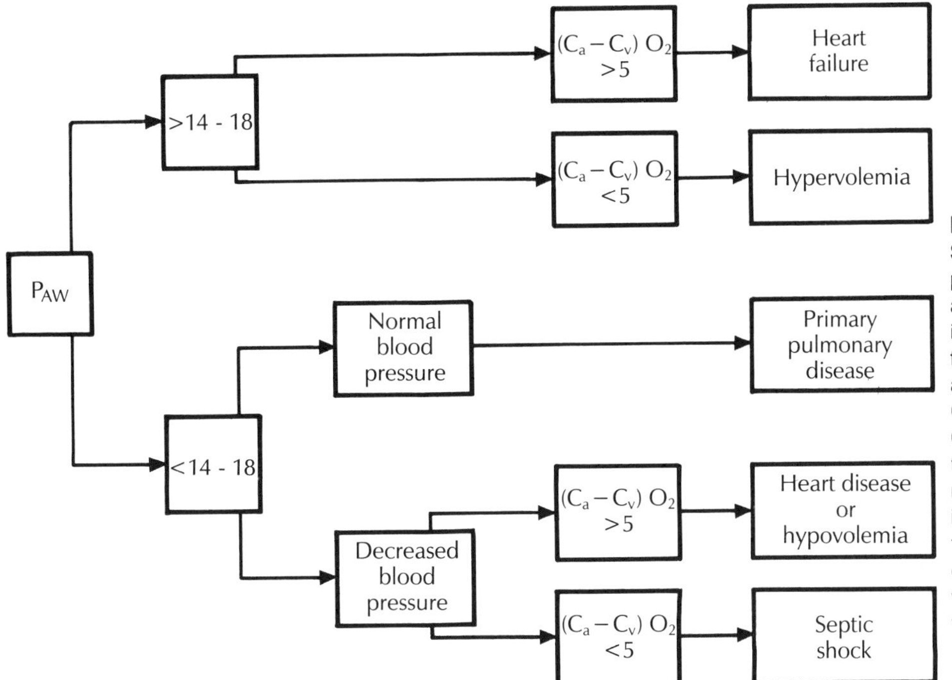

FIG 7–43
Scheme for assessment of causes of pulmonary edema. A high pulmonary artery wedge pressure (P_w) would indicate a hemodynamic cause either from heart failure, which should be associated with a low Q_T of high $(Ca-Cv)O_2$, or from hypervolemia when the Q_T is high and $(Ca-Cv)O_2$ is low. If the P_w is low and there is normal hemodynamics, it is likely ARDS. If P_w is low and blood pressure is low or the patient is in shock, $(Ca - Cv)O_2$ difference may help to determine whether it is due to heart failure, hypovolemia, or sepsis. (From Stevens PM: *Chest* 1975; 67:1. Used by permission.)

gastric tonometry,[131] direct monitoring of cerebral and myocardial O_2 sufficiency by using infrared technology,[132] or magnetic resonance spectroscopy may, in the future, obviate the problems of invasive monitoring, which is our current state of the art.

REFERENCES

1. Zwillich C et al: Complications of assisted ventilation. *Am J Med* 1974; 57:161.
2. American Thoracic Society: Standardization of spirometry 1987 update. *Am Rev Respir Dis* 1987; 130:1296–2009.
3. Lenfant C: Foreword, in *Guidelines for the Diagnosis and Management of Asthma.* U.S. Public Health Service Publication No 91-3042, Bethesda, MD, 1991.
4. Wright BM, McKerrow CB: Maximum forced expiratory flow rate as a measure of ventilatory capacity. *BMJ* 1959; 2:1041–1047.
5. Quakenboss JJ, Lebowitz MD, Krzyzanowski M: The normal range of diurnal changes in peak expiratory flow rates: Relationship to symptoms and respiratory disease. *Am Rev Respir Dis* 1991; 143:323–330.
6. Kacmarek RM, Cycyk-Chapman MC, Young-Palazzo PJ, et al: Determination of maximal inspiratory pressure: A clinical study and literature review. *Respir Care* 1989; 34:868.
7. Black LF, Hyatt RE: Maximal static respiratory pressure in generalized neuromuscular disease. *Am Rev Respir Dis* 1971; 103:641–650.
8. Black LF, Hyatt RE: Maximal respiratory pressures: Normal values and relationship to age and sex. *Am Rev Respir Dis* 1968; 99:696–702.
9. Smyth RJ, Chapman K, Rebuck AS: Maximal inspiratory and expiratory pressures in adolescents. *Chest* 1984; 86:568–572.
10. Tobin MJ: Respiratory monitoring in the intensive care unit. *Am Rev Respir Dis* 1988; 138:1625–1642.
11. Rochester DF, Arora NS: Respiratory muscle failure. *Med Clin North Am* 1983; 67:573–597.
12. Rochester DF, Braun NMT: Determinants of maximal inspiratory pressure in chronic obstructive pulmonary disease. *Am Rev Respir Dis* 1985; 132:42–47.
13. Marini JJ, Smith TC, Lamb V: Estimation of inspiratory muscle strength in mechanically ventilated patients: The measurement of maximal inspiratory pressure. *J Crit Care* 1986; 1:32–38.
14. Sahn SA, Lakshminarayan S: Bedside criteria for discontinuation of mechanical ventilation. *Chest* 1973; 63: 1002–1005.
15. Herrara M, Blasco J, Venegas J, et al: Mouth occlusion pressure ($P_{0.1}$) in acute respiratory failure. *Intensive Care Med* 1985; 11:134–139.
16. Sassoon CSH, Te TT, Mahutte CK, et al: Airway occlusion pressure: An important indication for successful weaning in patients with chronic obstructive pulmonary disease. *Am Rev Respir Dis* 1987; 135:107–113.
17. Murciano D, Aubier M, Lecocguic Y, et al: Tracheal occlusion pressure as an index of respiratory muscle fatigue during acute respiratory failure of COPD patients (abstract). *Am Rev Respir Dis* 1984; 129:34.
18. Montgomery AB, Holle RHO, Neagley SR, et al: Predic-

tion of successful ventilator weaning using airway occlusion pressure and hypercapneic challenge. *Chest* 1987; 91:496–499.

19. Tobin MJ: Noninvasive evaluation of respiratory movement, in Nochomovitz ML, Cherniack NS (eds): *Noninvasive Respiratory Monitoring 1986.* New York, Churchill Livingstone, 1986, pp 29–57.
20. Geddes LA, Baker LE: *Principles of Applied Biomedical Instrumentation* New York, John Wiley & Sons, 1968, pp 150–205.
21. Kubicek WG, Karnegis JN, Patterson RP, et al: Development and evaluation of an impedance cardiac output system. *Aerospace Med* 1966; 37:1208–1212.
22. Bernstein DP: Continuous noninvasive real-time monitoring of stroke volume and cardiac output by thoracic electrical bioimpedance. *Crit Care Med* 1986; 14: 898–901.
23. Konno K, Mead J: Measurement of the separate volume changes of ribcage and abdomen during breathing. *J Appl Physiol* 1967; 22:407.
24. Krieger BP: Ventilatory pattern monitoring: Instrumentation and applications. *Respir Care* 1990; 35:697.
25. Cohen C, Zagelbaum G, Gross D, et al: Clinical manifestations of inspiratory muscle fatigue. *Am J Med* 1982; 73:308–316.
26. Roussos CS, Macklem PT: The respiratory muscles. *N Engl J Med* 1982; 307:786–797.
27. Tobin MJ, Perez W, Guenther SM, et al: Does ribcage abdominal paradox signify respiratory muscle fatigue? *J Appl Physiol* 1987; 63:851–860.
28. MacIntyre NR: Respiratory monitoring without machinery. *Respir Care* 1990; 35:546.
29. Osborn JJ, Beaumont JO, Raison JCA: Computation for quantitative on-line measurements in an intensive care ward, in Stacy RW, Waxman B (eds): *Computers in Biomedical Research.* New York, Academic Press, 1969.
30. Marini JJ, Crooke III PS: A general mathematical model for respiratory dynamics relevant to the clinical setting. *Am Rev Respir Dis* 1993; 147:14–24.
31. Osborn JJ, Beaumont JO, Raison JCA: Measurement and monitoring of acutely ill patients by digital computer. *Surgery* 1968; 64:1057.
32. Fallat RJ, McQuitty JC: Bedside testing and intensive care monitoring of pulmonary function, in Clausen JL (ed): *Pulmonary Function Testing Guidelines and Controversies.* London, Grune & Stratton, 1984, pp 293–310.
33. Fallat RJ: Respiratory monitoring. *Clin Chest Med* 1982; 3:181.
34. Marini JJ: Monitoring during mechanical ventilation. *Clin Chest Med* 1988; 9:73–100.
35. Bone R: Thoracic pressure-volume curves in respiratory failure. *Crit Care Med* 1976; 4:148.
36. Sly PD, Bates JHT, Milic-Emili J: Measurement of respiratory mechanics using the Siemens Servo Ventilator 900C. *Pediatr Pulmonol* 1987; 3:400–405.
37. Pepe PE, Marini JJ: Occult positive end-expiratory pressure in mechanically ventilated patients with airflow obstruction. *Am Rev Respir Dis* 1982; 126:166.
38. Brown DG, Pierson DJ: Auto-PEEP is common in mechanically ventilated patients: A study of incidence, severity, and detection. *Respir Care* 1986; 31:1069–1074.
39. Aldrich TK, Hendler JM, Vizioli LD, et al: Intrinsic positive end-expiratory pressure in ambulatory patients with airways obstruction. *Am Rev Respir Dis* 1993; 147:845–849.
40. Grootendorst AF, Lugtigheid G, van der Weygert EJ: Error in ventilator measurements of intrinsic PEEP: Cause and remedy. *Respir Care* 1993; 38:348–350.
41. East TD: What makes noninvasive monitoring tick? A review of basic engineering principles. *Respir Care* 1990; 35:500.
42. Gilbert R, Keighley JF: The arterial/alveolar oxygen tension ratio: An index of gas exchange applicable to varying inspired oxygen concentrations. *Am Rev Respir Dis* 1974; 109:142–145.
43. Gilbert R, Auchincloss JH Jr, Kuppinger M, et al: Stability of the arterial/alveolar oxygen partial pressure ratio: Effects of low ventilation/perfusion regions. *Crit Care Med* 1979; 7:267–272.
44. Covelli HD, Nessan VJ, Tuttle WK: Oxygen derived variables in acute respiratory failure. *Crit Care Med* 1983; 11:646–649.
45. Maunder RJ, Hudson LD: Respiratory monitoring in the intensive care unit, in Shoemaker WC, Abraham E (eds): *Diagnostic Methods in Critical Care.* New York, Marcel Dekker, 1987, pp 33–45.
46. Stoller JK: Therapeutic manipulation of oxygen consumption and carbon dioxide production in acute respiratory failure. *Respir Care* 1993; 38:769–783.
47. Silberman H, Silberman AW: Parenteral nutrition, biochemistry and respiratory gas exchange. *JPEN J Parenter Enterol Nutr* 1986; 10:151–154.
48. van den Berg B, Stam H: Metabolic and respiratory effects of enteral nutrition in patients during mechanical ventilation. *Intensive Care Med* 1988; 14:206–211.
49. Askanazi J, Rosenbaum SH, Hyman AI, et al: Respiratory changes induced by the large glucose loads of total parenteral nutrition. *JAMA* 1980; 243:1444–1447.
50. Rutten P, Blackburn GL, Flatt JP, et al: Determination of optimal hyperalimentation infusion rate. *J Surg Res* 1975; 18:477–483.
51. Long CL, Schaffel N, Geiger JW, et al: Metabolic response to injury and illness: Estimation of energy and protein needs from indirect calorimetry and nitrogen balance. *JPEN J Parenter Enterol Nutr* 1979; 3:452–456.
52. Foster GD, Knox LS, Dempsey DT, et al: Caloric requirements in total parenteral nutrition. *J Am Coll Nutr* 1987; 6:231–253.
53. Weissman C, Kemper M, Askanazi J, et al: Resting metabolic rate in the critically ill patient: Measured vs. predicted. *Anesthesiology* 1986; 64:673.
54. Hunker FD, Burton CW, Hunker EM, et al: Metabolic and nutritional evaluation of patients supported with mechanical ventilation. *Crit Care Med* 1980; 8:628–631.
55. Browning JA, Linberg SE, Turney SZ, et al: The effects of a fluctuating F_{IO_2} on metabolic measurements in me-

chanically ventilated patients. *Crit Care Med* 1982; 10:82–85.
56. Kinney et al: A method for continuous measurement of gas exchange and expired radioactivity in acutely ill patients. *Metabolism* 1964; 13:205–211.
57. Severinghaus JW, Astrup PB: History of blood gas analysis vs. oximetry. *J Clin Monit* 1986; 2:270–88.
58. Clark JS, Vottieri B, Ariagno RL, et al: State of the art: Noninvasive assessment of blood gases. *Am Rev Respir Dis* 1992; 145:220–232.
59. Severinghaus JW: Historical development of oxygenation monitoring, in Payne JP, Severinghaus JW (eds): *Pulse Oximetry.* Berlin, Springer-Verlag, 1986, pp 1–18.
60. Eberhard P, Severinghaus JW: Measurement of heated skin O_2 diffusion conductance and Po_2 sensor induced O_2 gradient. *Acta Anaesthesiol Scand Suppl* 1978; 68:1–4.
61. Steinacker JM, Spittelmeister W: Dependence of transcutaneous O_2 partial pressure on cutaneous blood flow. *J Appl Physiol* 1988; 64:21–25.
62. Severinghaus JW, Stafford M, Bradley AF: $TcPco_2$ electrode design, calibration and temperature gradient problems. *Acta Anesthesiol Scand Suppl* 1987; 68:118–122.
63. Eletr S, Jinison H, Ream AK, et al: Cutaneous monitoring of systemic Pco_2 on patients in the respiratory intensive care unit being weaned from the ventilator. *Acta Anaesthesiol Scand Suppl* 1978; 68:123–127.
64. Severinghaus JW: A combined transcutaneous Po_2-Pco_2 electrode with electrochemical HCO_3 stabilization. *J Appl Physiol* 1981; 51:1027–1032.
65. McLellan PA, Goldstein RS, Ramcharan V, et al: Transcutaneous carbon dioxide monitoring. *Am Rev Respir Dis* 1981; 124:199–201.
66. Rahn H, Farhi LE: Ventilation, perfusion and gas exchange: The V/Q concept, in Fenn WO, Rahn H (eds): *Handbook of Physiology,* vol 1. Washington, DC, American Physiology Society, 1954, pp 735–766.
67. Luft UC, Loepky JA, Mostyn EM: Mean alveolar gases and alveolar-arterial gradients in pulmonary patients. *J Appl Physiol* 1979; 46:534–540.
68. Falk JL, Rackow EC, Weil MH: End-tidal carbon dioxide concentration during cardiopulmonary resuscitation. *N Engl J Med* 1988; 318:607–611.
69. Bland DK, Anholm JD: Arterial oxygen saturation during exercise: Erroneous results with ear oximetry (abstract). *Am Rev Respir Dis* 1988; 137:150.
70. Hansen JE, Casaburi R: Validity of ear oximetry in clinical exercise testing. *Chest* 1987; 91:333–337.
71. Smyth RJ, D'Urzo AD, Slutsky AS, et al: Ear oximetry during combined hypoxia and exercise. *J Appl Physiol* 1986; 60:716–719.
72. Ries AL, Farrow JT, Clausen JL: Accuracy of two ear oximeters at rest and during exercise in pulmonary patients. *Am Rev Respir Dis* 1985; 132:685–689.
73. American Society of Anesthesiologists: *Standards for Basic Intra-operative Monitoring.* ASA Directory of Members, Philadelphia, 1991, pp 670–671.
74. Conference report: Further recommendations for prescribing and supplying long-term oxygen. *Am Rev Respir Dis* 1988; 138:745–747.
75. Carlin BW, Clausen JL, Ries AL: The use of cutaneous oximetry in the prescription of long-term oxygen therapy. *Chest* 1988; 94:239–244.
76. Criteria for Medicare coverage of oxygen services in the home. *Fed Register* April 5, 1985, p 50.
77. Huch A, Huch R: Transcutaneous, noninvasive monitoring of Po_2. *Hosp Pract* 1976; 11:43–52.
78. Monaco F, Nickerson BG, McQuitty J: Continuous transcutaneous oxygen and carbon dioxide monitoring in the pediatric ICU. *Crit Care Med* 1982; 10:765–766.
79. Yahav J, Mindorff C, Levison H: The validity of the transcutaneous oxygen tension method in children with cardiorespiratory problems. *Am Rev Respir Dis* 1981; 124: 586–587.
80. Burki NK, Albert RK: Noninvasive monitoring of arterial blood gases. A report of the ACCP section on respiratory physiology. *Chest* 1983; 83:666–669.
81. Eberhard P, Mindt W, Schafer R: Cutaneous blood gas monitoring in the adult. *Crit Care Med* 1981; 9: 702–705.
82. Wyss CR, Matsen FA III, King RV, et al: Dependence of transcutaneous oxygen tension on local arteriovenous pressure gradient in normal subjects. *Clin Sci* 1981; 60:499–506.
83. Rome ES, Stork EK, Carlo WA, et al: Limitations of transcutaneous Po_2 and transcutaneous Pco_2 monitoring in infants with bronchopulmonary dysplasia. *Pediatrics* 1984; 74:217–220.
84. Durand M, Ramanathan R: Pulse oximetry for continuous oxygen monitoring in sick newborn infants. *J Pediatr* 1986; 109:1052–1056.
85. Bucher HU, Fanconi S, Baeckert P, et al: Hyperoxemia in newborn infants: Detection by pulse oximetry. *Pediatrics* 1989; 84:226–230.
86. Jones NL, McHardy GJR, Naimark A, et al: Physiological dead space and alveolar-arterial gas pressure differences during exercise. *Clin Sci* 1966; 31:19–29.
87. Hansen JE, Sue DY, Wasserman K: Predicted values for clinical exercise testing. *Am Rev Respir Dis* 1984; 129(suppl):49–55.
88. Rithalia SVS: Clinical application of transcutaneous carbon dioxide monitoring. *Intensive Care World* 1985; 2:3–6.
89. Mahutte CK, Michiels TM, Hassell KT, et al: Evaluation of a single transcutaneous Po_2-Pco_2 sensor in adult patients. *Crit Care Med* 1984; 12:1063–1066.
90. Williams R, Riker R, Narkewicz M, et al: Uses of an iridium-oxide electrode on adult surgical patients. *Crit Care Med* 1985; 13:848–850.
91. Greenspan GH, Bolck AJ, Halderman LW, et al: Transcutaneous noninvasive monitoring of carbon dioxide tension. *Chest* 1981; 80:442–446.
92. Swan HJG, Ganz W, Forrester J, et al: Catheterization on the heart in man with use of a flow-directed balloon-tipped catheter. *N Engl J Med* 1970; 283:447–451.
93. Marshall HW, Helmholz HF, Woods EH: Physiological consequences of congenital heart disease, in Hamilton

WF, Dow P (eds): *Handbook of Physiology,* vol 1. Washington, DC, American Physiological Society, 1962, p 417.
94. Geddes LA: *The Direct and Indirect Measurement of Blood Pressure.* St Louis, Mosby–Year Book, 1970.
95. Erlanger J: A new instrument for determining the minimum and maximum blood pressures in man. *Johns Hopkins Hosp Rep* 1903; 12:53–110.
96. Boehmer RD: Continuous, real-time, noninvasive monitoring of blood pressure: Peñaz methodology applied to the finger. *J Clin Monit* 1987; 3:23.
97. Molhoek GP, Wesseling KH, Settels JJ, et al: Evaluation of the Peñaz servo-plethysmomanometer for the continuous, noninvasive measurement of finger blood pressure. *Basic Res Cardiol* 1984; 79:558–609.
98. Gravenstein JS, Paulus DA, Feldman J, et al: Tissue hypoxia distal to a Peñaz finger blood pressure cuff. *J Clin Monit* 1985; 1:120–125.
99. Gardner RM, Chapman RH: Trouble-shooting pressure monitoring systems: When do the numbers lie? in Fallat RJ, Luce JM (eds): *Cardiopulmonary Critical Care Management.* New York, Churchill Livingstone, 1988, p 145.
100. Maloy L, Gardner RM: Monitoring systemic arterial blood pressure: Strip recording versus digital display. *Heart Lung* 1986; 15:627.
101. Cengiz M, Crapo RO, Gardner RM: The effect of ventilation on the accuracy of pulmonary artery and wedge pressure measurements. *Crit Care Med* 1983; 11:502.
102. Goldberg RJ: Risks and benefits of pulmonary artery catheterization. *J Intensive Care Med* 1988; 3:69–70.
103. Fallat RJ: Hemodynamic monitoring, in Clausen JL, Zarins LP (eds): *Pulmonary Function Testing Guidelines and Controversies.* New York, Academic Press, 1982, p 311.
104. Culver BH: Hemodynamic monitoring: Physiological problems in interpretation, in Fallat RJ, Luce JM (eds): *Cardiopulmonary Critical Care Management.* New York, Churchill Livingstone, 1988, p 165.
105. Donovan KD, Dobb GJ, Woods WPD, et al: Comparison of transthoracic electrical impedance and thermodilution method for measuring cardiac output. *Crit Care Med* 1986; 14:1038–1044.
106. Abrams JH, Weber RE, Holmen KD: Continuous cardiac output determination using transtracheal Doppler: Initial results in humans. *Anesthesiology* 1989; 71:11–15.
107. Clausen JP, Larsen OA, Trap-Jensen J: Cardiac output in middle-aged patients determined with CO_2 rebreathing method. *J Appl Physiol* 1970; 28:337–342.
108. Mahler DA, Matthay RA, Snyder PE, et al: Determination of cardiac output at rest and during exercise by carbon dioxide rebreathing method in obstructive airway disease. *Am Rev Respir Dis* 1985; 131:73–78.
109. Muiesan G, Sorbini CA, Solinas E, et al: Comparison of CO_2 rebreathing and Fick methods for determining cardiac output. *J Appl Physiol* 1968; 24:424–429.
110. Smith AS, Russell AE, West MJ, et al: Automated noninvasive measurement of cardiac output: Comparison of bioimpedance and carbon dioxide rebreathing techniques. *Br Heart J* 1988; 59:292–298.
111. Stetz CW, Miller RG, Kelly GE, et al: Reliability of the thermodilution method in the determination of cardiac output in clinical practice. *Am Rev Respir Dis* 1982; 126:1001–1004.
112. Shapiro BA: In-vivo monitoring of arterial blood gases and pH. *Respir Care* 1992; 37:165–169.
113. Gottlieb A, Divers S, Hui HK: In vivo applications of fiberoptic chemical sensors, in Wise DL, Wingard LB (eds): *Biosensors With Fiberoptics.* Clifton, NJ, Humana Press, 1991, pp 325–366.
114. Peterson JL, Vuerk GG: Fiber-optic sensors for biomedical applications. *Science* 1984; 224:123–127.
115. Brown EG, Krouskop RW, McDonnell FE, et al: A technique to continuously measure arteriovenous oxygen content difference and P_{50} in vivo. *J Appl Physiol* 1985; 58:1383–1389.
116. Gehrich JL, Lubbers DW, Opitz N, et al: Optical fluorescence and its application to an intravascular blood gas monitoring system. *IEEE Trans Biomed Eng* 1986; 33: 117–132.
117. Fallat RJ, Osborn JJ: Patient monitoring techniques, in Burton GG (ed): *Respiratory Care: A Guide to Clinical Practice.* Philadelphia, JP Lippincott, 1977.
118. Stevens PM: Assessment of acute respiratory failure: Cardiac versus pulmonary causes (editorial). *Chest* 1975; 67:1.
119. Suter PM, Fairley HB, Isenberg MD: Optimal end-expiratory pressure in patients with acute pulmonary failure. *N Engl J Med* 1975; 191:184.
120. Suter PM, Lindauer JM, Fairley HB, et al: Errors in data derived from pulmonary artery blood gas values. *Crit Care Med* 1975; 3:175.
121. Dorinsky PM, Gadek JE: Mechanisms of multiple nonpulmonary organ failure in ARDS. *Chest* 1989; 96:885.
122. Tuchschmidt J, Fried J, Astiz M, et al: Supranormal oxygen delivery improves mortality in septic shock patients (abstract). *Crit Care Med* 1991; 19(suppl 4):66.
123. Martin C, Saux P, Eon B, et al: Septic shock: A goal directed therapy using volume loading, dobutamine and/or norepinephrine. *Acta Anaesthesiol Scand* 1990; 34:413–417.
124. Tuchschmidt J, Fried J, Astiz M, et al: Elevation of cardiac output and oxygen delivery improves outcome in septic shock. *Chest* 1992; 102:216–220.
125. Danek SJ, Lynch J, Weg J, et al: The dependence of oxygen uptake on oxygen delivery in the adult respiratory distress syndrome. *Am Rev Respir Dis* 1980; 122:387–395.
126. Kruse JA, Haupt MT, Puri VK, et al: Lactate levels as predictors of the relationship between oxygen delivery and consumption in ARDS. *Chest* 1990; 98:959–962.
127. Vincent J-L, Roman A, De Backer D, et al: Oxygen uptake/supply dependency: Effects of short-term dobutamine infusion. *Am Rev Respir Dis* 1990; 142:2–7.
128. Ronco JJ, Phang PT, Walley KR, et al: Oxygen consumption is independent of changes in oxygen delivery in se-

vere adult respiratory distress syndrome. *Am Rev Respir Dis* 1991; 143:1267–1273.

129. Boyd KD, Thomas SJ, Gold J, et al: A prospective study of complications of pulmonary artery catheterization in 500 consecutive patients. *Chest* 1983; 84:245–249.
130. Robin ED: Death by pulmonary artery flow-directed catheter. Time for a moratorium? (editorial). *Chest* 1987; 92:727–731.
131. Gutierrez G, Palizas F, Doglio G, et al: Gastric intramucosal pH as a therapeutic index of tissue oxygenation in critically ill patients. *Lancet* 1992; 339:195–99.
132. Jöbsis FF. Noninvasive, infrared monitoring of cerebral and myocardial oxygen sufficiency and circulatory parameters. *Science* 1977; 198:1264–1266.

8

Cardiopulmonary Laboratory Instrumentation

MICHAEL SNOW, R.P.F.T.
ROBERT FALLAT, M.D.

OBJECTIVES

- Explain why it is important to be able to differentiate between the various types of cardiopulmonary instruments.
- Differentiate between the various methods for measuring airflow and lung volumes.
- Compare the instruments used in pulmonary function systems to analyze gases.
- Contrast the various pulmonary function systems presented in this chapter.
- Differentiate between the three types of body plethysomographs.
- Describe the methodology for measuring the heart-lung response to exercise.
- Distinguish between the various types of oxygen and carbon dioxide sensors presented in this chapter.
- Appraise the methodology for diagnosing sleep apnea.

Cardiopulmonary laboratories provide quantitative analysis of functional changes in the cardiovascular and pulmonary systems. Many of these measurements involve static testing of volumes and capacities. Others measure interrelationships of responses to external interventions such as exercise or bronchoactive agents. Specific patterns of functional impairment are usually associated with changes in pathology or the physiologic responses to these stimuli. Clinical treatment may be based on these inferred processes.

Distinct diagnostic instrumentation has been developed to reflect or drive our understanding of the interrelationship of these physiologic processes. Currently, cardiopulmonary laboratory instrumentation may be loosely grouped into five general categories: (1) pulmonary function testing, (2) cardiovascular and pulmonary stress testing, (3) blood gas analysis, (4) bronchoscopy, and (5) sleep disorders.

There is substantial commonality to many of the instrumentation used for the different categories. Despite this, the different applications have led to the development of numerous modifications to the basic sensor packages that improve performance for a specific application. Many of these changes are the result of technological advances, and others reflect adaptation of techniques originally designed for some other purpose.

As a result of this evolving technology and the widespread use of computers to control data acquisition, methodology, and presentation, differentiation between manufacturers may be very subtle. Accordingly, great emphasis is placed by manufacturers on differentiating their system from others. These differences may have a profound impact on test results or may make absolutely no significant difference. Accordingly, featured claims of improved technology should always have at least a plausible association with a clinically meaningful benefit or be recognized as packaging.

Ease of use and "user friendly software" are claims made by nearly every manufacturer. Hardware design certainly plays an important role, but ultimately the software user interface is probably the determining factor. Similarity to previous systems plays a role in determining how intuitive the interface is. Also, the closer the interface can mimic existing laboratory methodology and clinical practice, the more friendly a system will seem. There are an astonishing number of subtle nuances that affect the interface. All manufacturers have developed their software over several years—adding and streamlining features based on customer preferences. Ultimately, the only way to determine how easy a system is to use is to use it in your environment.

Various groups such as the American Thoracic

Society (ATS), American College of Sports Medicine (ACSM), and the American Heart Association (AHA) have promulgated recommendations for standardized terminology and procedures as well as equipment performance standards. Currently, procedural recommendations exist for spirometry, diffusing capacity, selection of lung function reference values, flexible endoscopy for pediatrics, and exercise testing.[1–6] A set of recommendations for lung volume determination is under development. Most commercially available systems meet or exceed these recommendations. Manufacturers will provide some documentation of their compliance if requested.

Evaluation of instruments for replacement of existing systems must include detailed understanding of the actual methodology used in the measurement as well as a comparison of results with the current system. Many newer systems use subtly different algorithms or technology, which can introduce a systematic error when comparing dissimilar equipment. For example, before the ATS recommendations for single-breath diffusion, systems did not always subtract apparatus and patient dead space before the calculation of alveolar volume. This is approximately a 200-mL correction. For a subject with a 2.0-L vital capacity (VC), this will cause a 10% difference depending on whether or not the dead space is subtracted not only for alveolar volume but also for diffusing capacity. Although these changes may be justifiable and even desirable, it is important to consciously decide to accept the resulting differences in data rather than discover them a year or so later.

Finally, caution should always be used when evaluating claims made by manufacturers without independent confirmation. The history of independent testing of spirometers showed that only 46% of the systems tested in 1979 met minimum recommended performance guidelines.[7] Eight years later, the tests were repeated with only slight improvement in the percentage of acceptable systems.[8]

As another example, when evaluating gas analyzers, accuracy or linearity specifications are frequently given as plus or minus a percentage of full scale or plus or minus a percentage of reading. These have totally different meanings. A claim of ±0.5% full scale on an oxygen analyzer, with a scale of 0% to 100%, would translate to a claim that when reading room air, the analyzer will display a value between 20.43% and 21.43%. This is clearly inadequate for any measurement of gas exchange. On the other hand, a claim of ±0.05% of reading would translate to a observed value between 20.92% and 20.94.0%.

Occasionally manufacturers resort to what may be called "specsmanship," i.e., emphasizing the best numbers while obscuring the meaning. An example of this would be comparing an accuracy claim of 0.03% O_2 with a claim of ±0.05% of reading. Superficially, it would seem that the first analyzer is more accurate since 0.03% is less than 0.05%. However, the 0.03% is an absolute accuracy for the scale of 0% to 100%. It implies that if the actual reading is 20.93, you will recover a value between 20.90 and 20.96. The analyzer with a specification of ±0.05% of reading would recover a value between 20.92 and 20.94. In fact, if you calculate the error as a percentage of reading, the stated ±0.03% O_2 specification would actually translate to ±0.14% specification.

PULMONARY FUNCTION TESTING SYSTEMS

Pulmonary function testing provides information on the lungs' ability to provide gas exchange. This process involves the movement of air into and from the lung, distribution of the inspired air to functional alveolar capillary units, and the transfer of oxygen and carbon dioxide between alveolar gas and the pulmonary capillary blood volume. Frequently, this evaluation is made in association with the administration of bronchodilators or bronchoconstrictive agents to evaluate the reactivity of the airways and the response to therapy. The patterns of dysfunction or responses provide a method of classification and a guide for therapeutic intervention.

Generally, classification of pulmonary function results are made into obstructive, restrictive, pulmonary vascular, or mixed patterns. Within each pattern, there are further categories such as bronchospasm, compression, or occlusive types of obstruction. Lung diffusion impairment may be associated with any of these patterns or may be manifested as a singular abnormality. Table 8–1 illustrates a typical classification scheme with associated functional impairments.

Pulmonary function systems typically provide the capability to assess flow and volume relationships, diffusing capacity for carbon monoxide, and static lung volumes. Airflow assessment is performed by using spirometry, either with flow-based or volume displacement devices. Diffusing capacity measurements are generally performed by using a single-breath technique. Lung volume determination is generally made by dilutional techniques such as nitrogen washout and helium dilution or by body plethysmography.

Spirometry and Airflow Assessment

Spirometry, originally described by Hutchinson[9] as a measurement of the respirable air, was modified by Tiffineau and Pinelli[10] and Gaensler[11] to include timed volumes. The addition of direct measurement of flow was

TABLE 8–1

Classification of Functional Impairments

Impairment	Flow	Volumes	Diffusion	Distribution
Obstructive				
Bronchospasm	Reduced, reversible	High	Normal/high	Abnormal
Airway compression	Expiratory collapse	High	Low	Abnormal
Upper airway	Inspiration reduced	Normal	Normal	Normal
Small airway	Terminal flows reduced	RV* high	Normal	Variable
Mixed	Collapse, partial reversibility	High	Low	Abnormal
Restrictive				
Parenchymal removal	Normal FEV_1/FVC*	Low	Low	Normal
Parenchymal infiltration	High FEV_1/FVC	Low	Low	Abnormal
Extrapulmonary	Normal FEV_1/FVC	Low TLC,* high RV	Normal	Variable
Reduced force	Reduced	Low TLC, high RV	Normal	Normal
Vascular				
Occlusion	Normal	Normal	Low	Normal

* RV = residual volume; FEV_1 = forced expiratory volume in 1 second; FVC = forced vital capacity; TLC = total lung capacity.

popularized by Hyatt et al.[12] The interrelationship of flow, volume, and time provides essential information regarding the elastic and resistive properties of the lung. Currently, the measurement of spirometry or flow-volume curves is the most common pulmonary function test. This test may be performed in the laboratory, in a private office, or at the bedside.

The instruments designed to make these measurements can be roughly categorized as flow-based or volume displacement devices. Most of the earlier pulmonary function systems involved volume displacement. As the flow technology advanced and the application for airflow assessment sensors expanded into screening spirometers, cardiopulmonary exercise systems, and metabolic carts, the trend has been increasingly toward flow-based systems. This trend has been accelerated by the concerns regarding cross-contamination between patients. Currently, the majority of systems being sold are flow based.

Volume Displacement Devices

As the name implies, movement of air into the device displaces a sensor, which provides a calibrated output. Originally, the sensing element was a cylindrical metal bell connected to a pen by a chain and pulley. As the bell rose, the pen would lower and provide a permanent record of the volume displaced. Over time, the metal bell and chain have been replaced by a directly connected pen and a lightweight plastic bell to minimize errors resulting from flexing of the chain and inertia of the metal bell. Other changes have incorporated a rolling dry seal instead of water. Newer designs changed the shape of the displacement device. Pistons and bellows were used in varying designs. All of these design changes were focused on minimizing the effects of inertia and resistance and reducing the size and weight of the device.

As technology changed, the transducer changed also. The pen gave way to an electrical output generated by a rotary potentiometer that was essentially a variable resistor. Linear displacement optical sensors using digital encoding increasingly replaced potentiometers, reduced noise, and increased precision. Regardless of the technological improvements, the devices remained conceptually faithful to the original design. The most common types of volume displacement devices are illustrated in Figure 8–1.

Whereas volume is measured directly, flow must be differentiated from the volume and time signals. The advantages of this approach are reliability, low cost, and simplicity. As the systems became more automated and complex, these advantages became less apparent. Perhaps the most important disadvantage of these systems is the inability to clean or decontaminate the device in a practical sense. It is very difficult to disassemble a piston or bellows device for cleaning. Although a water seal cylinder can be disassembled, draining the water is a cumbersome process that tends not to be done with regularity.

Flow Sensors

Laminar Flow Sensors

Most current flow sensors can be categorized as laminar or turbulent flow devices. Laminar flow devices, such as Lilly- or Fleisch-type pneumotachographs, are essentially a fixed-diameter tube designed to ensure laminar flow and incorporate a resistance that generates a differential pressure proportional to flow. The concept for this approach is the application of Poiseuille's

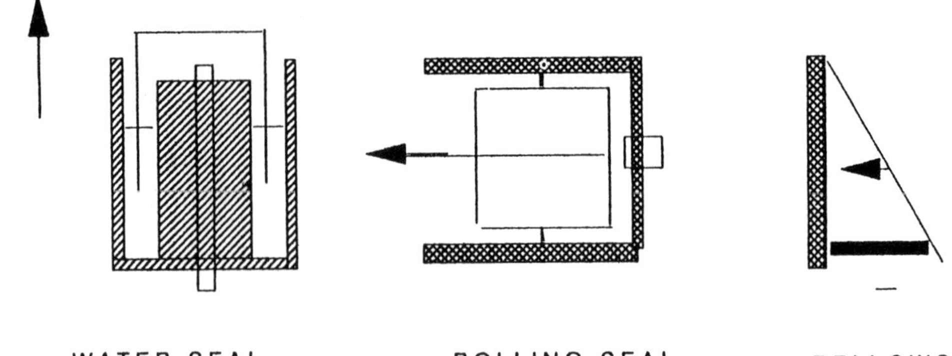

FIG 8–1
Volume displacement spirometers. (From Snow MG: Assessment of airflow In: *Foundations of Respiratory Care*, Churchill Livingston, 1992. Used by permission.)

principle. In general terms, flow through a tube occurs because of a difference in pressure between the two ends. Increases in this differential pressure will result in higher flows. An important consideration is the loading effect that too high a resistance can place on a patient's already impaired respiratory system. The resistive element varies depending on the type of pneumotachograph, but it is generally either a cluster of parallel capillary tubes (Fleisch) or a mesh screen (Lilly/Silverman). Figure 8–2 illustrates Lilly- and Fleisch-type pneumotachographs.

The Fleisch-type pneumotachograph tends to be more sensitive to upstream and downstream geometry and more susceptible to phase lags between flow and the differential pressure and has a more limited dynamic range. To accommodate a wide range of flows, Fleisch-type pneumotachographs are offered in a variety of sizes. The size selected depends on the maximal flows to be measured. The resistive element is susceptible to partial occlusion of the capillary tubes because of condensation or particle deposition. Generally, the resistive element is heated to minimize condensation, and the pneumotachograph is installed with tapered adapters to reduce turbulent flow patterns.

The Lilly-type pneumotachograph consists of three parallel screens mounted with pressure ports to measure the pressure drop across the middle screen. The outer screens serve primarily to produce laminar flow across the middle screen and to protect the middle screen. All three screens are heated to minimize condensation. The three screens, in conjunction with tapered connectors, tend to make this type of pneumotachograph less sensitive to airway geometry and give it a somewhat wider dynamic range. In pediatric applications, a single screen is used with a smaller cross section. Many screening spirometers use a single-screen disposable sensor.

Turbulent Flow Sensors

Turbulent flow sensors make no attempt to maintain laminar flow profiles and thus are less affected by circuit geometry. Turbulent flow sensors without resistive elements measure changes in differential pressure as a function of the square of flow. Perhaps the most common example of a nonresistive flow sensor is the Pitot tube. The Pitot tube measures airflow as a function of the difference between the impact pressure or velocity pressure and the static or downstream pressure. An example of a Pitot tube–type sensor is shown in Figure 8–3.

The fact that the flow sensors have a wetted surface

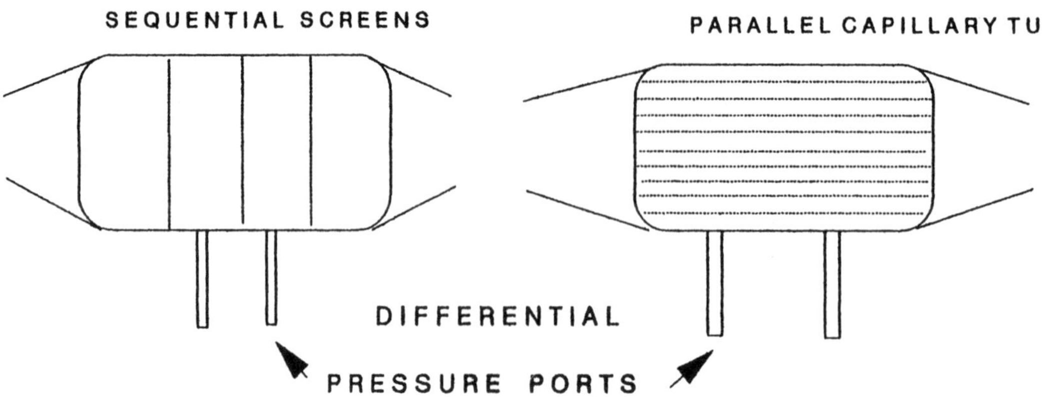

FIG 8–2
Lilly- and Fleisch-type pneumotachographs. (From Snow MG: Assessment of airflow In: *Foundations of Respiratory Care*, Churchill Livingston, 1992. Used by permission.)

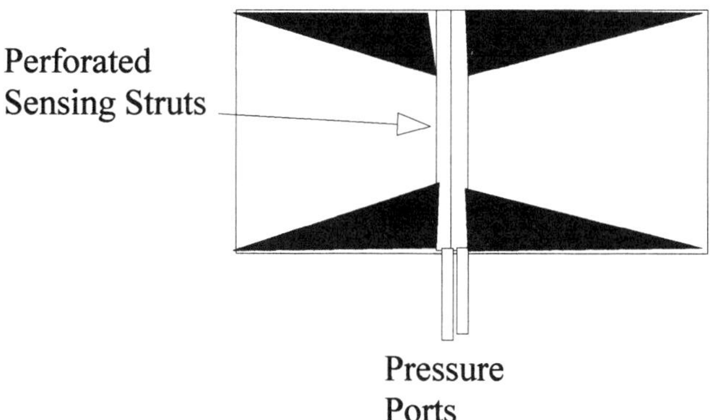

FIG 8–3
Pitot tube–type sensor.

means that the device must be replaced or decontaminated between patients. The resistive elements, since they are carefully constructed to ensure laminar flow, are typically a relatively high-cost item that may preclude single use. Decontamination, either by immersion in cold solutions or by gas sterilization, can be a time-consuming and inconvenient process.

Hot-Wire Anemometers

Another type of flow sensor is to equate flow to the convective cooling effect of airflow over a heated wire. The heat extraction is proportional to the mass of the gas flowing over the heated element. By measuring this extraction it is possible to assess the airflow. A more recent innovation in this technology is the introduction of the constant temperature/current ratio.

By this approach, two heated wires are placed in the flow path. The wires are heated to specific, different temperatures by a controller that monitors the current required to heat the wires. The ratio of the current for the two wires is established. As air flows across the wires, the wires will cool. The rate of cooling is a function of the airflow and the thermal conductivity of the gas mixture. The controller attempts to correct for the heat loss induced by the gas flowing over the surface of the wires by changing the current. The heat extraction from a single wire will be affected by air temperature changes. However, by comparing the ratio of the current required to maintain temperature on both wires, the device will measure convective cooling from airflow rather that artifacts resulting from air temperature changes.

This type of device is not sensitive to water vapor or the temperature or viscosity of the measured gas, but it is sensitive to moisture buildup as well as the adhesion of materials such as sputum or cleansing solutions. Periodic use of a high-temperature circuit provides a self-cleaning function to burn off foreign materials. A drawback to the use of hot-wire anemometers is the inability to determine flow direction. Convective cooling occurs regardless of flow direction, and the sensor records the magnitude of the airflow, not the direction. Some systems use a separate sensor to record direction; others isolate the anemometer with a nonrebreathing valve. Figure 8–4 shows a hot-wire anemometer.

General Considerations for Flow Sensors

The presence of condensation or accumulation of particulate matter on the sensing elements of any type of flow sensor can alter the resistance or the pressure/flow phase relationship. For this reason, it is important to visually inspect any reusable flow sensor periodically and to ensure that the screen is adequately rinsed after immersion sterilization. Condensation is generally not a problem during spirometry, and many screening spirometers are not heated. Condensation may be more of a problem during rebreathing tests, exercise testing, or extended metabolic measurements where heated screens cannot accommodate the increased moisture volume.

Pressure Transducers

The differential pressure produced by the pneumotachograph is measured by a pressure transducer. This device generally consists of a diaphragm that is deformed by the applied pressure. The amount of deformity is directly proportional to the magnitude of the applied pressure difference. Movement of this diaphragm is usually sensed as either a change in capacitance or

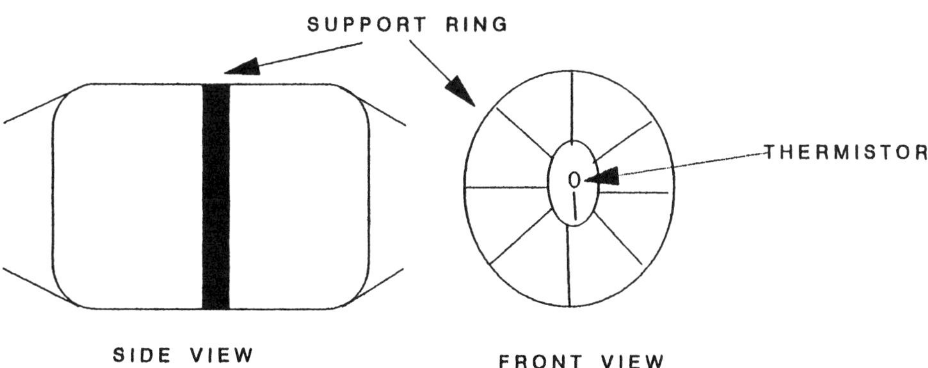

FIG 8–4
Hot-wire anemometer.

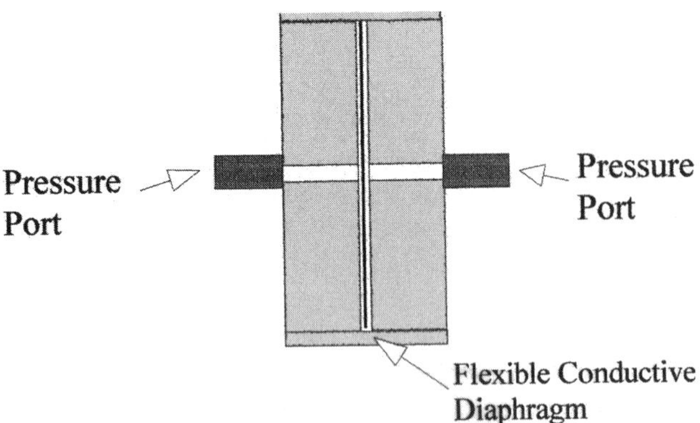

FIG 8–5
Differential pressure transducer.

reluctance. An example of a differential pressure transducer is shown in Figure 8–5.

A variable-capacitance transducer consists of two conducting surfaces, or plates, separated by a dielectric, or insulating, material. The magnitude of the capacitance varies directly with the area of the plates and inversely with their separation. In practice, pressure applied to one plate causes the separation to decrease. This change in capacitance is reflected as output voltage.

Variable-reluctance transducers consist of a conductive diaphragm mounted within a magnetic field. Application of pressure to one side of the diaphragm causes the diaphragm to deform away from the pressure. The movement of the conductive diaphragm through the magnetic field creates a current proportional to the applied pressure difference.

Most of the historical problems associated with pneumotachographs have reflected problems in the design of the pressure transducer rather than flaws in the pneumotachograph. Many transducers were originally designed for acoustic devices such as microphones. As such, these transducers were extraordinarily sensitive to vibration and therefore noise or movement. Devices with large internal volumes provided an ideal environment for incorporating noise onto the signal and mechanical damage to the diaphragm because of overpressure or nonuniform tightening around the periphery of the transducer. More recent designs incorporate very small internal volumes and provide a greatly improved common mode rejection of noise.

Pulmonary Function System Gas Analyzers and Applications

Helium Analyzers

All gases have a measurable capacity for conducting heat away from a heated object. Helium, in particular, has a relatively high capacity when compared with oxygen and nitrogen. This characteristic can be used to make quantitative measurements of helium concentration changes. Most modern helium analyzers incorporate a thermistor as the sensing element. A thermistor alters its electrical resistance in response to temperature changes. If a current is passed through the thermistor, heat will result. The gas around the thermistor will draw off this heat through convection. The resistance of the thermistor will reach a steady state for the current and the gas composition. If the gas composition is changed while the current remains constant, the thermistor's resistance will change.

The analyzer consists of two active sensing elements, reference and sample, connected to an electronic circuit called a Wheatstone bridge. When both elements are exposed to the same gas, the output sensed by the bridge is balanced, and the resulting signal is zero voltage. As one side is exposed to a different gas composition, the thermal characteristics of the gas cause one sensing element to be more or less efficient in drawing off the heat contained in the thermistor than the reference side. This creates an unbalanced condition that the Wheatstone bridge converts into an output proportional to the difference.

Helium Dilution Lung Volume Determination

In practice, a rebreathing circuit is established with a known volume and concentration of helium. At a predetermined point in the respiratory cycle, generally functional residual capacity (FRC), the patient is turned into the circuit and allowed to rebreathe until the helium concentration equilibrates. This equilibration occurs when the rebreathing circuit and the patient's lungs contain the same concentration of helium. The dilution of the initial helium concentration reflects the volume added by the patient. Since the system volume and initial and final concentrations of helium are known, the volume that the patient added to the circuit can be calculated. This is illustrated in Figure 8–6.

A stylized representation of a helium dilution circuit is shown in Figure 8–7. The principal components of the circuit include valving to control the directional flow of the respired air, chemical reagents to remove carbon dioxide and water before analysis, the helium analyzer, a source of oxygen, and a device for measuring volume.

Most differences in implementation relate to selection of the sensors. However, there are two distinct techniques related to ensuring adequate oxygen during rebreathing. The most common technique was described by Herrald and McMichael.[13] This technique involves continuously added oxygen to the circuit to maintain a constant volume. The other technique, described by Meneely et al.,[14] is to introduce a bolus of oxygen during

$V_1 \cdot C_1 = V2 \cdot C2$

$V_1 \cdot C_1 = (V_1 + V_{add}) \cdot C_2$	$5 \cdot 10\% = (5 + V_{add}) \cdot 6\%$
$V_1 \cdot C_1 / C_2 = V_1 + V_{add}$	$5 \cdot 10\%/6\% = 5 + V_{add}$
$(V_1 \cdot C_1 / C_2) - V_1 = V_{add}$	$(5 \cdot 1.667) - 5 = V_{add}$
Therefore	$V_{add} = 8.335 - 5 = 3.335,$

V_{add} = Volume added to the system
V_1 = Initial system volume = 5 L
C_1 = Initial helium concentration = 10%
C_2 = Final helium concentration = 6%

FIG 8–6
The volume added to the circuit by a patient can be calculated.

circuit setup to raise the oxygen concentration in the circuit. Rather than adding oxygen to match the subject's oxygen consumption, the circuit volume is allowed to decrease. The bolus is intended to provide sufficient oxygen to maintain the oxygen concentration above 21% during rebreathing. Both approaches can lead to errors unless adequate corrections are used.

In a constant-volume system, adding too much or too little oxygen will result in changes in the circuit volume that result in helium concentration changes since the volume of helium is fixed. The oxygen bolus approach permits dynamically changing gas concentrations for oxygen and nitrogen, which will affect the thermal conductivity of the sample gas. It is possible to correct for these effects, but the corrections may be imprecise.

The initial setup of the rebreathing circuit begins with the reference and the sample side of the analyzer exposed to room air. The analyzer is then zeroed by balancing the output voltage. Subsequently, any gas sample that contains a different gas composition than the room air seen by the reference will cause an offset voltage proportional to the different thermal conductivity.

A volume of helium is added to the circuit, and the new output will reflect the established helium concentration. Since there is more conductivity on the sample side containing the helium than on the reference side, an output voltage is created proportional to the difference in thermal conductivity. Assuming that all other gases remain constant, higher helium concentrations result in higher thermal conductivity on the sample side. After the

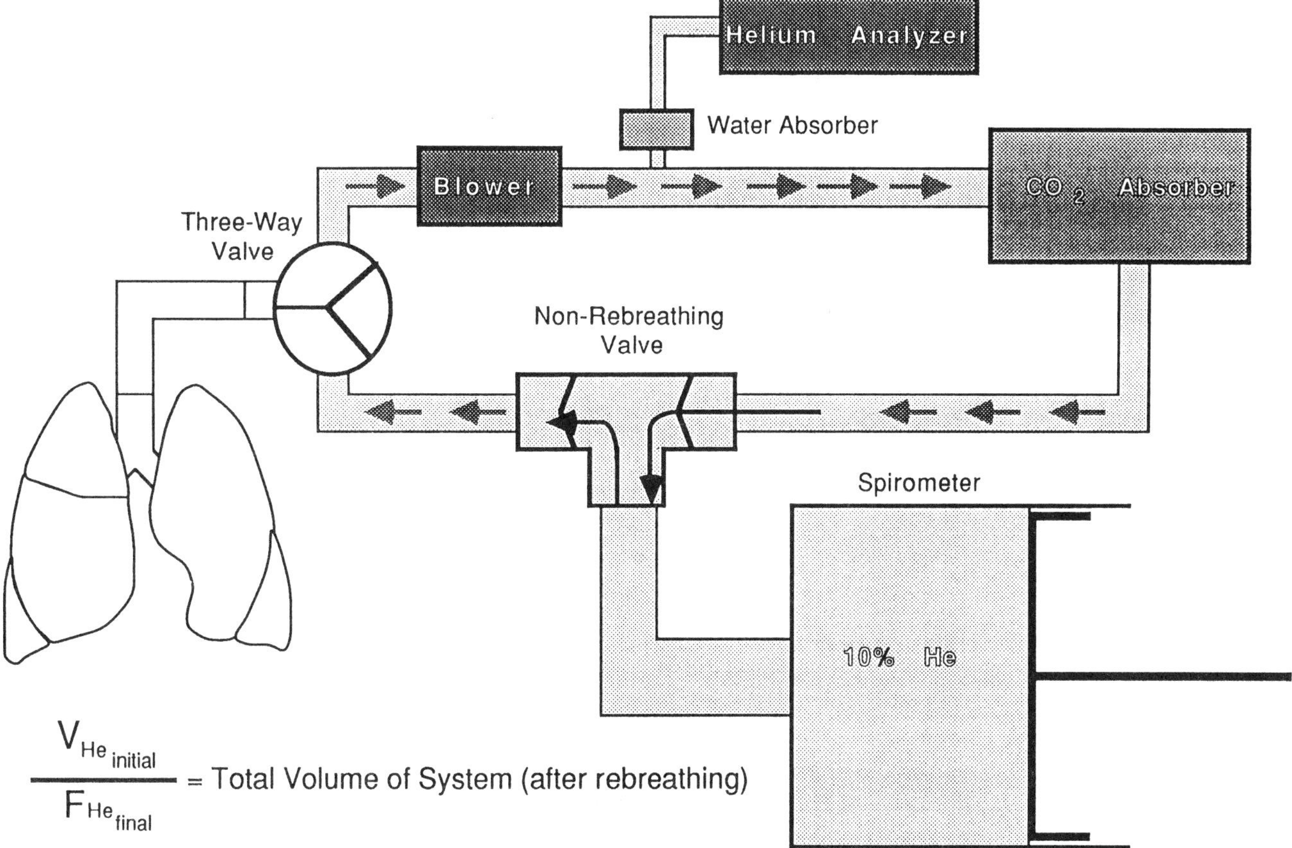

FIG 8–7
Helium dilution circuit. (From Snow MG: *Respir Care* 1989; 34:586–596. Used by permission.)

patient begins rebreathing on the circuit, the concentration will decrease as the helium equilibrates between the circuit and the patient's lungs. As the helium concentration decreases, the output voltage will proportionally decrease.

However, this thermal conductivity change is very nonspecific and reflects the characteristics of the overall gas mixture. If the gas composition contains other gases with significant thermal conductivity capability, changes in the concentration of these gases will also change the output. A primary assumption is that changes in thermal conductivity are a result of helium concentration changes only. Therefore, gases that also have relatively high thermal characteristics, such as carbon dioxide and water vapor, must be removed before analysis. As noted earlier, even changes in nitrogen and oxygen concentrations can induce errors unless some correction is made. Because thermal changes are due to convection and the rebreathing circuits are large relative to the measured volume, the response time of helium analyzers in this application is relatively slow.

The most common problem with helium dilution techniques, other than failure to replace chemical absorbers, is the presence of leaks in the circuit. Leaks commonly occur in the absorber containers during reassembly or at the patient connection. In some cases, the patient is the leak when the eardrum has been perforated. Leaks are nearly impossible to detect during the test because the effect of a leak is to slowly decrease the helium concentration. The failure to achieve equilibrium, which may also be due to severe air trapping, is the only indication during the test. Circuit leaks can easily be detected before the test by observing that the helium concentration remains stable for at least 1 to 2 minutes before switching in the patient. Patient connection leaks are usually only detectable through inference of inconsistent results.

Nitrogen Analyzers

Nitrogen analyzers function on the principle of emission spectroscopy. As gas is ionized, it emits a characteristic glow that contains a glow discharge band of colors or wavelengths over both visible and nonvisible light. Each gas component will contribute to the overall intensity, although at individualized wavelengths. The intensity of the specific wavelengths for each gas is proportional to the concentration.

To ionize the gas, a small sample of gas is pumped into a vacuum chamber. As the gas enters an optical chamber with photodetectors, a high voltage is applied across the chamber. Between the anode and cathode of the voltage circuit the ionized gas begins to glow. Within the glow discharge band, several dark regions also form.

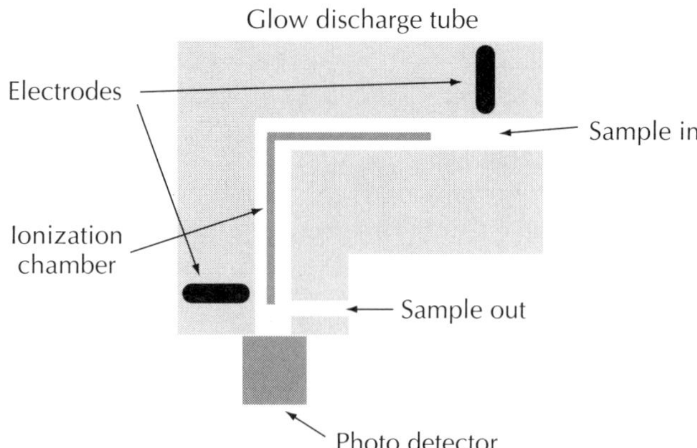

FIG 8–8
Nitrogen analyzer ionization chamber.

These regions move back and forth within the glow discharge as a function of vacuum variability. With laterally mounted photodetectors, movement of these dark regions can affect the stability of the output signal. For this reason, the stability of the vacuum is essential for accurate measurements. An illustration of the ionization chamber is shown in Figure 8–8.

Spectroscopy is used to measure the intensity of the discharge across the spectrum. Specific gases can be quantified by the presence and intensity of the glow in specific, well-defined wavelengths. Most gases actually emit multiple, scattered wavelengths, many of which overlap with other gases. The emitted light is filtered to pass only desired wavelengths. Selection of the wavelength to monitor must consider the potential for overlap. The filtered light is sensed by a photodetector that converts optical intensity into an output voltage.

Although nitrogen is the most common gas measured in this manner, with appropriate filters and detectors other respiratory gases can also be analyzed. The response time of this type of nitrogen analyzer is relatively fast, on the order of 150 ms, more than adequate for breath-by-breath applications. Typically, no preconditioning of the gas is necessary before analysis. However, with most currently used vacuum pumps, regular maintenance must include periodic oil changes since impurities in the oil and degradation from use will decrease the stability of the vacuum.

Nitrogen Washout Lung Volume Determination

This technique is generally an open-circuit method in which the patient inspires 100% oxygen and exhales into a collection/sampling circuit. The procedure continues until no appreciable nitrogen is left in the lung as determined by end-tidal nitrogen concentrations less than 1.5%. The volume of nitrogen exhaled during the washout represents approximately 80% of the volume in the lungs when the test began. This volume of nitrogen can be determined by collecting all exhaled gas or by integrating the volume from each breath.[15, 16] Nearly all commercially available systems integrate nitrogen on a breath-by-breath basis. Figure 8–9 shows a representative configuration for nitrogen washout determinations.

The patient is switched into the oxygen, typically at FRC, and allowed to breathe quietly for several minutes. The first exhaled breath will contain nearly 80% nitrogen; subsequent breaths will contain progressively less. Generally, nitrogen concentration is displayed vs. time to permit observation of the washout. System leaks are usually apparent because the display will show a sharp increase in nitrogen concentration during exhalation or a failure to reach zero during inspiration. However, some automated systems do not provide a display for inspiratory nitrogen concentration.

Perhaps more troubling is the insidious nature of vacuum fluctuations and alinearity on results. Occasionally, these problems will only be manifested with certain breathing patterns , which makes them extremely difficult to detect. Many problems with nitrogen washout can only be detected by trending physiologic standards such as normal staff members or through syringe dilutions.

Infrared Analyzers

Carbon monoxide (CO) analysis is most commonly accomplished by using a nondispersive infrared analyzer. In this technique, an infrared beam is passed through a chamber containing the sample gas. CO absorbs infrared in well-defined wavelengths. By measuring the intensity

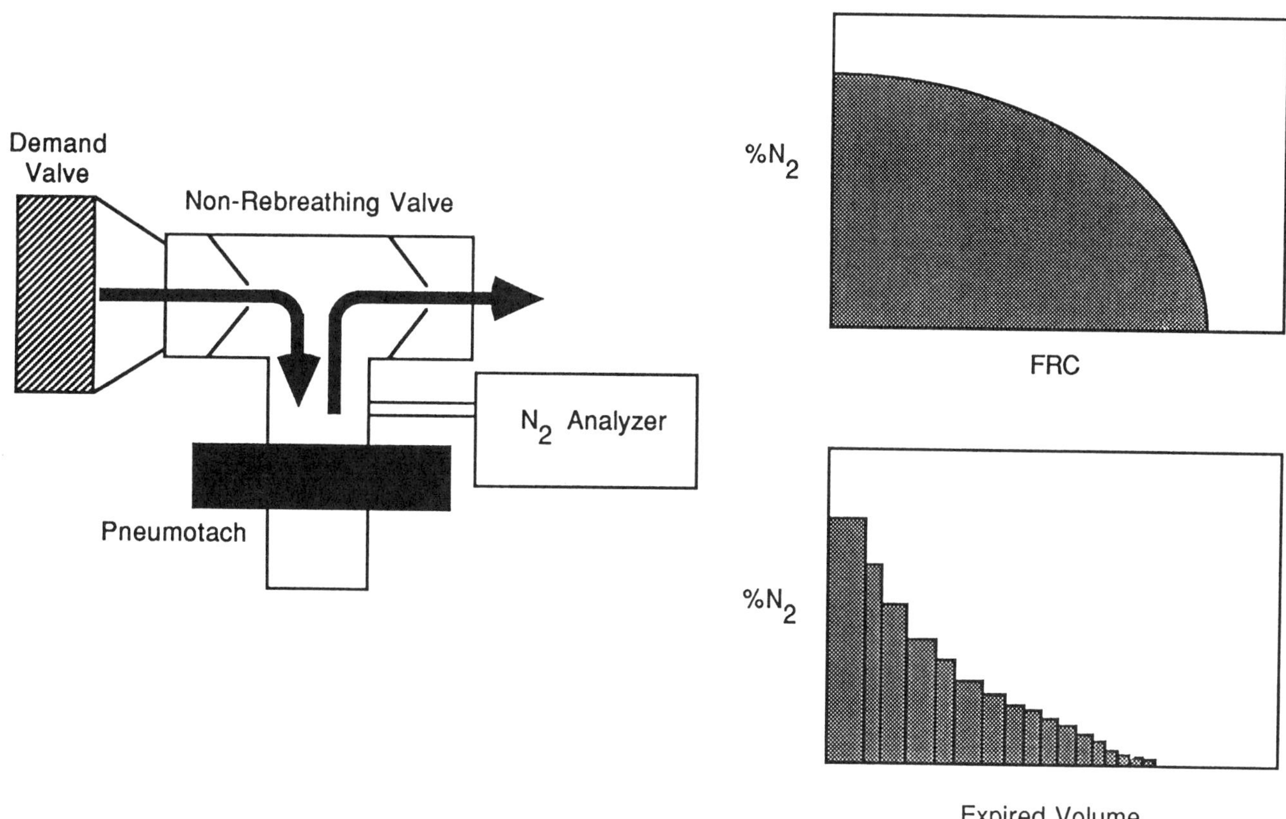

FIG 8–9
Nitrogen washout circuit. (From Snow MG: *Respir Care* 1989; 34:586–596. Used by permission.)

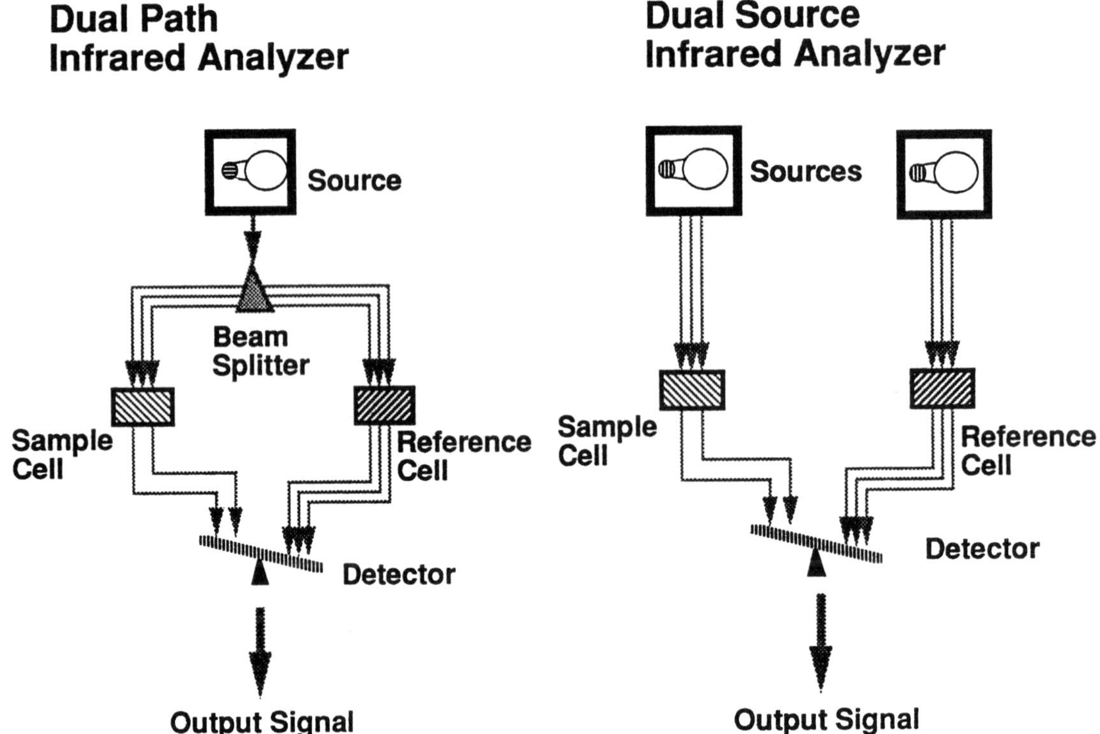

FIG 8–10
Carbon monoxide analyzer.

of the transmitted light and comparing this level with a reference containing no CO, a determination of the relative concentration can be made. A representative infrared CO analyzer is illustrated in Figure 8–10.

The cell consists of two parts, a measuring cell and a reference cell. The reference cell contains the environmental atmosphere against which the specific gas is to be compared. Thus, when the specific gas is present in the measuring cell, a larger amount of the transmitted light is absorbed in the measuring chamber than is absorbed in the reference cell. Inclusion of a chopper that interrupts the beam at specified intervals causes the detector to emit a pulsating dc signal proportional to the infrared absorbance of the gas being analyzed. There are two basic types of infrared analyzers, dual beam and dual path. The types differ primarily in the method by which the reference intensity level is obtained.

In a dual-beam type, two separate beams are used, one passing through the sample chamber and the other through the reference chamber. The intensity levels of the transmitted light of the two beams are compared, and the difference represents CO. Obviously the intensity of the two beams must be precisely matched and remain consistent. In the dual-path type, a single beam is passed through the sample chamber and the reference chamber alternately. The intensity levels associated with the two chambers are compared.

Infrared analyzers are not limited to CO. Any respiratory gas that absorbs infrared at defined wavelengths can be measured by this technique. Another common application for this technology is the analysis of carbon dioxide. Since carbon dioxide has an overlapping absorption, it must be removed before analysis. Additional gases such as methane and acetylene can also be evaluated by measuring the intensity at other specific wavelengths. Methane is an inert, relatively insoluble gas that can be used to measure the dilution caused by residual volume (RV). Acetylene is a highly soluble gas that is easily absorbed into blood. A multigas infrared analyzer, using acetylene, can be used to determine pulmonary capillary blood volume.

Gas Chromatographs

Gas chromatographs use two distinct principles for measurement. First, the sample is separated into its constituent gases by passing the sample through a filter of diatomaceous earth that selectively slows or blocks component gases on the basis of their size or affinity for the filter medium. Water and carbon dioxide, for instance, will not pass through a molecular sieve filter. Each sample is therefore separated into its constituent gases, with each individual gas appearing in a predictable sequence and timing. Smaller molecules appear first, and larger molecules are delayed. This permits each gas to be measured without the effect of any other component and precludes the need to precondition the gases by removing water and carbon dioxide.

The gas analysis is performed by thermal conductivity as in a helium analyzer. Helium, with its relatively high thermal conductivity, is generally used as a carrier or reference gas. Unlike the helium analyzer, the thermal conductivity of each component gas is assessed as it appears by comparing it individually with the reference gas. The relative concentration of each component gas is proportional to its thermal conductivity difference from the helium. The higher the concentration of nonhelium gas, the higher the conductivity voltage difference. A continuous recording of the conductivity output will show variations from baseline as the individual gases appear. The relative concentration of each gas is therefore measured without any background mixtures, which improves specificity.

For example, during the measurement of diffusing capacity for carbon monoxide (D_{LCO}), the CO in the diffusion gas inspired is compared with the reference gas. A voltage differential is obtained that is proportional to the concentration of CO. After the test, the patient sample is similarly compared. Since the patient has extracted CO from the sample, the CO concentration is reduced, which will be seen as a reduction in the output voltage. An illustration of gas chromatography is shown in Figure 8–11.

Single-Breath Measurement of Diffusing Capacity

Measurement of D_{LCO_2} consists of measuring the timed extraction of CO from a measured volume of inspired gas. CO is chosen in place of oxygen since the backpressure from CO in the pulmonary capillary bed is usually negligible and CO binds with hemoglobin similarly to oxygen.

In practice, this means analyzing the gas concentration of test gas to be inspired, determining the volume of test gas inspired, measuring the amount of time that the test gas was resident in the lungs, collecting a sample during exhalation, and analyzing the gas concentration of the sample. Additionally, dilution of the inspired gas by the RV, which is independent of diffusion, must be taken into account. This dilution is generally determined by the inclusion of an inert gas such as helium, neon, or methane in the test mixture. The dilution of the inert gas provides a reliable indicator of the CO available in the alveoli for diffusion. The functional components of Krogh's D_{LCO} measurements have not changed significantly from the original modifications of Forster, Ogilvie, and Jones and their colleagues.[17–20] An illustration of the circuitry is shown in Figure 8–12.

Procedurally, the patient exhales to RV, at which time the valve is activated to direct the subsequent full inspiration from the circuit containing the test gas. After full inspiration, the patient breath-holds for a preset lockout time, typically 7 to 9 seconds. After the lockout, the patient exhales into a collection circuit with the initial gas being discarded until an alveolar sample is ensured. This sample is analyzed and the results calculated.

Although the procedure is straightforward, the test has numerous possible sources of error. The ATS has published recommendations for standardization of the procedure.[2] This document thoroughly delineates the various sources of error and provides suggested corrections and methods. These sources of error include timing methodology, correction for hemoglobin and carboxyhemoglobin, adequacy of the inspired volume and exhaled discard volume, correction for sample volume changes because of removal of carbon dioxide and water, system

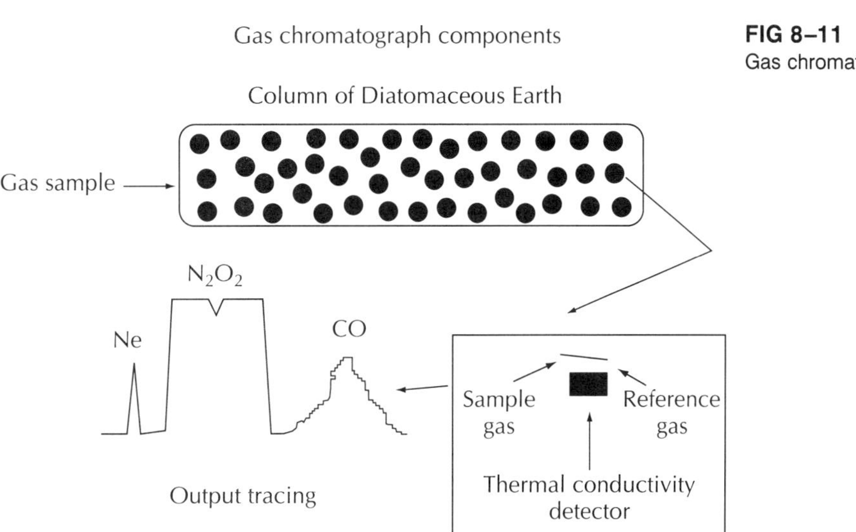

FIG 8–11
Gas chromatography.

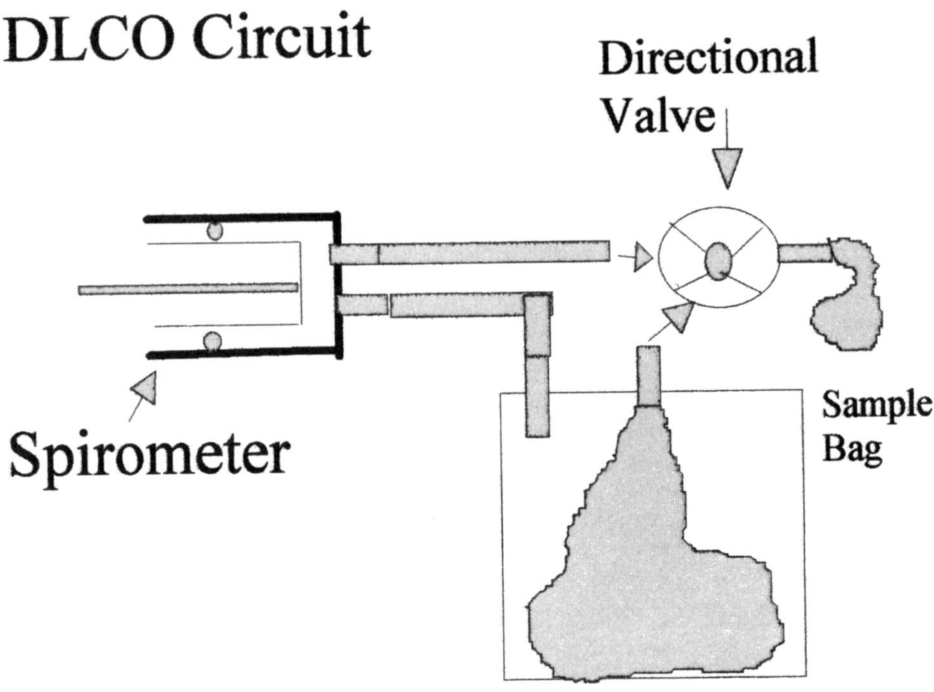

FIG 8–12
Single-breath DLCO circuitry

dead space, and the interval between determinations. It also recognizes the potential advantages of alternate methodology and requires that the alternate methodology be demonstrated to provide comparable results.

Examples of Pulmonary Function Systems

Warren E. Collins GS/Plus

The Collins GS system, shown in Figure 8–13, uses a volume displacement water seal spirometer, infrared CO analyzer, and thermal conductivity helium analyzer. A pneumatic breathing valve provides automatic sequencing for the testing. During diffusing capacity testing, the spirometer acts as a reservoir for the inspiratory test gas. This substitutes for the demand valves used in other systems.

During DLCO measurements after the patient has exhaled completely, the universal breathing valve switches inspiration to the spirometer reservoir. After full inspiration, the valve occludes to maintain breath holding. After breath holding, the breathing valve opens to permit the subject to exhale into the circuit. Once the preset exhaled volume has been met, the breathing valve switches the patient's continued exhalation into a collection circuit for sampling. After the preset volume has been collected in the circuit, the breathing valve opens to permit the remainder of the exhalation. The collected sample is then evacuated by a pump into the helium and infrared analyzers. The helium is used for the inert gas.

Lung volume determination is by closed-circuit helium dilution. The rebreathing circuit consists of the spirometer, universal breathing valve, and chemical scrubbers to remove carbon dioxide and water vapor. A blower assembly mixes the air within the rebreathing circuit. Oxygen is added to the circuit during the test to maintain a stable volume. The helium and oxygen concentrations are set up before testing in the spirometer. RV is determined by subtracting expiratory reserve volume (ERV) from FRC. Total lung capacity (TLC) is calculated by adding RV to VC.

Although complete flow-volume loops and spirometry can be performed with the volume displacement spirometer, a screen-type pneumotachograph is also provided to permit the user the choice of sensors. Spirometry is performed in accordance with ATS recommendations. The breathing circuit, including the universal breathing valve, spirometer, tubing, and blower housing, can be disassembled for cleaning. A barrier filter can also be inserted between the universal breathing valve and the patient.

Cybermedic Spinnaker Excel

The Cybermedic Spinnaker Excel, shown in Figure 8–14, uses both volume displacement and pneumotachograph technology for flow and volume measurements. The volume displacement device, a low-resistance, 9-L wedge bellows, is primarily used for lung volume and DLCO determinations. If the user desires, the wedge bellows can also be used for spirometry. The system has two Fleisch-type pneumotachographs for sensing flows. One no. 3 pneumotachograph is used for spirometry. The other is used to measure tidal breathing and the end-expiratory point to eliminate switch-in and sample size errors in FRC and DLCO. The helium analyzer is a linear thermal conductivity sensor, and the carbon monoxide analyzer is a linear, low-noise chemical fuel cell.

The system is computer driven with all calibrations controlled by software. The software is based on Microsoft Windows. This allows use of all Windows features, including true multitasking. For example, this permits actions such as analyzer calibration during forced vital capacity (FVC) testing and real-time error messages about patient or system performance.

The system has a built-in adapter for a disposable viral/bacterial filter optimized for low resistance and low dead space. This filter is used for all testing (FVC, maximum voluntary ventilation [MVV], slow vital capacity [SVC], FRC, and DLCO) to provide a barrier between the patient, the equipment, and the technician.

When FVC is performed, the heated Fleisch pneumotachograph is used with the display screen to show real-time volume-time and flow-volume graphics so that the operator can determine both forced and terminal efforts. The spirometry is performed using the current ATS recommendations with the system advising the technician whether the patient's efforts are acceptable or not and why.

The MVV is performed on the pneumotachograph, with the display showing both predicted and expected

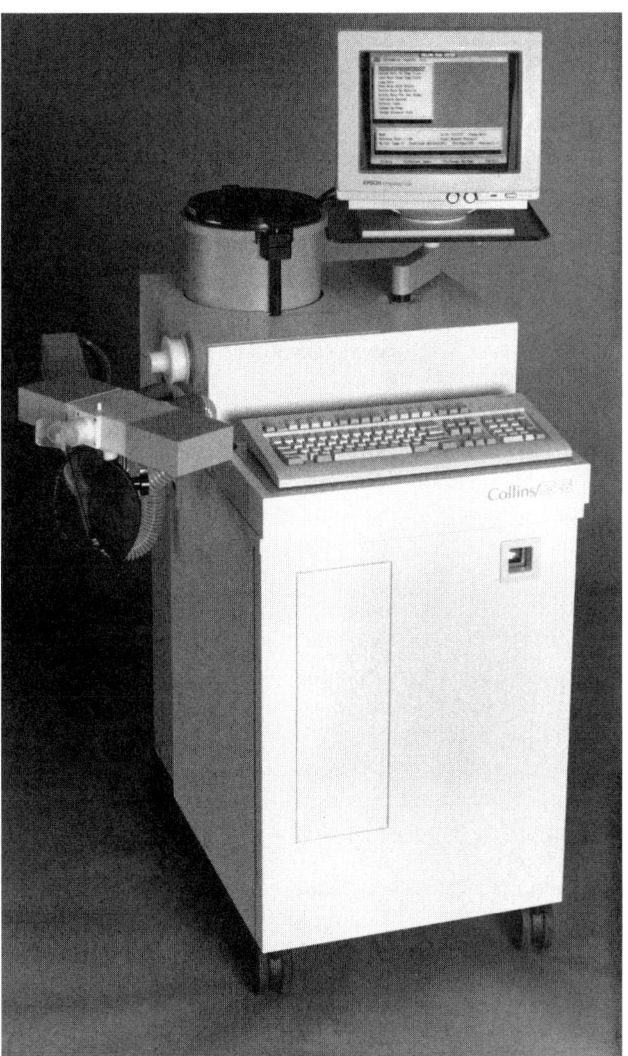

FIG 8–13
W.E. Collins GS system. (Courtesy of W.E. Collins, Braintree, Mass.)

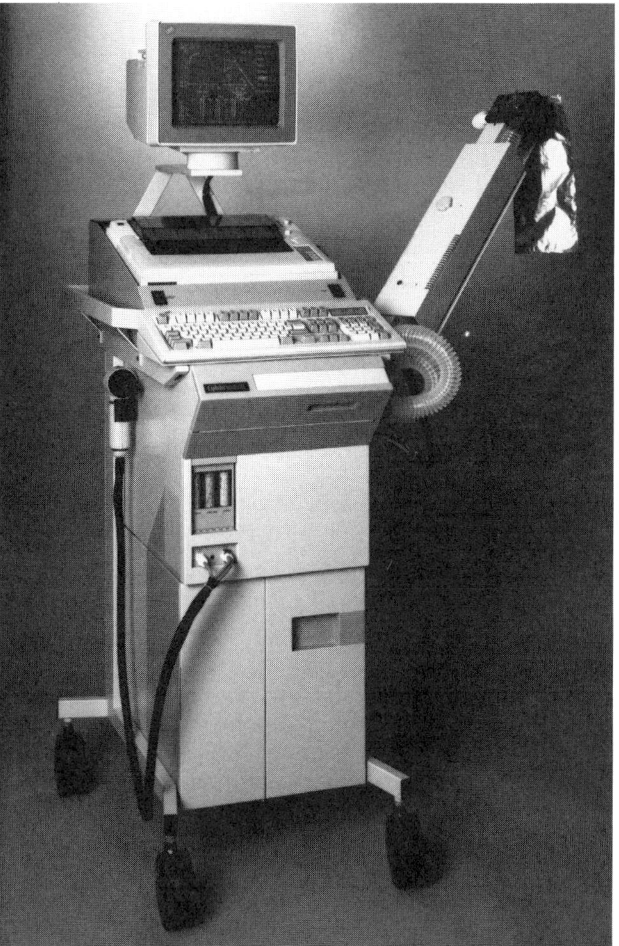

FIG 8–14
Cybermedic Spinnaker Excel. (Courtesy of Cybermedics Corp, Boulder, Colo.)

results from the forced expiratory volume in 1 second (FEV_1), the FVC having previously been performed.

The lung volume determinations are accomplished by using the helium dilution method. Setup of the system is automatic, and total system volume is determined before testing. At the beginning of the test the patient is connected to the patient valve, and before switching the patient into the closed circuit, the patient is monitored by the pneumotachometer so that the operator can determine that the patient is breathing and stable and at FRC. When the patient is stable, the operator touches the enter key, and the system waits for the next end exhalation and automatically switches the patient into the system. Once the patient is on the system, the patient's breathing is monitored, and after five breaths a baseline is drawn. When the breaths drift off the baseline because of oxygen consumption, oxygen is automatically added. SVC is performed after equilibration of the helium is reached and while the patient is still on the system.

The D_{LCO} measurement is performed by using the same circuit as the FRC. At the start of the test, the computer will display the SVC previously performed with a 90% target shown so that the operator can determine patient effort. Before testing, the patient's breathing is monitored by the pneumotachograph, and at any time during exhalation the technician presses the enter key; when the computer senses end exhalation, the patient is automatically switched into the system and inhales diffusion gas (CO and He) from the wedge bellows. After maximal inspiration, the patient valve closes and prevents the patient from prematurely exhaling. At the end of the breath holding time the valve opens and the washout volume is discarded; then the patient valve opens so that the sample can be collected in a nonpermeable Mylar alveolar sample bag. The technician can enter the hemoglobin and carboxyhemoglobin values before or after testing for corrections.

Medical Graphics PF/DX Systems

The MedGraphics DX system is shown in Figure 8–15. This system incorporates a disposable pneumotachograph and breathing circuit with a multiplexing demand valve. All patient contact surfaces are replaceable, thus simplifying decontamination between patients. The flow sensor can be used within the circuit for D_{LCO} and nitrogen washout studies or independently for spirometry. The MedGraphics PF/DX system uses a gas chromatograph for gas analysis and neon for the inert gas.

Directional control is achieved by two scissor valves and a solenoid that activates the demand valve. During spirometry, both scissor valves are open to permit the subject to breath straight through the circuit. Optionally, the flow sensor may be removed from the circuit for spirometric measurements. An illustration of the circuit is shown in Figure 8–16. Spirometry is performed in accordance with ATS recommendations.

During D_{LCO} measurements after the patient has exhaled completely, the back scissor valve closes, and the demand valve is activated. The inspiration is therefore from the demand valve through the flow sensor. After full inspiration, the forward scissor valve closes to act as a shutter while the back scissor valve opens. After breath holding, the forward scissor valve opens to permit the subject to exhale through the back of the circuit. Once the preset exhaled volume has been met, the back scissor valve closes and forces the patient's continued exhalation into the expiratory circuit for sampling. The expiratory circuit contains a rectangular mixing chamber and directional one-way valves that do not permit inspiration. After the preset volume has been collected in the circuit, the back scissor valve opens to permit the remainder of the exhalation to continue out the back. The expiratory circuit is then evacuated by a pump into the gas chromatograph for analysis. Since carbon dioxide and water do not pass through the molecular sieve, no conditioning of gas is necessary before analysis.

Lung volumes are performed by nitrogen washout with an open-circuit method. The subject inspires from a demand valve and exhales through the expiratory circuit. During nitrogen washout measurements, both scissor valves are open until the subject has demonstrated quiet, stable breathing. Simultaneously, the back scissor valve is closed and the demand valve activated for delivery of oxygen. Inspiration is from the demand valve, whereas exhalation is directed down the expiratory circuit. The directional one-way valves do not permit inspiration from the expiratory circuit. The total nitrogen exhaled in each breath is calculated and corrected for the initial concentration of nitrogen in the lungs. RV is derived by subtracting ERV from the measured FRC. TLC is calculated by adding RV and VC.

The breathing circuit and the flow sensor are designed for single patient use. The entire circuit may be discarded after testing. Replacement of the circuit is accomplished by pulling the tabs over the inspiratory and expiratory connections. The flow sensor disconnects from the pressure-sensing collar. A new sensor is snapped into place.

Jaeger Master Lab-Compact

The ML Compact system uses a screen-type pneumotachograph, infrared analyzer for carbon monoxide, and a helium analyzer. The system is shown in Figure 8–17. The helium analyzer is used for lung volume determinations and single-breath diffusion. Breathing

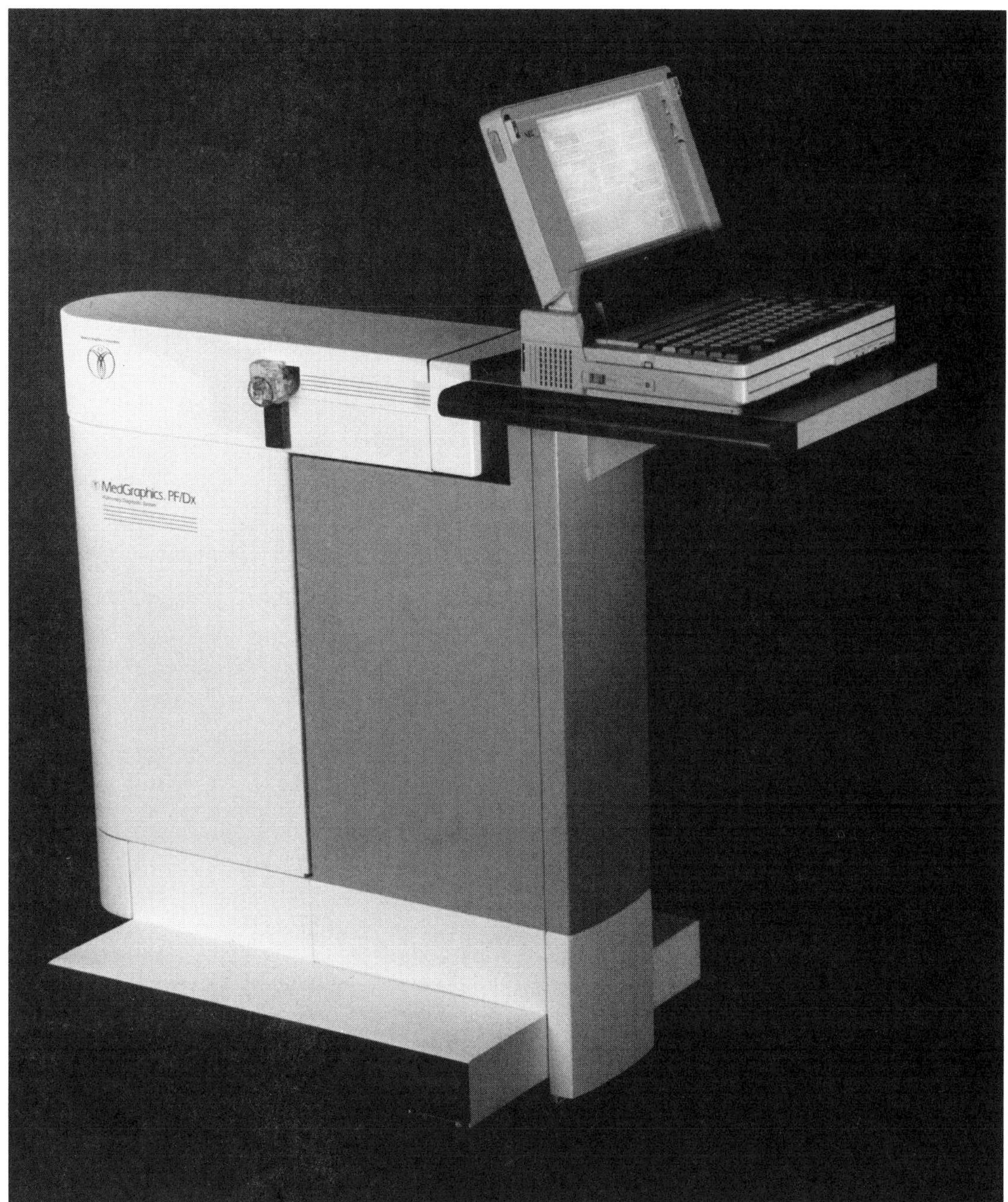

FIG 8–15
MedGraphics PF-DX System. (Courtesy of MedGraphics Corp, St Paul, Minn.)

circuitry is pneumatically controlled and permits software selection of ports. A key feature of this system is the breathing circuit design, which combines all directional control and shutter functions into a single clear acrylic block that is easily removed for cleaning as shown in Figure 8–18.

Calibration is performed on the pneumotachograph by using manual syringe injection and withdrawal. Flow is integrated and the resulting volume compared with the calibration signal. Individual correction factors are applied inspiratory and expiratory flow signals. Flow zero is automatically determined.

A second internal pneumotachograph is used to deliver preset volumes to the rebreathing bag for helium dilution lung volume determinations. Part of the calibration process includes adjustment of the preset volume

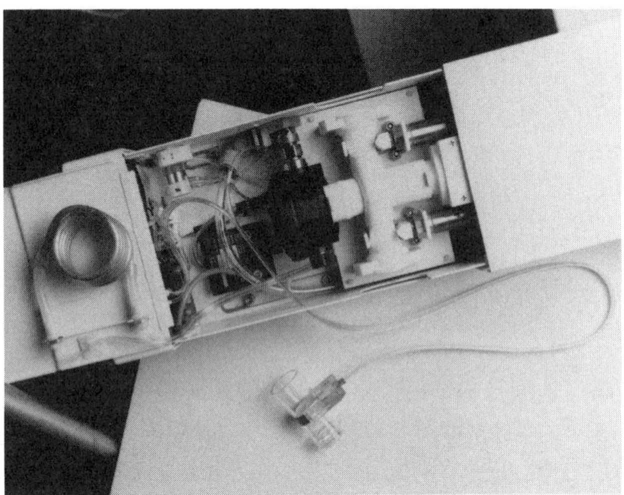

FIG 8–16
MedGraphics breathing circuit. (Courtesy of MedGraphics Corp, St Paul, Minn.)

and comparison of the internal pneumotachograph delivery of the FRC test gas (9% He/35% O_2/balance N_2) with the previously calibrated spirometry pneumotachometer.

The system contains helium, carbon monoxide, and oxygen analyzers, which are calibrated by sampling room air and then by sampling test gas mixtures. The system will adjust the amplification necessary to match the gas specifications. All corrections are stored for subsequent comparison and trending.

Spirometry and flow-volume measurements are made by using a screen-type pneumotachograph. The software functions with simple start and stop instructions. No additional interaction is necessary during testing. Switching between SVC, FVC, and MVV can be accomplished with a single mouse click. Up to five efforts may be saved. If a sixth effort is obtained, one of the five saved efforts must be deleted before proceeding.

Diffusing capacity measurements are made by using the single-breath technique, but the system also supports steady-state measurement and determination of membrane diffusing capacity. For the single-breath technique, helium is used as the inert gas to account for the dilution of the inspired gas by RV.

Before measurement of diffusing capacity, two metal or plastic foil bags are attached to the valve block. Both bags are emptied. Default discard and collection volumes and lockout time can be reviewed and changed at this point. One bag is flushed and filled with the test gas. A sample from this bag is analyzed as the inspiratory gas mixture.

During the diffusion test, the subject breathes through the pneumotachograph and the breathing

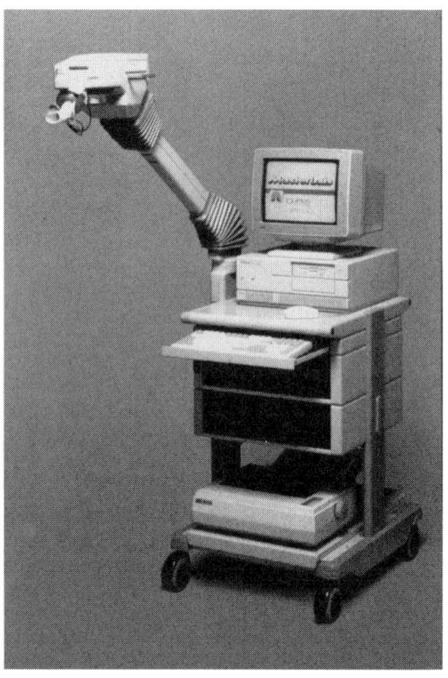

FIG 8–17
Quinton MasterLab ML Compact. (Courtesy of Quinton Instruments, Seattle, Wash.)

circuit. After exhalation, the pneumatic circuit switches the inspiratory path to the Mylar bag containing test gas for inspiration. At full inspiration, the pneumatic circuit seals the breathing ports for a preset time. After breath holding, the subject exhales through the circuit until a preset volume has been achieved, and the exhalation is then diverted into a expiratory port containing a separate Mylar sample bag. Once the bag has been filled, the pneumatic circuit again vents the expiratory path to room air. Analysis of the gas sample is obtained by using the

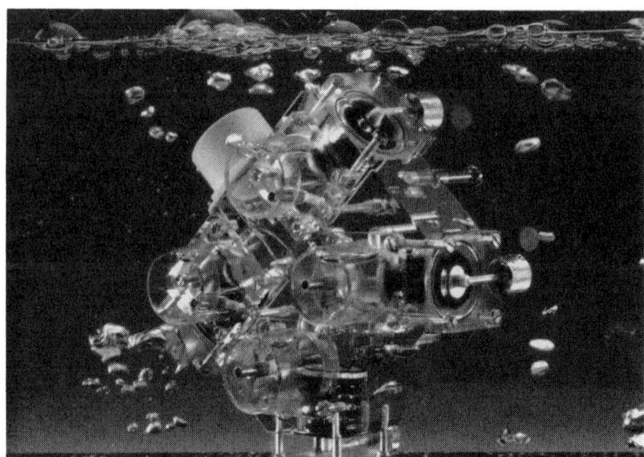

FIG 8–18
Quinton removable breathing circuit. (Courtesy of Quinton Instruments, Seattle, Wash.)

helium and infrared analyzers. Sample gases are conditioned with chemical reagents before analysis to remove carbon dioxide and water vapor.

Lung volume determination is performed by multiple-breath helium dilution. The system performs the measurement by using the oxygen bolus technique. The constant-volume technique can be optionally added. This adaptation is unusual in that the volume signal is derived from the pneumotachograph rather than a volume displacement device. Pneumotachographs are sensitive to changes in viscosity, and helium has a substantially different viscosity than room air. For this reason, most flow-based systems use the nitrogen washout technique. This system makes spirometric determinations on room air before rebreathing. The rebreathing circuit volume is determined by the internal pneumotachograph that was previously calibrated by using the test gas. During the rebreathing phase a viscosity-corrected volume signal and the helium concentration are displayed to aid in ensuring equilibration.

Procedurally, the rebreathing bag is attached to the valve block and filled with a preset volume of test gas (typically 10% helium, 35% oxygen, the balance nitrogen). The patient performs tidal breathing on room air to establish lung subdivisions and is switched into the rebreathing bag at FRC. After rebreathing until equilibration or the oxygen level falls below a previously set lower limit, typically 21%, the patient is switched out of the circuit. Without the optional addition of oxygen to maintain oxygen levels and an additional reagent container to remove CO_2, the test is generally limited to 2 minutes.

Since moisture and carbon dioxide are removed before analysis, the only changes in gas concentration relate to helium and oxygen. The relative effect of oxygen concentration on thermal conductivity can be calculated. Correction of the helium reading is made for the measured oxygen concentration in the gas sample. A correction is also made for the system dead space. FRC can be corrected for switch-in error. Calculation of TLC is made by adding inspiratory capacity to the measured FRC.

SensorMedics 2200

This instrument is also flow based and uses a pneumatically controlled breathing circuit. The system is shown in Figure 8–19. The flow sensor is a hot-wire anemometer that measures flow by changes in resistance caused by the thermal characteristics of the gas flowing across the element. Since the hot-wire anemometer cannot detect flow direction, a pressure drop pneumotachometer is employed to sense changes between inspiratory and expiratory flow. A representation of the 2200 patient circuit is shown in Figure 8–20.

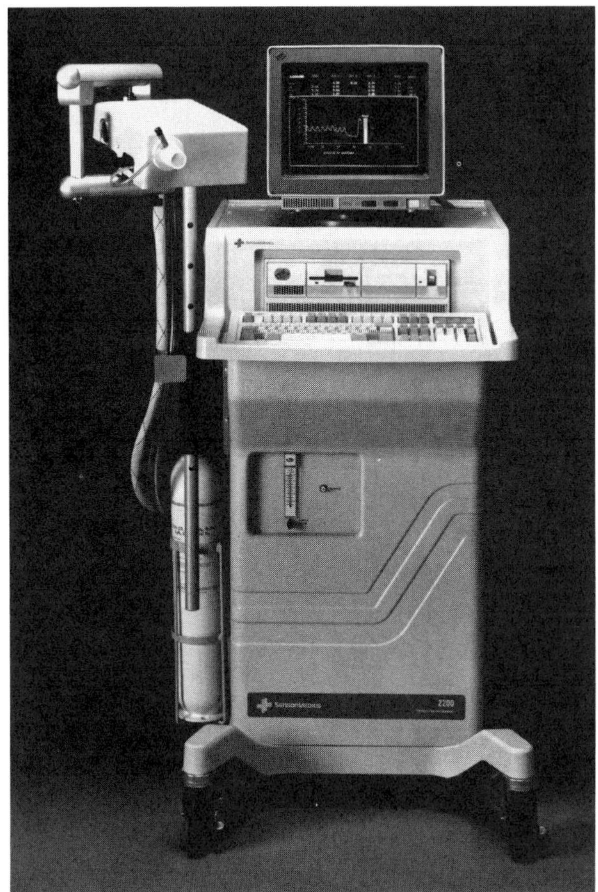

FIG 8–19
SensorMedics 2200 pulmonary system. (Courtesy of SensorMedics, Yorba Linda, Calif.)

Spirometry is performed according to ATS recommendations. Acceptability criteria are reviewed and displayed for each effort. Up to three efforts may be retained for both before- and after-bronchodilator testing.

The system performs diffusion studies by using a single-breath technique with a multigas infrared analyzer. The system does not collect a discrete expiratory sample but rather displays a continuous waveform of the expiratory gases and averages the concentrations over specified intervals. This permits selection of appropriate discard and sample volumes over a wide range of patients including pediatric patients. Since the system does not collect a fixed sample size, testing can theoretically be performed on any volume that substantially exceeds dead space. Other systems have a lower volume limit defined by the size of their collection circuit. The performance of the system for diffusing capacity was also evaluated by an independent laboratory and was judged to be in compliance with recommendations and comparable to other systems.

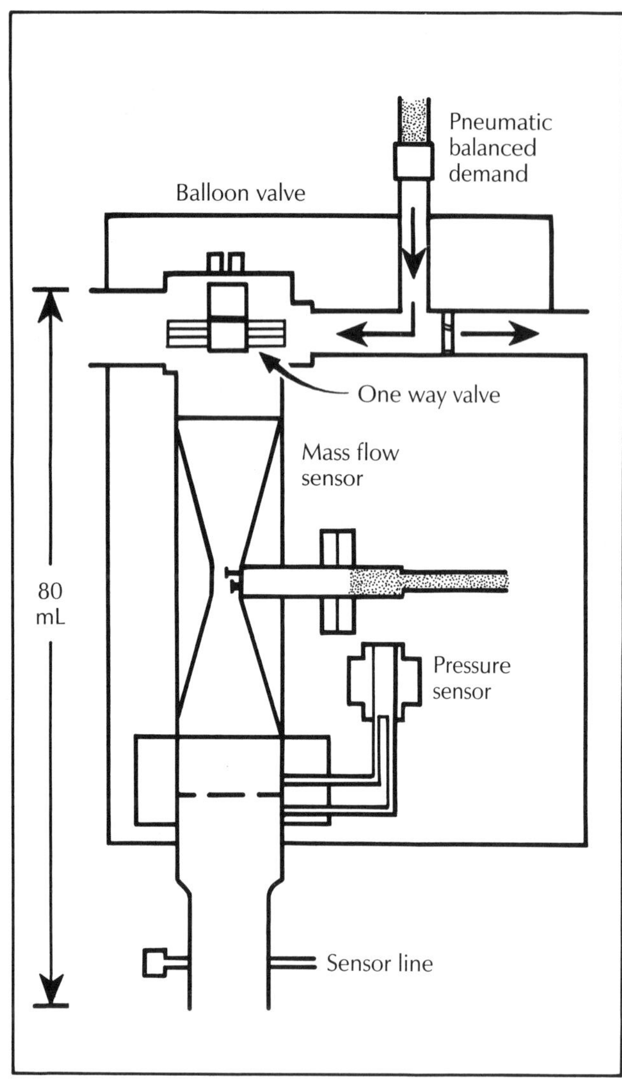

FIG 8–20
SensorMedics 2200 breathing circuit. (Courtesy of SensorMedics, Yorba Linda, Calif.)

During quiet breathing the patient breathes through the flow sensor and directional control valve. Selectively inflatable balloons control the airflow path. After exhalation, the expiratory port is occluded, and the patient inspires test gas from a demand valve that is purged before testing. Breath holding is assisted by occluding both balloon valves. After breath holding, the patient exhales through the flow sensor, and gas is analyzed continuously at the mouth. Default settings make the gas measurement by averaging the concentrations of a liter of exhaled gas after discarding the first 750 mL.

A unique aspect of this system is the rapid-response multigas infrared analyzer, which permits continuous analysis of carbon monoxide and methane during the exhalation. Methane is used as the inert gas to account for dilution of the inspired gas by RV. The continuous analysis provides assurance of dead space clearance since the software permits reselection of the portion of the carbon monoxide curve to be averaged within specific volume limits. Water vapor is removed before analysis by a sample tube that is semipermeable to moisture. This tubing equilibrates the sample gas with ambient humidity.

In addition, the inclusion of acetylene to the standard diffusion mixture permits a calculation of pulmonary capillary blood volume based on the acetylene uptake. Since pulmonary capillary blood volume plus shunt equals cardiac output, it is possible to provide an assessment of resting cardiac output. However, this technique may be less accurate in patients with distribution abnormalities and requires careful control over flows. Additionally, since acetylene is absorbed into the blood and only slowly excreted, adequate washout time between efforts is required.

Lung volume determinations are made by using a nitrogen washout technique. After observing several tidal breaths, the software switches the subject into the oxygen demand valve. The total nitrogen exhaled in each breath is calculated and corrected for the initial concentration of nitrogen in the lungs. RV is derived by subtracting expiratory reserve from the measured FRC. TLC is calculated by adding RV and VC.

SensorMedics 2600 Pediatric/Infant Pulmonary Cart

This system is functionally similar to the 2200 but uses a single-screen pneumotachograph rather than a hot-wire anemometer. The system is tailored for pediatric and infant applications. Different-size pneumotachographs are used for different flow ranges. Specific adaptations of the basic spirometry software provide capabilities for performing flow-volume loops in a tidal breathing mode, with a hugger device, or as forced efforts. Lung volumes are determined by nitrogen washout as in the 2200, except that the patient switch-in is manually performed. The 2600 system is shown in Figure 8–21.

Several pulmonary mechanics measurements can be performed. These measurements include Hering-Breuer reflex studies, pressure/volume curves, respiratory compliance, and resistance. Directional control of flow and shutter operations are achieved through the use of pneumatic balloon valves and a foot switch.

Pressure-volume loops are performed by using a mask or directly onto the endotracheal tube of ventilated patients. Four consecutive tidal breaths are recorded, and measurements of tidal volume, flow, airway pressures, and inspiratory and expiratory time are obtained. Lung distension is evaluated by observing the morphology of the loop, calculating the compliance of the terminal 20% of inspiration, and referencing this to the overall compliance for the entire breath. Since driving pressure during tidal breathing is a function of elastic recoil and is basically sinusoidal, expiratory flow is inversely proportional to airway resistance and directly proportional to driving pressure. The flow pattern will therefore be sinusoidal flow-time or oval flow-volume curves. A help screen provides on-line comparison for common flow-volume patterns.

Respiratory compliance and resistance are obtained by periodically occluding tidal breaths and recording the airway pressure plateau. Compliance is calculated from the total passive expiratory volume and the airway pressure plateau. Resistance is computed from the measured compliance and the time constant. Reference points are established at 65% and 90% of the tidal volume.

The Hering-Breuer reflex test is performed by recording three successive spontaneous tidal breaths and occluding the shutter at the end of inspiration. The

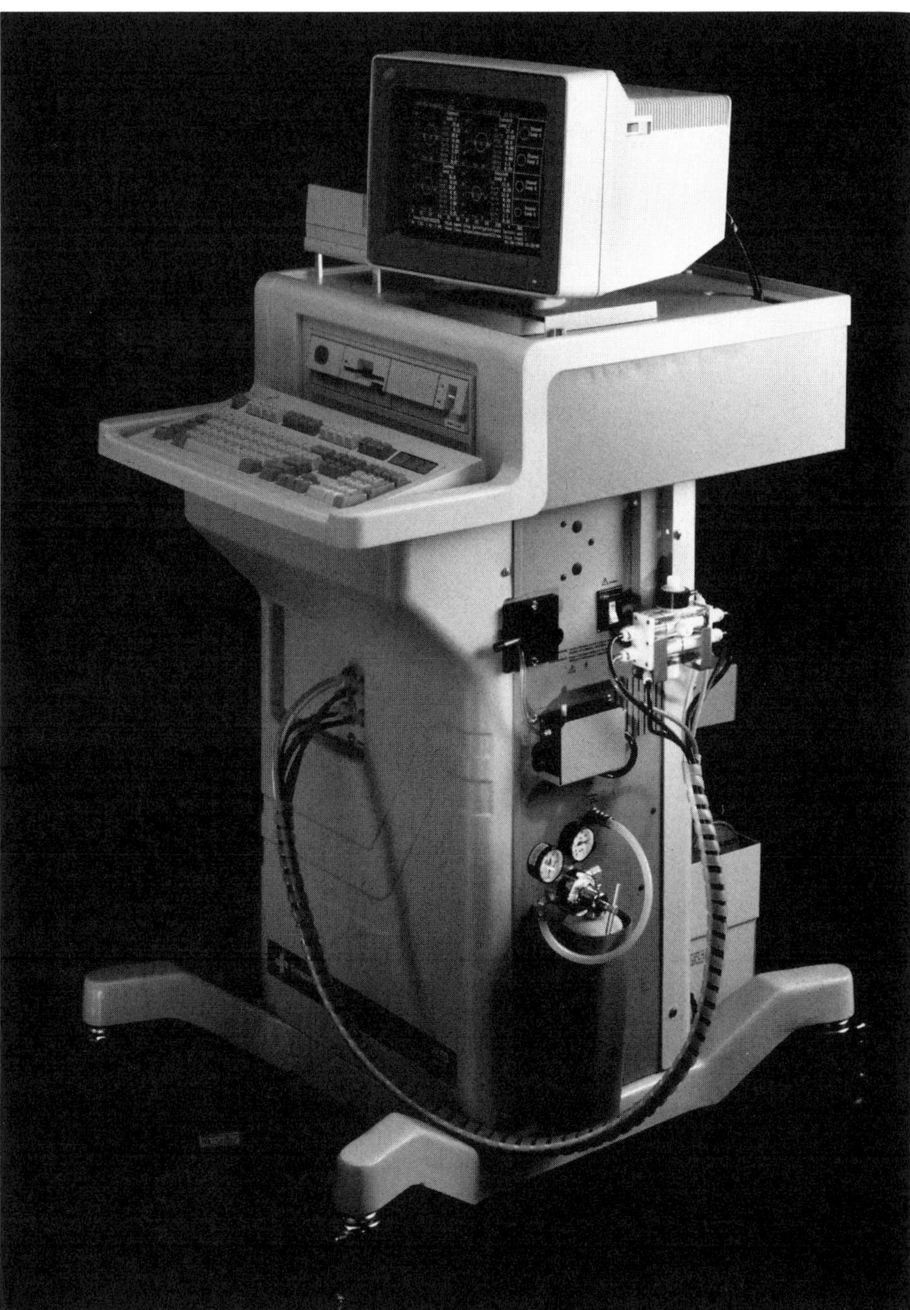

FIG 8–21
SensorMedics 2600 Pediatric/Infant Pulmonary Cart. (Courtesy of SensorMedics, Yorba Linda, Calif.)

shutter remains occluded until the next inspiratory effort. The average expiratory time for the preceding breaths is compared with the occlusion time.

Body Plethysmography

The original development of the plethysmographic technique dates back to Gad[21] and Pfluger's[22] independent work in the 1880s. Their original work described a technique for determining residual volume by forcibly applying compression and distension forces to a subject's lungs while the airway was occluded. Modern body plethysmography using voluntary compression and decompression in a clinically useful system was described by DuBois et al.[23]

Thoracic Gas Volume

Based on an application of Boyle's law, body plethysmography thoracic gas volume (TGV) measures all compressible gas within the thoracic cage regardless of the distribution patterns. Simply stated, volume varies inversely with pressure if the temperature is held constant. Therefore, the change in pressure within the lung as it is distended by a measured external volume change is a function of the lung volume. The complete derivation of the equation is shown in Figure 8–22.

By way of illustration, if two similar balloons are inflated, one with 500 mL of air and the other with 1,000 mL of air and both balloons are compressed the same amount, the balloon with the smaller volume will exhibit a greater internal pressure change than the larger one. In fact, the magnitude of the pressure change for any given compression volume can be predicted if the original volume and ambient pressure are known. Therefore, by measuring the ratio of the change in internal pressure and the change in external compression, the original volume of the balloon can be calculated. This is illustrated in Figure 8–23.

However, the issue of temperature stability is essential for accurate measurements, and the delay while awaiting cabinet equilibration can account for a large portion of the testing time. As temperature rises within a cabinet, the pressure will also increase. This problem applies to flow-type as well as pressure-type cabinets

FIG 8–22
Derivation of the thoracic gas volume equation.

Boyle's Law States that

$$PV = P'V'$$

if temperature remains constant. *P* is ambient barometric pressure and *V* is the volume to be determined

$$P' = (P + \Delta P) \text{ and}$$
$$V = (V - \Delta V)$$

where ΔP and ΔV are the changes in pressure and volume respectively.
Therefore,

$$PV = (P + \Delta P)(V - \Delta V) \text{ or}$$
$$PV = PV - P\Delta V + \Delta PV - \Delta P\Delta V$$

by subtracting *PV* from both sides, this becomes

$$PV - PV = PV - PV + \Delta PV - P\Delta V - \Delta P\Delta V \text{ or}$$
$$0 = P\Delta V - \Delta PV - \Delta P\Delta V$$

Since the product of the pressure and volume changes $\Delta P\Delta V$ is so small in absolute terms, it can be safely ignored; therefore

$$0 = P\Delta V - \Delta PV \text{ or}$$
$$\Delta PV = P\Delta V$$

By dividing both sides by ΔP the equation becomes

$$V = P\Delta V / \Delta P$$

Since *V* is the volume to be determined and *P* is barometric pressure, the only factor left to be determined is $\Delta V/\Delta P$, which is the measurement of airway pressure changes in association with the cabinet volume displacement by the patient's thoracic cage during the maneuver thus permitting calculation of the lung volume.

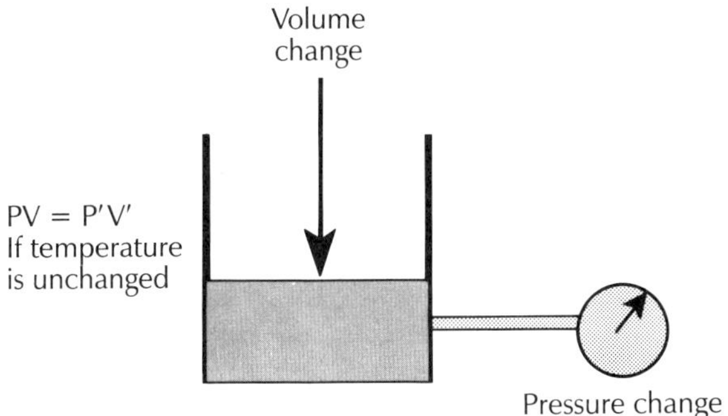

FIG 8–23
As the volume compresses, the pressure inside the chamber increases proportionally . Since the initial pressure is known, the initial volume can be calculated.

since the pressure increase causes flow out of the cabinet. There are three primary sources of heat in the cabinet. Exhaled air, being substantially warmer than ambient air, has a significant heating effect. Another source is heat radiating from the patient. A third factor is the heater element of the pneumotachograph, if present. These factors synergistically combine to rapidly raise the ambient temperature of the cabinet once a patient is inside with the door closed. This heating cycle is a function of the temperature difference between the ambient temperature in the cabinet and the heating source. Since the initial difference is great, the temperature rise is very fast early and slows as the gradient decreases.

Since it is difficult to distinguish between pressure shifts resulting from heating and those due to expansion of the thoracic cage, testing must not be performed during a period with rapid temperature changes. Typically, the operator observes the pressure signal and waits until thermal equilibrium is approached before testing commences. Most systems attempt to minimize this delay either by minimizing cabinet heating or by cabinet venting and dynamic referencing of the pressure transducer. Failure to wait for equilibrium is a common error and leads to inaccurate results.

Functionally, a subject enclosed within a rigid cabinet pants gently against a shutter while compressing and expanding his thoracic cage, which causes volume changes within the cabinet. The thoracic cage changes are equal to the volume changes seen by the alveoli. As a result of this thoracic movement, alveolar pressure changes concurrently. The ratio of these changes indicates the trapped thoracic volume for a given barometric pressure. Smaller alveolar pressure changes relative to cabinet volume changes indicate a larger TGV. Conversely, smaller TGVs lead to larger alveolar pressure changes.

There are two fundamental assumptions required for the measurement of TGV. The first assumes that the temperature in the cabinet is not changing significantly, and the second assumes that mouth pressure equals alveolar pressure in the absence of airflow. The assumption that mouth pressure reflects alveolar pressure is based on the physics of gases and liquids in rigid tubes and may not always be true given the nonrigid nature of the tracheobronchial tree. Also, it is possible to generate mouth pressure changes associated with cheek movement that are independent of the thoracic cage.

Several recent studies have demonstrated problems in measurement of TGV in subjects with severe obstruction. These problems have been attributed to inaccurate assessment of alveolar pressure. Studies with esophageal balloons led to the theory that there is preferential distribution of gas into the highly compliant extrathoracic airways instead of the more rigid intrathoracic airways.[24, 25] However, shifts in lung volume invalidate the assumption that esophageal pressure equals alveolar pressure. Further, pleural pressure contains both elastic and resistive elements, and failure to adequately control panting frequency would also invalidate the assumption.[26] Therefore, the results with esophageal balloons may be in error. The actual mechanism by which alveolar pressure would be inaccurate is unclear. Regardless of the mechanism, other studies have shown that reducing the panting frequency eliminates the overestimation of TGV.[27]

Dilutional techniques only measure areas of the lung that are ventilated during the dilution, and significant portions of the lung may ventilate so slowly they do not contribute to the dilution. Prolonged dilution times can improve the accuracy in patients with substantial airway obstruction, but this may be impractical. Since a single determination can take from 7 to 10 minutes and the patient may take at least that long to clear the helium or oxygen from his lungs, it may not usually be practical to perform repeat measurements.

Body plethysmography can make several measurements of TGV in a fraction of the time required for dilutional tests. This provides assurance that the result is reproducible. In addition, questionable results can be repeated after equipment checks and additional instructions to the patient.

Airway Resistance

By including airflow measurement with the airway pressure that represents the driving pressure, body plethysmography can provide a measurement of airway resistance (R_{aw}). Airway resistance, specific airway resistance (S_{raw}), and its reciprocals airway conductance (G_{aw}) and specific conductance (S_{gaw}) can provide a sensitive early indication of peripheral airway dysfunction, differentiate the site of obstruction, and monitor the response to bronchoactive drugs. Perhaps even more compelling, airway resistance measurements are largely effort independent.

Measurement of airway resistance requires an understanding of the interrelationship of pressure, flow, and resistance. The primary determinants of airflow are the driving pressure and the elastic and resistive properties of the airways that oppose flow. The driving pressure must exceed the resistance of a tube or airway for flow to occur. Basically, the relationship can be stated as

$$R_{aw}\ (\text{cm/H}_2\text{O}) = \text{Pressure (cm H}_2\text{O)/Flow (L/sec)}.$$

Therefore, if the flow and driving pressure can be measured, resistance can be calculated.

Functionally, flow is measured during gentle panting or quiet breathing, and then the airway is occluded and the pressure measured as the subject continues to pant or breathe quietly. With the airway occluded, the assumption is made that mouth pressure reflects alveolar pressure, at least initially. By this technique, several measurements of R_{aw} can be made in a very short time frame.

Methodology differences are numerous in R_{aw} measurements. In Europe, R_{aw} determinations during quiet breathing measurements are prevalent. Gentle panting is more typical in the United States. Adherents of quiet breathing frequently make the case that panting is more difficult for patients to learn. Panting advocates usually counter that gentle panting is not as difficult to learn as MVV or single-breath diffusing capacity measurements.

In the original description of the measurement, three reasons were given for panting: (1) the body temperature and pressure, saturated (BTPS) effect of inspiring cool, dry gas and exhaling heated, humidified gas; (2) phase alignment of the pressure and flow signals; and (3) minimization of the oropharyngeal resistance component by fixing the glottic aperture during panting.

Alternatives to panting for eliminating the BTPS effect have long been available. During the maneuver, this effect is seen as a volumetric shift between inspiration and expiration. An early method was to have the patient inspire from a reservoir containing heated humidified air. More recently, this correction has been made electronically. This offset can be removed by electronically adjusting the box volume signal.

Phase alignment of the pressure and flow signals can be accomplished by having the patient increase his resting respiratory rate slightly to approximately 30 breaths per minute, although this minimizes the patient cooperation advantage of quiet breathing measurements. Another approach is through the use of reference chambers that blunt the response of the cabinet pressure signal. This has the effect of slowing the pressure signal but will also slow the response to fast-changing signals. One alternative is to switch to the reference chamber only during quiet-breathing resistance measurements.

The third reason is the most difficult to resolve. Resistance determinations made during panting and quiet breathing measure distinctly different pathophysiology. To the extent that one is trying to assess *airway* resistance, panting is preferable. If one is trying to assess *total* resistance during normal breathing, quiet breathing would seem preferable. The ultimate answer probably devolves to personal preference. Fortunately, most newer, commercially available plethysmography devices offer both techniques.

Types of Plethysmographs

There are, potentially, three different types of body plethysmographs: volume displacement, flow, and pressure, as shown in Figure 8–24. The types are defined by

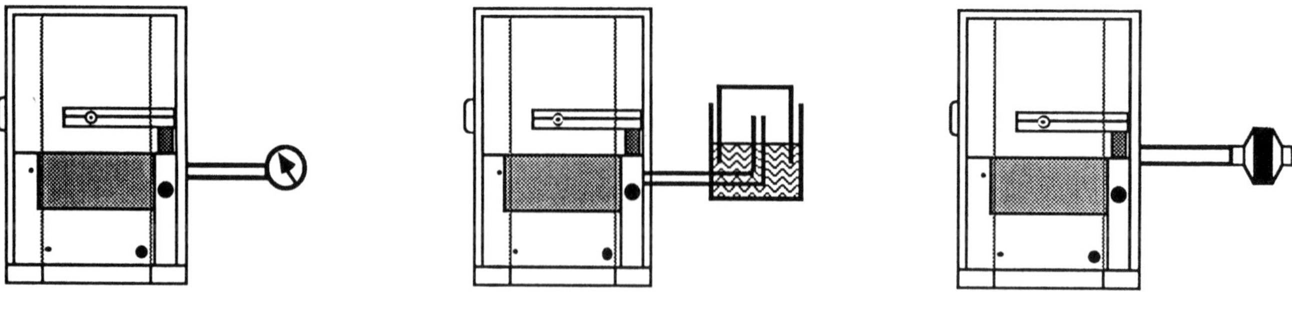

FIG 8–24
Different types of body plethysmographs. (From Snow MG: *Respir Care* 1989; 34:586–596. Used by permission.)

how they detect volumetric changes within the cabin. Volume- and flow-type plethysmographs measure volume changes as displacement either directly into a spirometer or as displacement through a flow sensor mounted in the cabinet wall. Pressure-type plethysmographs measure changes in cabinet volume by monitoring cabinet pressure. Since pressure and volume changes are inversely proportional, as a subject expands his thoracic cage, cabinet pressure will increase.

Volume displacement–type plethysmograph designs must be free of leaks since the volume change must cause physical displacement of the spirometer. Also, since the spirometer and the plethysmograph are a sealed system, temperature increases will cause displacement and can damage the spirometer. For this reason, volume-type plethysmographs are generally air-conditioned to prevent temperature increases. Additionally, since the displacement device has inertia, there will be a phase lag between a pressure increase in the cabinet and actual volume displacement. Typically, this is corrected by using a pressure transducer to provide a phase correction. Because of the relative complexity of this type of design, its use has largely been limited to the research setting.

The flow-type plethysmograph is also a volume device, although it uses a flow sensor to derive volume changes. Since the flow sensor is in effect a large leak in the cabinet, damage from pressure buildup is not possible. Therefore, air-conditioning may not be necessary as long as thermal equilibrium is achieved. As in volume-type plethysmographs, there can be a lag between the chest wall excursions and the movement of gas through the flow sensor. This can lead to the necessity of pressure-correcting the flow signal. In practice, flow plethysmographs are more technically demanding than pressure types for the measurement of TGV and R_{aw}.

Most commercially available plethysmographs are of the pressure type. This can also be referred to as a constant-volume, variable-pressure type of plethysmograph. The advantage to this approach is a higher-frequency response since the pressure signal responds immediately and is relatively tolerant of small leaks. Also, this type of cabinet tends to be very reliable. Some plethysmographs offer combined features that add a flow mode for specific measurements. Despite widespread belief to the contrary, all of the major manufacturers currently use a pressure-type plethysmograph mode when determining TGV and R_{aw}.

Compression Flow-Volume Loops

Much of the confusion regarding plethysmograph methodology stems from the measurement of compression flow-volume loops. This is a feature that flow- or volume-type plethysmographs offered as an inherent capability. Accordingly, when comparing flow-type with pressure-type plethysmographs, this was frequently a point of differentiation between manufacturers.

Essentially, this capability involves the ability to simultaneously measure airflow at the mouth and chest wall movement associated with a forced expiratory maneuver and provides an estimate of airway compressibility. During the maneuver, chest wall movement compresses the airways within the lung to some degree. The result of the airway compression is that flow assessed by chest wall movement will always be equal to or higher than airflow measured at the mouth. The magnitude of this compression can be estimated by overlaying the simultaneously obtained curves. The difference in absolute flow at specific points of exhaled volume reflect airway compression. In addition, the failure to achieve higher peak flows from chest wall movement than from mouth flow can be attributed to submaximal effort. The clinical utility of this measurement has not been established.

Some plethysmographs offer a combination of these approaches in that they use a pressure-type mode for TGV and R_{aw} determinations and switch to a flow-based mode for specific optional tests. There is nothing that inherently precludes a pressure-type plethysmograph from using an additional flow sensor in the wall of the cabinet and simultaneously processing flow signals obtained at the mouth and from chest wall movement. Most major manufacturers offer this as an option.

Examples of Body Plethysmographs

MedGraphics 1085/DL. The Medical Graphics system 1085, a standard constant-volume, pressure-type cabinet, is shown in Figure 8–25. Shutter control is a pneumatic scissor valve that compresses the disposable neoprene patient circuit. Door sealing is ensured by proximity electromagnets with release controls available both externally and internally. The system provides the ability to make standard TGV as well as R_{aw} measurements.

Diffusing capacity measurement is available by using the single-breath method and a gas chromatograph for gas analysis. Complete spirometry can be performed with the door open or closed. Additionally, maximal inspiratory/expiratory pressures can be determined. Spirometry and diffusing capacity measurements are identical to the MedGraphics PF/DX pulmonary function system and are more fully described in the pulmonary function section.

The hexagonal shape and cabinet pressure reference chamber facilitate fast thermal equilibration. Calibration is performed by using an automated manometer, a 50-mL sinusoidal pump, and a 3-L syringe. Data collection is time

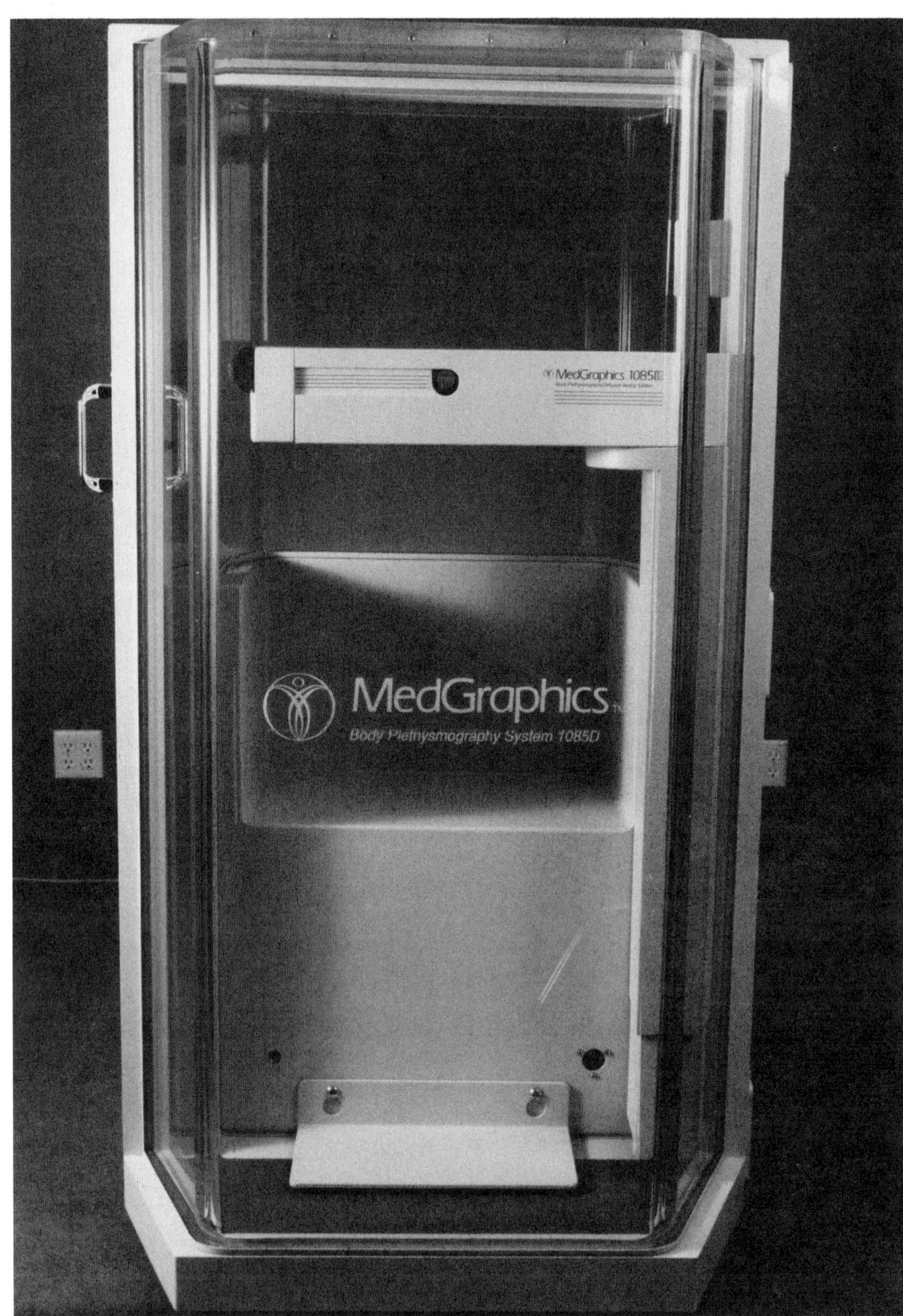

FIG 8–25
MedGraphics System 1085 Plethysmograph. (Courtesy of MedGraphics Corp, St Paul, Minn.)

driven or manually controlled. Up to ten efforts can be collected for TGV and R_{aw}, with manual correction of the computer selected angles. All data are automatically stored and available for review and selection after the patient has completed the testing. This raw data can also be stored onto a diskette.

Procedurally, for TGV determinations the patient breathes quietly to establish a stable end-tidal point; at end expiration, the shutter is closed and the patient pants gently. After collection, the patient may perform a VC maneuver for lung subdivisions. TLC is calculated by subtracting ERV from the measured TGV to obtain RV, which is added to VC. All efforts can be reviewed and averaged. R_{aw} measurements may be made with quiet breathing or panting maneuvers.

SensorMedics 6200. The SensorMedics plethysmograph, a combined pressure-compensated flow and constant-volume pressure-type cabinet, is shown in Figure 8–26. The patient generally breathes transmurally from the outside of the cabinet rather than rebreathing from within the plethysmograph. The transmural breathing delays the internal heating within the cabinet. By this approach, patient testing can commence earlier since heating is delayed. This does not, however, eliminate the heating effect within the cabinet. After a few minutes the temperature in the cabinet will rise and must be vented.

Complete spirometry can be performed by using a hot-wire anemometer. Lung diffusion testing can also be performed in the plethysmograph by using the breathing assembly and analyzers from the SensorMedics 2200 Pulmonary Function System. This capability is described more fully in the section on pulmonary function systems. Pressure measurements are made by using variable-reluctance transducers. Since hot-wire anemometers are not able to detect flow direction, a small differential pressure pneumotachograph is inserted into the pathway to provide the ability to separate inspiratory and expiratory flows.

During TGV and R_{aw} measurements the plethysmograph functions as a standard pressure-type instrument. The cabinet flowmeter is closed off to maintain a constant cabinet volume. Mouth pressure measurements made against a closed pneumatic shutter are displayed against pressure changes representing cabinet volume changes. Resistance measurements may be made either by tidal breathing or panting. During airway resistance measurements the patient does not breath transmurally. Inspiratory and expiratory airflow stays within the cabinet. Data acquisition consists of collecting four consecutive pants and displaying the tracings side by side. Any or all of the

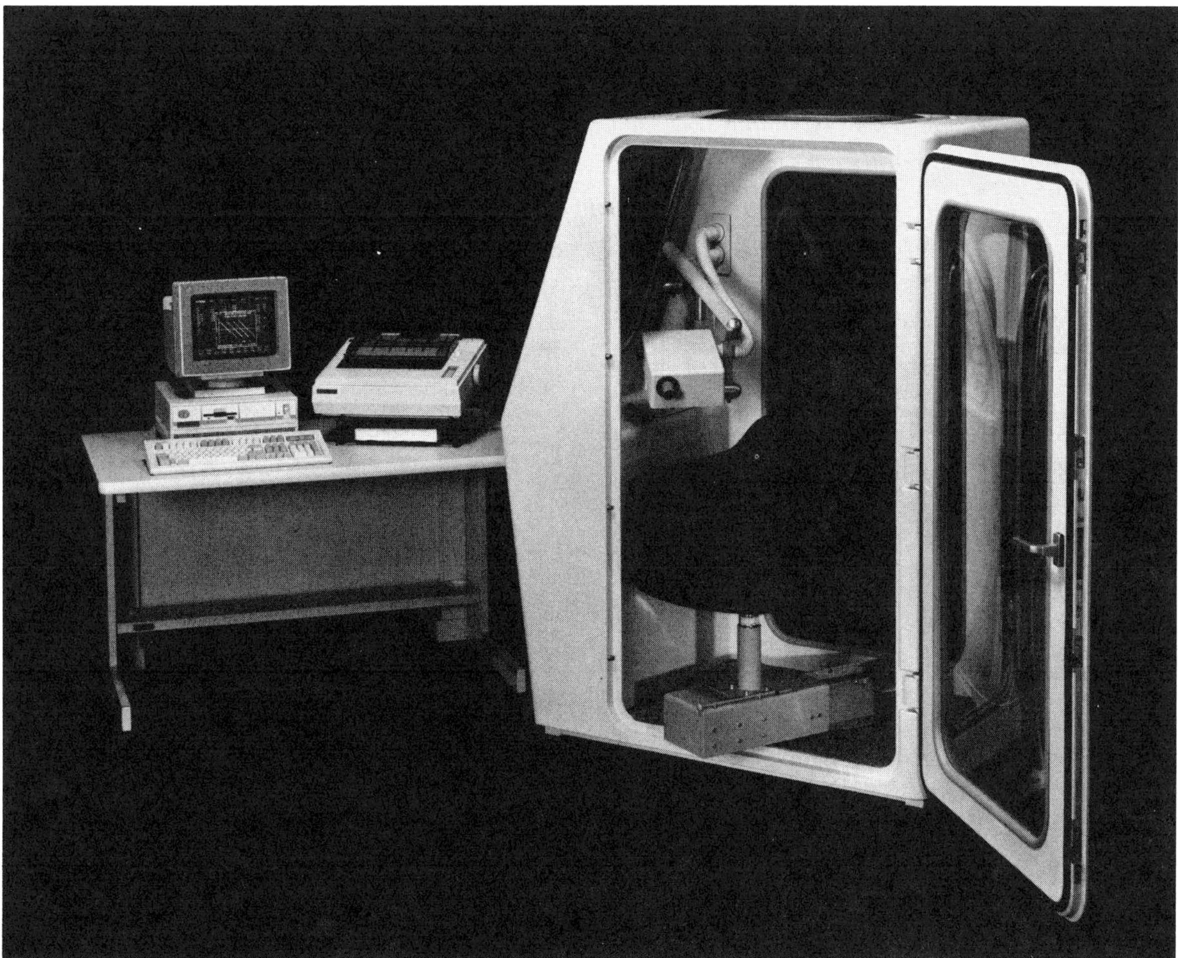

FIG 8–26
SensorMedics 6200 Plethysmograph. (Courtesy of SensorMedics, Yorba Linda, Calif.)

individual pants can be adjusted and included for the effort. Up to three efforts can be stored.

Procedurally, for TGV determinations the patient breathes quietly to establish a stable end-tidal point; at end expiration the shutter is closed, and the patient pants gently. After collection, the patient may perform a VC maneuver for lung subdivisions. After shutter closure for TGV measurements, the patient pants gently against the shutter. The last four panting excursions within the effort can be reviewed individually and included or excluded from the calculation.

During measurement of compression flow-volume loops, the pneumotachograph in the transmural breathing pathway measures the airflow from the mouth while the cabinet pneumotachograph measures chest wall excursions. Compression volume is calculated as the difference of chest wall and mouth flow. Additionally, the flow difference at specific lung volume points is provided.

CARDIOPULMONARY EXERCISE SYSTEMS

The delivery of oxygen and removal of carbon dioxide are the joint responsibility of the heart and lungs. The heart must provide adequate blood flow through the lungs and to the involved cells. The lungs must remove carbon dioxide and oxygenate the returning venous blood to provide an adequate supply of oxygenated blood for delivery. In the absence of adequate supplies of oxygen, the process can proceed anaerobically for a limited time with an increased output of carbon dioxide. Exercise rapidly consumes local stores of energy and creates an increased demand. The manner in which the cardiopulmonary system responds to this increased demand provides a mechanism for differential diagnosis of the functional limitation.

Pulmonary Response

Gas exchange is accomplished by matching blood flow in the pulmonary capillary bed with ventilation to form functional alveolar-capillary units. Because of pressure gradients between alveolar air and blood gases and as a result of chemical reactions in the blood, oxygen is transferred into the blood, and carbon dioxide is released. When blood perfuses capillaries without a matched ventilated alveoli, gas exchange cannot take place. This type of blood flow is termed a shunt. Ventilation that occurs without matched blood flow is termed wasted ventilation or "physiologic dead space." As metabolic requirements increase, additional alveolar-capillary units are recruited, which normally reduces ventilation/perfusion mismatching.

Insofar as these additional alveolar-capillary units are able to match the increased demand, metabolism is aerobic, which means that oxygen uptake ($\dot{V}O_2$) and carbon dioxide production ($\dot{V}CO_2$) will increase proportionately with work. At some point, demand will exceed supply, and anaerobic metabolism will increase. During anaerobic metabolism, carbon dioxide production will reflect both the aerobic and anaerobic components, and its rate of increase will exceed that of oxygen uptake. This relationship between $\dot{V}O_2$ and $\dot{V}CO_2$ is referred to as the respiratory exchange ratio (RER). The RER provides information regarding the relative contributions of aerobic and anaerobic metabolism as well as being a marker of maximal exercise.

Exercise performed above the anaerobic threshold results in progressive increases in blood lactate concentration. The ability to continue exercise decreases dramatically as anaerobic metabolism becomes predominate. Therefore, the anaerobic threshold represents the level of activity that can be sustained for long durations of time and is a reliable indicator of the degree of functional disability. Further, the anaerobic threshold is an objective measure to quantify the effect of exercise training for rehabilitation.

Minute ventilation increases are driven primarily by the need to excrete the increasing amounts of carbon dioxide produced by metabolism. During aerobic metabolism, minute ventilation will increase proportionally to both oxygen uptake and carbon dioxide production. As anaerobic metabolism increases, minute ventilation will continue proportional to carbon dioxide production but will be disproportionate for oxygen uptake. Ventilatory responses are achieved by altering the tidal volume and the respiratory rate in response to chemoreceptor stimulation resulting from changes in blood CO_2 or O_2 content.

Cardiac Response

The cardiovascular response to increasing levels of work is to increase delivery of oxygen. This is achieved by increasing both the total blood flow as well as the delivery to the working muscle groups. Cardiac output increases as a result of varying stroke volume and heart rate. Locally, blood flow is increased to working muscle groups by selective vasodilation resulting from increased temperature and lactic acidosis. Vasodilation reduces the capillary resistance and, when coupled with increased blood pressure associated with the increased cardiac output, controls the distribution of blood flow.

During maximal exercise, oxygen uptake and delivery will reach a plateau that results from a limitation in cardiac output and is a measure of maximal reserve of the cardiovascular system. This can be seen by examining the relationship between oxygen uptake and delivery as represented by the Fick equation:

$$\dot{V}O_2 = \text{Cardiac output} \times \text{Arteriovenous } O_2 \text{ difference}$$

or

$$\dot{V}O_2max = Qmax \times (CaO_2 - CvO_2$$

Cardiac output represents the maximal delivery of blood to the circulation. The A-VO_2 difference represents the local response of selectively redistributing blood flow to active skeletal muscle and away from regions of low extraction such as the splanchnic area and kidneys. It also reflects, to a lesser degree, the effect of shifts in the oxyhemoglobin dissociation curve. Since this redistribution is highly efficient, the maximal systemic A-VO_2 difference is relatively constant. Accordingly, differences in $\dot{V}O_2max$ primarily reflect differences in cardiac output rather than oxygen extraction.

Rhythm disturbances may alter the heart rate response, whereas myocardial contractility or valvular dysfunction will limit the stroke volume response. Further examination of the Fick equation provides evidence for a noninvasive method of following stroke volume response. Since cardiac output is stroke volume times heart rate and since the A-VO_2 difference is relatively constant,

$$\dot{V}O_2 = \text{Stroke volume} \times \text{Heart rate} \times \text{A-}VO_2 \text{ difference}$$

$$\dot{V}O_2/\text{Heart rate} = \text{Stroke volume} \times \text{A-}VO_2 \text{ difference}$$

or

$$\dot{V}O_2/\text{Heart rate} = \text{Stroke volume}$$

As exercise increases, the consumption of oxygen by myocardial tissue increases as well. Oxygen extraction from arterial blood will increase as a means of enhancing oxygen supply. The inability to provide adequate oxygenated blood to the heart muscle will result in ischemic changes in the area of blood flow limitation. Ischemia will cause changes in the propagation of electrical impulses through the myocardium. These changes will initially be seen as ST segment or T wave changes. Arrhythmias, particularly those that are exercise induced, are also associated with the incidence of myocardial ischemia. Coupled ventricular premature contractions (VPCs) are of special concern since they may precede more serious lethal arrhythmias such as ventricular fibrillation. Some subjects have occasional VPCs at rest or with low work levels, but these ectopic beats are surpressed as the work load increases. The most serious ventricular ectopic beats may sometimes be seen during the immediate recovery phase. The development of conduction abnormalities or ectopic beats during exercise is strong evidence for underlying coronary artery disease.

The initial response to exercise is an increase in stroke volume as well as in heart rate. The stroke volume response peaks early during relatively low levels of work, with subsequent cardiac output increases resulting primarily from heart rate increases. High heart rate responses early in exercise could indicate that stroke volume increases are compromised. This response is also seen in deconditioned subjects. ST segment depression at low work levels that increases with the heart rate and continues into the recovery phase may indicate multivessel coronary artery disease.

Systolic blood pressure increases dramatically with increasing work from a normal 120 mm Hg to approximately 200 to 250 mm Hg. Diastolic blood pressure typically rises only slightly (10 to 15 mm Hg) or not at all. The increase in systolic blood pressure is due to increases in cardiac output, primarily stroke volume. Although cardiac output may increase nearly fivefold, systolic blood pressure only doubles because of the substantial decrease in peripheral vascular resistance. This decrease in resistance is predominantly due to vasodilation in the working muscle groups.

Abnormal blood pressure responses also provide indications for terminating the exercise. Increases in systolic pressure in excess of 250 mm Hg or abrupt decreases in systolic or diastolic values with increasing work levels are abnormal and should be grounds for stopping the exercise. However, it should be realized that variations in blood pressure during exercise may be caused by respiratory efforts. Wide pressure swings of as much as 30 mm Hg can be seen between inspiration and expiration in patients with pulmonary disease.

In summary, the cardiopulmonary response to work provides direct, noninvasive information about a patient's clinical condition. The pattern of responses provides information regarding the type of impairment, whereas the magnitude of the response quantifies functional impairment. The cardiac response provides information about oxygen delivery and specifically about the cardiovascular system's ability to provide increased delivery on demand.[28–32]

The ventilatory response provides similar information about the lungs' ability to adequately oxygenate the blood. Diffuse airway obstruction limits the flows necessary to adapt respiratory rate, whereas restrictive processes limit tidal volume increases. Ventilatory limitations will cause arterial desaturation. Ventilation-perfusion mismatching will cause high wasted ventilation or prevent effective recruitment of additional functional alveolar-capillary units.

Gas Exchange Measurement

The difference in gas concentrations between inspiratory and expiratory gas is a result of extraction of oxygen and excretion of carbon dioxide. Ideally, measurement of the volume of oxygen and carbon dioxide inspired would be compared with the volume expired. This measurement would involve measuring the inspired and expired volume and the fractional concentrations for oxygen and carbon dioxide.

$$\dot{V}O_2 = \dot{V}I\ (FIO_2) - \dot{V}E\ (FEO_2)$$

and

$$\dot{V}CO_2 = \dot{V}E\ (FECO_2) - \dot{V}I\ (FICO_2)$$

In practice, measurements of the differences between inspired and expired volume are extremely difficult to make accurately. This difference is a result of the difference between oxygen uptake and carbon dioxide production. For example, assuming a minute ventilation of 10 L/min and an RER of 0.8, if the $\dot{V}O_2$ is 250 mL/min, the $\dot{V}CO_2$ would be 200 mL/min. The difference between inspiratory and expiratory minute ventilation would be 50 mL. If the respiratory rate is 10 breaths per minute, the difference for each breath would be 5 mL. This is beyond the resolution limits of most flow sensors. Therefore, most commercially available systems measure the expired volume and apply the Haldane transformation to correct it.

The Haldane transformation assumes that there is no net shift in nitrogen and that the only gases exchanged are oxygen and nitrogen. Therefore, the fractional concentrations for nitrogen can be calculated as

$$FEN_2 = 1 - FEO_2 - FECO_2$$

and

$$FIN_2 = 1 - FIO_2 - FICO_2.$$

Therefore

$$\dot{V}I = (FEN_2/FIN_2)\ \dot{V}E.$$

Including this correction in the general equation for $\dot{V}O_2$ results in

$$\dot{V}O_2 = \dot{V}E \frac{1 - FEO_2 - FECO_2}{1 - FIO_2 - FICO_2} (FIO_2 - FEO_2)$$

and

$$\dot{V}CO_2 = \dot{V}E\ (FECO_2 - FICO_2)$$

By collecting all expired gas over a time interval and analyzing the sample for gas concentrations and volume, it is possible to calculate the average volume of oxygen uptake ($\dot{V}O_2$) and carbon dioxide produced ($\dot{V}CO_2$) as well as the minute ventilation ($\dot{V}E$). By convention, these measurements are reported as milliliters or liters per minute. Primary measurements for gas exchange systems include oxygen, carbon dioxide, and flow.

Data acquisition and display can make significant differences in the quality of the data presented. Data sampling is acquired either breath by breath or at specified time intervals from a mixing chamber.[31] Breath-by-breath measurements reflect substantial variability between breaths. For example, a sigh interspersed with tidal breaths will cause variability in the measured minute ventilation as extrapolated from a single breath. This variability reflects physiologic changes as well as measurement "noise." Although breath-by-breath results offer advantages when studying the kinetics of gas exchange in response to incremental exercise, the data are usually averaged for presentation.

A mixing chamber minimizes the variability seen with a breath-by-breath mode by averaging several breaths over a fixed amount of time. The mixing chamber volume must be flushed to accurately represent the subject's expired air. The initial gas entering the mixing chamber will be diluted by the resident room air. As successive breaths enter the chamber, the resident gas will gradually begin to reflect the average of multiple breaths. This has the effect of damping or slowing the observed response but may make it easier to select a representative value. However, depending on the size of the mixing chamber, it may require a large number of breaths to flush the chamber and obtain accurate results.

In theory, averaging breath-by-breath data over a specific time interval should provide the same information as that collected from a mixing chamber and therefore provides the advantages of both. However, there is ample evidence that accurate breath-by-breath measurement is not a trivial accomplishment.

Several factors must be taken into account to support the calculation. These factors include the accuracy and response time of the sensors, phase delay between sensors, and temperature and humidity changes between inspiratory and expiratory gases. All of these factors and their interrelationships must be handled correctly. It should be noted that these same factors also apply to mixing chamber systems.

Accuracy

Accuracy may be defined as how close an observed value will be to the expected value. Thus, accuracy is a reflection of the expected error of the measurement. By using the analogy of a target, a high degree of accuracy will bring the shots closer to the target center as shown in Figure 8–27. When combined with high precision, high

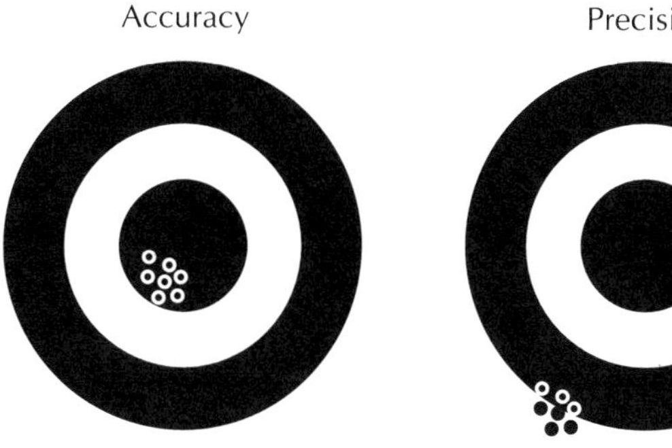

FIG 8–27
Incorrect phase alignment.

levels of accuracy will consistently bring all shots closer to the target center.

The importance of accuracy can easily be demonstrated by example. Table 8–2 illustrates the effect on oxygen uptake and carbon dioxide output of various errors in the analysis of oxygen and carbon dioxide. As can be seen for typical measurements of 16.00% oxygen and 4.00% carbon dioxide, the error for oxygen uptake can vary from 3.9% to 24.4%.

However, accuracy may be limited to only a portion of the needed range. If the accuracy changes over the full scale, the analyzer is said to be alinear. Linearity is just as important as absolute accuracy and precision. In essence, if a device is linear, the accuracy will be the same throughout the full scale of the analyzer. Many analyzers are alinear at the extremes of their ranges. Figure 8–28 illustrates an alinear analyzer that is linear within the clinical range.

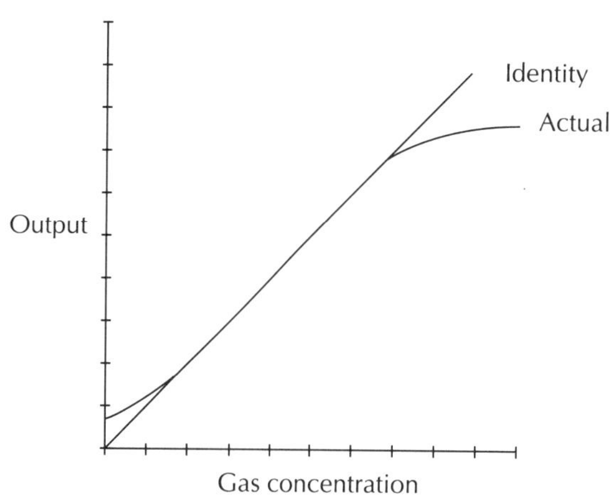

FIG 8–28
Analyzer alinearity.

Phase Alignment

When making breath-by-breath measurements of respiratory gas exchange, the breath-by-breath volume of CO_2 and O_2 exchanged is calculated by multiplying the integral of gas flow by the fractional concentration of CO_2 and O_2. Since all of these waveshapes are changing with time, it is essential that the points to be integrated represent simultaneous data points within the breath stream. For example, if the gas analysis for CO_2 lags behind the flow sufficiently that after flow has apparently ceased the gas concentration is still rising, then the cross-product of zero flow times the highest gas concentration will give zero CO_2. Obviously this will underestimate the actual volume of CO_2 for that breath. This is shown in Figure 8–29.

TABLE 8–2
Effect of Errors on V_{O_2} and V_{CO_2}

Error (%)	F_{EO_2} (%)	V_{O_2} (mL/min)	Error (%)	F_{ECO_2} (%)	V_{CO_2} (mL/min)	Error (%)
1.00	17.00	587	24.4	5.00	750	25.0
0.50	16.50	688	13.9	4.50	675	12.5
0.10	16.10	732	5.9	4.10	615	2.5
0.05	16.05	740	4.6	4.05	608	1.3
0.03	16.03	743	4.2	4.03	605	0.8
0.02	16.02	745	4.0	4.02	603	0.5
0.015	16.015	746	3.9	4.015	602	0.3

$\dot{V}_{CO_2} = V_E\ (STPD^*) \cdot F_{ECO_2}$

$$\dot{V}_{O_2} = V_E\ (STPD) \cdot \frac{1 - F_{EO_2} - F_{ECO_2}}{1 - F_{IO_2} - F_{ICO_2}} (F_{IO_2} - F_{EO_2})$$

V_E STPD	15.0 L
F_{IO_2}	0.2093
F_{ICO_2}	0.0
F_{EO_2}	0.16
F_{ECO_2}	0.04
$\dot{V}_{O_2}$	776
$\dot{V}_{CO_2}$	600

* STPD = standard temperature and pressure, dry.

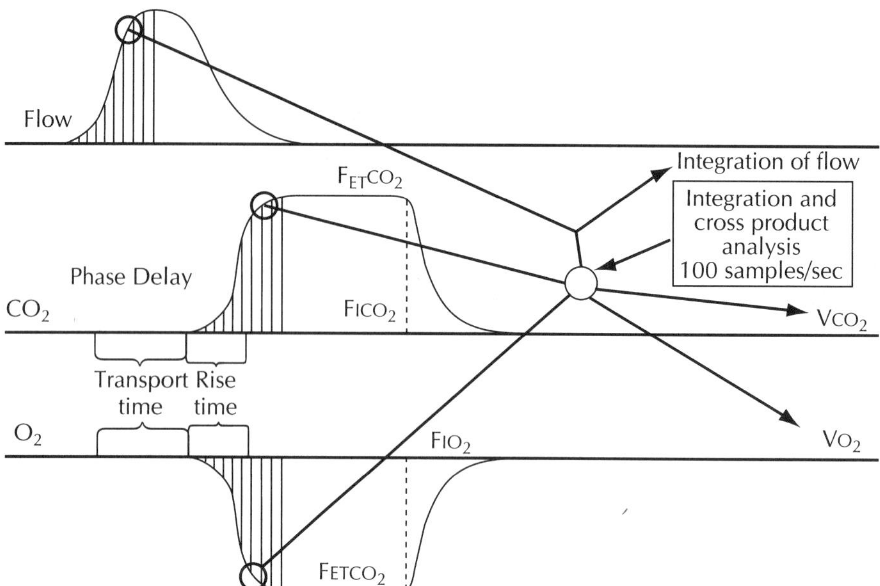

FIG 8–29
Phase delay with its constituents.

Flow and gas concentration are sensed independently, and each sensor has its own response characteristics. Gas flow is propagated at the speed of sound and may be considered instantaneous for our purposes. Gas analysis lags behind the actual event by a finite amount of time equal to the transport time plus the analyzer response time. It is necessary to adjust the flow signal until time alignment with the gas concentration signal is achieved.

Transport time. The time required to move the gas from the tip of the sample line to the analyzer is termed the transport time. The transport time is very reproducible, barring any occlusion, and may be accurately measured by imposing a step change in gas concentration and simply measuring the delay before onset of the analyzer response. The transport time is important only in that it must be predictable and unchanging during the analysis. Relatively long transport times can be tolerated as long as the system can phase-align the gas analysis with the flow signal.

Response time. Any analyzer requires some amount of time to make an analysis once the sample has been introduced. This will differ between analyzer types and even within a specific model. Analyzer response time is generally specified as the time required to achieve 50% or 90% of the final value. The time required to achieve 90% of the final reading is a useful check on analyzer performance and provides an indication of sensor degradation. Obviously, the more prolonged the response, the less applicable an analyzer is for making rapid measurements. All analyzers' performance degrades over time as sample paths become occluded or the sensors physically deteriorate.

Phase delay adjustment. The point at which the flow and gas concentration signals are aligned is critical.[33] The signals cannot be aligned with the onset of the respective changes since the leading edge of the gas concentration signal is diluted by dead space. Alignment at this point would introduce significant error of overestimating $\dot{V}CO_2$ and underestimating $\dot{V}O_2$.

Typically, breath-by-breath systems are aligned at a percentage of the maximal response, which ensures clearance of dead space, generally 50% or 66%. This position is derived mathematically by evaluating the concentration change as an exponential. In an exponential shape where the signal duration is large in comparison with the time constant and the valve dead space is cleared quickly at the start of expiration, the trailing edge of the waveform will contribute to the integral. The minimum error will correlate with the rise time to one half the maximum amplitude.

Errors in gas exchange measurement resulting from the misalignment of flow and gas concentration signals are linearly related to the magnitude of the misalignment with exponential signals. For every 10-ms alignment error, there will be a corresponding 1% error in the calculated gas exchange. In situations where the waveshape has been distorted, such as by insertion of water absorbers, the simple model is no longer accurate. The integrals in gas exchange measurement are quite sensitive to the waveshape. The distortions introduced by absorbers will vary with time and cannot be compensated by calibration. Figure 8–29 illustrates the concept of phase delay with its constituent times.

Temperature and Humidity Changes

Inspired room air is typically approximately 23°C and 50% saturated. Expired air is generally 100% humidified and approaches 37°C, although cooling occurs quickly once the gas exits the mouth. Ventilation is reported at body temperature and pressure, saturated (BTPS), whereas oxygen uptake and carbon dioxide production are reported at standard temperature and pressure, dry (STPD). In order to make these corrections, it is necessary to know the temperature and saturation of the measured gas.

The temperature of expired gas changes rapidly once it leaves the mouth and is typically corrected by allowing it to cool to room temperature and applying a static correction, by correcting each breath via an empirical factor based on the respiratory rate and flow, or by dynamically measuring the temperature and adjusting the correction factor appropriately. Most computerized gas exchange systems use an empirically determined factor. These factors can introduce errors at very high minute ventilations.

Corrections for humidity are more complicated. Since both inspired and expired gas samples must be measured, it is important to correct both appropriately. For this purpose it is simplest to measure both inspired and expired gas samples at the same saturation by conditioning the gas before analysis.

The technique used with older mixing chamber systems was to pass the gas to be analyzed through chemical reagents that remove all moisture. This dries both inspired and expired samples. However, this process disrupts the gas wave front and cannot be used with the breath-by-breath method.

Humidity is related to temperature to the extent that complete saturation will occur at 37°C. Once saturated, a gas remains saturated even as it cools, although the cooling will cause condensation. Some systems attempt to prevent condensation by heating the sample line above 37°C. The effect of heating the sample line can lead to unpredictable errors since the expired sample may no longer be fully saturated and the inspired gas must now be assumed to be saturated as well. Since exhaled air is fully saturated even if cooled, it can be corrected by applying a wet/dry correction factor.

Alternatively, by using recently developed moisture-permeable sample tubing, it is possible to condition the gas without affecting the gas wave front. This tubing provides very efficient transfer of moisture between the gas sample within the tubing and ambient air surrounding the tubing. Two versions of this approach are currently used.

The first equilibrates both inspired and expired gas samples to ambient conditions. The permeable tubing permits moisture within the gas sample to pass through the wall of the tubing until it equilibrates with ambient air. The drawback to this approach is that ambient conditions are neither dry nor fully saturated. This leads to a correction that involves assumptions regarding the actual moisture volume.

The second involves equilibrating the gas samples to a known, dry condition. This is accomplished by encasing the permeable tubing within a second sheath. A dry gas passed within the sheathing causes the gas sample to give up its moisture completely. The dry gas is created by pumping ambient air through a chemical reagent. Since the gas sample does not have to pass through the reagent, the wave front is undistorted.

Types of Sensors

Oxygen Analyzers

Oxygen analysis can be made by several techniques that make use of the unique properties of oxygen. These techniques include zirconia cells, mass spectrometers, and paramagnetic analyzers. Zirconia fuel cells are the most widely used method for exercise since they provide the fast response required for breath-by-breath measurement at a reasonable cost. Mass spectrometers, although they provide excellent characteristics, are not commonly used in commercial systems because of the high cost of the instrument. Paramagnetic analyzers generally do not have the response time necessary for exercise but are used in metabolic carts.

Zirconia cell analyzers. Zirconia is a ceramic material that is semipermeable for oxygen at high temperatures. The zirconia element is typically stabilized with yttria to produce a cubic crystal structure that is stable from room temperature to its melting point. This process creates vacancies in the crystal lattice structure that are sized for oxygen ions, which makes the zirconia element essentially a semipermeable membrane for oxygen. Electrically, zirconia is a very effective nonconductor; however, at high temperatures it passes oxygen ions readily.

The exposed surfaces of the zirconia element are coated with platinum to form an electrode. One side of the electrode is exposed to a reference gas such as room air while the other side is exposed to the sample gas. Figure 8–30 illustrates a zirconia cell oxygen sensor. The migration of oxygen ions across the electrode creates a voltage proportional to the oxygen concentration differences. This relationship is described by the Nernst equation:

$$E = KT \cdot \log P_{O_2}\ (\text{reference})/P_{O_2}\ (\text{unknown}),$$

where T is the temperature and K is a constant describing the characteristics of the electrode. Temperature is

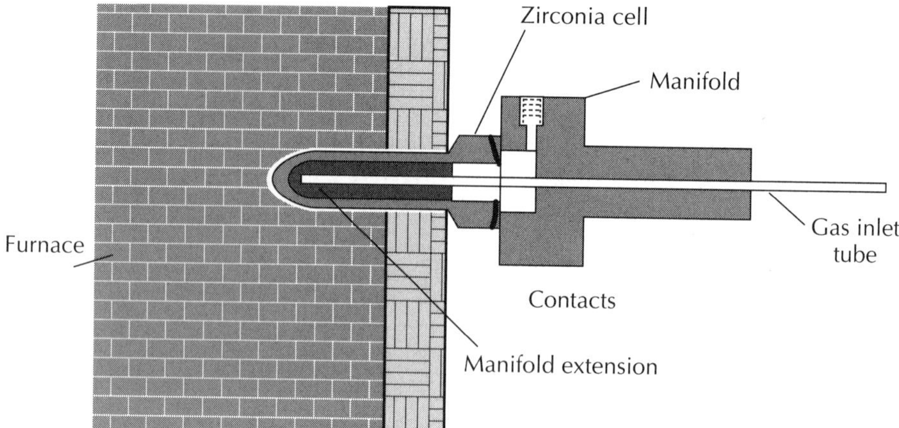

FIG 8–30
Zirconia cell oxygen sensor.

usually held constant at approximately 700°C. The high temperature requires adequate insulation to maintain a constant temperature. From a cold start, the analyzer will require a substantial warm-up period.

Since zirconia cells measure the partial pressure of oxygen, fluctuations in ambient pressure will also cause variations in the oxygen readings. It is necessary that the ambient pressure on both sides of the electrode be equal. This can present difficulties if the sample side is exposed to variable pressures, as may be generated by mechanical ventilation. Zirconia cells are also flow dependent at sample flows above 200 mL/min. This effect is probably due to temperature changes induced by the variations in flow. To maintain accuracy at higher flows, the sample flow must be tightly controlled. At lower sample rates, variations in flow are not as critical.

Combustible gases in the sample will also cause erroneous oxygen readings, as a portion of the oxygen in the expired sample will be used to support the combustion. Water vapor will dilute the sample, thus creating an offset error. Further, it is obvious that a high-temperature analyzer should never be used in an explosive environment.

Paramagnetic analyzers. Because of their molecular structure, gases can be influenced by magnetic fields. Most respiratory gases are diamagnetic and are repelled by a magnetic field. Some gases, most specifically oxygen and nitric oxide, are strongly attracted to a magnetic field. This property of paramagnetism can be used to measure variations in oxygen concentration. The most common approach is to suspend a freely rotating dumbbell within a nonhomogeneous magnetic field. The dumbbell is filled with a diamagnetic gas such as nitrogen and will align itself toward the strongest part of the magnetic field.

As oxygen or nitric oxide molecules enter the chamber, they will be drawn to the center of the field. This will cause a displacement of the dumbbell proportional to the concentration of oxygen. This displacement can be detected optically by directing a light onto a small mirror attached to the dumbbell and sensing the reflected light with photocells.

Another approach is to inject the sample gas and a reference gas into a space between the poles of an electromagnet separated by a transducer diaphragm. Switching the magnet on and off will mix the gases within the field and create a differential pressure proportional to the difference in magnetic susceptibility and therefore the gas concentration.

Paramagnetic analyzers are sensitive to pressure changes, moisture, and the presence of high concentrations of diamagnetic gases such as nitrogen. Generally, the analyzer is zeroed with background gas, such as room air, and then spanned with an oxygen concentration similar to the expected sample. Smaller concentrations of diamagnetic gases such as 0% to 5% carbon dioxide will not appreciably affect the reading. Figure 8–31 illustrates a paramagnetic oxygen analyzer.

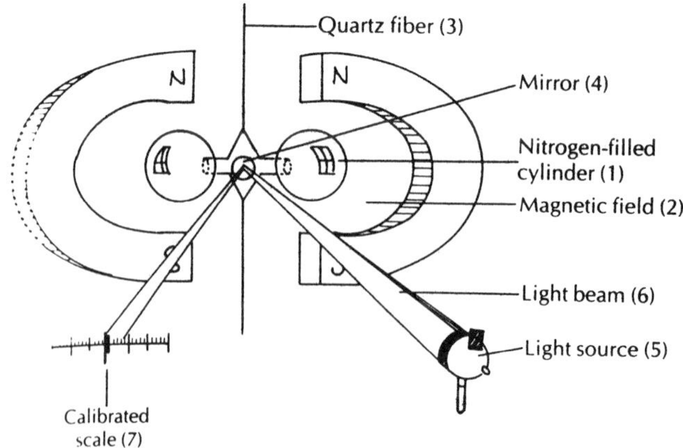

FIG 8–31
Paramagnetic oxygen analyzer. (From Eubanks DH, Bone RC (eds): *Comprehensive Respiratory Care: A Learning System,* ed 2. Eubanks DH, Bone RC: Oxygen analyzers, 363, St Louis, Mosby–Year Book, 1990.)

Carbon Dioxide Analysis

By far the most common type of carbon dioxide analyzer uses nondispersive infrared analysis. This technique is common to the carbon monoxide analyzer that was discussed in detail earlier in the pulmonary function section. As in the carbon monoxide analyzer, the infrared beam is passed through a chamber containing the sample gas. By measuring the intensity of the transmitted light a determination of the relative concentration can be made.

Cardiovascular Monitoring

Electrocardiographic (ECG) monitoring during exercise is typically made with at least 3 chest leads and more commonly 12 leads. Standard precordial lead configurations (V_1 through V_6) are commonly used. Limb leads are generally moved to the torso to minimize motion artifact. Also, vectorcardiographic leads are sometimes used to display initial forces and phase relationships as well as improve sensitivity for detection of rear wall ischemia.

Common parameters for cardiovascular stress monitoring include calculation of averaged or median beats for all leads, determination of ST levels and slopes and J point changes, and arrhythmia detection. Comparison with preexercise values is automatically made. Algorithms to remove respiratory and motion artifacts are commonly added.

Examples of Exercise Systems

MedGraphics CPX

The CPX uses a disposable flow sensor, zirconia cell oxygen analyzer, and infrared carbon dioxide analyzer. The system consists of a computer, monitor, and two hardware modules and is shown in Figure 8–32. A gas analyzer module contains the oxygen and carbon dioxide analyzer and associated electronics. The flow module includes the flow sensor and waveform analyzer, which controls the data acquisition and signal processing. The system can be mounted into a mobile cart with a printer or used as a desktop system. A 12-lead ECG capability can also be added. Additional software provides the capability to perform noninvasive cardiac output by using CO_2 rebreathing, anaerobic threshold detection, and exercise interpretation. These results are combined into consolidated reports.

The system can be interfaced with a variety of external devices such as ECG monitors, oximeters, treadmills, ergometers, and automated blood pressure monitors. The outputs from these devices can be incorporated into a consolidated report. With input from indwelling arterial sensors, the software will calculate cardiac output from the Fick equation and various rate-pressure products. Treadmills and ergometers can be controlled by the CPX system to automate exercise protocols and provide the capability of continuous ramping.

Operationally, the system software is menu driven, and data collection can be as straightforward as pressing the space bar to start and stop the study. Manual measurements and comments can be added to the data during the exercise without stopping the data collection. All measurements are made breath by breath, but the operator has the ability to select averaging routines for graphic display and data calculations. Exercise protocols, graphic data displays, and tabular reports can be scripted in advance by the operator and selected by name.

Using the disposable flow sensor eliminates the need for a nonrebreathing valve and large-bore collection tubing. Flow is measured at the mouth, and the flow sensor contains a sample port for the gas analyzers. The flow sensor is a turbulent flow–type device that uses differential pressure to monitor the flow. The pressure transducers are contained in the flow module, and a small umbilical connects the sensor to the transducers as well as provides the gas sample line. The gas sample line connects to the gas analyzer module and contains a moisture-permeable section that completely dries the sample. This provides a known reference for calibration and calculations.

SensorMedics 2900

The 2900 uses a hot-wire anemometer flow sensor, zirconia cell oxygen analyzer, and infrared carbon dioxide analyzer. The system consists of a computer, monitor, signal processing board, and two gas analyzers and is shown in Figure 8–33. The 2900 uses a moisture-permeable sample line to equilibrate both calibration and sample gas to ambient humidity.

The system can be purchased as a mobile cart or on a free-standing pedestal. A 12-lead ECG capability can also be added. Additional software provides the capability to determine noninvasive cardiac output by using CO_2 rebreathing, anaerobic threshold detection, and exercise interpretation. These results are combined into consolidated reports.

Menu-driven software permits the addition of manually entered results and selection of preconfigured protocols. The flow sensor is placed in the expiratory breathing path by using a low-resistance nonrebreathing valve. The system offers two modes, breath by breath and dynamic switching mixing chambers.

The mixing chamber is actually three fixed-size chambers (1, 5, and 7 L) that can be software-selected based on the minute ventilation. Adequate mixing in a chamber is a function of the size of the chamber and the amount of ventilation. Generally, the rule of thumb is that to adequately flush a chamber requires ventilation five times the chamber volume. Therefore, a large chamber will take longer than a small chamber to flush. During exercise, the minute ventilation may increase from approximately 10 L/min to over 100 L/min at maximal exercise. A single-size chamber will be inadequate to rapidly measure ventilatory changes, which may change by an order of magnitude.

Marquette MAX-1

The MAX-1 has a 15-lead input capability for standard 12-lead displays as well as vector displays and late-phase potentials. The MAX-1 provides automatic or manual treadmill control. The system can also interface with an ergometer. In addition to standard demographics, physician impressions can be entered directly by using the keyboard. Menu and function control is combined with a single selector, and a test control keypad mounted just below the display provides convenient access to operations during the exercise test. The MAX-1 is shown in Figure 8–34.

The system permits selection of preconfigured summary reports that can be user defined. The reports can be stored onto diskettes. Marquette also offers an information management system based on a local area network. This system stores tests and provides remote access to the data at several different workstations simultaneously by using bar code retrieval. This network

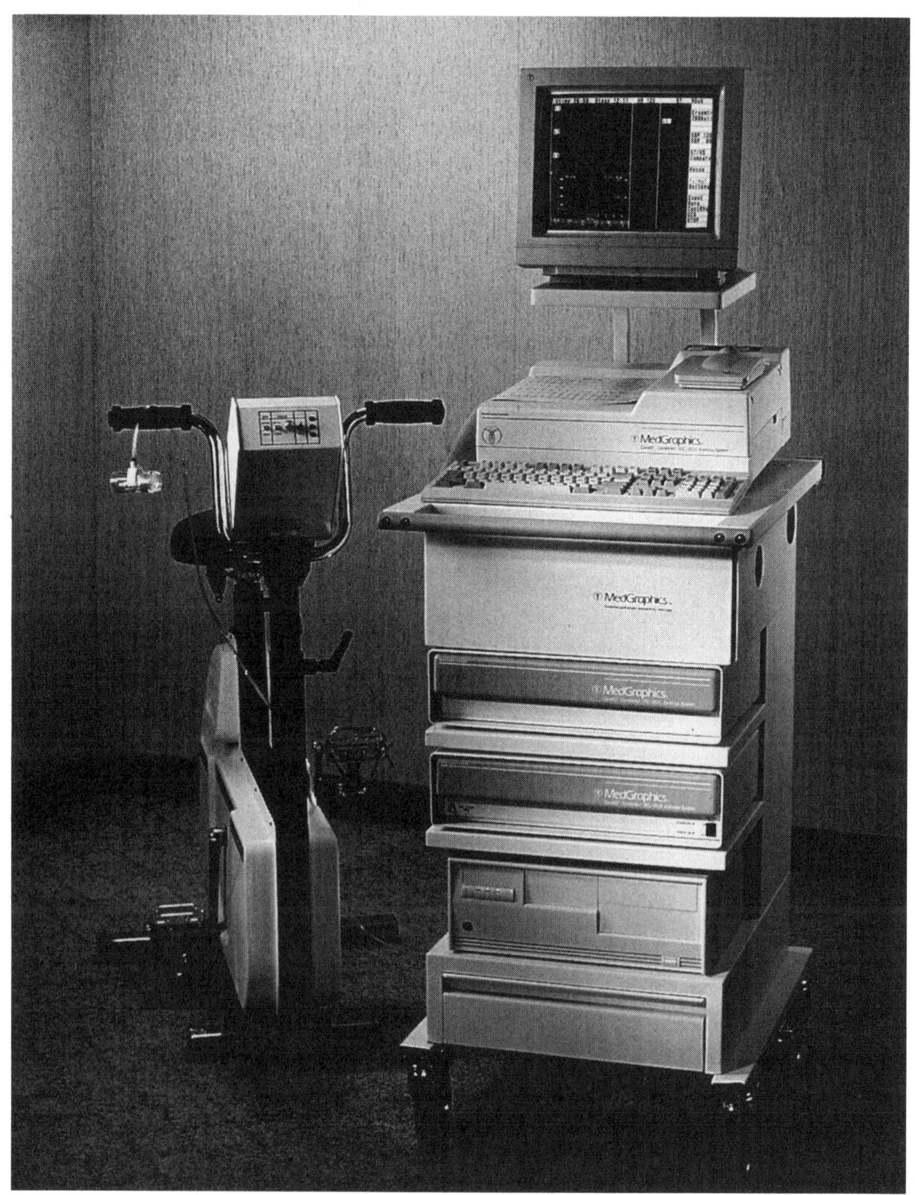

FIG 8–32
MedGraphics CPX Exercise System. (Courtesy of MedGraphics Corp, St Paul, Minn.)

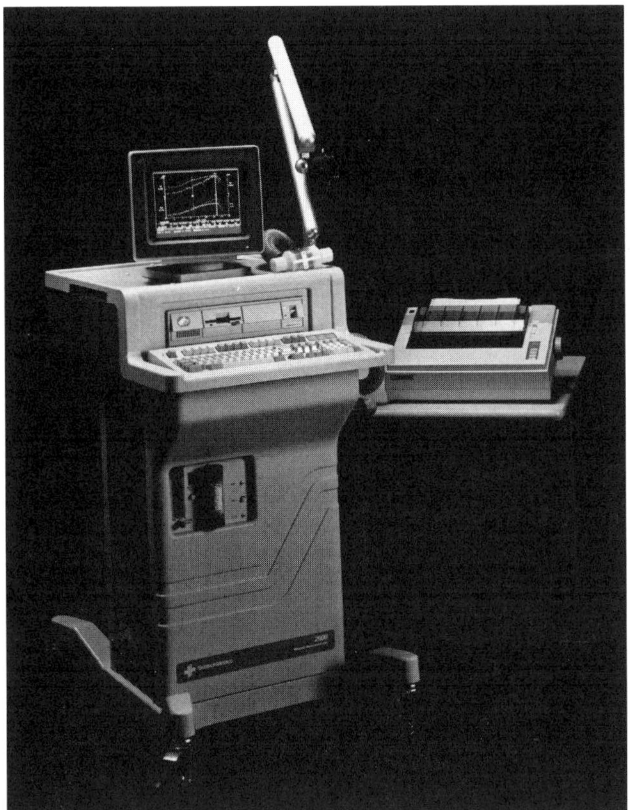

FIG 8–33
SensorMedics 2900 Exercise System. (Courtesy of SensorMedics, Yorba Linda, Calif.)

can also be interfaced with a hospital information system.

Quinton 4500

The 4500 is a personal computer–based system that provides standard 12-lead displays and configurable protocols. Dual filtering reduces baseline wander and muscle artifact. The 4500 offers user-configurable data acquisition screens that permit the combination of nine different trend graphs in combination with real-time display. Configurations are made by using pull-down menus.

The system provides considerable flexibility for report configuration. Final reports can be customized to automatically extract data and add text for protocol, patient age, maximal-stage heart rate and blood pressure, and various ECG calculations such as ST levels and slopes for any lead and worst case. This text can be customized for individual physician impression. Additionally, the system provides the capability to pre-edit the physician impression during recovery, which speeds up report turnaround time. The Quinton 4500 is shown in Figure 8–35.

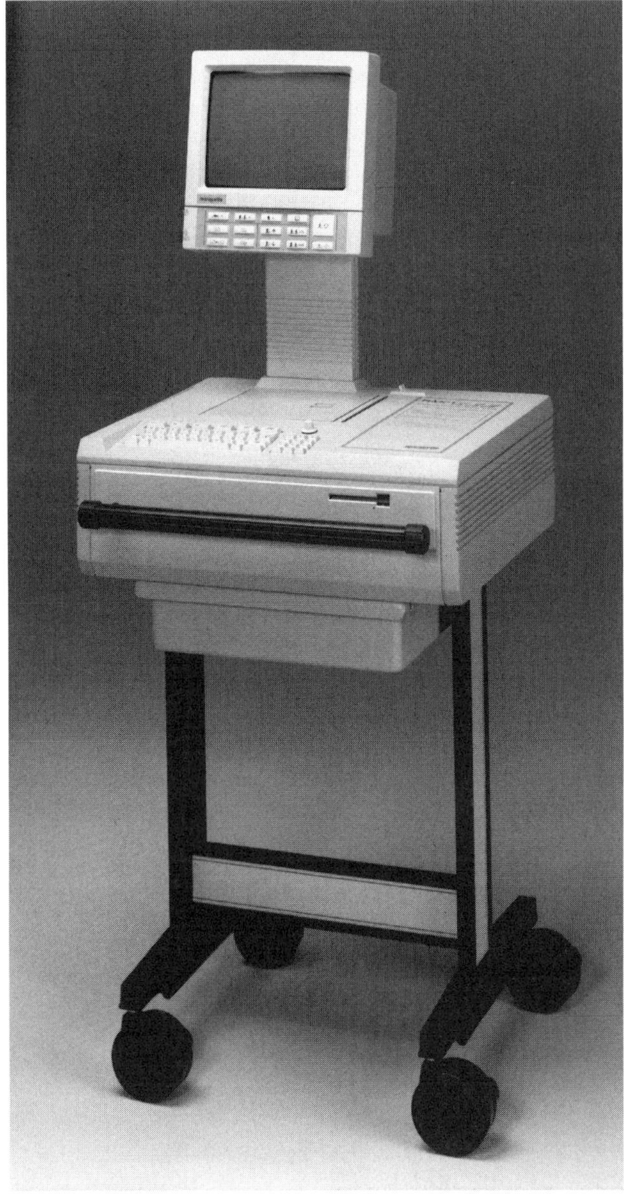

FIG 8–34
Marquette MAX-1 Cardiac Stress System. (Courtesy of Marquette Electronics, Milwaukee, Wisc.)

BLOOD GAS ANALYSIS

Estimation of oxygenation, acidosis, and ventilatory failure before the development of arterial blood gas (ABG) electrodes was largely based on clinical evaluation. It was recognized in the 1950s that the diagnosis of cyanosis by physicians was poor unless the oxygen saturation was less than 80%[34] and the Pa_{O_2} was less than 50 mm Hg as measured by the tedious Riley bubble method or by the Scholander technique, which was only available in research laboratories.

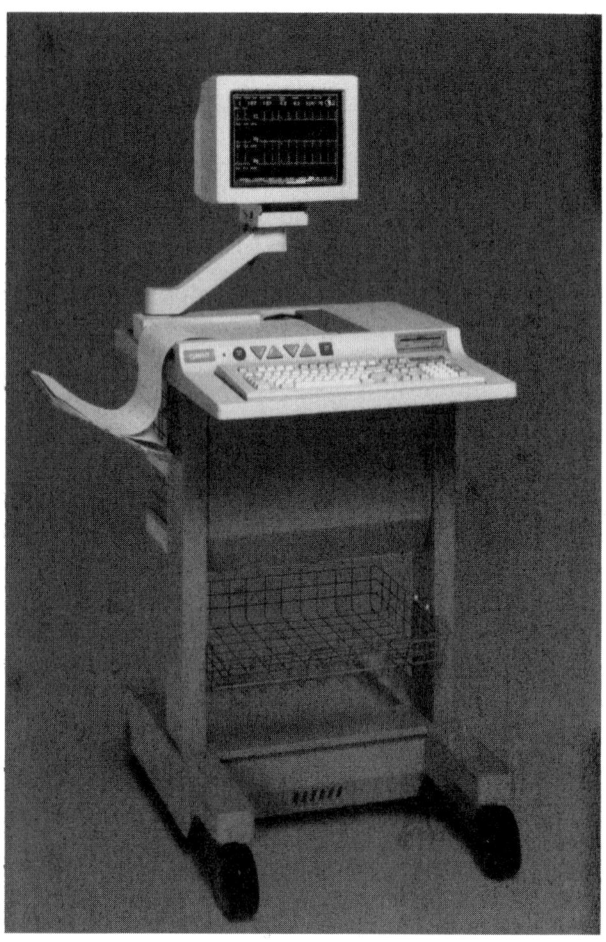

FIG 8–35
Quinton 4500 Cardiac Stress System. (Courtesy of Quinton Instruments, Seattle, Wash.)

The measurement of O_2, CO_2, and pH in arterial blood is commonly referred to as ABGs. The pH electrode was first developed in 1922, and use was limited to chemistry laboratories. The development of electrodes suitable for use with blood was popularized in the 1950s by Astrup. This electrode not only measured pH but also P_{CO_2} by detecting the change in pH when an unknown blood sample was equilibrated at two different known P_{CO_2} values. Nomograms were constructed to then calculate the P_{CO_2} from the two measured pH values.

The P_{CO_2} electrode was originally proposed by Stow et al.[35] and modified in 1958 by Sevringhaus and Bradley.[36] The electrode consisted of a pH electrode mounted in a bicarbonate solution and sealed with a Teflon membrane that allowed CO_2 to diffuse into the solution. This altered the H^+ concentration, which was then measured by pH-sensitive glass. The P_{O_2} polarographic sensor was originally discovered in 1897, but the first feasible design was made by Clark in 1953[37] and modified by Sevringhaus and Bradley in 1958.[36] Clinical use of these electrodes started in the 1960s and was quickly accepted as a mainstay in clinical pulmonary and critical care medicine.

ABGs have been prescribed as a touchstone in pulmonary and critical care medicine. Major decisions are made at boundaries determined by clinical experience. For example, the current medicare mandate is that continuous oxygen prescriptions are indicated when arterial Pa_{O_2} is below 55 mm Hg on room air at sea level. The presumption is that the measurement is an accurate representation of a patient's status. Yet, the acceptable error in Pa_{O_2} is ± 4 mm Hg. Further, in many patients with chronic obstructive pulmonary disease (COPD), hyperventilation, coughing, or exercise will improve Pa_{O_2} by 5 mm Hg or more. Yet another factor is that normal values decrease with age to about 70 mm Hg at 70 years of age. In this situation, the same criteria may not apply. Clearly, the Pa_{O_2} is but one factor in the complex decision of committing a patient to a lifetime of tethering to an O_2 line.

The major disadvantage of ABGs is well demonstrated by this example. Since it is an invasive and costly test, it is not reasonable to obtain multiple samples under different conditions when the patient is at her best, which would require an indwelling catheter. It is here that pulse oximetry has had such value and yet created a new set of problems. This was experienced in the late 1980s regarding the question of long-term oxygen prescriptions. Sa_{O_2} measurements by pulse oximetry (Sp_{O_2}) can be made readily during exercise or sleep when values may well decline. The critical decision was that an Sp_{O_2} of 85% was approximately equivalent to a Pa_{O_2} of 55 mm Hg. Yet it was subsequently shown that 40% of patients would be erroneously judged to need O_2 with an 85% cutoff; so guidelines were changed to 88%. The accuracy of Sp_{O_2} is less than Pa_{O_2}.

ABGs are most frequently necessary and depended upon in the critical care setting. The need for intubation and mechanical ventilation is frequently decided on the basis of low Pa_{O_2} (less than 50 to 60 mm Hg on maximal Fi_{O_2}) or respiratory acidosis (pH of 7.25 to 7.30 with a Pa_{CO_2} greater than 50 to 60 mm Hg). Yet a study of stable, endotracheally intubated patients on a fixed Fi_{O_2}, with measurements of ABGs made 50 minutes apart, revealed a coefficient of variation of 5% for Pa_{O_2}, 3% for Pa_{CO_2}, and a mean range for pH of 0.03 units. The Pa_{O_2} varied by as much as 45 mm Hg or 30% over this relatively short interval. The Pa_{CO_2} had a range of 8 mm Hg or 17% over the interval. Clearly, therapeutic decisions should not be made on single determinations of ABGs but rather from trends and clinical correlations.

The above examples assume good technique in blood sampling, delivery to the laboratory, and accurately

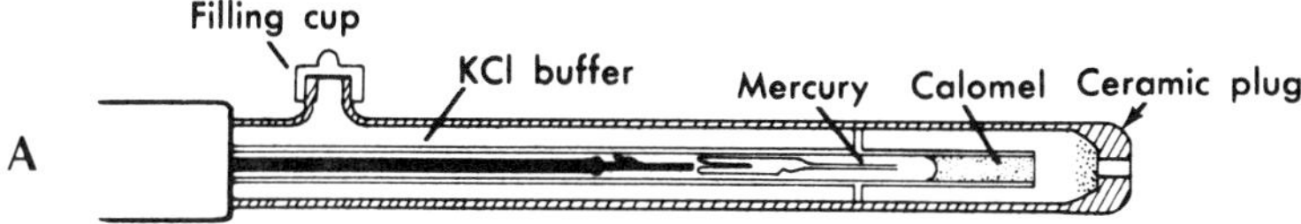

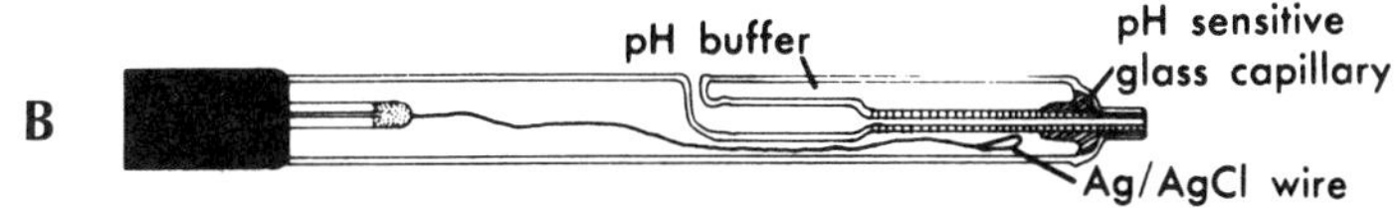

FIG 8–36
A and **B,** pH electrode. (From Ruppel G: *Manual of Pulmonary Function Testing,* ed 5. St Louis, Mosby–Year Book, 1991, p 227. Used by permission.)

calibrated electrodes. In a study of blood gas proficiency monitoring for 580 instruments, 1 SD for pH, P_{CO_2}, and P_{O_2} was reported as 0.014, 2.05, and 6.49 respectively. The same group reported that out of 894 instruments and 450 laboratories, only 4 instruments failed to meet model-specific targets for pH, 2 failed P_{CO_2}, and only 3 failed P_{O_2}. These results give a good indication that the blood gas analyzers have a remarkably good record of accuracy. Those few that failed could be characterized as underutilized, isolated laboratories. Proficiency testing programs are useful and are currently mandated by federal regulations (Clinical Laboratory Improvement Act of 1988 [CLIA-88]).[38]

Theory of Operation

pH Electrode

The measurement of pH involves a special pH-sensitive glass electrode assembly containing two distinct elements. A reference electrode is interfaced with the blood sample through a liquid junction or salt bridge and maintains a constant potential. The sample electrode is composed of pH-sensitive glass and measures the difference in hydrogen ion concentration between a sealed reference solution within the glass and the blood sample. The movement of hydrogen ions into the glass electrode creates an electrical potential between the two sides proportional to the pH. The relationship between pH and voltage is described by the Nernst equation, and for each pH unit difference there is a voltage difference of approximately 60 mV. A pH sensor is illustrated in Figure 8–36.

Carbon Dioxide Electrode

The Stow-Sevringhaus P_{CO_2} electrode is in reality a modified pH sensor. As modified, the pH-sensitive glass does not actually come into contact with blood. A thin-film bicarbonate solution surrounds the pH-sensitive glass. A membrane permeable to CO_2 separates the solution from the blood sample. As CO_2 diffuses into the bicarbonate solution, a hydrolysis reaction takes place that results in the production of hydrogen ions. The resulting pH change is proportional to the partial pressure of CO_2 in the solution. An illustration of the Stow-Sevringhaus electrode is shown in Figure 8–37.

Oxygen Electrode

The Clark P_{O_2} electrode is a polarographic sensor. The basic components of the sensor include an external battery or power source to provide a polarizing voltage, an ammeter or display, and a silver silver-chloride anode and platinum cathode immersed in an electrolyte solution. The negatively charged platinum cathode attracts oxygen molecules, which react with water and are consumed. This consumption draws replacement electrons from the silver silver-chloride reference electrode into the electrolyte solution. The reaction at the platinum cathode is as follows:

$$O_2 + 2\ H_2O + 4e^- = 4\ OH^-$$

while at the anode:

$$4\ Ag + 4\ Cl^- = 4\ AgCl + 4e^-$$

The result of these reactions is the flow of current between the anode and cathode. This current generated is proportional to the amount of dissolved O_2 in the solution. Protein deposits on the electrode alter its electrical characteristics. Clark's modification of the electrode separates the blood from the cathode with a semipermeable membrane that selectively allows oxygen to diffuse through the membrane and into the electrolyte. The measurement consumes O_2, which must be trans-

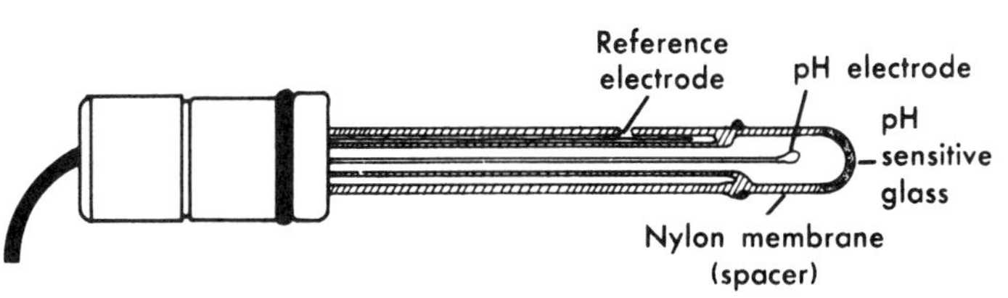

FIG 8–37
Stow-Sevringhaus P_{CO_2} electrode. (From Ruppel G: *Manual of Pulmonary Function Testing,* ed 5. St Louis, Mosby–Year Book, 1991, p 227. Used by permission.)

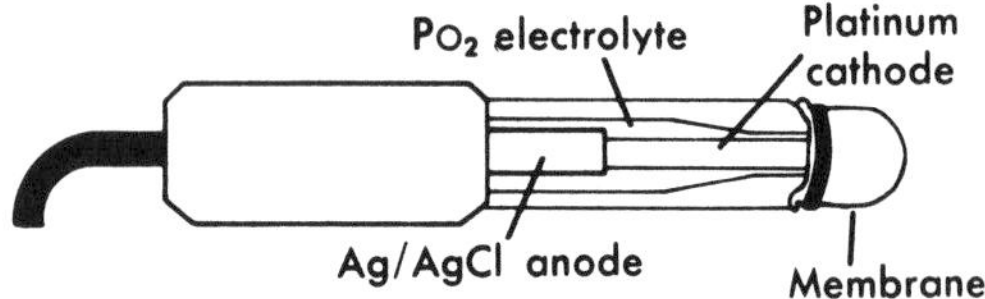

FIG 8–38
Clark Po_2 electrode. (From Ruppel G: *Manual of Pulmonary Function Testing,* ed 5. St Louis, Mosby–Year Book, 1991, p 227. Used by permission.)

ported through the membrane and diffused into the electrolyte. This process accounts for the prolonged response time, which can vary from 30 to 360 seconds depending on the membrane and electrode design. An illustration of the Clark polarographic electrode is shown in Figure 8–38.

Bedside or Point-of-Care Systems

ABGs are now universally used in hospitals. There now are available "point-of-care" instruments that simplify the technology to the point that not only ABGs but also electrolytes and other studies can be done conveniently with small samples of blood at the bedside. These systems currently use standard ABG technology, but miniaturized with specifically designed disposable, single-use cartridges that automate the calibration and sample as shown in Figure 8–39. The electrochemical sensors are "Clark"-style polarographic electrodes for O_2, Stow-Sevringhaus electrodes for CO_2, and ion-selective technology for pH and electrolytes. Because the systems are automated and used by personnel who are not trained laboratory technicians, quality control has been emphasized by the manufacturers. These requirements are mandated by CLIA-88.

In addition, microelectrodes with new technology allow continuous measurement of ABGs via intravascular catheters. However, it must be recognized that ABGs are limited because they are invasive and are greatly influenced by the mode of ventilation, hemodynamics, and pulmonary and nonpulmonary factors, as discussed in Chapter 7.

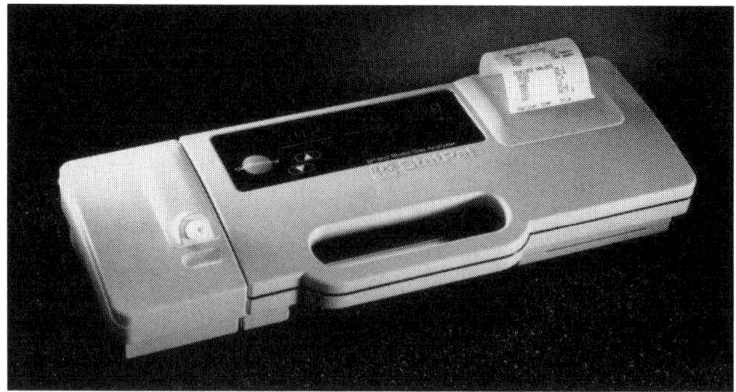

FIG 8–39
PPG StatPal point-of-care analyzer. (PPG Industries, La Jolla, Calif.)

Examples of Arterial Blood Gas Systems

Corning 238/278/280/288

This series of blood gas systems differs primarily in the level of automation and the provision for measuring electrolytes and hemoglobin in addition to blood gases. The 238 is designed for point-of-care usage for blood gases, whereas the 288 is a combined blood gas, electrolyte, and hemoglobin measurement system. The systems provide automatic calibration at operator-selected frequencies and can run up to 35 samples per hour. A feature of this series is maintenance-free electrodes. The electrodes are simply replaced on a periodic basis. Automatic quality control tracking calculates

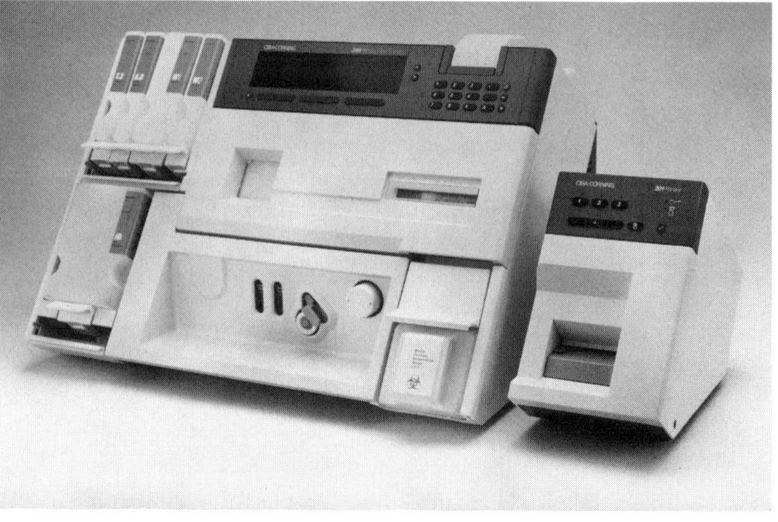

FIG 8–40
Corning 288 Arterial Blood Gas Analyzer. (Courtesy of Corning Instruments.)

means, standard deviation, and coefficients of variations for quality control materials. A Corning 288 is shown in Figure 8–40.

BRONCHOSCOPY

Bronchoscopy was originally developed in the late 1890s as a means of removing foreign bodies from the airways. The original device was a rigid metal tube that allowed the use of special instruments to reach into the bronchus. Later advances added a light system and a stylet for suctioning, which led to the technique of bronchial lavage for the removal of purulent secretions in bronchiectasis. Rigid bronchoscopes have largely been replaced by flexible fiber-optic bronchoscopy.

Flexible fiber-optic bronchoscopy was introduced in Japan by Ikeda in the early 1960s. Commercial availability in the late 1960s made a profound impact on the diagnosis of indeterminate pulmonary disease. Widely used in a variety of localized and diffuse lung diseases, flexible fiber-optic bronchoscopy is used not only for diagnostic endoscopy but also for the therapeutic management of airway disorders.

Several biopsy techniques are available with fiber-optic bronchoscopy. These include forceps biopsy, brush biopsy, needle biopsy, and bronchoalveolar lavage (BAL). These techniques permit both cytopathologic evaluation of neoplasms and bacteriologic evaluation of bacteria, mycobacteria, fungi, and viruses. Additionally, the suction tip can be used to relieve atelectasis secondary to retained secretions and mucous plugs.

Application of bronchoscopy can be divided into diagnostic and therapeutic uses. Diagnostic uses include evaluation of lung lesions, assessment of airway patency, evaluation of problems with endotracheal tubes, and evaluation of hemoptysis. Therapeutic uses include removal of foreign bodies, mucous plugs, and retained secretions as well as assisting in difficult intubations. BAL fluid analysis can also be useful in evaluating the deposition of aerosolized pharmacokinetic agents.

Theory of Operation

The bronchoscopy setup generally has several components. A flexible bronchoscope is coupled with a light source. Attachments are available, such as dual viewing for training. A variety of instruments for biopsy and foreign body removal are usually associated with the setup. For BAL and suctioning, a suction pump or wall vacuum must be provided. Additionally, an optional camera or videocassette recorder can be used to document the findings.

The fiber-optic bronchoscope usually consists of a sheathed bundle containing wire guides for controlling the tip and three independent channels. Two of the channels are used for fiber-optic glass fibers, one fiber-optic channel for illumination and a separate channel for visualization. A third operating channel is used for suctioning and passing instruments. In some instruments, a fourth channel is available to permit independent suctioning and passing of instruments.

Bronchoscopes are classified according to the diameter of their distal ends. These sizes range from 4.9 to 6.0 mm for adults and 2.2 to 3.7 mm for children. The smallest-diameter scopes (pediatric scopes and laryngoscopes) have diameters that are too small to permit passing of instruments or suctioning and are only used for visualization.

At the head of the scope is the viewing lens, which also provides the option of attaching a camera or a video camera. The angle of visual field varies by brand and model and ranges between 75 and 120 degrees. Also part of the bronchoscope head is the focus adjustment, the fingertip suction control, and the lever to control motion of the bronchoscope tip. The tip can be flexed a variable amount in two directions, again depending on the brand and the model. The range of flexion is from 100 to 130 degrees down and 160 to 180 degrees up, usually with more flexion in one direction than another. Finally, the diaphragm valve that allows passage of an instrument into the suction channel without losing the ability to suction is located further down below the handgrip. There are also available bronchoscopes with two hollow channels, one for suctioning and one for instrumentation.

Light sources are available in different sizes and intensity. Xenon provides the greatest intensity, but more affordable is the halogen light source. Smaller, portable light sources are also available. If photographing or video is anticipated, the brighter light sources with flash capability are preferred. Each bronchoscope company manufactures a companion light source to their bronchoscope, but most can be interchanged with other brands.

Videobronchoscopy arrangements with or without computer interface are available. These systems allow live video viewing on a TV size monitor as well as the option of making a videotape for permanent reference. The computer systems allow for still shots that can be edited and printed on a laser color printer.

Instruments used through the bronchoscope include biopsy forceps, brushes, and aspiration needles. Forceps come in various sizes and configurations (e.g., with or without a serrated edge). Brushes are available with or without a protective plug, which allows uncontaminated specimens to be obtained from the distal airways. Aspiration needles come in a variety of lengths and diameters designed to facilitate aspiration of either proximal or distal masses. These needles protrude from a protective sheath after being passed through the bronchoscope.

Bronchoscopy Procedures

The bronchoscopy procedure varies depending on the status of the patient, the diagnostic needs, and individual preference of the physician. After informed consent is obtained, the patient is usually sedated with some combination of benzodiazepine, opiate, and/or sometimes an anticholinergic agent. Local anesthesia of the upper airway is generally obtained with the use of some combination of the following agents: 1%, 2%, and/or 4% lidocaine (nebulized, sprayed, applied with gauze, etc.); viscous lidocaine to the nose; cocaine; and benzocaine spray.

The bronchoscope may be passed through the nares or the mouth (with a protective bite block in place). It may also be passed through an endotracheal tube by using a special diaphragm valve to maintain pressure if the patient is on a ventilator. The scope is positioned above the vocal cords, which are then anesthetized with 2% or 4% lidocaine. The scope is then passed into the trachea, and further local anesthesia is obtained with 1% or 2% lidocaine as needed to suppress coughing. The tracheobronchial tree is inspected for endobronchial lesions or abnormal secretions.

Biopsy samples of endobronchial lesions can be obtained under direct vision by using forceps. Endobronchial lesions can also be brushed for cytologic study. Transbronchial biopsies can be performed by passing the forceps toward the edge of the lung (frequently with fluoroscopic guidance) and sampling alveolar tissue. This procedure carries the risk of hemorrhage and pneumothorax. An aspirating needle may be passed through the tracheal wall into a lymph node or directly into a visualized lesion to obtain a specimen for cytologic examination.

Bronchoalveolar lavage is performed by wedging the scope into a selected bronchus and injecting saline through the channel. Volumes injected range from 20 to 240 cc (usually around 60 to 100 cc in 30 to 60-cc aliquots). After each injection, the lavage fluid is aspirated back into the syringe. Bronchial wash is a similar technique, but the specimen is obtained by putting a trap in the line with the suction.

Depending on the status of the patient, the amount of sedation, and the extent of the procedure, monitoring of the patient during and after the procedure may be appropriate. This may include monitoring of blood pressure, heart rate, respirations, and oxygen saturation. After any transbronchial biopsy, a chest x-ray should be performed to ensure that a pneumothorax is not present. Some physicians like to obtain x-ray studies several hours later as well to catch late-developing pneumothoraces.

The bronchoscope should be completely cleansed following use. This would include immediate rinsing of the channel with water and passing a brush through the suction channel. By using the suction control, alternately aspirate the detergent and water solutions and then aspirate air to remove residual water. The outside surface of the bronchoscope should be wiped with alcohol. The bronchoscope should be carefully inspected for damage, especially at the tip. Angulation should function smoothly to the full range of deflection. The bronchoscope should

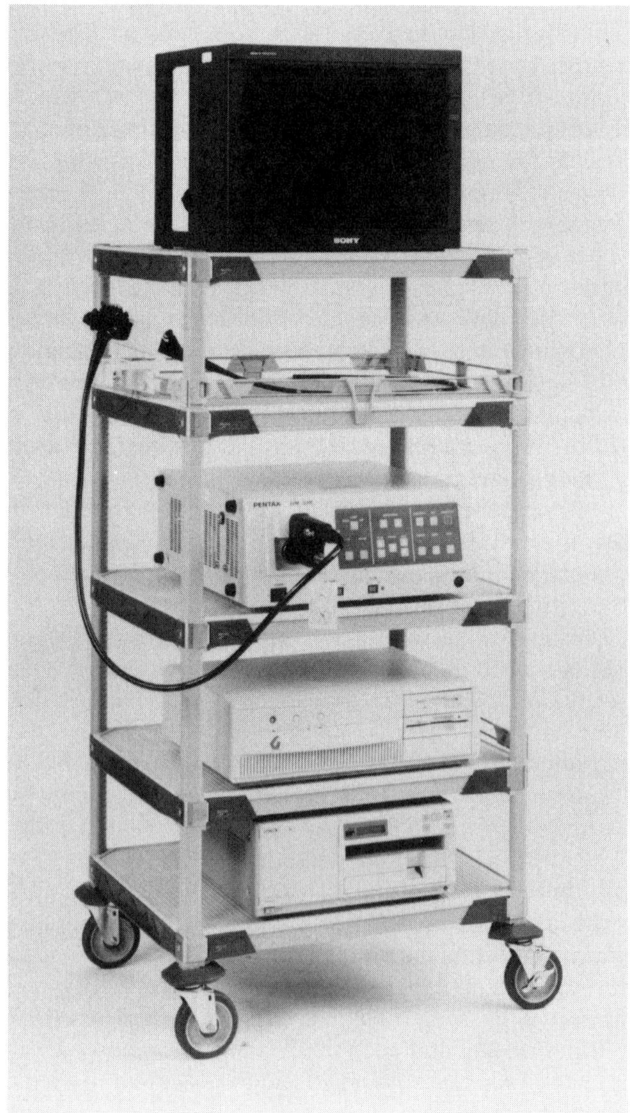

FIG 8–41
A bronchoscopy system.

be leakage-tested regularly to ensure the function of the seals. Finally, the bronchoscope should be cold-sterilized either with glutaraldehyde or alcohol in accordance with manufacturers' specifications.

Differences between bronchoscopes are subtle since each manufacturer provides an array of models ranging in size and function. Since patients vary in size and applications range from BAL and biopsy to imaging, institutions generally have several bronchoscopes with overlapping usage. Many of the variations between manufacturers ultimately involve subjective factors such as ease of use, comfort, and a generic sense of image quality. Unlike other types of instrumentation, there generally are no specific differences in the function or method of operation. It is common practice to mix light sources, video recorders, and accessories with different bronchoscopes. A bronchoscopy system is illustrated in Figure 8–41.

SLEEP

The awareness of sleep disorders as a clinical problem has received widespread recognition in the past 15 years. Substantial segments of the population suffer from some form of sleep disorder. Laboratories performing diagnostic evaluation of these disorders have grown accordingly, expanding from traditional electroencephalography (EEGs) into gastric reflux, arterial oxygen desaturation, respiratory muscle function, and ventilatory drive studies.

Treatment modalities have changed dramatically with the advent of nasal continuous positive airway pressure (CPAP) and intraoral devices as an alternative to pharmacologic and surgical interventions. A newer development that has helped with patient tolerance and compliance is nasal bilevel positive airway pressure (BiPAP). This is a similar machine with a nasal mask but has two levels of pressure, a higher inspiratory pressure and a lower expiratory pressure. Again, the pressure settings should be determined by titration during polysomnography (PSG).

These devices have revolutionized therapy for obstructive sleep apnea since they are essentially curative. Tracheostomies are now rarely if ever indicated for obstructive sleep apnea. The nasal CPAP and BiPAP machines are small, portable, and relatively quiet. Oxygen can be bled into the system if necessary. Many patients will require a nasal decongestant to avoid congestion resulting from the positive pressure. Appropriate use of these alternatives has reemphasized the need for an accurate differential diagnosis.

Sleep disorders include several different types of dysfunction. From the standpoint of the cardiopulmonary department, the interest usually focuses on apeic episodes during sleep, which may be defined as a cessation of breathing that exceeds 10 seconds. Hypopnea is another sleep disorder characterized as airflow reductions of at least 50% that last for at least 10 seconds and are associated with oxygen desaturation. These events are usually terminated by a brief arousal from sleep. Clinically important changes can accompany either prolonged apnea or increased frequency of apneas/hypopneas.

Sleep disorders may be divided into three distinct categories: central, obstructive, or mixed. Central apnea is defined as the absence of both respiratory effort and airflow either for prolonged periods or with increasing frequency during sleep. Central apnea becomes more frequent with age. Recent evidence has shown that in subjects over 60 years of age, more than 25% of individuals may experience some degree of breathing disorder during sleep. In most cases, the problem does not present clear-cut sequelae.

Obstructive sleep disorders may include both apnea or hypopnea and can be categorized as obstructive or mixed. Obstructive apnea is characterized by cessation of airflow in the presence of respiratory effort, whereas in mixed apnea respiratory effort is generally absent at the beginning of the apneic phase but becomes apparent just before the return of airflow. There is evidence that hypopneas have similar sequelae to complete apneas. Accordingly, obstructive apneas and hypopneas are usually considered together.

The site of obstruction is generally the upper airway and oropharynx. Frequently, the obstruction progressively narrows until the airway completely closes followed by an apneic period. Even without complete closure, the obstruction may be sufficient to cause oxygen desaturation or multiple transient arousals. The consequences of this desaturation and arousal pattern are the clinical reactions.

The clinical problems associated with sleep disorders include excessive daytime sleepiness, frequent nocturnal awakening, insomnia, loud snoring, morning headaches, systemic and/or pulmonary hypertension, arrhythmias, and intellectual deterioration accompanied by personality changes. These clinical features may also not be associated with obstructive sleep apnea. Various protocols have been developed for screening patients short of a complete overnight PSG.

Methods of Detection

Perhaps the simplest test is monitoring nocturnal oxygen saturation and heart rate. Pulse oximeters provide the capability to store 8 to 10 hours of continuous saturation and heart rates and then subsequently print these trends.

Nocturnal desaturation represents a positive test for clinically significant sleep apnea but does not provide a means for differentiating between central and obstructive apneas or for sleep staging. Moreover, it is possible to have significant apeas that are not associated with desaturation, particularly when the apeic events are numerous but not prolonged. Therefore, the nocturnal saturation study can generate false negative results. This technique also cannot distinguish between central and obstructive apneas. However, the convenience with which nocturnal saturation studies may be made on inpatients contributes to its popularity despite the reduced sensitivity.

Four-channel apnea studies provide important additional information regarding respiratory effort. Typically, these recorders include heart rate, respiratory effort, nasal airflow, and oximetry. The addition of respiratory effort and nasal airflow offers a means of differentiating central from obstructive events. Additionally, these studies quantify the severity of the episode and the number of occurrences. As with simple saturation monitoring, this approach will not stage the sleep and may therefore result in some number of false negative studies when patients do not reach rapid eye movement (REM) sleep.

The most reliable diagnostic test is the overnight study, with PSG providing the capability for sleep staging as well as monitoring multiple physiologic parameters. In addition to heart rate, respiratory effort, nasal airflow, and oximetry, these studies record EEG, electro-oculography (EOG), and electromyography (EMG) as well. Generally, 16 channels of data are recorded for review. Recent innovations include the computer storage of full-disclosure tracings to minimize the need for large amounts of paper recordings and computer-assisted scoring of the studies.

Representative Example of Sleep Systems

Vitalog provides up to 23 data input channels for EEG, ECG, EMG, and other operator-defined inputs. Additionally, the system provides both on-site and remote monitoring capability.

SUMMARY

Understanding how systems work is essential for appropriately selecting and maintaining equipment. Maintaining equipment includes not only repairs but also assessing result quality over time. As instrumentation ages, the sensor quality may degrade subtly, which can best be detected by analysis of trends. A formal, regular system for monitoring instrument performance that takes into account specific instrument operating characteristics is critical for ensuring quality control.[39]

A frequently overlooked source of changes in results is software upgrades from the manufacturer. Software or hardware upgrades are frequently provided as an enticement to maintain service contracts. These upgrades may provide desirable improvements but may also introduce subtle changes in results either through intentional or inadvertent alterations in methodology and actual calculation errors. Many changes cannot be easily detected, and the changes will only become apparent when comparing trends. It is useful to maintain an equipment logbook in which all changes are documented. With computerized instrumentation, the device is the result of software and hardware interaction and must be considered a new device if either is modified. Just as a new system would not be used clinically without testing, altered systems must be evaluated carefully.

REFERENCES

1. American Thoracic Society: Standardization of spirometry: 1987 update. *Am Rev Respir Dis* 1987; 136:1285–1298.
2. American Thoracic Society: Single breath carbon monoxide diffusing capacity (transfer factor). Recommendations for a standard technique. *Am Rev Respir Dis* 1987; 136:1299–1307.
3. American Thoracic Society: Lung function testing: Selection of reference values and interpretative strategies. *Am Rev Respir Dis* 1991; 144:1202–1218.
4. American Thoracic Society: Flexible endoscopy of the pediatric airway. *Am Rev Respir Dis* 1992; 145:233–235.
5. American College of Sports Medicine: *Guidelines for Graded Exercise Testing and Exercise Prescription,* ed 3. Philadelphia, Lea & Febiger, 1986.
6. Hellerstein HK, Brock LL, Bruce RA: *Exercise Testing and Training of Apparently Healthy Individuals: A Handbook for Physicians.* New York, Committee on Exercise, American Heart Association, 1972.
7. American Thoracic Society: Snowbird workshop on standardization of spirometry. *Am Rev Respir Dis* 1979; 119:831–838.
8. Nelson SB, Gardner RM, Crapo RO, et al: Performance evaluation of contemporary spirometers. *Chest* 1990; 97:288–297.
9. Hutchinson J: On the capacity of the lungs and on the respiratory functions, with a view of establishing a precise and easy method of detecting disease by the spirometer. *Med Chir Soc Trans* 1846; 29:137–252.
10. Tiffeneau R, Pinelli A: Regulation bronchique de la ventilation pulmonaire. *J Fr Med Chir Thorac* 1948; 2:221–244.
11. Gaensler EA: Analysis of the ventilatory defect by timed

capacity measurements. *Am Rev Tuberc* 1951; 64:256–278.

12. Hyatt RE, Schilder DP, Fry DL: Relationship between maximum expiratory flow and degree of lung inflation. *J Appl Physiol* 1958; 13:331–336.
13. Herrald FJC, McMichael J: Determination of lung volume, a constant volume modification of Christie's method. *Proc R Soc Lond* 1939; 126:491–501.
14. Meneely GR, Ball CO, Kory RC, et al: A simplified closed circuit helium dilution method for the determination of residual volume of the lungs. *Am J Med* 1960; 28:824–831.
15. Light RW, George RB, Meneely GR, et al: A new method for analyzing multiple breath nitrogen washout curves. *J Appl Physiol* 1980; 48:265–272.
16. Brunner JX, Wolff G, Cumming G, et al: Accurate measurement of N_2 volumes during N_2 washout requires dynamic adjustment of delay time. *J Appl Physiol* 1985; 52:1378–1382.
17. Krogh M: The diffusion of gases through the lungs of man. *J Physiol (Lond)* 1914; 49:271–300.
18. Forster RE, Fowler WS, Bates DV, et al: The absorption of carbon monoxide by the lungs during breathholding. *J Clin Invest* 1954; 33:1135–1145.
19. Ogilvie CM, Forster RE, Blakemore WS, et al: A standardized breathholding technique for the clinical measurement of the diffusing capacity of the lung for carbon monoxide. *J Clin Invest* 1957; 36:1–17.
20. Jones RS, Meade F: A theoretical and experimental analysis of anomalies in the estimation of pulmonary diffusing capacity by the single breath method. *Q J Exp Physiol* 1961; 46:131–143.
21. Gad C: Ueber Grosse und Bedeutung des Residualluftraumes. *Versamml Gesell Dtsch Naturforsch Aerzte* 1881; 54:117–119.
22. Pfluger E: Das pneumonometer. *Pflugers Arch* 1882; 29:244.
23. DuBois AB, Botelho SY, Bedell GN, et al: A rapid plethysmographic method for measuring thoracic gas volume: A comparison with a nitrogen washout method for measuring functional residual capacity in normal subjects. *J Clin Invest* 1956; 35:322–326.
24. Brown R, Ingram RH, McFadden ER: Problems in plethysmographic assessment of total lung capacity in asthma. *Am Rev Respir Dis* 1978; 118:658–692.
25. Rodenstein DO, Stanescu DC: Reassessment of lung volume measurement by helium dilution and body plethysmography in chronic airflow obstruction. *Am Rev Respir Dis* 1982; 126:1040–1044.
26. Hida W, Suzuki S, Sasaki H, et al: Effect of ventilatory frequency on regional transpulmonary pressure in normal adults. *J Appl Physiol* 1981; 51:678–685.
27. Shore S, Milic-Emili J, Martin JG: Reassessment of body plethysmographic technique for the measurement of thoracic gas volume in asthmatics. *Am Rev Respir Dis* 1983; 126:515–520.
28. Wasserman K, Whipp BJ: Exercise physiology in health and disease. *Am Rev Respir Dis* 1975; 112:219–249.
29. Weber KT, Janicki JS: Cardiopulmonary exercise testing for evaluation of chronic cardiac failure. *Am J Cardiol* 1985; 55:22–31.
30. Weber KT, Kinasewitz GT, Janicki JS, et al.: Exercise testing in the evaluation of the patient with chronic cardiac failure. *Circulation* 1982; 65:1213–1223.
31. Sullivan M, Froelicher V: Maximal oxygen uptake and gas exchange in coronary heart disease. *J Cardiac Rehabil* 1983; 3:549–560.
32. Jones NL: Exercise testing in pulmonary evaluation: Rationale, methods and the normal respiratory response to exercise. Parts I and II. *N Engl J Med* 1975; 293:541.
33. Beaver WL, Wasserman K, Whipp BJ: On-line computer analysis and breath-by-breath graphical display of exercise function tests. *J Appl Physiol* 1973; 34:128–132.
34. Comroe JH: *Physiology of Respiration,* ed 2. St Louis, Mosby–Year Book, 1974.
35. Stow RW, Baer RF, Randall BF: Rapid measurement of the tension of carbon dioxide in blood. *Arch Phys Med Rehabil* 1957; 38:646–650.
36. Sevringhaus JW, Bradley AF: Electrodes for blood Po_2 and Pco_2 determination. *J Appl Physiol* 1958; 13:515–520.
37. Clark LC: Monitor and control of blood and tissue oxygen tensions. *Trans Am Soc Artif Intern Organs* 1956; 2:41–48.
38. Hansen JE: Participant responses to blood gas proficiency testing reports. *Chest* 1992; 101:1240–1244.
39. Snow MG: Standardization in the pulmonary function laboratory. *Respir Ther* Oct/Nov 1991.

INDEX

I